OXFORD MEDICAL PUBLICATIONS

Community Nutritional Assessment

Frontispiece. Xerophthalmia: due to severe vitamin A deficiency, showing main clinical signs, which are always bilateral (see p. 265). (Photographs by the late Professor H.A.P.C. Oomen, courtesy of Helen Keller International, New York.)

Know the Signs and Symptoms of Xerophthalmia

Xerophthalmia is the term used to describe the eye signs of vitamin A deficiency.

It is a childhood blinding disease which is caused by a lack of vitamin A in the diet.

The first symptom often is night blindness, followed by the occurrence of Bitot's spots on the conjunctiva.

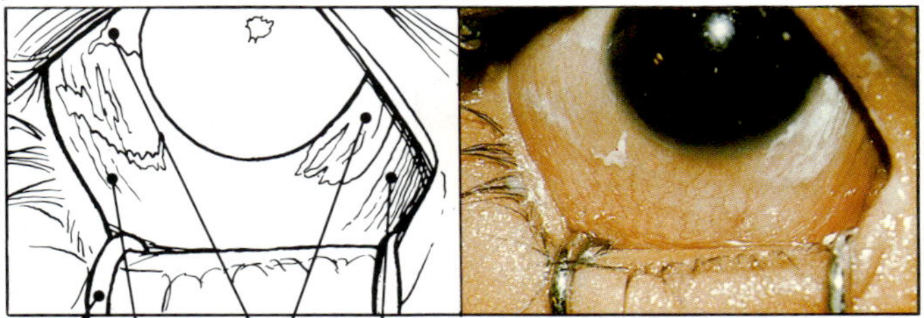

Although Bitot's spots differ somewhat in size, location and shape, they have a similar appearance.

They are accumulations of material on the conjunctiva, often in association with other signs of xerophthalmia.

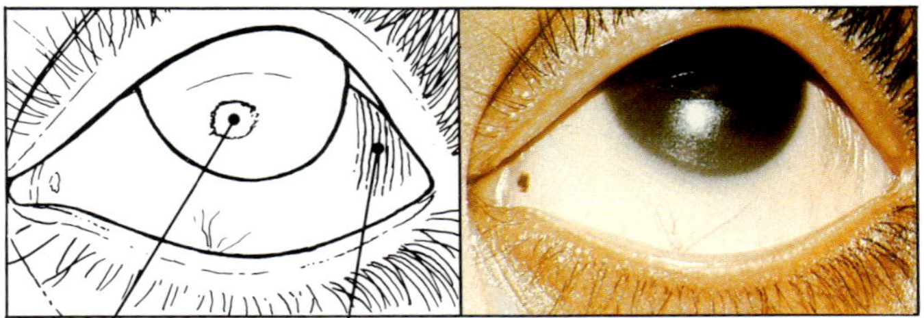

Corneal dryness (xerosis) may develop if the disease is not treated.

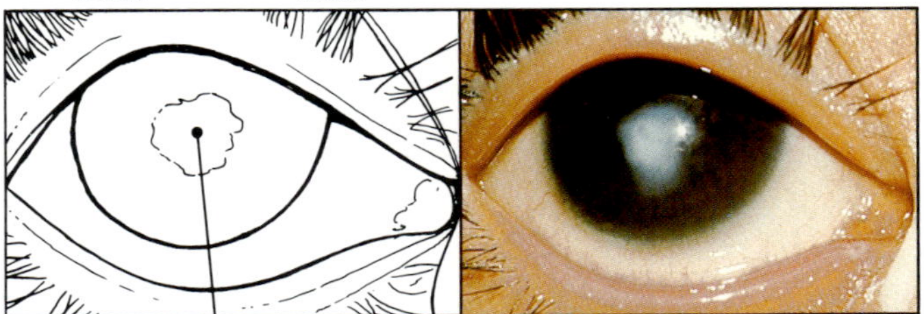

As the nutritional status of the child worsens, or the child develops an infectious disease, the cornea may become increasingly damaged.

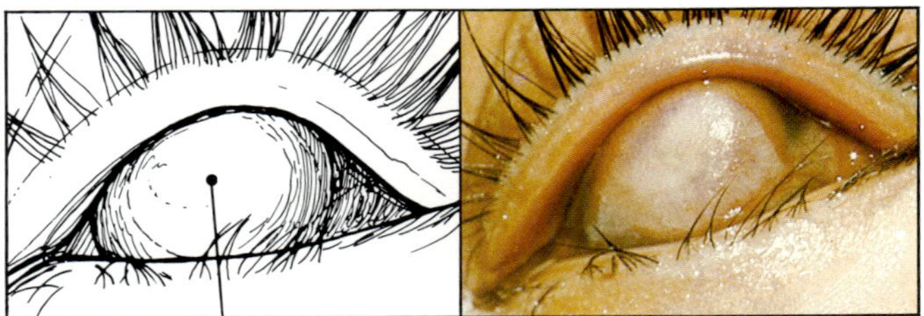

Bulging staphyloma of left eye.

If xerophthalmia is not treated, or is treated too late, it may result in severe damage and permanent blindness.

A scar of the cornea impairs its transparency and interferes with vision, while a perforated eyeball shrinks and leads to complete blindness.

For further information, please contact

Helen Keller International, 15 West 16th Street, New York, N.Y. 10011

Photographs by Prof. H.A.P.C. Oomen

Community Nutritional Assessment

with special reference to less technically developed countries

DERRICK B. JELLIFFE
Professor of Public Health and Pediatrics

and

E. F. PATRICE JELLIFFE
Lecturer and Researcher,
School of Public Health

in collaboration with

Alfred Zerfas
Formerly Director, Nutrition Assessment Unit
School of Public Health

and

Charlotte G. Neumann
Professor of Public Health and Pediatrics,
University of California, Los Angeles

Oxford New York Tokyo
OXFORD UNIVERSITY PRESS
1989

Oxford University Press, Walton Street, Oxford OX2 6DP
Oxford New York Toronto
Delhi Bombay Calcutta Madras Karachi
Petaling Jaya Singapore Hong Kong Tokyo
Nairobi Dar es Salaam Cape Town
Melbourne Auckland
and associated companies in
Berlin Ibadan

Oxford is a trade mark of Oxford University Press

Published in the United States
by Oxford University Press, New York

British Library Cataloguing in Publication Data
Jelliffe, D.B. (Derrick Brian)
Community nutritional assessment. — New ed.
1. Developing countries. Man. Nutrition
I. Title II. Jelliffe, E.F. Patrice
(Eleonore Florence Patrice) III. The
assessment of the nutritional stutus of
the community (with special reference to
field surveys in developing regions of
the world)
613.2'09172'4
ISBN 0-19-261218-2

Library of Congress Cataloging in Publication Data
Jelliffe, Derrick Brian.
Community nutritional assessment: with special reference to surveys in less technically developed countries/Derrick B. Jelliffe and E.F. Patrice Jelliffe, in collaboration with Alfred Zerfas and Charlotte G. Neumann.
(Oxford medical publications)
Bibliography Includes index.
1. Nutrition surveys. 2. Nutrition surveys — Developing countries.
I. Jelliffe, E.F. Patrice. II. Title. III. Series.
TX359.J45 1989 363.8'2 — dc 19 88-22631
ISBN 0-19-261218-2

Set by Graphicraft Typesetters Ltd., Hong Kong
Printed in Great Britain by St. Edmundsbury Press
Bury St. Edmunds, Suffolk

Contents

1

Scope

All proofs are incomplete from the viewpoint of formal logic. ... Professedly rigorous proofs usually have holes which are covered over by intuition. .... The bases on which predictions are made are many: experience, reason, intuition, chance, 'hunches' and the advice of experts.

P.J. Davis and R. Hersch (1986)

Nutrition has to be considered as an applied science with methods of assessment and any action taken as a result guided (but not dominated) by metabolic minutiae and mathematical precision. In particular, methods of classifying malnutrition have to be useful for assisting communities using primary health care services — the majority of the world.

Despite the more than 20 years since this book's predecessor,[1] much that was emphasized in 1966 continues unchanged. The main foci remain the most common and most socially significant, potentially preventable nutritional deficiencies. These are found predominantly in the physiologically, culturally, and economically vulnerable populations of less technically developed countries, and, as in the past, mainly involve young children and women (Tables 1.1 and 1.2).

There is a continuing, increasingly recognized need for simple affordable methods of detecting less severe degrees of malnutrition. These must provide rapid results which are not only biologically and statistically valid, but also easily understood by scientists, administrators, and the general population, if advocacy of inter-sectoral nutrition programmes is to be acceptable.

At the same time, during the past two decades much has altered. In particular, a large array of new techniques and perspectives has evolved which need to be incorporated into practical activities, without creating unworkable overcomplexity.

Nutrition has been defined as 'the process by which the (human) organism utilizes food' (McLaren 1981). 'Nutriture' (more usually termed 'nutritional status') is the state of the body produced by this process as a result of eating, digestion, absorption, transport, storage, and metabolic effects at the cellular level (McLaren 1981). Conversely, malnutrition has

[1] D. B. Jelliffe (1966). *The assessment of the nutritional status of the community.* WHO Monograph No. 53.

Table 1.1 Approximate estimates of total persons affected by currently preventable major forms of malnutrition in the world today, with special relation to less technically developed regions. (LTDC) (*Modified from Latham, personal communication*)

Deficiency	Main morbidity due to malnutrition	Prevalence	Age group affected	Mortality per year	Prevention
(1) **Localized distribution**					**Theoretically straightforward:**
Vitamin A (xerophthalmia)	Blindness	6 million	Young children	750 000 (associated)	Nutrition education for mothers and young children; vitamin capsules; prevention of diarrhoea and infections
Iodine	Goitre	150 million	Adults (especially women)	?	Iodized food (usually salt); intramuscular iodized oil
	Cretinism	6 million	Newborn		
Vitamin D	Rickets	Uncertain numbers	Young children	?	Ultra-violet light for mothers and young children; vitamin D fortification; vitamin capsules
(2) **World-wide distribution**					**Complex, variable:**
Iron	Anaemia	350 million	Women 18–45	?	Nutrition education Iron supplements
	? Limitation on learning ability	Uncertain numbers	Young children	?	Treat hookworm
Protein and energy	Stunted growth and wasting	500 million	0–6	10 million	Nutrition and health education (breast feeding, weaning foods)
	Kwashiorkor and marasmus	1 million	1–4	?	Prevention of infections Nutrition supplements
Western-type diet: sucrose	Dental caries	Millions (LTDC: increasing)	All ages	Nil	Nutrition education; Fluoride and early management

Table 1.2 Main forms of malnutrition in young children: size of problem, social significance, and preventability. *(Modified from Beaton and Bengoa 1976)*

Condition	Size of problem	Social significance	Preventability
PEM (Protein-energy malnutrition)	+++	+++	+
Iron deficiency anaemia	++	++	++
Xerophthalmia (vit. A)	++*	+++	+++
Iodine deficiency disorders	++*	+++	+++
Rickets (vit. D)	+*	+	+++

* Relatively limited geographical distribution.

been given the following broad definition: 'a pathological state due to a deficient availability of essential nutrients at the cellular or basic level during a prolonged period; it manifests itself by physical, psychological and biochemical abnormalities. (Mata 1978).

However, community nutritional assessment needs to include not only the direct human 'end results', but also 'ecological variables' (particularly the categorization and measurement of causes, especially those that are preventable and/or amenable to intervention). Such information is needed if practical programmes are to be devised aimed at local 'risk factors' (p. 453) and evaluated using available resources, with the greatest chance of benefiting the largest number at risk of the consequences of malnutrition at the least cost. Such forgetting has become especially apparent in harsh situations, such as famines, refugee camps and urban slums.

Organization of book

The first section of this book deals with the direct assessment of nutritional status (pp. 13–126), that is information obtained by examination, selected laboratory tests, and anthropometric measurements of individuals in a population or singly. Such data, however, need, whenever possible, to be complemented by information from other sources, particularly suggesting causes. This especially includes enquiry into dietary intake (p. 187).

Subsequent sections cover possible assessment from health statistics (p. 128) (previously termed 'indirect assessment'). These can include, for example, age-specific mortality rates and death rates from certain infections, such as measles. The assessment of 'ecological variables' follows (p. 142) (including investigation into the relative significance of risk factors, such as socio-economic, environmental, and cultural influences, contributory infections, 'food considerations', and other circumstances, which may be either 'associated' or, in varying degrees, 'causative').

The need for the interpretation in different age-groups (p. 226) is covered later. This is followed by sections on channels for assessment (p. 355), sequence and range of activities (p. 384), and suggestions for stimulating action (p. 449) to improve the nutritional level of communities.

New specialized knowledge

In recent years, a flood of new knowledge has emerged as a result of the awakening awareness of the significance of nutrition to human health, and from practical experience both in more and less technically developed countries. The results of surveys and epidemiological studies of many different types and levels of complexity (p. 362) have covered, for example, attempts to evaluate the effectiveness of nutritional and other community programmes, the assessment of relief operations during natural and man-made disasters (such as famines and refugee camps), individual appraisal in hospitalized patients, and the definition of functional outcomes or consequences of malnutrition, especially less severe degrees.

At the same time, a large amount of detailed anthropometric investigation, laboratory research, and other fundamental studies have been undertaken[2] (e.g. information collected by scientists concerned with precise measurement of human growth and development (auxologists), with biological variation in body morphology in different genetic groups of mankind (physical anthropologists), and with the estimation of body composition using modern technology as a part of sophisticated hospital management of some seriously ill patients).

Many different specialists have become involved increasingly with nutritional assessment, or at least with some of the methods often used, most

[2] Numerous practical and theoretical reviews of nutritional assessment are available, including earlier works: Bigwood (1939), and ICNND (1963); and more modern accounts: Christakis (1973), Kanawati (1976), Frankle and Owen (1978), Graitcer (1981), *Proc. Nutr. Soc.* (1982), and the *Am. J. Clin. Nutr.* (1982).

commonly with anthropometry. These include a wide range of disciplines and interests, including surgeons and other clinicians in the hospital 'nutritional support' movement (p. 348), bariatricians (as some experts in obesity have labelled themselves), and others concerned with Western-world 'feeding problems' (such as anorexia nervosa and bulimia) (p. 329). In addition, investigations have been made by those working in sports medicine, in the care of handicapped children, in aerospace medicine, in pharmacokinetics, and even those concerned with highway safety (in relation to the design of equipment, such as bicycles and automobile safety belts for children). Although their purposes, detailed methods, and technological resources are usually far removed from those in Third World countries, information has become available from many different sources. What is more, it is to be hoped that these different groups will realize that they can learn from each other. For example, detailed hospital investigations using sophisticated equipment can be (or ought to be) helpful in testing the significance of uncomplicated field methods used in primary health care services. These include, for example, technological methods where arm circumference measurements can be validated by estimates of muscle mass.

Examples of disciplines with a relatively new, or much increased, interest in nutritional assessment include epidemiology, anthropology, sociology, geography, agriculture (FAO 1982), economy, and development planning. In theory and, ideally, in practice, this means that consultation and collaborative team work is indicated more than ever, and, in the present publication, relevant references to such endeavours are included. However, in practice, this collaboration may be difficult. Problems can arise in such interdisciplinary activities because of the conflicting (or lighly specialized) terminology, theories, methods, and emphases used by the different branches of science (Van Esterik 1984).

As a result of a multitude of activities, a large amount of literature continues to be published, widely scattered in a bewildering range of professional and technical journals, and/or drawn together for various purposes in chapters in books and in reports of international meetings, including those held under the auspices of WHO, FAO, UNICEF, USAID, and other agencies. The limited and selective bibliography in the present book is itself indicative of the volume of recent literature. It is very far from complete and is intended to focus on more relevant past and recent work. (Also see: Bibliography 1988, p. 611.)

This ferment of new knowledge has had a variety of different effects — simplifying matters on one hand and, on the other, the making them more complicated. Technically, these include, for example, increased emphasis on the assessment of materno–fetal nutrition, on the realization of the wide public health and social significance of iodine deficiency disorders as one of the leading causes of mental deficiency in some Third World countries (p. 272) (Hetzel 1983), on the significance of lesser degrees of deficiency of iron (p. 263), zinc (p. 263), and vitamin A (p. 265), on the rising incidence of dental caries in urbanized areas (p. 348), on the significance of calories as the commonest limiting (or surplus) nutrient (p. 273) in many circumstances, and on the realization of a much greater normal biological variation in nutrient needs and physiological adaptations than previously appreciated (p. 126).

From a public health point-of-view, recent decades have focused attention on the importance of identifying communities, families, or individuals at high risk of malnutrition (Backett *et al.* 1984) (p. 453), and the social significance of what Bengoa (1970) termed 'surviving children,' following, for example, prolonged moderately severe protein–energy malnutrition (p. 273). In Gopalan's words (1983), the long-term 'qualitative dimension' (p. 443) caused by widespread community nutrition in mothers and young children needs to be given adequate consideration in planning, in addition to the immediately obvious morbidity and mortality.

Most significantly, reappraisal of the relative usefulness of methods has taken place in recent decades. There has been a decreased emphasis on biochemical tests (p. 31) and on clinical signs (p. 14). The latter trend has perhaps led to a negative stage where previously well-known signs have become quite unfamilar and not readily recognized by recently trained health professionals (e.g. angular stomatitis in elderly people in nursing homes or vitamin B12 deficiency in a vegan (exclusive vegetarian).

Ingenious new 'appropriate technology' has been introduced to aid primary health care workers in screening (p. 361) or in assisting in the assessment of national 'development' (WHO 1981) or the standard of living (Martorell 1982). At another level, sophisticated investigations have been developed to test for impaired immunocompetence (p. 139) and decreased work performance (p. 50), which can result from different forms of nutritional inadequacy.

From a negative point-of-view, this large volume of information, derived from different disciplines, and its interpretation can result in communication problems. Similar technical terms may be used by different professions to mean various things. Among nutritionists, it has lead to differences of opinion and to various schools of thought. Examples include the usefulness of, or potential need for, different 'standards' (or reference data) in anthropometry in dissimilar ethnic groups, in systems of categorization and labelling of children with less severe protein–energy malnutrition (p. 272), and in determining the immediate and long-term functional significance or outcome as regards mortality and morbidity in various forms of under- or overnutrition (p. 124).

This information explosion is in real danger of causing increasing complexity and confusion, less certainty, and even 'analysis paralysis' in which action cannot be taken because of conflict of opinion. Nevertheless, there is a need to include the most recent work, and **modern information concerning each section of the book is summarized in Addendum 1988** (p. 604).

Areas of general agreement

Fortunately, some trends and areas of general agreement appear to be emerging and these need to be firmly grasped as the basis for practical guidance in nutritional assessment in developing countries. Most important is *the recognition of the difficulties, imperfections, and approximations of all methods and reference levels*, including food composition (p. 212), recommended dietary allowances (p. 212), anthropometric data (p. 122), etc. In turn, this emphasizes the importance of trying to obtain confirmatory information from several sources (Gopalan 1987), and the absurdity of over-elaborate mathematical manipulation of useful, but necessarily approximate, data. Seeking, probably unattainable, 'perfect' interpretations may delay the 'good' that is feasible with less refined approximations.

Other realizations include a greater awareness of the considerable range of variation in normal levels in most indicators measured; the need for *practical*, basic mathematical guidance in sampling and analysis; the use of feasible epidemiological techniques (e.g. case control studies (p. 158) and the investigation of 'positive deviants' (p. 359); and an increased reliance on anthropometry (p. 64), despite its recognized limitations and need for caution in interpretation (p. 126) (Gopalan 1987).

This book attempts, therefore, to highlight such areas of consensus, drawing on the relevant recent technical information to guide methods which can be used in Third World countries. At the same time, it is based considerably on the authors' personal experience and opinions. The emphasis is directed towards: (1) being as useful and uncomplicated as possible for practical work in less technically developed communities; (2) basic scientific soundness (according to present knowledge);[3] and (3) having as much international agreement as practicable.

Among other developments, it has become increasingly apparent that methods of nutritional assessment have to be varied to suit local needs, resources, and other circumstances. Standardization and uniformity of the methods and reference data used in different studies are undoubtedly ideal, especially for international comparisons. This has been reiterated

[3] As selection of a limited number of most useful tests or measurements always has to be made, their epidemiological 'sensitivity' (proportions of truly positive identified) and 'specificity' (proportion of truly negative identified) need to be known and understood (Appendix 4).

for decades, but often cannot be achieved. This is partly due to the individual views and biases of all investigators. It is also due to variation in local needs and to the use of locally necessary modifications and adaptations. This makes it important that the procedures, methods, and reference data used are clearly described when results are reported (p. 443). At the same time, techniques should be selected to permit as much comparability as possible with similar studies elsewhere. However, *local usefulness must always take precedence over comparability.*

Situations considered

The present book differs from its predecessor (Jelliffe 1966) in several ways. It continues to give major attention to the huge, dominant, and sometimes increasing public health nutritional problems in less technically developed countries, mainly affecting mothers and young children. At the same time, the scope has been widened to include some consideration concerning other high-risk groups, such as adolescents (p. 329) and the elderly (p. 352). Some appropriate references are given to newer publications in these fields. However, they are not covered in detail.

Nutritional assessment in specially vulnerable groups is covered fully, notably in early childhood (p. 259) and pregnancy (p. 226). Likewise, the sorting out of at-risk communities, families, and individuals (p. 453) is presented. Brief mention is made of some nutritional problems of more affluent areas, such as obesity (p. 343), 'failure to thrive' (p. 57) in young children, and malnutrition in severely ill patients in hospitals with extensive laboratory facilities available (p. 348). These are also world issues, although with varying levels of numerical priority. In fact, nutritional disorders of affluence occur in some percentage of all populations, as can problems of 'malnutrition minus' (such as protein–energy malnutrition) in disadvantaged minorities in rich countries.

Guiding principles

Avoiding discontinuity

The present publication attempts to identify, highlight, and compare major trends in different forms and methods of nutritional assessment, and then to dovetail them as smoothly as possible with previously described views and practices that have become established routine in many areas in the past two decades. This has not been easy and was not always possible. However, it is hoped that confusion due to discontinuity and needless change has been minimized, so that comparisons with results from earlier studies can be made, at least approximately. This particularly concerns changes related to more recently accepted anthropometric reference data (p. 110).

Scientific precision, practicality, and appropriate technology

Another major concern remains the search for a harmonious bridging of the gap between the refinements of precise scientific research (such as the ultrastrict mathematical application of statistical and epidemiological principles) and practical, albeit approximate, procedures which can give valid and useful information, and which can be carried out rapidly and effectively with limited resources, especially in poorer communities. Key examples remain the selection of body measurements to be included (p. 105) and the anthropometric equipment to be used (p. 64).

With increasing involvement of workers from the more numerate fields such as epidemiology and biometrics, it is important to find a balance between much-needed statistical guidance and the real danger of unnecessary, unexplained complexity — producing a 'Babel' of technical neologisms ('mystifying by mathematics') (Miller 1979), sometimes needing a 'verbal autopsy' with assistance from a specialized dictionary (Last 1983).[4] Indeed, the unnecessary use of highly technical terminology (e.g. Z-scores, 'normative reality', meta-analysis, type II errors, commensability, etc.) can have the effect of inhibiting uninitiated workers, including health professionals without particular training in, or knowledge of, what has the risk of becoming a 'priestly' in-language, frequently used instead of available everyday words.

From the opposite extreme, the practical utility of visual observation is being rediscovered — in some special circumstances — as the ultimate in simplified 'appropriate technology' (p. 361). This has long been emphasized (correctly) as subjective, imprecise, and biased by the investigator's recent and past experience. However, it is interesting and even rather comforting in the era of the computer to note that clinical inspection ('eye-balling') continues to be useful as a rough screening procedure in emergency situations among refugees (p. 366), in judging which individuals are probably obese and need further fatfold or other measurements (p. 343), and in deciding subjectively which slightly 'underweight' infants appear healthy, vigorous, and otherwise 'normal' (p. 294).

Similarly, the value of appropriate technology, particularly for use by community health workers, in nutritional assessment has come to the forefront. This has been most noticeable in anthropometry (p. 64) in which low-cost, culturally appropriate, uncomplicated equipment has

[4] Some commoner terms are given in Appendix 4.

come increasingly into use. Such items as colour-coded arm tapes (or bands) (p. 94) which can be used to categorize individuals and indicate the need for certain actions to be taken, can give results which are scientifically based and clearly understandable, even by illiterate workers. Reference to different forms of appropriate technology recur as a constant theme throughout this book. Mostly, they are economical tools for use on a wide scale in primary health care services. However, appropriate technology may also include the use of programmable calculators, microcomputers, aerial photography for population sampling, and satellite sensing as part of an early-warning system in drought or other potential famine situations.

Widening perspectives

In retrospect, this book's predecessor (Jelliffe 1966) was oversimplistic (as were the times) and also gave the impression that nutritional assessment was only, or mainly, the clinical responsibility of health workers, especially physicians. Indeed, the publication actually emerged from a 1963 *WHO Expert Committee Report on the Medical Assessment of Nutritional Status*. It had as its distant international precedessor a rather little known 1939 League of Nations Health Organization monograph by Bigwood entitled, *Guiding principles for studies on nutrition of populations*. This focused on dietary surveys and on numerous, often complex anthropometric indices, all of which were subsequently abandoned. These were exclusively devised by individual clinicians, with little mathematical awareness, for circumstances in Europe and the USA prior to World War II.

In retrospect, it is clear that the 1963 WHO Expert Committee mainly reflected the views of physicians with some experience in community work, but with little statistical or epidemiological training or awareness. Understandably, their main frame of reference was based subconsciously on the clinical and laboratory diagnosis of severely malnourished individuals whom they had encountered in hospital practice in less technically developed countries, so that these physicians had limited knowledge of the situation in the community. In modern terminology, they were 'clinicians' in the process of becoming 'clinical epidemiologists'.

Consequently, earlier investigations into the nutritional status of communities in Third World countries often had a heavy emphasis on clinical signs. These evolved in subsequent years into combined studies based on clinical signs, anthropometry, simplified estimates of dietary intake, and varying, usually very limited, laboratory investigations. However, most were not designed to be statistically rigorous and, in present-day epidemiological terms, would be considered as descriptive rather than analytical.

However, as Gordon (1963) pointed out, early nutritional epidemiology was itself a more precise, analytical development of what was then termed 'geographical pathology' — that is, the 'observation and measurement of diseases in their natural setting'. Modern epidemiological assessment not only attempts a more precise statistical estimate of the commonness and distribution of diseases, including malnutrition, but also tries to differentiate (and rate the significance of) causes from non-causal associated factors. This is usually a complex task, needing statistical assistance. Also, the same considerations as in the past may make the mathematical guidance of descriptive studies difficult to achieve. These almost always include lack of resources, changing circumstances, difficulties with definitions, and often such logistical considerations as terrain and inaccessible widely scattered populations.

In the present publication, the emphasis has been widened to cover not only those activities traditionally considered as appropriate for health services, but also to give some attention to newer methods of collecting and to include information on conditions related to the nutritional situation in a community, such as economics, food availability, and cultural attitudes (p. 165). In particular, it is recognized that a clearer picture can be given by *combining* 'quantitative' and 'qualitative' methods that have evolved from authropological techniques (Scrimshaw and Hurtado 1987).

However, almost all aspects of life can have a direct or indirect effect on the nutritional status of a community (Williams, *et al.* 1986), ranging from considerations of food production through to cellular metabolism ('from the combine harvester to the ribosome') (Rivers 1979). This means that a recurrent and universal problem in community nutritional assessment always remains practicality. This is dominated by the selection of a limited number of the most locally useful indicators of complex community forces and biological determinants (and their consequences). The collection of such information is always constrained by limited time, money, staff, and the resources needed for analysis. However, the selection process has been made more important as the *inaccuracies, approximations, and difficulty of interpretation of all methods* have become more obvious, making corroboration by information from several sources increasingly necessary. This remains a perennial paradox, which can be guided statistically, but ultimately rests with 'common sense' combinations, which also can be fallible.

With the easy wisdom of hindsight, it is now obvious that many previous attempts at nutritional assessment of communities, especially surveys, were sometimes isolated medical or research exercises. There was usually little involvement of the community nor was there realization of the need for speedy follow-up activities to channel the information obtained as rapidly as possible and present it to both the policy-makers at governmental and local levels, and, if possible, to the community itself as well as to fellow nutritionists. The recognition of these ill-perceived blindspots is endorsed by the recently increased emphasis on nutritional surveillance (p. 551), with its intended continuous monitoring of a community's nutritional situation, as it fluctuates with changing circumstances. This is based on the feedback of basic information affecting nutritional status, including selected, relevant ecological variables (e.g. food prices, abnormal rainfall, locust damage, etc.), which can permit timely action to be taken, when indicated and if funding and political support are available (p. 449).

International comparability versus local usefulness

Last, it is now apparent that the nutritional status of a community (or an individual) is the result of many interacting forces which vary greatly in type and degree in different cultural, geographical, socio-economic, and genetic circumstances in various parts of the world. In community studies, therefore, it is desirable, whenever possible, to consider information collected both in a form that allows international comparability, and, at the same time, in a way that is realistically practicable and geared to local circumstances, needs, and possibilities. Both are important but, of the two, information in a form which has the greatest practical usefulness for improving the local situation plainly should have priority.

This book necessarily covers a very wide range of topics, methods, and approaches. It is not intended as a universal guide, but has to be used selectively by different workers to meet their particular needs.

Action research

The practical assessment of nutritional status and its causation needs assistance from different types of scientists working in fundamental research. They can suggest new techniques and test the significance of existing field methods.

However, from a community health point-of-view, fundamental research is usually a lesser objective, and 'action research' should be the aim. *The purpose of nutritional assessment should be appropriate action to attempt nutritional improvement, when indicated, using methods which appear to be feasible and concerned with local priorities.*

2

Direct assessment of nutritional status

What was once relatively straightforward, seems lately to have become more confusing.

J. Lindenbaum (1983)

A classification is a man-made tool, not something existing of itself. Classifications differ, therefore, for different purposes. Chemistry manuals put diamond and graphite in the same chapter. Jewellers, however, put diamonds and emeralds together, although these are chemically different. The jeweller's customers are interested in different criteria and so the jeweller must choose a classification that is helpful in his trade.

I. Finch (1983)

Introduction

The term 'direct assessment' refers to methods in which individuals or communities are investigated directly. Theoretically, this can include a sequence of examinations ranging from tests for biochemical changes to visible or palpable anatomical abnormalities in the form of clinical signs, and/or anthropometric or biophysical changes (Table 2.1). However, some tests may not be available to detect abnormalities, or, if available, may not be feasible because of lack of funds or of laboratories and facilities such as refrigeration, via an effective 'cold chain', and transport (p. 31). Also, the interpretation of normal limits of, say, biochemical tests is often far less clear than previously considered in relation to lesser abnormalities and to 'functional significance' (p. 124), biological variation, age, and the particular laboratory method employed. In addition, differentiation has to be made to reflect recent food intake and chronic depletion (p. 443). Thus, the neat and orderly systematic progressions (from diet to body levels to clinical abnormalities) often presented are useful only as theoretical guides (Table 2.2).

While special tests may be called for (e.g. for zinc deficiency), the assessment of nutritional status needs, of necessity, to focus on major world-wide public health problems, such as nutritional anaemia (mostly due to iron deficiency), xerophthalmia, iodine deficiency disorders, and protein–energy malnutrition in less technically developed countries, and obesity in more affluent communities (Table 2.3).

Table 2.1 Methods available for the direct assessment of nutritional status

Clinical signs
Laboratory tests:
Biochemical
Haematological
Parasitological
Biophysical methods
Anthropometry

Table 2.2 Clinical malnutrition — classical considerations on its development and evaluation. (*From Krehl and Hodges 1965*)

Primary dietary deficiency ↘		Secondary deficiency (infections, etc.) ↙	Inadequate intake Poor absorption Decreased utilization Increased excretion Destruction Increased requirements
	Gradual tissue desaturation of nutrients ↓		Evaluated by blood, urine and tissue analyses
	Biochemical lesions ↓		Reduction in enzyme activity, altered metabolite level
Clinical trial of therapy →	> Anatomic lesion or sign of deficiency disease (i.e. scurvy, pellagra, etc.)	←	Clinical evaluation

Clinical signs

This is an age of complex tests, but all tests are not available everywhere, so it behooves us to keep our five clinical senses.
J. Willocks (1977)

Clinical examination has always been, and remains, a widely used practical, direct method for trying to assess the nutritional status of individuals

Table 2.3 Nutritional disorders partly related to deficiency or chronic excess of certain nutrients. (*Modified from Miller 1979*)

Deficiency	Nutrient	Chronic-excess
Marasmus	Energy*	Obesity
Constipation	Fibre	Malabsorption
Wasting	*Protein	Gout
Anaemia	Iron	Siderosis
Cramps (muscle)	Sodium	Stroke
Goitre	Iodine	Thyrotoxicosis
Dental caries	Fluorine	Fluorosis
Xerophthalmia	Retinol (vitamin A)	Hypervitaminosis
Rickets	Calciferol (vitamin D)	Hypercalcaemia
Scurvy	Ascorbic acid (Vitamin C)	Renal stones

* Various syndromes of protein–energy malnutrition (p. 273).

and communities. This stems, in part, from the fact that clinical health workers, especially paediatricians, have usually been involved in this type of work at an early stage. They see the end-results — that is severe malnutrition in children in hospital.

Clinical signs are obviously more useful in community studies where the nutritional situation is seriously abnormal. However, some selected signs are usually included in assessment anywhere, including well-to-do countries (Christakis 1973). They also need to be considered and recognized in modern at-risk groups, especially the elderly, who may be both undernourished and on several therapeutic drugs. Signs possibly suggestive of overnutrition may be looked for in adults, such as xanthomata and a well-marked corneal arcus suggesting possible atheroma, and prominent perinasal veins suggesting excessive alcohol intake.

Essentially, assessment by clinical signs is based on examination for changes believed to be related to inadequate or excessive nutritional intake, that can be seen or felt in superficial epithelial tissues, especially the skin, eyes, hair, and mouth, or in organs near the surface of the body, such as the thyroid, and the skull (craniotabes). It often also includes signs due, in part, to the local effect of the diet in the mouth rather than malnutrition. These include dental caries, and dental hypoplasia in young children (Sweeney *et al.* 1971; Jelliffe and Jelliffe 1971), and dental attrition and/or periodontal infection (pyorrhoea) in adults. These may also be recorded because of their secondary nutritional consequences resulting from difficulties in chewing because of pain or loss of teeth (Geissler and Bates 1984).

In addition, clinical examination can include the observation and recording of more obvious signs of some nutritionally important conditioning or contributory infections (p. 139). These particularly include acute diseases, such as measles, severe acute diarrhoea, and whooping cough, especially if an outbreak is occurring. However, chronic infections can also have nutritional significance. These range from minor, but irritating conditions such as scabies, to debilitating severe illness, such as tuberculosis, to chronic disabling infections, for example, tropical ulcers or Guinea worm.

This method has understandable appeal to those with clinical training. It also has the obvious advantage of relatively low cost, as neither elaborate equipment nor an expensive laboratory are needed. Furthermore, with careful training and continuing supervision, junior personnel, village workers, older children, and parents themselves can be taught to recognize certain crucial clinical signs (p. 23) when screening in primary health care services or in surveys for specific deficiencies, such as avitaminosis A. Indeed, some signs and symptoms of xerophthalmia, notably Bitôt's spots (p. 265) and night blindness (p. 265), may be recognized and given special vernacular names in some cultures.

Clinical assessment of an individual or of a community alone can sometimes give valuable, if approximate, objective information to the health worker. This is especially so in regions of the world where some forms of severe malnutrition, and hence more clear-cut, marked nutritional signs, are widespread. The value of the method decreases as the nutritional level of the community improves. Also, in some communities, actual clinical signs of malnutrition may be uncommon, although anthropometry may demonstrate that protein–energy malnutrition is widespread. In addition, in certain acute nutritional disorders, such as infantile beriberi (p. 260), clinical examination can play little or no part in cross-sectional prevalence surveys as the condition is usually either rapidly fatal or speedily cured.

The cheapness and relatively easy organization of nutritional assessment by means of clinical examination has sometimes led to the assumption that the method is simple, quickly mastered by the beginner, and yields results that are easy to interpret. This is not the case. As with other methods of assessment, clinical examination has its own limitations, which must be recognized, if benefit is to be obtained from its use (Table 2.4). Certain common problems, difficulties, and potential errors, due to incorrect procedures and observer bias (which are often insufficiently appreciated) need to be emphasized. These include, for example, mistakes caused by boredom and monotony (if large numbers of people are examined), the subconscious changing of criteria (if positive signs are frequent or rare) (p. 21), and the degree of training and experience of the observers, including lack of agreed definitions and inadequate testing for 'quality control' (proficiency of the examiners) (p. 410).

Table 2.4 Clinical signs: considerations in community nutritional assessment in less technically developed countries

Advantages	Disadvantages	
Very inexpensive (no equipment)	Subjective (less marked signs)	Standardization problems Experience of examiner Findings in particular survey
Fast	Limited diagnostic certainty	Nutrient Non-nutrient
Highly qualified staff not needed	*Well-trained* staff needed Often wrongly assumed to be easy	
Non-invasive	Many signs only in severe cases May be no signs early on (e.g. protein–energy malnutrition)	

Lack of specificity

While a few physical signs are completely diagnostic of specific nutritional deficiency syndromes, such as the 'flaky-paint' rash in kwashiorkor, this is usually not the case. Various non-nutritional environmental influences can sometimes be responsible for similar appearances. For example, the clinical picture of angular stomatitis, often incorrectly considered as diagnostic of riboflavin deficiency, can result from fungal infection with *Monilia*. In parts of India the excessive chewing of betel nut preparations (*pan*) containing large amounts of irritant lime can produce a similar result. In other words, the 'final common path', leading to a clinical sign can be reached by nutrient deficiency, local irritation, or infection. Another common sign, conjunctival pallor, may be due to non-nutritional anaemia — for example, from malaria or sickle cell disease.

Almost all the signs usually recorded lack complete nutrient specificity. Glossitis can be seen in niacin, folic acid, vitamin B12, or riboflavin deficiencies. Phrynoderma appears to be caused by deficiency of essential fatty acids, and/or vitamin E more often than avitaminosis A (Nadiger 1980).

Many signs of malnutrition are not specific to the lack of one nutrient. Furthermore, dietary deficiency is rarely caused by one nutrient alone. Some signs may have complex origins , and the nature of the underlying factors and interrelationships remains unknown. Some signs can vary between different age-groups, sometimes different ethnic groups, and probably with the previous nutritional history — that is whether the malnutrition is chronic or acute. For these reasons, they cannot usually be pigeon-holed easily, as can a few signs found in some infectious diseases, such as Koplik's spots in the mouth in measles. Other signs may be markers or indicators of previous malnutrition. Such 'inactive' signs can include corneal scars, healed angular cheilosis, and bow-legs.

The association of signs with known dietary inadequacy, and/or with biochemical and other tests may help to identify the lacking nutrient or nutrients responsible for a given clinical sign. However, it is common to find a deficiency of several nutrients in any one diet and this often makes the final, specific diagnosis difficult. It is in such instances that small-scale therapeutic trials may be useful, especially if they can be carried out under controlled conditions, preferably 'double-blind'.

Apart from suggesting nutritional deficiency, some signs may also be considered as indicators of probable future survival. For example, a study in Indonesia demonstrated that pre-school age children with mild xerophthalmia had a mortality rate at least four times as high as unaffected children (Sommer 1984).

Nutritional relevance of commonly recorded signs

In the past, a large number of ill-defined signs have often been recorded in the course of different types of nutritional assessment. Recent experience in different parts of the world has suggested that some of these are not related to malnutrition at all, while others are seen only in serious hospitalized cases. Over 25 years ago, the report of the WHO Expert Committee on Medical Assessment of Nutritional Status (1963) suggested the classification of signs often recorded at that time into three groups:

Group 1. Signs that are considered to be of value in nutritional assessment, as, according to present evidence, they indicate with considerable probability deficiency of one or more nutrients in the tissues in the recent past;

Group 2. Signs that need further investigation, but in whose causation malnutrition, sometimes of a chronic nature, may play some part, together with other factors. They are found more commonly in people with low standards of living than among more privileged groups;

Group 3. Signs not related to nutrition, according to present knowledge, but which, in some instances, have to be differentiated from signs of known nutritional value in Group 1.

Modern reconsideration of this type of classification (Appendix 1) suggests its obvious limitations and vagueness. It can sometimes assist in choosing the most useful selection of signs to record in a particular survey. Recognition and elimination of signs unrelated to nutrition (Group 3) will decrease confusion in interpretation and save time and effort (Figs.

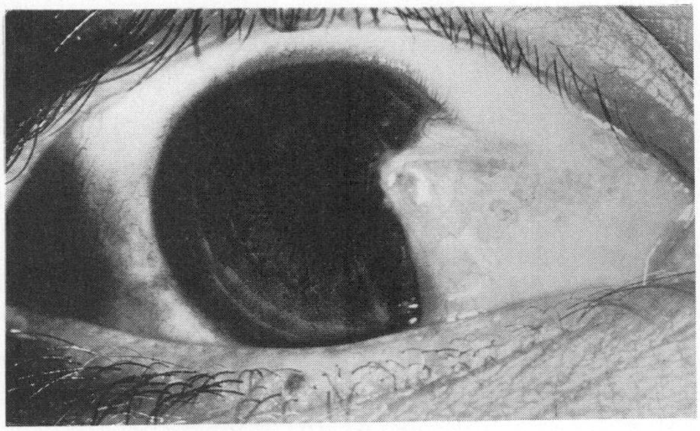

Fig. 2.1 *Signs not related to malnutrition.* Pterygium: wing-shaped double fold of conjunctiva growing across eye from medial side; mainly related to prolonged exposure to sun glare and wind. (Courtesy of Helen Keller International.)

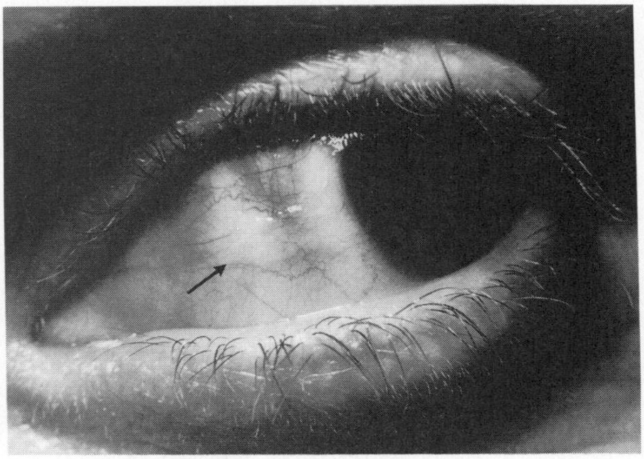

Fig. 2.2 *Signs not related to malnutrition.* Pingueculum: fibro-fatty deposit in lateral conjunctiva. (Courtesy of George Kurz and Helen Keller International.)

2.1 and 2.2). If early experience in an investigation suggests it, additional clinical signs can be included.

As a generalization, it is preferable to limit the signs sought to those considered essential (p. 23). Experience suggests that over-all accuracy and reliability is often inversely proportional to the number of signs included.

Future investigations may, of course, show that the significance of some of the signs listed has to be reappraised. Similarly, newly recognized signs considered to be related to malnutrition will be discovered in the future and may need to be included. For example, it is now clear that signs suggestive of neonatal cretinism, such as a large tongue, dry skin, and sparse hair, as well as of fetal iodine brain damage (p. 272) due to material iodine deficiency need to be clarified, so that they can be differentiated from infants and young children with other types of mental deficiency (Hetzel 1983; Hetzel *et al.* 1986).

Definition and standardization

The physical signs recorded must always be defined as precisely as possible. Otherwise, the meaning of data from various parts of the world remains in doubt, and comparability between the results of different observers or between the findings of the same investigator at different times is impossible. However, as noted by a well-known philosopher, the clinical signs of nutritional deficiency, especially when less marked, will always, like beauty, be to some extent 'in the eye of the beholder.'

Standardization of definition of commonly employed physical signs is obviously especially important for international comparison, and a descriptive list is therefore given in Appendix 1. It was originally based on the 1963 report of the WHO Expert Committee on Medical Assessment of Nutritional Status, but has been expanded and modified to give fuller descriptive detail in light of more recent experience.

As well as carefully written definitions, clear unambiguous photographs or colour slides[5] are helpful, both for training purposes and also as practical guides, especially during actual field work. The basic problem is that such illustrations are almost always of advanced, obvious examples. In reality, it is the early or doubtful signs which are hard to recognize, to photograph, and to agree upon. Some illustrations may need to be made for the particular ethnic group being investigated, particularly skin or hair changes (pp. 471, 483).

The definitions of the signs to be used need to be available in written form for investigators. Before carrying out a survey, the team must be given instruction and practical visual training in their recognition in order to ensure uniformity of judgement and understanding. As well as the use of colour transparencies, observation of clinical patients in hospital and, when feasible, practice pilot field tests are important for standardization (p. 410). Staff members working under close supervision can have their techniques and results reviewed and standardized by some form of quality control testing (p. 410).

Earlier practices of general grading of subjects into 'good', 'fair', or 'poor' by physical inspection in pre-World War II investigations (Bigwood 1939) is obviously even more difficult to assess objectively. It is based on

[5] Series of slides of different stages of xerophthalmia are available from Helen Keller International, 22 West 17 Street, New York 10011.

numerous factors, such as the amount of muscle and subcutaneous fat present, the posture, pallor, and behaviour. Furthermore, it is often influenced subconsciously by the examiner's own body build, the investigator's recent experiences in the field of nutrition (including the present investigation), and cultural concepts of a desirable body build in the particular community. Still more difficult is the assessment of the nutriture of schoolchildren using such indefinite subjective features as 'carriage — erect, slack, or slovenly', as was used in the 1930s (Bigwood 1939). More recently, malnutrition could not be identified adequately by clinical examination alone (e.g. inspection and palpation) in hospitalized surgical patients, but also needed anthropometric 'objective assessment of nutritional depletion'. Nevertheless, rough categorization by inspection can play a role in, for example, initial screening in emergency refugee situations and famines, and in interpretation of the condition of young children with slowing of growth on weight charts (p. 294).

Another well-documented, serious difficulty in survey work is that the observer is subconsciously prone to interpret signs on the spot, and to change the criteria from time to time, depending on the group being examined. If, for example, a sign is found to be common in a certain group, but rare in the one previously examined, there is a tendency to alter the diagnostic criteria without appreciating it, and to record more severe degrees of the sign. For example, standards of judgement of 'normal physique' were noted to change rather rapidly in a lean or an obese population (ICNND 1963).

In the past, the problem of standardization was aggravated by understandable, but ill-advised, attempts to grade the signs recorded into different degrees of positiveness (e.g. 0 to +++). Under field circumstances, and with some exceptions (as with thyroid enlargement and oedema), it is usually not only impossible, but also time-consuming, frustrating, and pseudoscientific, to attempt to differentiate degrees of severity of the physical signs noted. A record of a positive or a negative is usually the best that can be achieved.

Theoretically, it has often been suggested that certain signs can be estimated quantitatively and objectively using mechanical instruments. For example, the gums have been tested for bleeding by the use of a spring-loaded probe that can exert a standard pressure. A special apparatus has even been devised to measure knee jerks quantitatively (ICNND 1963), and an 'epiphysometer' has been suggested to gauge wrist enlargement in rickets (Jelliffe 1971). Similarly, an apparatus has been devised to test for oedema. In practice, however, such mechanical approaches are neither feasible nor worthwhile.

In addition to the standardization of definition, it is important that details of the examination should be described. If a full-scale examination for all clinical signs is intended, theoretically the skin of the whole body should be examined, as some lesions are found most commonly on the buttocks or perineum. This is usually neither practicable, nor culturally acceptable, nor needed. However, a note should be made concerning the extent of the examination. Anyway, in present-day studies, only a limited number of signs is usually looked for (p. 23). Both full-scale and limited clinical assessment must always be carried out with good illumination, preferably with indirect sunlight. Care needs to be taken to avoid fatigue in the observer brought on by excessive, continuous, repetitive, ultimately boring work.

Strongly suggestive clinical signs

A descriptive list of clinical signs that have been used is given in Appendix 1. Clinical diagnosis of individuals with severe nutritional deficiency, such as those who are likely to be hospitalized, will usually be based on the presence of 'groupings' of signs (Appendix 1).

In recent work, clinical examination has focused on a limited number of what may be termed 'strongly suggestive' signs. In some ways, this dates back to the concept of the 'key sign', introduced by Jolliffe in the 1950s (Jolliffe 1962). This was based on the association of a particular sign with a supposed lack of a given nutrient — such as angular stomatitis and riboflavin deficiency. As noted earlier, this is no longer regarded as completely valid, because of the lack of specificity of the signs recorded and because it is unusual for the diet of a community to be deficient in one nutrient only. Nevertheless, experience in community work in the past two decades has in effect reintroduced the Jolliffe concept, in a modified, limited form, and with a less definite emphasis. Certain signs can be considered as 'strongly suggestive' of a particular nutrient deficiency (Table 2.5 and Figs. 2.3–2.12).

The fact that most clinical signs are non-specific does not preclude their selective use in nutritional assessment. The frequent occurrence of one particular sign may give a lead to further investigations. Its association with other related signs increases the likelihood of its nutritional significance, both in an individual and in a community.

The interpretation of particular clinical signs may then be reinforced by discovering 'multiple signs' which can occur with deficiency of a particular nutrient, especially in some conditions, such as vitamin D deficiency or severe protein–energy malnutrition. However, often only one clinical sign may be present. In addition, moderately severe protein–energy malnutrition in young children may or may not show one or more clinical signs. Usually, it will be detected by anthropometry (p. 273).

The clinical patterns on which these groupings of 'multiple signs' are based differ in detail, or in the most prevalent combinations of signs, in various parts of the world, depending upon the degree, duration, and

Table 2.5 Commonly recorded clinical signs 'strongly suggestive' of dietary deficiency or excess

Sign*	Suggested nutrient abnormality
Deficiency	
Pale conjuctiva	Anaemia (iron/folic acid/B12)
Bitôt's spots	Vitamin A
Angular stomatitis	Riboflavin
Spongy, bleeding gums	Vitamin C (after infancy)
Thyroid enlargement	Iodine
Oedema (both lower legs) (young children)	Protein–energy malnutrition
Epiphyseal enlargement (both wrists)	Vitamin D
Excess	
Mottled enamel	Fluoride
Dental caries (cavities, etc.)	Sugar (sticky forms; direct oral effect)

* For illustrations see Fig. 2.3–2.12.

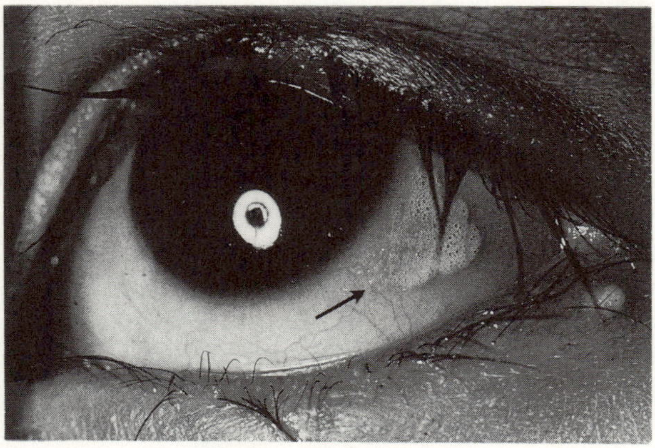

Fig. 2.3 *Strongly suggestive clinical signs.* Vitamin A deficiency: Bitôt's spot (left eye) — large, dry, white or silvery 'foamy' area on lateral conjunctiva, roughly triangular, usually bilateral (Indonesia). (Courtesy of the late Professor H.A.P.C. Oomen.)

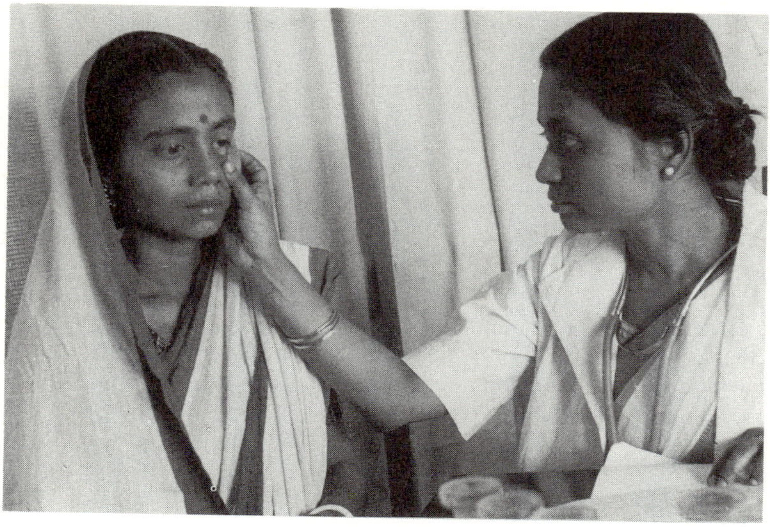

Fig. 2.4 *Strongly suggestive clinical signs.* Nutritional anaemia: pallor of the conjunctiva — examination of multiparous pregnant lacto-vegetarian Hindu mother (Calcutta, India).

speed of onset of malnutrition. Other factors influencing the clinical picture can include details of the prevailing diet, genetic background, the age and activity of the person, and the environment in which they live, as regards both hygiene, climate, exposure to infection and parasitism, and 'stimulation' (care, love, and attention), especially in young children.

Age plays a particularly important part in the clinical signs produced by nutrient deficiency. This is shown by the different pictures produced in young children and in adults as a result of ascorbic acid lack or protein–energy malnutrition. Furthermore, age plays a significant, though not fully understood, part in determining the incidence and nature of the eye manifestations of vitamin A deficiency, where signs in early childhood often appear to differ from those seen in schoolchildren and adults (McLaren 1963; Sommer 1982).

Patterns of clinical signs associated with specific nutrient deficiencies cannot be standardized precisely for all areas of the world, although there is always a substantial agreement on the major features encountered. For example, the clinical picture of kwashiorkor varies in detail from one region to another. At the same time, a core of four clinical features seem recognized universally — oedema, mental change, wasted muscles (with some remaining subcutaneous fat), and growth retardation (as judged initially by inadequate weight gain) (p. 278).

Sometimes, examination for selected signs may be all that is required in a rapid 'focused' screening survey (Zerfas *et al.* 1982). Thus, the examina-

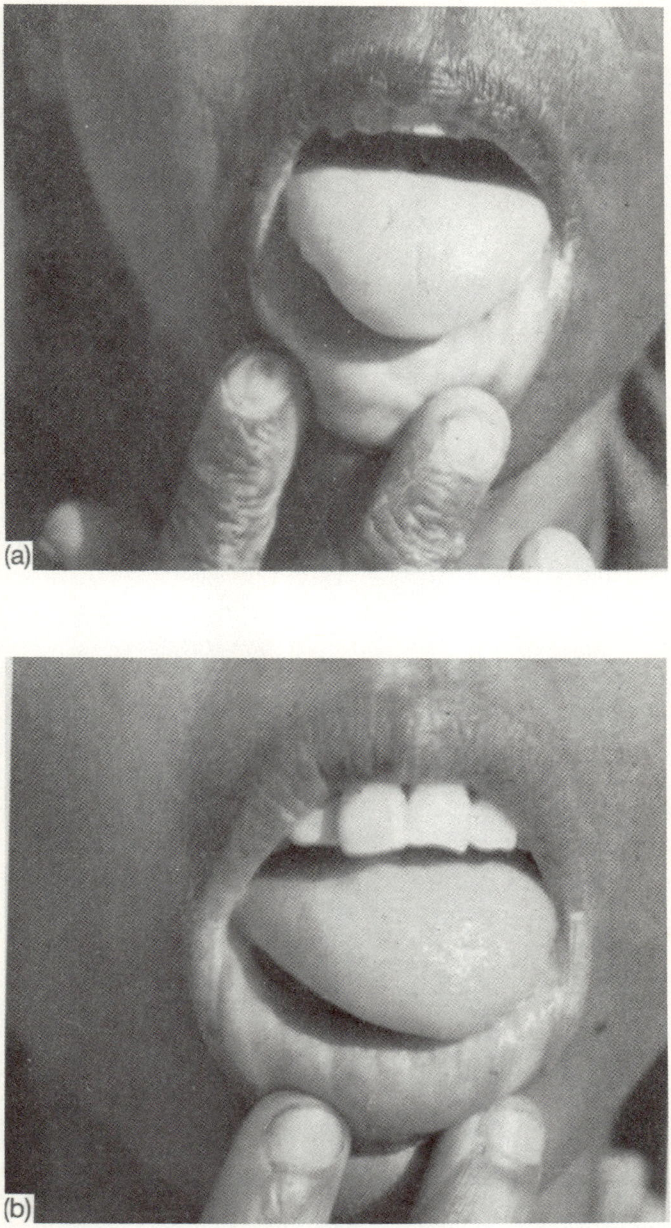

Fig. 2.5 *Strongly suggestive clinical signs.* Nutritional anaemia: mucosal and nailbed pallor: present in (a), compared with normal (b). (Courtesy UNICEF, New Delhi, India.)

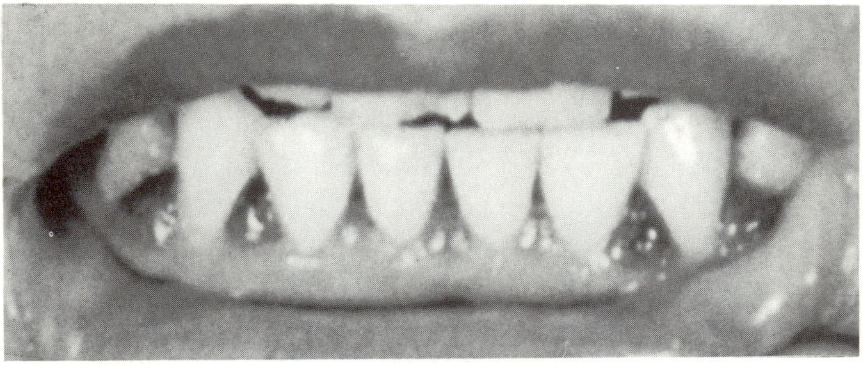

Fig. 2.6 *Strongly suggestive clinical signs.* Vitamin C deficiency (scurvy): swollen, spongy, bleeding gums.

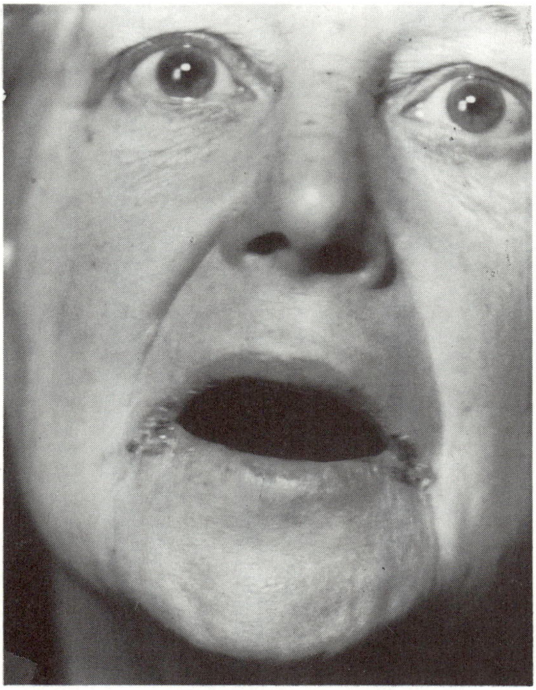

Fig. 2.7 *Strongly suggestive clinical signs.* Riboflavin deficiency: sodden excoriated fissures at the angles of the mouth. (Courtesy of the Burroughs Wellcome Museum, London.)

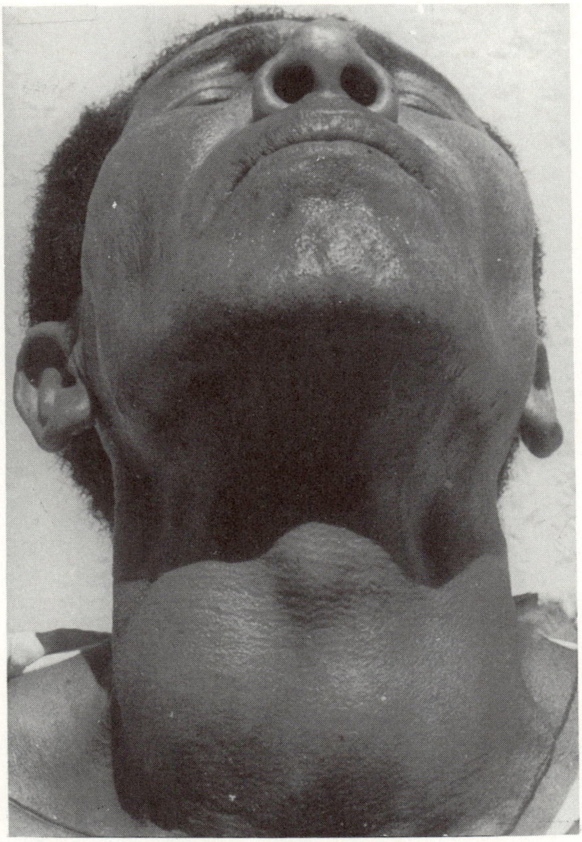

Fig. 2.8 *Strongly suggestive clinical signs*. Iodine deficiency disorders (IDD): enlarged thyroid (goitre) (WHO Stage 1-B) (p. 482)

tion for epiphyseal enlargement at the wrist will give a rough indication of the prevalence of clinical rickets. However, surveys and other studies based on clinical signs need confirming, whenever possible, by: (1) investigation of the local diet, particularly by food consumption surveys (p. 189): (2) appropriate anthropometric measurements to detect protein–energy malnutrition (p. 64); and, when feasible, (3) selected laboratory tests (p. 31), possibly on a subsample. Each of these methods is imperfect and incomplete. Used together, in locally relevant and practicable combinations, they can give more complete information on nutritional situations, both in individuals and in communities, especially if combined with 'qualitative' observations (Scrimshaw and Hurtado 1987).

In some circumstances, therapeutic trials can be a useful extension of clinical assessment where the need is to establish the cause of a deficiency

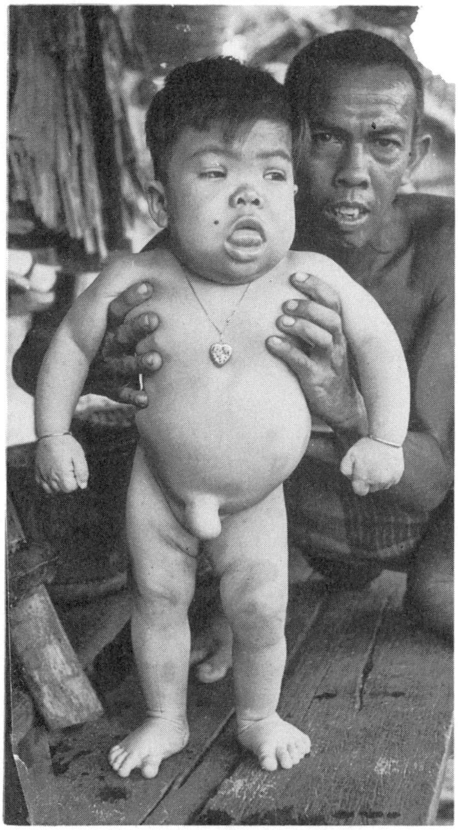

Fig. 2.9 *Strongly suggestive clinical signs.* Iodine deficiency disorders: endemic cretinism with mental and physical retardation and other characteristic signs (including large tongue, distended abdomen, etc.). (Courtesy of Dr Elaine Field.)

syndrome or to clarify the specificity of a clinical sign. They can, for example, be of value in defining the nutritional aetiology of anaemia, as judged by haematological response, including a rise in the reticulocyte count and haemoglobin level following the administration of different nutrients (e.g. iron, folic acid, etc.). This type of investigation can sometimes be carried out at the end of a survey or as part of a follow-up on a limited number of affected persons. Such therapeutic trials will also be guided by biochemical and dietary findings. Therapeutically effective doses of the single nutrient being investigated are given to the selected persons for what is judged to be a sufficient time to produce results. For example, a recent therapeutic trial in Liberia (Jackson and Latham 1982) clearly demonstrated the predominant role of iron deficiency in anaemia of pregnancy there. Conversely, a therapeutic trial in the Gambia (Pren-

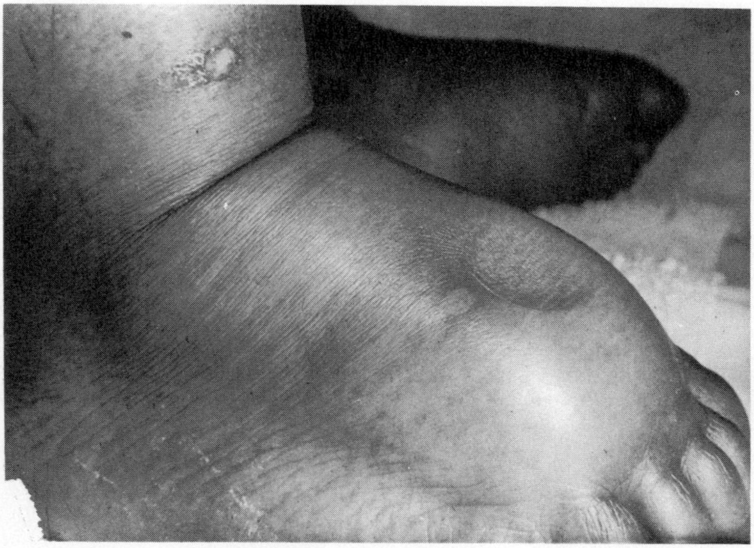

Fig. 2.10 *Strongly suggestive clinical signs.* Kwashiorkor (severe form of protein–energy malnutrition): pitting oedema — bilateral in 15-month-old African child.

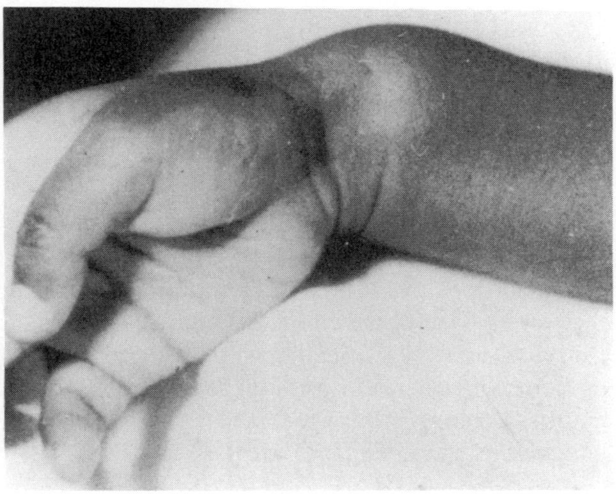

Fig. 2.11 *Strongly suggestive clinical signs.* Vitamin D deficiency (rickets): epiphyseal enlargement (wrist joint) in one-year-old infant — bilateral, painless.

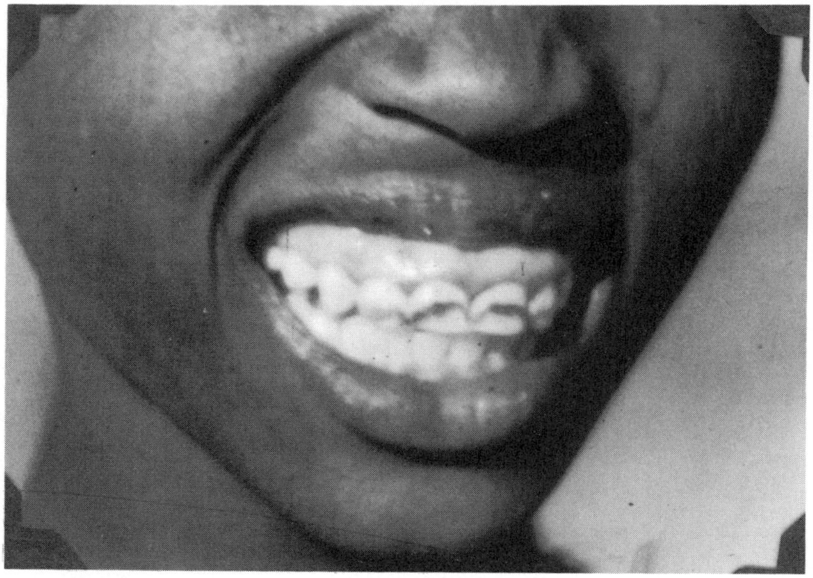

Fig. 2.12 *Strongly suggestive clinical signs.* Flouride excess (fluorosis): mottling of teeth in young man (rural Tanzania) whose only water supply had a very high fluoride content.

tice *et al.* 1983) showed no relationship between bleeding gums with gingivitis and vitamin C deficiency.

If the nutrient is given by mouth, biochemical tests to ensure that absorption has occurred are desirable, but not usually practicable. If practicable, a control group with similar clinical features should be given a placebo in order to control for spontaneous improvements, such as those due to seasonal differences. Ideally, the trial should be 'double-blind' in that the observer should not be able to differentiate between nutrient and placebo until after the trial is completed. Statistical guidance as to sufficient sample size is desirable (p. 405).

Clinical changes need to be critically evaluated, preferably quantitatively, by measurements of the size of a lesion, or by before-and-after photographs, preferably in colour, supported, when possible, with the results of appropriate biochemical or haematological tests.

Conclusions

In retrospect, too much was expected from a complex range of difficult-to-define clinical signs of uncertain aetiology in surveys and other investigations undertaken two to three decades ago. Some inherent difficulties and advantages of clinical signs were noted earlier and are summarized in Table 2.4. These signs represented a rather haphazard mixture of features noted by clinicians (usually paediatricians) whose patients were most often hospitalized and severely ill, and of signs found in community studies where less marked malnutrition would be more usual. For example, a 'Casal's necklace' (p. 483) is diagnostic of severe clinical pellagra, but would be very uncommon in population surveys. As mentioned, hospitalized cases of severe deficiency are more likely to show several of the signs indicated (Appendix 1).

However, clinical signs do need to be remembered and taught to medical, nursing, and nutrition students if they are not to go unrecognized or be overlooked in occasional individuals with marked dietary inadequacy, including those in technically more developed countries. These signs may occur in the elderly, the mentally ill, the urban homeless poor, or in individuals, including adolescents, voluntarily consuming very restricted 'fad' diets, or with anorexia nervosa. Also, if any less usual signs are noted during a community investigation, they need to be noted in the report.

From recent experience, it has become increasingly appreciated that clinical signs should be sought for selectively. Those to be included will depend on the purpose of the investigation, including the age-group and the likelihood of different nutrient deficiencies being present in the community under study, as judged by evidence from health services data and by existing knowledge of the local diet.

In addition, clinical signs may sometimes help in describing the general picture of nutrition in a particular community, particularly if protein–energy malnutrition is common in young children. More specifically, some signs are *strongly suggestive* of certain deficiencies, such as those of iodine, vitamin A, rickets, or riboflavin (Table 2.5). In addition, dental caries may be included by means of the DMF (decayed, missing, filled) score and by some form of questionnaire enquiring about the amount and type of sucrose preparation consumed (p. 189).

Such limited, selected signs can also be helpful in individual clinical diagnosis. They are particularly useful in rapid surveys (p. 364) or for village health workers in primary health care services. Most usually, they are potential clues, needing corroboration by information from other sources.

Laboratory tests

> *Interest in biochemistry as an aid to nutritional assessment stems from the belief that biochemistry should provide the earliest possible indication of change in nutritional status.*
>
> Alleyne *et al.* (1977)

The main laboratory tests of nutritional significance can be considered in three groups: biochemical, haematological, and parasitological. They will not be reviewed separately here, as the purpose of some of these investigations overlap. This is especially the case, for example, with anaemia (p. 31).

Biochemical estimations[6] of nutritional significance have been carried out on a variety of body tissues, including liver (by biopsy or at autopsy), muscle (Heymsfield *et al.* 1982, 1983), bone (Klepinger 1984), hair, nails, and subcutaneous fat (Smith *et al.* 1986). In practice, especially in community studies, tests are at most confined to two relatively easily obtainable body fluids: blood and urine. Hair has been used recently for some estimations on an experimental basis, especially for estimation of trace elements (Manson and Zlotkin 1985).

Problems

The number of biochemical tests and techniques that have been used for assessing malnutrition is considerable. A more extensive range can often be feasible for hospitalized subjects in more technically developed countries Micro-methods are available for most tests, but only in well-equipped laboratories.

Conditions in Third World countries greatly limit their practical application. Such limitations include the question of using single-specimen samples rather than the collection of 'timed' specimens or the use of loading tests; the impossibility or great difficulty in securing venous blood from young children; and the limitation of laboratory facilities, including skilled technicians.

If laboratory tests are under consideration, details concerning up-to-date information on methods, significance, reliability, and cost of biochemical tests need full discussion with colleagues who have an understanding of the local limitations and practical problems of processing, preserving, and storing samples, and the public health priority (or otherwise) of various tests.

Criteria

Ideal criteria for biochemical tests suitable for field work, include easily collectable samples (such as a finger-prick specimen of blood, or a random specimen of urine), stability during transport (preferably not requiring refrigeration), an inexpensive, uncomplicated laboratory technique, unaffected by a recent meal or by water intake, and capable of giving easy-to-interpret information of high sensitivity,[7] and specificity not

[6] This section was originally based largely on the report of the WHO Expert Committee on Medical Assessment of Nutritional Status (1963), and on the manual prepared by the ICNND (1963). In its revisions, the reviews by Alleyne *et al.* (1977), Christakis (1973), Kanawati (1976), National Academy of Sciences (1978*b*) *Proc. Nutr. Soc.* (1982), the *Am. J. Clin. Nutr.* (1982), Woods (1982), and Sauberlich (1983) have been invaluable. They should be consulted for further details, including laboratory procedures, and information on other more complex tests.

[7] Definition given in glossary of commoner epidemiological terms (Appendix 4, p. 508).

already available from non-biochemical sources (including clinical signs and/or anthropometry) (Whitehead 1965). Ideally, laboratory tests should be useful for objective quantitative assessment, or as a screening procedure in communities. In well-equipped hospital circumstances, they may be used as indicators of severity and prognosis.

Specimens

Blood tests may be carried out with macro-methods, although the relatively large quantities required can be obtained in field circumstances only with great difficulty, even from adults or school-age children, if at all. Cultural attitudes (p. 165) and understandable apprehension may make this impossible. Micro-methods, using finger-prick samples, can be used for tests for some nutrients and are obviously especially suitable for young children.

When required, venous samples should be taken with disposable plastic syringes to avoid any risk of virus infection, especially hepatitis and now AIDS. A vacuum tube (such as the Vacutainer) may be employed instead, but cannot be used in malnourished young children with fragile easily collapsible viens.

Conclusions

Biochemical tests are usually costly and time-consuming to carry out. Lack of suitable laboratories, as is usual in most Third World countries, may be an absolute limiting factor. In all surveys, the expected value of results to be obtained from selected biochemical tests in the assessment of nutritional status must be weighed against the problems of collection, transport with refrigeration ('cold chain'), laboratory analysis, and interpretation. In addition, while a few tests are of considerable assistance, many still have as yet uncertain 'standards' (reference data) or cut-off points for less advanced degrees of malnutrition, when they are most needed, especially for young children (Table 2.6).

Laboratory tests expressed numerically can also have the paradoxical disadvantage of giving a scientific aura that is not usually justified by the reliability of the analysis or its actual biological meaning. In fact, numerous useful nutritional surveys of limited scope have been undertaken with a small team using clinical examination, anthropometry, and dietary inquiry, with no laboratory investigations, other than haemoglobin estimations.

Selection

The selection of appropriate biochemical tests depends on the type of investigation or study contemplated, and the nutrient deficiencies sus-

Table 2.6 Laboratory tests: considerations in community nutritional assessment in less technically developed countries

Advantages	Difficulties		
May precede other evidence	Expensive		
Objective	Difficulties with specimens	Collection Preservation Transportation	Technical Cultural
Gradable	Absence of laboratories		
	Reference Data	Technique 'Normal' range Age differences Genetic	
	Unwarranted numerate 'certainty' (cultural)		

pected. In some circumstances, adult serum cholesterol levels may be included (US Department of Health and Human Services 1985). However, for a nutrition survey to produce useful information, it is not necessary to have the funds, time, relatively large number of trained personnel, and quantities of equipment required for a wide range of biochemical test to be undertaken. This is rarely desirable and makes a survey less feasible financially.

Sometimes laboratory investigations may be practicable on a limited sample of people, the specimens from whom may be air-freighted to a central or regional laboratory. Selection of those to be tested may be by statistically-guided subsampling (p. 405) or by choosing contrasting subjects considered, on clinical evidence, to be likely to span the extremes of 'normal' through to the obviously nutritionally deficient. Thus, more detailed haematological tests may be carried out on a small percentage of those found to be definitely anaemic by clinical assessment or by haemoglobin level. Likewise, vitamin 'loading' tests with riboflavin may sometimes be possible in a sample of persons with angular cheilosis and other suggestive signs of ariboflavinosis. Serum retinol concentrations in samples of clinically unaffected children can be compared with those with Bitôt's spots (p. 475) in the same community. More detailed studies of iodine metabolism may be undertaken in areas where populations are affected by iodine deficiency disorders (p. 272).

By contrast, the use of some biochemical tests in severely ill patients in sophisticated hospitals with well-equipped laboratories has increased in recent years. Frequently, they have been used to determine which patients are likely to die, which will need special forms of nutritional support, including parenteral feeding (Woods 1982), and as indicators of improvement or deterioration.

As with all methods of assessment, the nutritional significance of the results of biochemical tests has to be considered together with all other evidence, including clinical examination, anthropometric measurements, and estimates of dietary intake.

Collection of specimens

Numbers

When the appropriate laboratory tests for a particular community study have been decided upon, a decision must be made as to the number of specimens that can be collected and processed. Obviously, this will determine the required amount of collecting equipment. In surveys, the number of specimens will depend on statistical sampling considerations (p. 405), in relation to the total number of persons examined clinically in the field, and on practical limitations imposed by facilities for transport, storage, and analysis. A subsampling technique will normally be required (p. 405). The type of specimen of blood or urine, and methods of collecting are outlined later (Appendix 2).

Laboratory considerations

Site

The various laboratory tests differ in complexity with respect to the staff and facilities required, and the time within which they have to be performed, once the sample has been taken.

In surveys, one, or all, of three laboratory sites have to be considered:

1. Survey site facilities, at least for taking, labelling, and packaging samples;
2. A field laboratory adjacent to, or not far distant from, the survey site. Adequate bench or table space should be available, as well as a water supply, a refrigerator, cylinders of gas, and, if possible, electricity;
3. A base, or central, or regional laboratory, often situated in a central institution, such as a nutritional institute, a medical school, or an agricultural research station.

The most suitable arrangement for a given study depends upon the tests envisaged, the availability and location of existing laboratories, the distances and transport involved, and the funds available. These, in turn, will depend on the purpose of the whole investigation.

In most developing countries, laboratory services are very limited, especially outside main centres, and plans must be made to take most of the samples back at the end of a survey, or to send them at intervals during the field work, depending on local circumstances. The necessary funds for staff, including drivers, and for equipment (Mitchell *et al.* 1983), including continous refrigeration ('cold chain'), must be included in the budget.

In many surveys, it is easier and more economical to make it a rule that, whenever possible, specimens should be collected in the field, preserved or refrigerated suitably, and ultimately taken back to the base laboratory at the end of the survey. This usually applies to the two main samples often obtained in less technically developed countries — blood for haemoglobin and malarial parasites, and faeces for ova and cysts.

Equipment

Initial and recurrent equipment needs must be calculated as far as possible by estimating the number of samples likely to be collected and their possible storage and transport. A 10 per cent excess is desirable for field work to cover breakage, loss, and any initial underestimate of attendance. The use of latex or rubber gloves may be indicated when taking blood samples in areas where AIDS is known to be common.

Supplies should be standardized, as far as possible. Containers should be labelled prior to the field work and be ready for use (e.g. with anticoagulants already in them). They should be as strong as possible and shaped so as to make packing easier and minimize breakage (e.g. sturdy, flat-bottomed, thick-glass, or plastic, screw-capped vials). If thick films are to be taken for the detection of malarial parasites, particular attention needs to be given to the cleanliness of the slides.

Techniques

Laboratory techniques must be selected for their accuracy, sensitivity, specificity, reproducibility, and practicability (Appendix 4) within the technical resources available. In all cases, the method employed must be described in reports, and, if it is a modification of a standard procedure or a new technique, details of any innovation given.

In subsequent reports, details must also be given of procedures used in the collection, transport, and storage of specimens, including, if relevant to the particular tests, the date and time when the specimen was taken, possible exposure to sun, heat, and air, and the period between collection and testing.

Interpretation

The significance and accuracy of results of laboratory tests are related to methods of collection, transport, and storage (including possible exposure to sunlight or heat, and shaking), the actual technique employed (including laboratory supervision using control sera), and the condition of those tested (e.g. age, time of day, fasting).

The interpretation of results varies with knowledge of the unique metabolism of each particular nutrient, including the effect of recent ingestion, the extent to which it is stored in the body, the possibility of synthesis, and the mode and speed of excretion.

The tests employed usually assess one of three aspects of nutritional adequacy. First, a biochemical investigation may give information on the dietary supply to the body by reflecting the concentration of nutrients in a particular tissue, most often the serum (e.g. ascorbic acid). However, the concentration of an essential nutrient in a body fluid may be reduced as a result of recent dietary deficiency, poor absorption, impaired transport (as can result from the decreased plasma proteins in protein–energy malnutrition), abnormal utilization, interaction with a therapentic drug, or a combination of these. The possible presence of haemoconcentration, as in dehydration, or of haemodilution, as in pregnancy, needs to be taken into account. Thus, while the measurement of nutrients in the serum may suggest the possibility of malnutrition, in some cases (e.g. ascorbic acid) it does not indicate the presence, or define the degree, of nutritional adequacy, but more often reflects recent dietary intake.

Second, some biochemical tests can be undertaken that reveal metabolic changes resulting from decreased tissue function due to inadequate supplies of essential nutrients, often of long duration. These include, for example, decreased production of serum albumin (p. 38) by the liver in severe protein–energy malnutrition.

Third, biochemical tests can give an estimate of the amount of nutrient stored in the body — for example, iron in the bone marrow or vitamin C in red or white blood cells.

The advantage of some biochemical tests is that they may give information concerning nutritional status, before the appearance of clinical or anthropometric changes.

Concentrations of nutrients in the body have to be compared with 'reference data' appropriate for the age and sex of the person under study, when these are available. Often such data will have been constructed from a 'normal' range of results obtained from supposedly well-fed healthy groups, contrasted with a range of results from patients obviously clinically ill with a particular form of malnutrition. In such circumstances, findings have often been sorted into various highly tentative groups, with descriptive labels, such as 'deficient', 'low', and 'acceptable'. This is helpful, although such value-laden labels inevitably tend to be regarded as more certain and absolute than justified. In addition, there is considerable need to determine ranges of 'normal' for different age-groups, based on better understanding of their effects on short- and long-term 'functional significance', although this represents a formidable task.

Often, however, reference values are not known, especially for children.

The results then are often necessarily expressed in relation to whatever data are available, even though the age-group is inappropriate. A recent compilation of a 'normal' range of values for children is given later (Appendix 2, p. 501) (Neumann *et al.* 1982).

The effects of such physiological events as pregnancy (p. 226) and ageing (p. 352) need consideration; as do possible drug–nutrient interactions, with, for example, antimalarials and isoniazid.

Whether there is sufficient information to sort into specific 'labelled' groups or not, results should always be reported mathematically as well. Such information should include the number of samples examined and the results expressed as means (averages) and standard deviations, as well as in numbers and percentages, in appropriate groups, defined numerically and sometimes given labels judged to be appropriate according to current practical information (e.g. 'low' or 'deficient', etc.).

Certain biochemical tests are used more commonly, and these are discussed below. Those employed less frequently are commented on later (Appendix 2), together with general notes on methods of collecting samples.

Protein and energy[8]

In practice, tests for protein adequacy are usually considered in relation to the different forms and degrees of severity of protein–energy malnutrition. As detailed later (p. 273), protein–energy malnutrition occurs most commonly in young children. It can affect any age-group and much attention has recently been given to its significance in hospitalized patients in technically more developed countries (p. 348). The severe syndromes — kwashiorkor and marasmus — are clinically obvious. It is with the identification of less severe degrees of protein–energy malnutrition that both biochemical tests and anthropometry (p. 56) have been mainly concerned.

In the past 20 years or so, numerous biochemical tests were developed in attempts to assess four aspects of protein nutrition in protein–energy malnutrition:

1. Diminished synthesis and depletion of stores;
2. Growth retardation;
3. Metabolic changes due to tissue malnutrition;
4. Relative adequacy of dietary intake.

Of these, only serum albumin — as an indicator of decreased liver function — has been widely used in some community studies. Other tests

[8] Detailed consideration of these biochemical tests were given by Alleyne *et al.* (1977) in *Protein–energy malnutrition.*

Table 2.7 Interpretation of serum albumin concentrations in malnourished children (*Alleyne* et al. *1977*). (Probably of practical relevance only in kwashiorkor-endemic areas)

Concentration (g/dl)	Interpretation
≥ 3.5	Normal
3–3.4	Subnormal
2.5–2.9	Low
< 2.5	Pathological

of various aspects of protein metabolism have been employed and can be useful in some circumstances (Appendix 2).

Plasma proteins Various plasma proteins, especially albumin, are much reduced in kwashiorkor (p. 276), but not nearly so markedly in marasmus (p. 282). This is the result of a combination of depleted body reserves and decreased hepatic synthesis. However, it seems generally agreed that the body's ability to synthesize serum albumin is affected relatively late, and that the primary effect of protein lack is depletion of the least metabolically vital protein store — muscle tissue. Concentrations of total plasma protein are even more difficult to evaluate in many developing countries, as raised globulin levels, due to infections, including chronic malaria, are likely to influence the results.

Investigations in Third World countries in the 1960s indicated that the concentration of serum albumin falls significantly only in severe protein depletion, thus serving 'only as a confirmation of a condition already clinically evident' (Arroyave and Wilson 1961), and that it is not of value for detecting 'marginal', mild–moderate cases (Waterlow 1978).

More recent studies show that the serum albumin is of help in indicating the severity of established kwashiorkor (Olusi *et al.* 1975), but confirm that it is usually of little value in identifying less severe protein–energy malnutrition with certainty. An exception perhaps in those regions of the world where kwashiorkor is the most common severe syndrome in the community, as in some parts of Africa. The normal range for serum albumin is 3.5–5.0 g/dl, and, in kwashiorkor areas, Alleyne *et al.* (1977) suggest the interpretation given in Table 2.7. Some marasmic children show 'low normal' levels.

Serum albumin is 'not an index of body wasting', but, in regions where kwashiorkor is endemic, low concentrations have been considered to 'aid detection of children who are at risk of an oedematous episode' (Whitehead *et al.* 1971). The serum albumin test has had the advantage of being simple and inexpensive, and it is likely to be available even in moderately equipped biochemistry laboratories. However, recent technical methods allow pre-albumin and transferrin to be estimated as easily as albumin, and have the advantage of giving an indication of more recent metabolic disturbance.

Paradoxically, serum albumin has been widely used in the 'nutritional assessment profile' in recent years, with severely ill hospital patients in some Western countries. A low serum albumin (3.5 g/dl) in combination with a low total lymphocyte count (p. 349) is an indicator of immunocompetence in so-called 'instant nutritional assessment' (Seltzer *et al.* 1981). However, it has not been found to be useful everywhere (Force and Shizgal 1980) and it may be that the low concentrations seen in hospitalized individuals are in part a response to associated infections, injuries, and/or other serious illness (Merritt *et al.* 1983).

Vitamins[9]

Assessment of vitamins are most commonly undertaken for retinol, vitamin D, and ascorbic acid.

Vitamin A or retinol[10] This is stored in the liver, and a direct assessment of body reserves can be made on liver biopsy material, but this is neither practicable nor ethical. However, hepatic stores have been measured at autopsy (McLaren 1963).

The most useful biochemical test for survey work is an estimation of serum vitamin A (retinol), especially in young age-groups. However, because of the substantial amount of this vitamin stored in the liver, a low serum concentration reflects not only an inadequate recent intake, but also the exhaustion of liver reserves. It is therefore related to prolonged severe dietary deficiency — probably of up to 1 year in adults and of up to 4 months in young children.

It has been shown that low levels of serum vitamin A are found in acute infections (McLaren 1963) and in kwashiorkor. These low levels are probably due in part to liver dysfunction and in part to impaired blood transport of the vitamin, notably a lowered retinol-binding protein (Pirie *et al.* 1976). Caution may therefore be required in interpreting results in populations among whom lesser degrees of protein–calorie malnutrition are common. High concentrations of beta-carotenoids may interfere with the estimation of serum vitamin A, depending on the analytical method.

In young adult males, a concentration of < 10 μg/dl serum retinol was thought to indicate deficiency (ICNND 1963), and this level has been found useful in many field surveys (Sommer 1982). In recent studies in young males 30 μg/dl has been considered suggestive (Sauberlich 1983).

[9] Biochemical tests for other vitamins are given in Appendix 2.

[10] One International Unit (IU) of vitamin A is equivalent to 0.3 μg of retinol.

The serum response to a known dose of retinol has been tried in population studies (retinol dose–response tests) (IVACG 1982; Leavell 1987).

In all investigations due attention must also be given to correlation with food-consumption studies, with clinical signs suggestive of avitaminosis A, and, in older children and adults, with results of dark-adaptation tests, if practicable. It seems probable that low serum vitamin A levels and abnormal dark-adaptation tests usually antedate the appearance of clinical signs as community indicators of inadequate vitamin A nutrition. Some appropriate practical village level tests for dark adaptation are given later (p. 268), and mothers' reports can be helpful in cultures where this condition is well-recognized in everyday life (p. 269).

The ocular (conjunctival) cytology test has recently become recognized as a feasible, low cost test for pre-clinical xerophthamia (Hatchell and Sommer 1984.) (Also see: Addendum, 1988).

Serum carotene estimations are of less value, as they reflect the dietary intake of carotene-containing foods and their digestion and absorption by the body. They are not directly indicative of vitamin A nutrition as such, particularly as some cannot be used by the body (McLaren 1963). At best, low concentrations are related to a low intake of carotene-containing foods — often important in tropical populations whose diet is deficient in expensive vitamin A (retinol).

Vitamin D Adequacy of vitamin D nutrition is never related to dietary intake alone, because body synthesis can produce part or all for the daily needs, provided that the skin is exposed to sufficient sunlight. In fact, vitamin D can best be considered as a hormone secreted by one of the body's largest organs — the skin. Severe shortage of vitamin D usually results in rickets in young children and osteomalacia in adults, frequently multiparous women. In these conditions, excessive, though incomplete, bone formation is associated with an increase in the serum concentration of the enzyme alkaline phosphatase prior to the onset of clinical signs (Hojer *et al.* 1977; Pettifor *et al.* 1980).

In young children, normal serum alkaline phosphatase ranges between 5 and 15 Bodansky units/dl, but, in clinical rickets, it usually rises to above 20 units.[11] Similarly, in osteomalacia in adult women, the serum alkaline phosphatase concentration rises above the usual 3 to 5 Bodansky units, to about 15 units (Sauberlich 1983).

Serum alkaline phosphatase levels have been shown to be reduced in kwashiorkor and appear to be affected in lesser degrees of protein–energy malnutrition. However, atypically studies in Ethiopia showed raised concentrations in marasmic young children with vitamin D deficiency

[11] Usual upper limits in King–Armstrong units are 20 units for children and 13 units for adults.

(Hojer *et al.* 1977). Individual diagnosis in children should be based on a combination of clinical signs, serum alkaline phosphatase levels, and radiological examinations (p. 54). In surveys, subsamples of the population at-risk should be examined biochemically and radiologically, when possible. In specialized studies, circulating vitamin D (25-hydroxycholecalciferol) can be assayed and has been shown to be low in elderly people in parts of the USA and Europe (Bouillon *et al.* 1987), who have been receiving little exposure to sunshine and have a diet low in vitamin D.

Ascorbic acid The simplest biochemical test for inadequate vitamin C nutrition measures serum ascorbic acid. Unfortunately, this mainly reflects recent dietary intake. Even a complete absence of serum ascorbic acid is not necessarily diagnostic of scurvy, as volunteers on a vitamin C-free diet had an absence of serum ascorbic acid for some three months prior to developing clinically evident disease. For young adults, 0.10–0.19 mg/dl is regarded as 'low', and under 0.10 mg/dl as 'deficient'. In highly specialized laboratories, leucocyte ascorbic acid can be estimated to determine tissue concentrations (Schorah *et al.* 1978).

Minerals and trace elements

With the exception of iron (pp. 227, 263), minerals and trace elements have not often been included as part of nutritional assessment. Recently, numerous special studies of zinc have been undertaken, including measurement of its concentration in white cells (Prasad 1985) and in hair (Dorea *et al.* 1982). However, hair analyses for zinc are considered unreliable for the assessment of nutritional status of individuals, although they may have some use for population studies. Samples have the advantages of being 'non-invasive', not requiring refrigeration, and being capable of being sent through the post. They require zinc and iron-free collecting containers. Also, difficulties with hair analyses have become apparent, including the effects of air pollutants and hair dyes. It is certain that investigations concerning trace elements will increase, especially for zinc, selenium, and copper.

Iron, folic acid, and vitamin B_{12} Anaemia can result from many non-nutritional mechanisms, singly or in combination. Examples include chronic haemorrhage (as with hookworm infection), and/or haemolysis (as with malaria). It can also occur if a person is deficient in various nutrients required for normal blood production, again either singly or in combination. The principal nutrients are iron, folic acid, and vitamin B_{12}.

Iron deficiency is by far the most common cause of nutritional anaemia and is a very large problem all over the world (Royston, 1982). Iron deficiency may exist in the body as a result of inadequate dietary intake, poor absorption (sometimes made worse by high phytate diets), or excessive loss (for example, as a result of severe hookworm infection, especially in children in developing countries), or a combination of these. It is more common in women, because of menstrual losses and the drain of repeated pregnancies. It is particularly likely to happen in early childhood and during pregnancy (p. 226) when the iron needs are high and the diet lacking, sometimes as a result of cultural restrictions (p. 165).

Iron deficiency results in the depletion of body stores, ultimately leading to the low haemoglobin of iron deficiency anaemia. Plasma ferritin concentrations (below 10 ng/ml) seem most widely recognized as indicative of iron depletion. Unfortunately, this test is often not feasible in less technically developed regions, for reasons mentioned earlier (p. 33).

Haemoglobin 'standards' have to be laid down for different age-groups, high altitudes, and possibly ethnic groups. These can be based on function and effect, or on distribution in the supposedly well-fed, non-iron deficient (Garn *et al.* 1980; Garn and Keating 1981).

Methods of haemoglobin estimation Methods used for estimating the concentration of circulating haemoglobin can be undertaken: (1) colorimetrically, as haemoglobin is the main pigment in the blood; (2) volumetrically, by measuring the erythrocyte volume (packed cell volume or haematocrit); or (3) densimetrically, measuring the specific gravity of blood.[12]

Despite its possible multiple causation, a colorimetric estimation of haemoglobin is undertaken in many types of assessment of individuals and communities, including surveys and surveillance. It is a relatively easily determined, objective, inexpensive, effective, and acceptable screening procedure. Owing to this, much emphasis continues to be given to devising methods of estimating haemoglobin employing 'appropriate technology' (p. 232) which will still give sufficiently accurate results for the particular purpose of the study, usually screening.

The haemoglobin can be estimated in various ways, usually based on colorimetry, employing, for example, the grey wedge photometer, the Spencer haemoglobinometer, the battery-operated haemoscope, the Dare haemoglobinometer, or the Dow haemoglobin analyser.

However, these instruments are relatively costly and WHO and organizations concerned with 'appropriate technology' continue to explore the development of cheap, technically uncomplicated photometers, which can be battery-operated, use standard reagents, are shock-proof and tropicalized to stand up to high temperatures and humidities, and give least opportunity for growth of moulds. Those tested include the POTLAB (potentiometer Laboratory Colorimeter — user's cost US$50) and MONA (Monochromatic Absorptiometer — user's cost US$250) models

[12] A detailed, standardized methodology for performing haemoglobin and haematocrit determinations is available on request from the Center for Disease Control, Atlanta, Georgia, USA.

(WHO 1979), together with the Swizzle Stick diluting device (Rideout *et al.* 1978), and the 'Hemocue' (Bridges *et al.* 1987).

A cyanmethaemoglobin method[12] has often been used, especially when specimens are collected in the field. In this method, 0.02 ml of blood, obtained by finger- or heel-prick without squeezing, is added to 4 ml of Drabkin's cyanide–ferricyanide solution. This acts as a preservative, if protected from the sunlight, and allows the resulting cyanmethaemoglobin (haemiglobincyanide) (WHO 1986) to be estimated colorimetrically with an electrical photometer at leisure on return to base, or even days later. If kept over 3 weeks, however, flocculation or fungus infection can occur. The photometer used requires careful testing and calibration. Some models can be powered by a car battery or have a built-in battery (Nicolson *et al.* 1977).

The 'Hemocue' is a simple portable battery-operated colorimeter, which is rechargeable. Blood obtained by finger-prick is collected in a micro-cuvette containing a quantity of dry chemicals which convert haemoglobin to haemiglobinazide, which is measured colorimetrically (Bridges *et al.* 1987; Yip *et al.* 1987). Unfortunately, the current user's cost is US$500 and a new microcuvette (US 80 cents) is needed for each test. However, the simplicity of the procedure makes it ideal for field testing of 'appropriate technology' types of direct colour comparison instruments, which can be used as 'categorizers' by community health workers.

The use of dried blood samples on standard discs of Whatman filter paper for subsequent estimations of haemoglobin and haematocrit has been revived recently as a method of transport requiring no refrigeration (Feraudi and Mejia 1987).

Other tests have been used for screening purposes or to categorize people into broad groups. Of these, the Talqvist and Sahli methods are too inaccurate to be recommended, and the results expressed in figures give a false impression of scientific precision.

The Van Slyke method (Van Slyke *et al.* 1950) has been revived. In this, the specific gravity of a finger-prick drop of blood is compared with that of a known solution of copper sulphate. In India, the method was not found to be adequate (Gammon and Baker 1977). However, preliminary results from Jamaica have been promising (Gurney 1983). In the Jamaica programme, blood is screened at concentrations of 10 g/dl (specific gravity of copper sulphate solution = 1.0477); if the haemoglobin is less than 10 g/dl, another drop of blood is screened (the specific gravity of copper sulphate solution = 1.0435).

Andrianasolo *et al.* (1979) summarized earlier Jamaican experience

[12a] Available from Hemo Diagnostics AB, S–251 09 Helsinborg, Sweden (US Distribution Centre: Medical Equipment Designs Inc., Laguna Hills, California , USA).

with the Van Slyke method, used in antenatal clinics by nurses and midwives, as follows: (1) the copper sulphate method can screen patients into categories of anaemia accurately enough to enable a decision to be made about management and treatment; (2) false negatives or false positives are few and confined to subjects whose haemoglobin concentrations are close to the cut-off points, in which case error has little practical significance; (3) the copper sulphate method is simple to use in clinics and can be carried out by nurses and midwives; (4) the copper sulphate method provides a result in 1 or 2 minutes so that the patient can be informed of her anaemia status (providing motivation) and given health education and treatment with iron tablets according to an agreed schedule; and (5) the method is cheap.

The specific gravity method of haemoglobin determination has also been tested in Nicaragua (Shumaker 1978). Solutions of copper sulphate with specific gravities corresponding to whole blood with haemoglobin levels of 12, 10, and 8 g/dl were prepared in a small regional Nicaraguan hospital. At the village level, an unskilled volunteer was easily trained in the specific gravity method and tested 115 people with 87 per cent agreement when values were compared to those obtained on a battery-powered, colorimetric haemoglobinometer. From the results of this work, it was concluded that the specific-gravity method of haemoglobin determination could be an accurate, reliable, economic, and simple means of anaemia screening that could be effectively employed at the village level. However, the practicality of this method in general use seems doubtful. For example, problems will occur with maintaining the concentration and hence the specific gravity of the copper sulphate solution in hot climates.

A new low-cost colorimetric instrument has been introduced — the Carib Haemoglobin Comparator. Initial results suggest that it is accurate, simple to use, and portable (Stone *et al.* 1983). Practical comparisons between this instrument and other methods were given by Stone *et al.* (1983) (Tables 2.8 and 2.9). However, it is still not generally available.

Anaemia can also be detected by 'appropriate technology' (p. 232) comparing the colour or pallor of the tongue, lower lip, and nails with the appearance on the anaemia recognition card (produced by the Voluntary Health Association of India and supplied by UNICEF) (Fig 2.5). The card has a picture of an anaemic woman on one side and a normal one on the other, contrasting the colour of tongue, lower lip, and nails.

Difficulties occurred with haemoglobin concentrations between 9 and 11 g/dl, among whom only half were correctly diagnosed. However, most patients with haemoglobin values below 9 g/dl were easily identified. As with all eye-estimation of colour comparisons, the question of varying degrees of colour-perception or even colour-blindness of the observers may need consideration (Vorster and Milner 1979). However, the anaemia recognition card can be used as a screening method for detecting

Table 2.8 Some colorimetric methods for measuring haemoglobin (*Stoner* et al. *1983*)

Method	Pipetting necessary	Light source	Approximate cost to buy in US$ (1983)	Special equipment
Dare haemo-globinometer	No	Battery (C size)	119	Lancet, etc. Model with disposable chamber needs replacements
Lovibond comparator	Yes	Daylight	64	Lancet, etc. Concentrated ammonia, distilled water
Sahli	Yes	Daylight	45	Lancet, etc. Hydrochloric acid
A.O. Spencer haemoglobin-ometer	No	Battery (C size)	123	Lancet, etc. Saponin sticks needed for haemolysing blood
Swizzle Stick technique	Simplified	Integral battery		Lancet, etc. Drabkin's reagent and cuvettes
Cyanme-thaemoglobin	Yes	Mains or car battery	300 (minimum)	Lancet, etc. Diluting fluids
Carib haemo-globin comparator	No	Daylight	20 (estimate)	Lancet, etc. Saponin sticks needed for haemolysing blood

moderate-to-severe anaemia in a population where medical facilities are scarce. It also has important advantages of adding to the technical prestige of the village health worker.

Haematocrit estimation These are practical in some studies, including surveys, especially if micro-methods are used. However, in recent community studies for iron deficiency anaemia, haemoglobin estimations have been found to be more useful than the haematocrit or other more expensive and complex methods (Graitcer *et al.* 1981; Hershko *et al.* 1981).

Technically, a capillary tube of blood is centrifuged at 3000 r.p.m. on

Table 2.9 Methods for assessing anaemia not based on laboratory colorimetry (*Stoner* et al. *1983*)

Method	What is measured	Light source	Equipment
Observation of tongue, lower lip, and nails	Paleness	Any	Colour chart
Talqvist	Colour of dried blood	Any	Lancet, etc. Blotting paper, colour chart
Copper sulphate	Specific gravity of blood	Any	Lancet, etc. Copper sulphate solutions at cut-off points desired
Erythrocyte volume fraction (packed cell volume or PCV; haematocrit)	Volumetric proportion of whole blood made up by cells	Any	Lancet, etc. Capillary tube, centrifuge

Table 2.10 Packed cell volumes (PCV) (haematocrit) indicating iron deficiency anaemia (*WHO 1968*)

Age (years)	Sex	PCV* (per cent)
0.5–4		32
5–9		33
10–14		37
Adults	Male	42
	Female	36
	Pregnant female	30

* Iron deficiency anaemia at or below these levels.

an electrical micro-haematocrit which can, if required, be run off a car battery. Alternatively, a hand-operated centrifuge may be used. With young children, when fresh blood is used from a finger-prick, this has to be done as soon as possible. Thus a separate 'station' with one or two persons is required to carry out the centrifuging and to measure the results. Haematocrit (or packed-cell volume readings) suggestive of iron deficiency anaemia are given in Table 2.10.

Table 2.11 Suggested criteria for the diagnosis of anaemia (*WHO 1968; Royston 1982*)*

Determination	Levels considered anaemic or iron-deficient†
Haemoglobin (g/dl)	
Children aged 6 months to 6 years	< 11
Children aged 6 to 14 years	< 12
Adult males	< 13
Adult females; non-pregnant	< 12
Adult females; pregnant	< 11
Serum iron (μg/dl)	
Adults	< 50
Transferrin saturation (%)	
Adults	< 15

* Serum ferritin has been used more recently to estimate iron stores (p. 500).
† Modification in haemoglobin levels needed if living at high altitude.

Reference data Data showing the haemoglobin concentrations suitable for particular age-groups[13] will have to be applied, while adjustment may be required for altitude. Suggested concentrations of haemoglobin are shown in Table 2.11 and of packed cell volumes (haematocrit) in Table 2.10. Other causes of anaemia, such as malaria, sickle cell disease, and thalassaemia may need to be considered in some parts of the world. The possibility of ethnic variation of normal haemoglobin levels, unrelated to nutrition, economics, or other environmental factors, has been suggested by analysis of data collected in the Ten-State Survey in the USA (Garn *et al.* 1975). For reasons unknown, Garn *et al.* (1980) found haemoglobins 0.8 g/dl lower in black Americans than in other ethnic groups of similar socio-economic level. Such ethnic differences are in dispute, and need further clarification and investigation.

Results of community surveys can be expressed in relation both to 'anaemia levels' (Table 2.11) and/or to spaced concentrations of haemoglobin — for example, up to 4 g/dl; 4.1–7 g/dl; 7.1–10 g/dl; 10.1–12 g/dl; over 12 g/dl. At times, it may also be useful and practicable to

[13] Centile curves for both haemoglobin and red cell volume have been prepared from 'normal' children (Dallman and Siimes 1979).

classify different levels of haemoglobin 'functionally.' This is in relation to their practical effect on the individual's function, particularly the ability to undertake physical activity, and on the type of management required, if any, ranging from oral iron to blood transfusion.

Other haematological tests used in more detailed nutritional assessment to differentiate between various causes of anaemia are given in Appendix 2. In addition, at a simpler level, a stained thin blood film may give useful information suggesting the type of anaemia (micro- or macrocytic, hypochromic, etc.), provided a skilled laboratory technician and a microscope are available.

Some comments on parasitological tests are given later (p. 159).

Conclusions

The rationale behind the search for laboratory tests for the practical assessment of nutritional status has been well expressed in the quotation at the beginning of this section by Alleyne *et al.* (1977), who were involved in pioneering many innovative methods.

Unfortunately, biochemical tests have certain inherent disadvantages. Subjects may object to the drawing of blood or the collection of urine, especially from young children, for cultural and other reasons (p. 165). Transportation of samples to a central laboratory may be impossible without deterioration. Techniques may vary from one laboratory to another. Normal ranges for most tests are wide and uncertain. Borderlines between categorizing 'poor' and 'low', 'fair' and 'normal', and 'excess' have not been clarified satisfactorily, nor has their functional significance been defined (Kanawati 1976). In addition, such tests are expensive and depend upon the availability of sophisticated laboratories, which are rarely present, except in research centres.

With inflationary costs rising world wide and with a move towards an increasing reliance on primary health care services, laboratory tests (with the single exception of haemoglobin estimations) can only be undertaken in less technically developed countries in two situations. The first would be investigations, based on clinical signs and/or dietary intake, into major public health problems, notably rickets (serum alkaline phosphatase), xerophthalmia (serum retinol), and scurvy (serum ascorbic acid). The second would be in the classification of the main cause(s) of some common community findings of uncertain aetiology — for example, angular cheilosis or, most commonly, anaemia.

The results of laboratory tests performed over the past 20 years for the detection of less severe degrees of protein–energy malnutrition in the community have, regretfully, been 'full of potential, but subject to too many variables . . . to be applied and interpreted with absolute confidence in all circumstances.' (Alleyne *et al.* 1977). With the possible exception of serum albumin in areas where kwashiorkor is the predominant form of frank protein–energy malnutrition, community assessment in less technically developed countries has to be based on anthropometry, supported by information concerning the diet, clinical signs, and indirect statistical evidence (p. 128).

Conversely, biochemical tests may be more useful in the assessment of the nutritional status of individuals, especially in well-equipped hospitals in technically more developed countries. The selection and value of such tests as 'high-risk' indicators have been the subject of much investigation and debate in recent years, and continue to be so. In addition, an important by-product of laboratory and radiological investigations, such as those currently feasible in the nutritional evaluation of surgical patients in some hospitals in industrialized countries (p. 348), can be the testing and validation (or otherwise) of simpler, 'low-technology' methods of assessment that can be undertaken in out-patients or at village level, including anthropometric measurements (p. 64).

Above all, as noted by Chandra (1982), with biochemical tests, as with other measurements of nutritional status, 'static "standards" are of limited use and we should define thresholds that separate normal function from dysfunction'. Such ranges of reference level need to take into account possible individual and community variation, and adaptability, age differences, particularly including the elderly, the effects of one deficiency on another, and the influence of concurrent drug therapy (i.e. antimalarials and isoniazid). The effects of associated non-nutritional disease have to be considered, including degenerative disease in the elderly, or parasitic and microbial infections in young children in developing countries.

Biophysical methods

Nutritional assessment may occasionally include selected biophysical methods — that is, using non-biochemical methods to measure functional ability of biological tissues (physical, physiological, or cellular), or alteration of structures inaccessible to clinical examination, especially the skeleton.

Functional ability

Many tests have been devised in the past to assess alterations in function associated with different forms of inadequate nutrition. These have included objective assessment of capillary fragility, nerve conduction, muscle co-ordination, etc. Most of them have an uncertain value and have never been used in practice. Exceptions are tests of physical performance (work capacity and energy expenditure) and of night blindness (dark adaptation). Skeletal muscle function has been tested in research studies (Russell *et al.* 1983; Spurr *et al.* 1984).

Work capacity and energy expenditure

Physical work capacity has been defined by WHO as 'the potential for an individual to engage in activities involving muscle action'. However, assessment is not easy, especially in children. Many factors need to be considered. These include the form and duration of the work, the degree of motivation, 'training', practical skill, general health, and nutritional status. Plainly, differences must be expected between results obtained by treadmill studies and in natural circumstances (Spurr *et al.* 1984).

In recent years, the need to emphasize the significance of nutrition programmes to 'development' in economic terms has directed increased attention to this difficult task, especially in relation to dietary calorie levels (Horton 1982) and to the deleterious effects of anaemia (Viteri and Torun 1974).

Such studies usually play no part in community nutritional assessment. Methods used have included (1) *direct physical measurement*, using the step test, employing oxygen usage (respirometer) and cardiac rate while performing different tasks (both natural or mechanically contrived, such as with a bicycle ergometer) (Gabbard and Patterson 1980) and (2) *continued observation* ('time allocation method') (Johnson and Behrens 1982), time spent during the day in various activities with known energy expenditures (e.g. weeding, sitting, walking, etc.) (Durnin and Ferro-Luzzi 1982). The latter are described in detail by Scrimshaw and Hurtado (1987).

Mechanical devices employed for direct physical measurement may pose practical cultural problems. For instance, the bicycle may be quite unfamiliar. Thus the time allocation method has generally been used by anthropologists who are often resident and accepted in communities. Such a study was reported by Montgomery (1978) among the Machuenga Indians, who are gatherer--hunters, with limited agriculture, in the Amazon rain forest. A diary of observed, timed activities enables the energy used to be assessed for each sex and for different seasons. Such studies obviously have to be highly individualized for different cultures. For example, one Arctic investigation had to take into account the energy used in cutting a hole in the ice for fishing.

Energy expenditure estimations need to be compared with the RDAs (Recommended Dietary Allowances) (p. 220) for calories, both as regards under- and over-nutrition. There are obviously special technical and motivational considerations to be taken into account when estimating various activities and, hence the energy expenditure in different cultures. Investigations of young children, especially babies, present special problems (Edelman and Maller 1982). Problems with selecting appropriate RDAs are considered later (p. 220).

Acheson *et al.* (1980) reviewed two of the most commonly used methods — electrical monitoring of the heart rate and time 'activity budgets' recorded as they occur by the subject or, more usually, an observer. The battery-operated SSR apparatus has been used experimentally for collecting this data (Lozoff and Brittenham 1977), but expense usually limits these studies to the straightforward recording of actual activities.

Night blindness (Dark adaptation)

It is currently considered that night blindness is the earliest detectable evidence of avitaminosis A (Sommer 1982). However, classical dark-adaptation tests are not possible in field circumstances, especially in young children.

In Indonesia, night blindness is recognized as a condition by the population and has a local name — *buta ayam* (chicken vision). Sommer and colleagues (1980) found that night blindness recognized by relatives in young children correlated well with clinical signs of conjunctival xerosis and low serum retinol concentrations. If the guardian or relative was unsure of the meaning of the term, the signs were described — for example, the child refusing to walk or crawl about the village or house at night, or unable to find his food or toys after dusk. This interesting practical approach seems likely to apply only to regions where night blindness is common, and, thus, well-recognized. Helen Keller International has recently suggested 'night blindness games' to enable older children to detect this condition in younger siblings (p. 268).

If facilities permit, a rapid (5-minute) test has been suggested in which the sorting of coloured discs (white, blue, red) is timed in a dim light (Thornton 1977). This needs further investigation, as one recent study in southern Brazil did not find it useful (Favaro *et al.* 1986).

Alteration of structure

Clinically accessible tissues

The physical properties of some easily accessible live tissues have been tested in relation to protein–energy malnutrition in young children. These have included: increased hardness of finger nails (Robson and El–Tahawi 1971); decreased tensile strength of hair; diminished elasticity of ear cartilage (Brown and Jelliffe 1967); and skeletal muscle function as measured by a strain gauge after electrical stimulation of the ulnar nerve (Lopes *et al.* 1982). Such investigations usually show marked differences between normal subjects and those with severe malnutrition. However, less severe degrees of protein–energy malnutrition always appear difficult to differentiate. Although none of these techniques has been used in community investigations, some may occasionally play a role in assessment in severely ill hospitalized subjects, including testing skeletal muscle function (Lopes *et al.* 1982).

Four very different methods of *estimating cellular activity* may, for convenience, be included under this heading — immune response, buccal smear cytology, ocular impression cytology, and hair root morphology.

Immune response A great deal of recent work has been carried out on the effect of protein–energy malnutrition on immunocompetence, particularly cell-mediated immunity, which is considerably affected (Cunningham-Rundles 1982). This new knowledge does not appear suitable for use in investigations on population groups. However, it is employed increasingly in nutritional assessment in hospital patients (p. 352), particularly as an indicator of the potential risk of post-operative sepsis (Chandra and Scrimshaw 1980; Cunningham-Rundles 1982).

This is indicated by delayed cutaneous hypersensitivity (anergy) to various intradermal antigens (Chandra 1982) and a low total lymphocyte count (< 1500 cm).

Buccal smear cytology The examination of stained epithelial smears obtained from the buccal mucosa was suggested originally by Squires (1965). Initial results in malnourished children and experimental animals suggested that the percentage of cornified cells increased with the degree of protein–energy malnutrition present. Cornified and non-cornified cells were considered to be differentiated by the colour reaction to Schorr's stain. Buccal smears from healthy children showed 60–70 per cent non-cornified cells, while in severe protein–energy malnutrition this proportion dropped to about 20 per cent or less (Squires 1965).

Subsequent testing of this method has shown it to be unsatisfactory (Wiersinga and Korte 1970). Both the technique of scraping and the staining method are difficult to standardize. Other conditions such as febrile illnesses, dehydration, and vitamin A deficiency appear to alter results.

Ocular impression cytology This has been introduced recently, using gentle impression on the conjunctiva with special filter paper and staining to estimate the presence or absence of mucin-secreting 'goblet cells' (Natadisastra *et al.* 1987. See also: Addendum 1988.)

Hair root morphology In the last 20 years, Bradfield has introduced and investigated the microscopic examination of the hair root for the assessment of protein–energy malnutrition of children in the community. The hair follicle is of interest because it is a site of intense protein synthesis and it is highly accessible. The normal high rates of mitotic and synthetic events which occur within the hair follicle are 'operative only under optimal conditions' (Bradfield 1974). Nutritional deficiencies in different forms of protein–energy malnutrition provoke distinct morphological changes in hair roots and growth which have been suggested as a practical field measure of nutritional status.

Abnormally loose hair roots have been recognized for decades, leading to sparseness (p. 471) and easy 'pluckability' (p. 472). An apparatus to measure the latter objectively has been described recently (Smelser *et al.* 1982).

The hair roots of children with kwashiorkor are very different from those of normal children. The number of growing bulbs (anagens) is about half, and those present are usually abnormally formed and exhibit severe atrophy and depigmentation. The extent of atrophy is indicated by the mean bulb diameter — approximately one-third that of normal values, and approximately the same size as the hair shaft itself. The number of bulbs in the resting phase (telogens) increases significantly. There is also a marked reduction of both the internal and external hair sheaths. When present, the external sheaths are frequently stripped back along the shaft or are shredded (Bradfield 1974).

Difficulties with interpretation of examinations of hair root morphology in identifying different degrees of protein–energy malnutrition have been described by Bradfield (personal communication), who concludes:

> As with other methods being used for assessment of nutritional status, the hair root method cannot be regarded as one of quantitative assessment. However, the ease and speed of sampling, the simplicity of examination, and the possible use of the method under adverse climatic and other physical conditions make it more attractive for population studies in lesser developed, tropical areas.

Clinically inaccessible tissues

Radiographic examination Radiological signs can occur in various severe clinical forms of malnutrition, such as beriberi (enlarged heart), osteomalacia (deformity and marked loss of density of bones, especially the pelvis), osteoporosis (decreased calcification), and advanced fluorosis (increased density of bones, calcification of ligaments, etc.). However, these changes do not occur reliably in early deficiencies and are essentially part of hospital diagnosis. For example, high-technology methods are available for measuring bone mass in osteoporosis (Johnston 1982).

Radiographic investigation will usually only play a part in community assessment in Third World countries for confirmation of serious cases referred to hospital, which can be helpful in corroborating other less clear evidence of the particular form of malnutrition in the population. In community studies, economic considerations, including the costs of apparatus, film, technician, transport, also make this type of approach impossible.

However, radiographic examination commonly has a 'supportive role' in community assessment concerned with only one condition — rickets (p. 270). Such surveys are usually based on clinical signs (p. 29) (guided

Table 2.12 Special roles for laboratory and biophysical tests

Role	Example	Test
Identification of cause* (clinical sign or syndrome)	Angular stomatitis	Riboflavin, etc.
	Anaemia	Haematology; parasitology
	Endemic mental deficiency (cretinism)	Iodine; thyroid function
Corroboration of community diagnosis	Rickets (clinical signs)	X-ray; serum alkaline phosphatase
Meaning of anthropometric measurement	Arm circumference	X-ray; urinary creatinine
Community screening†	Suspected problem	

* Often it is helpful to contrast results from marked, obviously seriously clinically deficient with apparently normal with no clinical signs initially. Results suggest the range of levels to be expected and included.
† Subsample statistically selected.

by a knowledge of the frequent occurrence and clinical picture of severely affected children), with tests for serum alkaline phosphatase (p. 271) and X-ray examinations carried out on subsamples.

In rickets, the following X-ray appearances are characteristic:

1. Active: widened concave (cupped), rarefied, frayed distal ends of long bones, usually the radius and ulna.
2. Healed: concave line of increased density at distal ends of the long bones, usually the radius and ulna.

However, radiological changes usually occur after those in the blood, and results can be influenced by technical factors, such as the type of apparatus and positioning of the child. In community studies into rickets, radiographic examination of a subsample of subjects is desirable. As with other forms of malnutrition, combined evidence is always preferable — clinical, dietetic, biochemical, radiological, and cultural, including information on limitations of exposure of mothers and young children to sunlight. However, the earliest change is biochemical — raised serum alkaline phosphatase (p. 271).

Conclusion

As with laboratory tests (p. 31), biophysical tests are only occasionally practicable, although ocular impression cytology needs further testing as an economical, easily transported test for pre-clinical xerophthalmia (p. 265) However, some potential uses are given in Table 2.12.

Anthropometry: general

Is the goal of nutrition (in young children) to produce muscle-men, geniuses, giants, dwarves, or Methusalehs?

L.A. Barness and P. György (1962)

Growth, development, and body proportions

Growth is the gradual increase in size of the body and its organs and tissues from conception through childhood and adolescence to adulthood. It is evident that growth velocity varies at different stages of life, as does the increase in size and complexity of the organs and tissues, including the relative proportions of muscle and fat. For example, during the pre-pubertal growth spurt, there is an extremely rapid growth in height and marked changes in muscle, fat, and organ development, followed by sexual maturation. In assessing the adequacy of growth, it is, therefore, necessary to compare any data (height, weight, etc.) to the expected rate of increase and to the body proportions appropriate to the subject's age and ethnic group.

In the present context, the term 'development' refers to the increase in the range and performance of skills by children, mainly as a result of maturation of the central nervous system, especially the brain. Although not measured by anthropometry, development is mentioned here, as it parallels growth in healthy children. Clinically, paediatricians have long considered growth and development together and, in the last few years, WHO has re-emphasized this association in recent reconsideration of methods of assessing child health throughout the world (Shah 1984).

Influences on growth

Growth can be influenced by a variable mixture of many factors. These can be roughly classified as *internal* (biological, including genetic influences) and *external* (including nutritional status) (Table 2.13). Inadequate or excessive growth can often be caused by several factors acting together or in sequence. For example, subnormal fetal growth and a low birth weight can result from obstetrical problems (such as placental insufficiency) or inadequate maternal nutrition, or both. The fact that those in lower socio-economic groups tend not to grow as much also reflects the combined effects of a mixture of external factors, such as diet and infection, and, in some communities, genetic influences as well.

The degree of attention and the priority given to the factors which can influence growth (Table 2.13) will depend on the presumed commonness of different conditions in the particular population being investigated; the perspective, training, and technical 'conditioning' of the investigator; and the purpose of the investigation.

Table 2.13 Some internal (biological) and external factors, including nutrition, which can influence growth

Factors	Examples
Internal	
Genetic	Individual (familial; parental size)*
	Ethnic group
	'intrauterine environment' (e.g. placental insufficiency)
Obstetrical	Low birth weight — birth order
	twins
Sex of individual	
External	
Diet	Fetus (maternal diet: protein-calories; iodine)
	Infants (breastfeeding or artificial feeding)
	Children (protein-calories; iodine; zinc, vitamin D; folic acid)
Drugs	Alcohol, tobacco, other addictive drugs ('substance abuse'); various medicines
	Altitude (? genetic)
Environment	Climate (including season)
	? Overcrowded housing
Diseases	
Endocrine	Pituitary growth hormone
Infections	Acute and chronic bacterial, viral, and parasitic
Congenital	Sickle cell anaemia, inborn errors of metabolism, etc.
Severe chronic illness	Cancer, intestine (malabsorption), heart, kidney, liver
Psychological	Emotional deprivation

* Parental size is influenced by genetics *and* the external influences, including nutrition, that occurred in the parents' childhood.

For example, in specialized growth clinics in Europe and North America, consideration of endocrine disorders may figure prominently. In paediatric practice in such areas, training is likely to set in motion a series of laboratory and radiological investigations for 'failure to thrive' (growth failure), sometimes without sufficient initial enquiry into possible external factors, notably the diet and emotional deprivation from parental neglect.

In such specialized growth (auxology) clinics in Europe and the USA, parents also may be concerned with their children's excessive tallness or shortness, or obesity, because of anxieties concerning possible ultimate appearance and cultural acceptance in society.

On a world-wide basis, growth is mainly influenced by genetic programming and external influences, notably the level of nutrition due directly to dietary intake and the deleterious effects of infective, parasitic, toxic, and/or psychological stresses. This is so, for example, in kwashiorkor — one of the two principal forms of severe protein–energy malnutrition in early childhood (p. 273). This condition is almost never exclusively dietary in origin, but rather the result of other cumulative stresses as well. These can include the nutritional ill-effects of intestinal helminths, bacterial and viral infections (such as whooping cough, measles, acute diarrhoea, chronic malaria, tuberculosis, etc.), the psychological trauma associated with weaning, and possible food toxins. In a similar way, multiple factors are usually ultimately responsible for xerophthalmia (p. 265).

The effects of the environment, such as altitude and climate, also need consideration. Such modifications may represent genetic adaptations evolved over many generations although an increase in growth rate has been shown to occur in the summer months in the Northern Hemisphere (Marshal and Swan 1971).

A major consideration in assessing growth, both in individuals and populations, frequently concerns the relative significance of 'nature' — that is, genetic influences — and 'nurture' — that is nutritional adequacy.

Genetic influences Genetic factors influence the growth of individuals and different ethnic groups (Eveleth and Tanner 1976; Marshall 1981). This genetic programming involves not only the ultimate adult height and weight, but also the sequence and tempo of change and final body proportions, including, for example, trunk–leg lengths and the distribution of subcutaneous adipose tissue (fat patterning).

Probably the most spectacular example of genetic influence is shown by the Pygmies, among whom birth weight and growth in childhood are somewhat below Western levels. However, their small adult size seems mostly due to the fact that no significant growth spurt accompanies puberty, so that they remain near their prepubertal body size (Mann *et al.* 1962).

The monumental global analysis of scientific evidence by Eveleth and Tanner (1976) clearly emphasizes the considerable variation in growth and body proportions in different genetic groups of humankind. This is scarcely surprising since there are innumerable other indications of genetic diversity, including blood groups, pigmentation, facial features, etc.

The influence of genetic variation is most clearly demonstrated by contrasting extremes. For example, the very tall, slender, long-legged Nilotic peoples, such as the Dinka of the Southern Sudan, are strikingly dissimilar to the geographically adjacent Pygmies of East-Central Africa. Over the centuries, they seem to have adapted genetically to their very different environments. Indeed, the small body size, shorter legs, and longer arms of the Pygmies appear to represent the 'optimum adaptation of the human species to the rain forest' (Ghesquière and Karvonen 1981).

The most clear-cut and explicit ecological influence on anthropometry seems to be altitude. However, at least in part, the short broad-chested physique seen, for example, in the Bolivian Andes, is a long-term genetic adaptation to hypoxia (Haas 1981). A more direct effect is indicated by the increase in low-birth-weight babies in high altitudes among populations who have not been resident for generations, as in Denver, Colorado.

As another example, the Pima Indians of Arizona seem to have an exceptional, possibly innate, tendency to obesity. It has been suggested that they may have a 'thrifty gene', which makes it easier for them to lay down fat stores (Daniels *et al.* 1982). This could have been an advantage in the past, helping survival at a time characterized by frequent food shortages and an active way of life. This characteristic may be somewhat similar to the pre-migratory deposition of fat in some species of birds or in bears before hibernation. However, with a more constant food supply and a less strenuous existence, this may have become a genetic burden.

External influences The potential influence of external forces in limiting or aiding genetically endowed growth potential is well illustrated by the marked differences seen in the size of children of the well-to-do compared with children of the poor of the same genetic group (Tanner, Whitehouse, and Takaishi 1966). This can result in positive or negative 'secular trends' in various communities over periods of years, due to a changed 'quality of the social and physical environment', particularly nutritional adequacy.

From early records of military recruits in Norway, it appears that an upward secular trend in height began in the 1830s. As a whole, there has been an increase in adult height of about 1 cm per decade in Western Europe and the USA in the past century, although this seems to have ceased or slowed very markedly from the late-1960s onwards (Bakwin and McLaughlin 1964). A similar positive secular trend towards increased stature has also been described in post-World War II Japan (Suzuki 1981), in China (Chinese Academy of Medical Sciences 1977), in Jamaica (Ashcroft and Lovell 1965), and in other countries.

In Japan, this largely post-World War II secular trend also appears to be slowing (Suzuki 1981; Takaishi 1986). Moreover, Tanner *et al.* (1982) note that presumably optimal Japanese adults are still less tall than similar groups in Northern Europe, mainly due to different body proportions, notably shorter leg-length. Differences in body proportions also need consideration when making comparisons between other groups of the human species.

Conversely, in some areas a secular trend has not been observed. For example, in rural Gambia continuous growth records from 1951 to 1975 showed no change, presumably because conditions have not altered significantly (Billewicz and McGregor 1982).

A secular trend of this type can be downwards, reflecting a deterioration. Modern Peruvian peasants seem to have a smaller stature compared with their pre-Conquistador ancestors. Graham (1966) suggests that this may be due in part to dietary change and, in particular, the abandonment of nutritioils *quinoa* (*Chenopodium quinoa*) as the main staple. More recent and well-documented historical examples include the decrease in height and weight of schoolchildren in Paris and Japan following prolonged dietary restriction and the stresses of World War II.

Historically, one of the earlier applications of anthropometry was as part of the examination of military conscripts. The discovery of stunted adult male recruits in industrialized countries, such as Britain, was, in turn, a most significant stimulus to trying to ensure a nutritionally adequate diet, especially during childhood and pregnancy.

Bengoa *et al.* (1959) suggested that the heights of groups of 7-year-old schoolchildren recorded at intervals of several years, could provide a rough guide to the state of child health and nutrition in a given area (p. 332). At 7 years of age, children would often be entering school. This would be prior to the pubertal growth spurt and their heights could be taken to reflect their cumulative nutritional and health experience up to that time. The approach has recently been confirmed in Central America (Valverde *et al.* 1985; Parillon *et al.* 1987).

Dietary intake also may be influenced by seasonal change or by relocation. For example, growth in West African children varies with the seasons (Billewicz and McGregor 1982), owing to decreased food supplies during the 'hungry season,' and to changes in the patterns of infectious diseases, such as diarrhoea, at different times of the year. Similar seasonal variations in maternal weight gain in pregnancy and in neonatal birth weight were considered to reflect annual cycles of agriculture, as reflected by food availability and physical activity in the fields (Adair and Pollitt 1983).

Improvement in the environment, including nutrition, can result from relocation. Children of Mexican migrant workers showed accelerated growth during summer residence in the USA (Dewey 1982). In Sweden, adopted young children from less developed countries showed increased growth, so that after 3 years they approximated Swedish levels (Magnusson and Proos 1980).

The problem of disentangling genetic factors from external influences, especially nutritional adequacy, is increased as it may require optimal nutrition for more than one generation for full genetic potential to be achieved. As Eveleth (1979) notes:

> Because of the overwhelming effect of adverse conditions on growth, it is frequently difficult to see the genetic target. A poor environment is most likely not

to be limited to one generation in its effects. Only recently have we been seeing that the effects may be witnessed in succeeding generations...

Thus, in Shanghai, a considerable increase in Chinese children's height was recorded between 1975 and 1981. However, 7-year-old boys were about 5 cm shorter than their US counterparts (Yi-Ling and Bei-Jun 1982). Future studies are needed to determine if this is partly genetic or not, and whether further changes will occur.

A basic and universal difficulty lies in defining *optimal growth*, including the upper limits, in any genetic group. This is more readily associated with calorie intake and fat stores. Moreover, diminished growth may also be due to deficiencies of previously less emphasized nutrients, such as iodine, iron, and zinc (Prasad 1985). Conversely, it may be speculated that the high calcium intake in milk-drinking groups (e.g. in North America and West Europe) may even be excessive resulting in an increase in the length of the long bones.

Such difficulties become especially relevant when nutritional assessment is undertaken in a country with two distinct ethnic groups. Examples include Fiji, with both Melanesian and Indian populations, and Bolivia, where the majority of the rural population is Amerindian while the majority of townsfolk are of European descent.

As will be discussed later when considering the selection of anthropometric reference data (p. 110), genetic factors regulating growth potential seem more important in certain age-groups than others. As a practical generalization, the influence of genetic programming on growth in early childhood seems less than that of environmental factors, especially nutrition. Genetic influences seem to become more dominant in older children and adults.

Practical considerations

Anthropometry is the most commonly used direct method for the assessment of two of the most wide-spread nutrition problems in the world: (1) protein–energy malnutrition, especially in young children and pregnant women in less technically developed countries, and in severely ill hospitalized patients; and (2) obesity in all age-groups.

Put another way, anthropometric measurements can be used to monitor normal or abnormal growth in childhood, pregnancy, and fetal life, as well as the pathological 'overgrowth' of obesity and the pathophysiological alteration of body dimensions in the elderly (p. 352). As with all methods, anthropometry has advantages and disadvantages (Table 2.14).

The measurements usually employed are weight and height (stature) (or length in infants and young children up to 2 or 3 years of age). The arm circumference and triceps fatfold are also commonly measured, and can give an indication of any decrease (or increase) in calorie stores (subcutaneous fat) and/or severe depletion of protein stores (muscle).

Table 2.14 Anthropometry: considerations in community nutritional assessment in less technically developed countries

Advantages	Disadvantages	
Relatively inexpensive (basic measurements)	Obtaining relevant reference data	Source Optimal (definition) Genetic influences
Fast	Potential errors	Equipment Observer Recording
Objective		
	Limited scope	Growth: Children, Pregnancy Excess → Obesity Deterioration → Age Malnutrition (Protein–energy malnutrition, calories)
Gradable	Numerate 'certainty' (cultural disadvantage)	
Non-invasive		

Measurements may be made at one time or serially, as when recorded graphically in growth charts for young children (p. 294) or pregnant women (p. 227). Serial measures plainly provide a dynamic insight into actual growth, or changes due to other causes, such as the increase or decrease in weight seen in some severe non-nutritional illnesses (e.g. oedema in heart failure or sudden marked weight loss in acute dehydration).

Advantages

Anthropometric measurements are: (1) relatively economical to carry out; (2) objective; (3) understandable by the population at large; (4) give results which can be numerically graded; and (5) supply information concerning adequate growth, early protein–energy malnutrition and obesity not easily or economically obtainable by other methods.

Disadvantages

Conversely, anthropometry has four potential disadvantages: (1) considerable potential for inaccuracy of measurement; (2) the need for reasonably precise ages in young children; (3) limited nutritional diagnostic relevance (mainly, but not exclusively, to protein–energy malnutrition); and (4) problems with the selection of appropriate reference data and of cut-off points above or below levels suggesting abnormality. In a few cultures, such as in parts of India, the weighing of young children may be refused as inauspicious or likely to expose a baby to the possible influence of the 'evil eye' (p. 68).

Inaccuracy of measurement Much anthropometry is carried out with relatively simple, every-day apparatus, such as a weighing scale or a tape measure, so that it may have little scientific mystique. At the same time, anthropometric measurement can be made inaccurately with unreliable instruments and expressed as numbers with decimal points. These instantly acquire a false and undeserved air of mathematical precision.

Errors made by the measurer (observer error) are often the most important source of inaccurate information and can be due to faulty technique (lack of training, carelessness, poor motivation, tiredness, boredom), and/or mistakes in recording, which are more likely if transcribing to the metric system is needed (e.g. inches to centimetres).

The equipment used needs frequent checking for accuracy through the range likely. Observer error can be minimized by emphasis on the need for proper technique and care, together with 'quality control' (p. 410) prior to (and during) a survey, and by the checking of results during any investigation.

Need to know precise age In young children when rapid growth is normal, a reasonably precise knowledge of age is necessary. However, most cultures do not attach importance to exact age, as it has no social significance. Thus, a means of estimating the age may be necessary, e.g. constructing a local calendar of past events (p. 318). Alternatively, measurements or indices (ratios) may be used which are independent of knowledge of the *exact* age (p. 326) (e.g. arm circumference (p. 307, weight-for-height (p. 311)).

Limited nutritional relevance Anthropometry is usually used in nutritional assessment to measure: (1) growth in young children; (2) weight gain in pregnant women; (3) prevalence of low-birth-weight babies; or (4) loss or gain in weight, due to deficient (or increased) stores of calories (body fat) and/or protein (muscle) in all age groups.

Changes in these measurements are currently considered to be mostly related to diets deficient in calories and protein (protein–energy malnutrition (p. 294), often with infections or infestations, or to excessive intakes of calories (obesity). With the exception of limited areas of the world where severe deficiencies of vitamin A, iodine, iron, or zinc occur in young children, growth retardation is not usually given any practical or specifically selective value as an indicator of deficiency of other nutrients (e.g. vitamins and minerals). At the same time, protein–energy malnutrition is usually accompanied by deficiencies of one or more other nutrients.

Selection of reference data For anthropometry in all age-groups, it is necessary to compare results with appropriate reference data. This is plainly critical. For example, it is possible, on paper, to eliminate severe protein–energy malnutrition in young children in a community or to greatly increase the prevalence of obesity, merely by changing the reference data and diagnostic criteria used.

Ways to improve the accuracy and usefulness of anthropometry in nutritional assessment are covered in the following sections on methods (p. 64), selection of measurements (p. 105), reference data (p. 108), and cut-off points (p. 122).

Anthropometry: methods

Nothing is measured with greater error than the body
Beneke 1878 (Quoted by Bastow 1982)

Assessment of growth, health, or disease by means of anthropometry is an ancient practice. Older methods include *general inspection*, particularly a subjective judgement of 'thinness' or 'fatness', a *single measurement*, for example, height, in the selection of military recruits, or *serial measurements*, e.g. using weight to monitor the growth of children.

In its most scientific application (auxology), anthropometry requires a well-organized research centre, elaborate and expensive equipment, and sophisticated mathematical knowledge. Simplified versions of techniques based on information from such centres have been used extensively in the last 20 years, in many regions of the world, especially for young children. Anthropometry also plays a considerable part in the assessment of obesity (p. 345), and, more recently, in nutritional support services in hospitals in some industrialized countries. It has long been a detailed tool of the physical anthropologist.

However, the interpretation of findings anywhere is always complex and often controversial. The 'normal' well-fed human body in any ethnic group can vary so much that interpretation of the nutritional significance of smaller differences in body size and proportion is peculiarly difficult. Questions concerning the significance of genetic variation and the additional widespread problem of lack of knowledge of the precise age of young children in most countries are detailed elsewhere (pp. 315–25). Also, measurements made at one time can reflect very differing past histories, including previous episodes of malnutrition of variable and severity, 'plurality of nutrient deficiencies' and inter-acting infections (Gopalan 1987).

Nutritional anthropometry is concerned with the measurement of the variations of the dimensions, proportions, and some aspects of the gross composition of the human body at different ages and at different levels of nutrition. Despite some difficulties, nutritional anthropometry has the advantages of being objective, relatively inexpensive to obtain, and understandable by both professionals and the public. It is most useful in young children where growth should be rapid and among whom protein–energy malnutrition occurs most commonly.

The present account, together with subsequent sections dealing with the interpretation of results (p. 443) and with special problems in different age-groups (p. 226), includes some mention of the nutritional assessment of the individual. However, it focuses mainly on methods that will supply useful, if approximate, information concerning the nutritional status of communities, which can be used to guide the development of nutrition policy and programmes (p. 449). Special emphasis is given to methods that can be carried out speedily with few staff and little equipment, or, in some cases, even by trained members of communities.

The methods and the measurements employed in anthropometry can vary greatly in number and complexity. Obviously, those for children will depend on the purpose, objectives, and level of accuracy needed in the particular survey, study, or investigation, and on the resources available. Some statistical and epidemiological considerations concerning the selection of measurements are given later (p. 395). Detailed, elaborate, and time-consuming techniques and analyses, such as refined scientific procedures for estimating body composition, can only be carried out by the laboratory research worker. Nevertheless, they can be valuable in that they help in the understanding of the meaning, limitations, and validation of simpler methods suitable for use both in community investigations and in the clinical assessment of individuals.

For the practical nutritionist, the problems are:

1. To select the minimum number of the least complex methods that can give useful, albeit approximate information for an individual and for a community;
2. To understand thoroughly the techniques involved and be able to carry them out accurately;
3. To interpret the results and express them in ways that are understandable by governmental authorities, by the community, by the individuals assessed (or their parents), and by other nutritional investigators elsewhere in the world.

In developing countries, anthropometry appears to be of the greatest use in the detection of growth failure and undernutrition, principally from lack of calories and protein. In particular, the often numerous but less severe forms of protein–energy malnutrition in early childhood are only detected objectively as a slowing of the usual rapid-growth characteristic of this age group (e.g. a declining or flattening growth curve (p. 296), a

Table 2.15 Major anthropometric measurements

Measure	Components	Tissues of major interest
Stature	Head, spine, pelvis, legs	Bone
Weight	Whole body	All tissues (especially fat, muscle, bone, and water)
Arm circumference	Subcutaneous fat, muscle, bone	Muscle (in LTDC*) Fat (in MTDC*)
Fatfold	Subcutaneous fat, skin	Fat

* LTDC: less technically developed countries; MTDC: more technically developed countries.

low body weight, or 'subnormal' height) and by a depletion of protein and calorie (energy) stores, as indicated by a decreased muscle mass and diminished subcutaneous fat (Table 2.15). Similar measurements have recently been incorporated as part of hospital nutritional assessment (p. 348) in severely ill individuals in some technically more developed countries, and, from the opposite point-of-view, as part of the monitoring of obesity (p. 343).

The methods used in anthropometry need to be considered in relation to instruments (equipment), techniques, standardization and quality control, and age assessment. The difficult decisions involved in the selection of appropriate 'reference data' for different measurements and age-groups are considered later (p. 110), together with the interpretation of anthropometric findings (pp. 126, 443).

Equipment: general[14]

The selection of suitable instruments is obviously important[15]. For survey work, they must be sufficiently accurate for the particular study, simple to use, easy to read, affordable, and, for fieldwork, 'readily portable and rugged enough to withstand severe handling'. Maintenance and replacement costs need consideration. Instruments require careful pre-testing and frequent checking and calibration. Details of suitable instruments for various practical procedures are given later. The design and type of anthropometric equipment needs to be related to its proposed use. A

[14] Information on some appropriate instruments is available in the UNIPAC Catalogue, UNICEF, Copenhagen, Denmark. (Also see Addendum 1988.)

[15] Further details concerning anthropometric equipment and techniques of measurement are given by Griffiths (1985), Burns (1986) and Shorr (1986). Information on availability of equipment can be obtained from TALC (P.O. Box 49, St. Albans, Herts, UK), AHRTAG (85 Marylebone High Street, London W1M 3DE, UK) and UNICEF (UNIPAC, Copenhagen, Denmark).

variety of different instruments are available with varying degrees of mathematical exactness — the cost usually increases greatly with higher levels of precision. However, community nutritional assessment lends itself particularly to the concept of low-cost 'appropriate technology' (p. 361) capable of 'categorizing for action' rather than measuring with great precision. Comparative costs of instruments are often the most important consideration.

Techniques: general

Of the almost unlimited number of possible body measurements,[16] those selected should be the simplest and quickest to take, the most acceptable to the subjects concerned, and the easiest to replicate that will, nevertheless, give the maximum information concerning the particular nutritional problem under investigation. They should employ affordable equipment and in developing countries should be easy to use by primary health care workers, including trained members of the community. In less technically developed regions of the world, this will almost always focus on the problem of protein–energy malnutrition, which cannot be detected practically in less severe forms by other means. This will mainly be in young children and pregnant women, but may include adults and school-age children. By contrast, in both North America and Europe, investigations have centred on obesity and excessive weight gain, but have recently become more concerned with inadequate nutrition in hospitalized individuals (p. 348), in the elderly (p. 352), and in the poor and homeless.

If many people are to be examined in surveys, sufficient personnel should be available to permit rest periods. Otherwise, the repetition, monotony, and physical strain of making large numbers of careful measurements, especially on uncooperative young children, lead to fatigue, boredom, carelessness, and inevitable error. Last, the average time required to carry out each procedure must be known in order to determine how many subjects can be dealt with at each session. An underappreciated cause of delay is the time spent removing clothes. It is preferable if young children can be undressed ahead of time.

The investigator can record immediately, or can dictate each measurement to a recorder, who repeats aloud the figure as it is given. The most efficient and accurate method varies in different circumstances and needs pre-testing. It should be appreciated that major errors in taking measurements are caused by mistakes in reading the scales and writing down the results.

In all published reports, full details of the methods used must be clearly

[16] 28 were recommended in the International Biological Programme (Weiner and Lourie 1981) while 87 were included by Snyder *et al.* (1977) in the Highway Safety Study in the USA.

stated. For example, the precise technique used for weighing must be set down, including the scales used, whether clothes were worn or not, etc. Perfunctory weighing of out-patients wearing varying clothes and shoes on never-checked scales is common in even the most sophisticated hospitals. The need for calibration of weighing machines and for 'quality control' (p. 410) for such a simple-seeming, non-technical measurement is often not appreciated.

Measurements should be made and recorded in the metric system. However, in areas where the only available weighing machines record in pounds and ounces, measurements may be taken in these units and later converted into metric units prior to comparison with standards of reference. Plainly, every effort must be made to use metric equipment as it avoids a time-consuming procedure, which is both unnecessary and a common additional source of error.

Major measurements

The most usual measurements are those made to assess: (1) *body mass*, as judged by weight; (2) *linear dimensions*, especially height (or length); and (3) *body composition and reserves* of calories (energy) and protein, as reflected by the principal accessible soft tissues — subcutaneous fat and muscle. All measurements may be carried out singly, or serially, when they are often recorded on different types of growth charts.

Body mass

Weight is the most used anthropometric measurement and is a time-honoured, basic indicator in clinical practice, especially paediatrics. Although instrument and observer errors easily occur, the potential value of weighing, especially for children, is appreciated not only by health personnel, but by patients and parents, for whom weight changes can also be useful as a part of health and nutrition education. However, in some areas, such as parts of India, weighing may be disliked and avoided for various cultural reasons (Gopalan and Chatterjee 1985).

In developing regions, the occurrence of protein–energy malnutrition appears to be best indicated by growth failure in children, demonstrated by inadequate weight gain as judged by serial measurements recorded on growth charts (p. 296). In Western countries, 'failure to thrive' in young children (p. 57) and obesity in children and older age-groups can be detected by serial growth measurements. More precise analyses have been employed to demonstrate 'growth velocities' — that is, rate of change over time (Tanner *et al.* 1966; Wiersinga and Van Rens 1973). This is obtained by calculating gains over known periods of time or by plotting on incremental (velocity) growth charts.

Weight estimations can be made on single occasions, as in cross-sectional prevalence surveys, or repeated at intervals, as at Young Child (or Under Fives) Clinics, pre-natal clinics, hospitals, schools, in the community, or in individuals. Serial measurements also form an integral part of longitudinal surveys.

Difficulties with the interpretation of single measurements have become increasingly obvious in recent years. As emphasized by Gopalan (1987), measurements made on a single occasion give no indication of the child's past history. Similar results may occur as a result of many different sequences (e.g. low birth weight, episodes of dietary inadequacy, infections etc).

The evaluation of the significance of measurements of body weight also must take into account the influences of body build and composition, especially length (height), breadth (in adults), and the relative proportions of fat, muscle, and bone, and the possible presence of pathological weight due, for example, to oedema or, in young children in some tropical areas, to very heavy roundworm infection or a greatly enlarged malarial spleen.

Accordingly, the interpretation of weight should be combined with clinical inspection and, whenever possible, with considerations of other appropriate measurements, especially height (length) (p. 77) in all age-groups and ideally, with breadth, in adults (p. 83). In some circumstances an assessment of subcutaneous fat and muscle may form a valuable part of what can be termed 'sequential anthropometry' (p. 109). Despite its subjectivity, clinical inspection can be helpful as a rough visual check of the significance of the results obtained.

By contrast, serial weight measurements give a more dynamic picture of growth and its failure (or excess). Early growth failure in protein–energy malnutrition has been the main reason for the development and use of growth charts (p. 296) for young children in Under-Fives Clinics, or as part of community assessment. Special considerations, such as devising growth charts for pregnant women, are considered later (p. 236).

Equipment

The choice of scales is a matter of importance, but will depend on various needs: the degree of mobility envisaged — stationary at a clinic or transportable on foot, vehicle, plane, etc, age-groups to be included, etc. The following criteria also need to be considered: 'sufficient' accuracy for particular purposes; clear readability; appropriate weight range; weighing surface suitable for age group (e.g. small babies versus adults); cost; simplicity (including repairs); possible transportability (weight, shape); sturdiness; a capacity for reliable and reproducible recordings under different climatic conditions over an extended period of time; and, for young children, a non-frightening appearance (Jelliffe and Jelliffe 1971*b*). Reliability may be preferred over great precision. For example, in the young child, day-to-day variability in weight may be as much as 0.2 kg due to food and fluid intake, and defecation and micturition. A fundamental point is whether *precise* weighing is the purpose or the *categorization* (as with some scales devised for trained birth attendants to detect underweight newborns) (p. 256). A review of scales has been undertaken by WHO (1986*d*).

Recent awareness, especially in India (Gopalan and Chatterjee 1985), that weighing was being done inaccurately in many primary health care services has led to a reconsideration of the scales used. A monograph by Burns (1986) on 'scales technologies' is a very comprehensive modern evaluation of weighing scales based on six criteria: *fundamental design* (maintenance, safety, durability, portability, 'universality' (e.g. age range covered)); *acceptability* (operator, mother, child); *potential for scale error* (accuracy, linearity (e.g. ability to weigh over range of weights), precision, sensitivity, unobvious damage, 'fatigue'); *potential for operator error* (accuracy, tare (ability to return to zero after weighing), complexity of use, damping (accuracy of reading with child in motion) self-contained); *general* (cost, packaging, potential for manufactured, instructions on use); *acceptability of the procedure* (operator, mother, child). A similar practical analysis is needed for other commonly used anthropometric equipment.

Burns (1986) based his publication on the detailed analysis of scales in India with these criteria in mind. He noted that confusion often existed. For example, the term 'Salter scale' was widely used for many dial scales, some of an inferior, less accurate type.

A major recommendation of this study (and with a workshop) (Burns 1986) was that engineers need to be consulted further, together with manufacturers and large organizations, notably UNICEF, to undertake the research and development which could lead to the manufacture of a sturdy scale with the other characteristics indicated, but with a large enough volume of sales to keep the price low. This is currently the case with the TALC scale (p. 306) and the PATH electronic scale mentioned later (p. 76).

Whatever model is used needs to be employed carefully and frequently re-checked for accuracy. This can be undertaken, for example, at the beginning of each session, after each transportation, and, ideally, after every 20 weighings. Weighing machines based on two different principles are commonly available: beam-balance and spring scales. More expensive devices based on other principles have been used, such as hydraulic pressure or strain-gauge digital read-out (Garn 1978). They do not usually have widespread practical usefulness, because of cost and fragility.

Relatively low-cost weighing machines are available that record up to 16–25 kg with increments of 10–20 g (1/2–1 oz) for young children and up to 140 kg with increments of 100 g (1/4 lb) for older children and adults. However, Salter scales for young children cost ±US$35 (1988) which is cheap for survey work, but impossibly expensive if needed for serial weighing in primary health care in hundreds of thousands of villages. In these circumstances, more economical scales and other methods are currently being tested (pp. 252–8). General scales are available for neonates measuring up to 10 kg with increments of 10 g. Expensive models, with a precision of 1–5 g are also available and can be used for the test-weighing of babies in estimating milk intake (p. 260). Scales should be checked for zero reading and through their expected range of weight after travel and several times during sessions when many individuals are measured. Appropriate accurate test weights should be available and should be easily transportable for survey work. Economical test weights can be stones of known weight or large plastic containers, marked so that they can be filled with water or sand to known weight marks in the village (e.g. 5, 10 litres, etc.). In some countries, standard weights may be purchasable (e.g. 5 and 10 kg, etc.),[17] but are usually expensive. Checking of weighing machines, preferably through the full range of expected use is just as necessary in hospital or clinic practice, but rarely undertaken.

Newborn Recent re-awakening to the awareness of the importance of recording birth weight (p. 252) has led to a search for a small, accurate, easy-to-read scale for midwives, which is also inexpensive and weighs up to 5 or 10 kg, at intervals of 100 g.

The Salter 'Super Samson'[18] tubular spring balance has these features and zero adjustments can be made, if needed (Fig. 2.13). However, midwives and community health workers may find the scale difficult to read. A colour-coded scale of a similar type has been devised for use by illiterate indigenous midwives for categorizing newborn babies by weight (Alisjahbana *et al.* 1984) (p. 255). Unfortunately, most scales of appropriate accuracy and compactness are much too expensive for widespread use in developing countries. Recently, a cheap, nationally produced scale has been reported in India (Kumar and Walia 1986), which can have a colour code taped on. This needs further testing as to durability in very humid environments, as does a similar cheap PATHweigh sale (estimated cost with in-country production US$4, see p. 76, footnote).

Young children

Beam-balance scales are accurate, if carefully looked after. Their accuracy depends, however, on the integrity of the balancing part or fulcrum. Many suitable models are available in different parts of the world. In clinics, frequently used scales have often been of the familiar Detecto[19]

[17] In the USA, available from the Toledo Scale Company, Toledo, Ohio.

[18] 'Super Samson,' Salter Abbey Weighing Machines Ltd, St. Botolph's Lane, Bury St. Edmonds, Suffolk, England.

[19] Detecto Scales Co, Cambridge Scientific Instruments, P.O. Box 265, Cambridge, Maryland, USA.

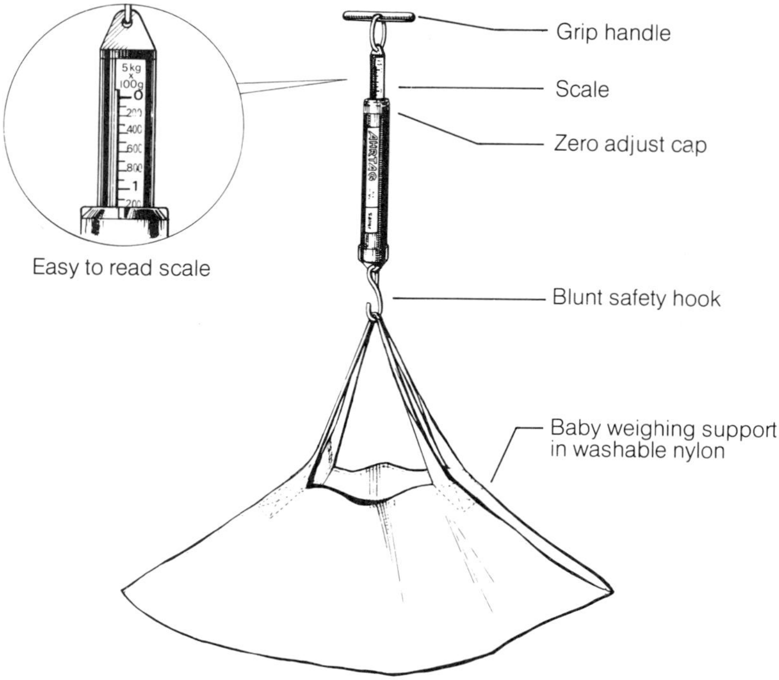

Fig. 2.13 Salter 'Super Samson' (AHRTAG) scale for weighing newborns. (Cost: approximately US$ 28 in 1987.)

type supplied by UNICEF for young children, measuring up to 16 kg (35 lb) at intervals of 0.1 kg. In the USA, the Homs[20] platform scale has been used, but is expensive, difficult to transport, and can become mechanically inaccurate after being jolted on a rough road. Thus, the use of a locking device or a wedge to hold the moving parts in place before journeys is advisable. They must be used on a firm, non-tilted surface and checked before use. Some models for young children are somewhat unstable and care needs to be taken to prevent an infant from falling off. For field work, the Detecto baby scale compares unfavourably with the Salter scale (see below) because: (1) the child must be properly centred in the pan and be perfectly still; (2) the knife edge requires checking; (3) there is no direct read-out dial (Zerfas 1979); and (4) it is relatively heavy and difficult to transport.

Another general type of scale, employing the beam-balance principle, is the butcher's steelyard, which is an ancient, simple, and inexpensive weighing apparatus. It is compact and can be easily transported, usually

[20] Douglas Homs Company, Inc., Burlingame, California.

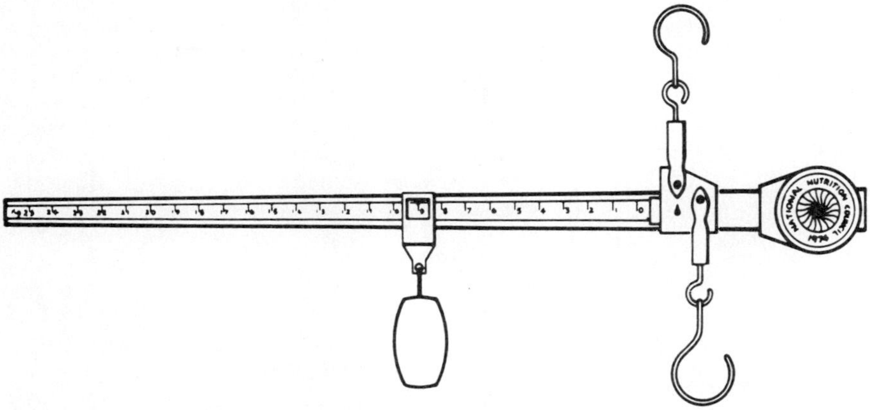

Fig. 2.14 Philippine bar scale, widely used in markets. (Courtesy of Director, Nutrition Centre of the Philippines.)

weighing up to 20 kg (44 lb) with an accuracy of up to 0.1 kg. It has to be suspended from the branch of a tree or roof beam, but can be read accurately, as there is little oscillation. In some places, the local traditional scale or steelyard used in the market may be appropriate and available, as with the *dacin* in Indonesia (Rohde *et al.* 1975) and the Philippine bar scale ($22.50) (Fig. 2.14).

In the past, various types of spring scale have been used, but could not be recommended as they easily became stretched and inaccurate from frequent use or as a result of the expansion of the spring in unduly hot weather. In recent years, the Salter scale (Portable Baby Weigher) (Model 235 B)[21] has been widely used in different parts of the world (Fig. 2.15). It is reliable for field work, sturdy, easily transportable, and relatively inexpensive, especially in relation to its durability compared with imitations (Burns 1986). It is a hanging scale with a stable teflonized spring, which is not significantly affected by temperature or frequent weighing. Its use together with growth charts has been well-tested (King *et al.* 1972). Either a basket or cloth (or plastic lined) trousers (pants) may be used for the children and can be readily and cheaply made locally. It is suggested that where pants are being used, several should be provided for waiting children, to speed up the procedure. The scale markings are available in metric or Imperial units (e.g. ounces) or both. They are usually graduated in 0.1 or 0.2 units for regular use. Such are required when weights taken are to be plotted on growth charts as they correspond approximating with lines on the weight graph. Scales are available for 25 kg and 50 kg ranges. In the field, there is usually little problem in using a

[21] CMS Weighing Equipment Limited, 18 Camden Road, London NW1 0JH, England.

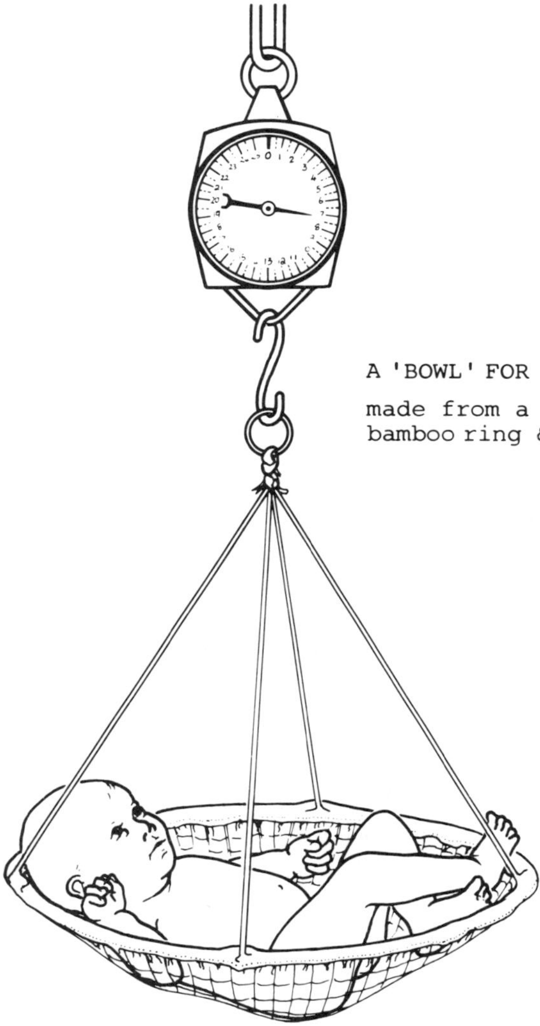

Fig. 2.15 Salter scale in use with bowl for baby. (Courtesy of Professor David Morley.) (Cost: approximately US$ 35 in 1988.)

horizontal branch, beam, or other structure for hanging the scale. Even in desert or similar treeless conditions, two assistants can support a length of bamboo or wood on their shoulders for the purpose of weighing during home visits. Such a length should have a central notch to avoid slippage of the attached rope or hook. Alternatively, a locally made transportable tripod can be used.

The need for better, simplified training in the use of Salter scales has been emphasized in recent years by UNICEF whose New Delhi office has produced an instruction booklet (UNICEF 1984). Also, Shorr (1986) has published a very detailed, step-by-step illustrated guide to accurate measurement of weight, height, and arm circumference. Training in measurement of growth has received attention recently from WHO, UNICEF, and IUNS (WHO 1985*a*; Jelliffe and Jelliffe 1989*b*).

Modifications of the Salter scale include practical technical improvements in suspension and the addition of a needle on the reverse face which shows health and nutrition education messages (or stages of development) appropriate for different weights (Morley and Cutting 1983).

Recently, the very inexpensive TALC[22] weighing scale (US$15 in 1987) has been introduced (Morley 1984, personal communication). This is essentially a spring with a backboard into which a growth chart can be inserted. By this means, it is hoped that the weights may be recorded directly on to growth charts by community health workers. Currently, plotting is one of the major difficulties in growth monitoring (p. 304).

Older children and adults The adult Detecto scale is suitable for weighing older children and adults and is often used in health centres and similar facilities. Its range is 140 kg with intervals of 0.1 kg. However, it is expensive, very heavy, and not easily transported. If used for community field work, checking and calibration before each weighing session and after each journey is recommended. It also contains a sliding rod for height measurement, which should not be used, especially for young children, unless nothing else is available, as it is not very accurate. The Homs hand carrying scale (No. 300 or 150 k) is more expensive. It is a sturdy compact model, but is very heavy, weighing 16 kg. The metric model (150 k) measures up to 150 kg by 5 kg increments on the main indicator scale and 50 g intervals on the fractional bar. The scale is near ground level and requires repeated stooping to read.

Spring bathroom-type scales are not recommended, unless nothing else is available. They are not sufficiently accurate, are fragile, and problems with parallax can occur. They may sometimes have to be used in situations where cost, portability, and availability are the most desirable requirements, such as in emergency or disaster situations in practice, they are still found in many health centres. Frequent calibration and checking with known weights are important during weighing sessions — preferably after 20 measures. A firm, flat surface is also important. However, the 'better' bathroom scales are not necessarily cheap; some costing more than US$30.

A CMS portable type field survey beam-balance scale has been devised to weigh all ages, including babies. It is small, flat, compact, relatively

[22] TALC, P.O. Box 49, St. Albans, Herts, UK.

light (with a carrying handle), easily read, and with a locking device (Morley 1978). Unfortunately, it is too expensive for widespread use.

Miscellaneous Many other scales are in use in different parts of the world. Their suitability for use in nutritional assessment needs checking with the criteria mentioned earlier (p. 70). Their availability, cost, ease of repair, and familiarity are important considerations. However, recent investigations indicate that some low-cost scales can be inadequately accurate and have a short 'life-span' (Burns 1986).

Recently, the low-cost PATH[23] electronic solar-powered Sensor scale has been devised. This can weigh *both* infants and older individuals. It has a digital read-out and is under trial in various parts of the world.

Techniques

Young children should be weighed nude, when permissible. Consideration needs to be given to a comfortable temperature, as mothers may be understandably reluctant to undress babies in cold or very sunny surroundings. In some cultures, weighing young children at all may pose difficulties, especially if nude, because of the belief that misfortune due to the 'evil eye' may be attracted or because the 'swaddling' of infants (especially the newborn) is considered important protection against various culturally-defined diseases (p. 165). If bells or heavy charms are worn, as in some rural African communities, they can be removed if practicable and permitted by the parents. Otherwise, due allowance should be made for their weight. Reliable scales which measure to the nearest 0.1 kg or less are desirable for young children, especially for serial measurements.

With due attention to technique, relatively passive infants can be weighed on most of the scales mentioned. The problem is more difficult with larger, more active pre-school children. As elsewhere in the world, it may be necessary to use an adult platform beam-balance scale to weigh the mother (or assistant) alone, and then weigh her carrying her child. The advantage of this method is that the child is calmed by the mother, so that time is saved and accurate recordings can be made. The disadvantage is that two weights have to be recorded and the risk of clerical error is doubled. It is a mistake to record only the differences in the measures. Both measures should be recorded as well as the final subtracted result. The result can then be checked later. This problem may be eliminated if the PATH Sensor electronic scale is found to be suitable for field work. The ground or 'stand-on' model allows the mother to be weighed, the

[23] PATH (Program for Appropiate Technology in Health), 4 Nickerson Rd, Seattle, Washington, 98109, USA (or) 200 West Mercer St, Suite 307, Seattle, Washington 89119, USA.

scale reset to zero, and the infant to be weighed directly in the mother's arms.

For older children and adults, undressing poses problems of modesty and has to be carried out separately for both sexes. Lightweight underpants, drawers, or shorts, or other minimum clothing of known weight will usually be retained. If clothing of significant weight is necessary, the weight of 'standard garments' should be discovered and subtracted from the individual's weight. Details should be included in the final report. It also may be noted that variation in weight of 0.2 kg or more can occur in pre-school-age children depending upon the recentness of a meal and/or defecation and micturition. Theoretically, weighing should not be done after a full meal, nor with a full bladder. However, such precautions are impossible to carry out in field studies.

Linear measurements

The basic linear measurement is that of *height (length) or stature*, and reflects skeletal growth. Other linear, mainly bony, measurements may be used for special purposes — for example, the length of the upper arm or foot. Also, *body breadth* (or *frame size*) may be graded by lateral or transverse measurements, such as biacromial width or elbow breadth (p. 84). In practice, this is rarely done.

Height

The height of an individual is principally a measure of skeletal bony tissue. It is made up of the sum of components: legs, pelvis, spine, and skull. For detailed scientific auxological studies of body proportions, all of these different measurements are required. For nutritional assessment, usually only the total height (or length) is measured routinely, or a substitute bony measurement, considered to be roughly proportional.

Body height decreases in old age and also to a small extent in other age-groups at the end of the day (about 1 cm). For example, in elderly bed-ridden persons, the arm length has been suggested as a 'proxy' or substitute measurement for height (Mitchell and Lipschitz 1982). Foot length has been used for this purpose in the newborn (Ramachandran 1986*b*).

Equipment For older children and adults, a vertical measuring rod or a scale or a non-stretch tape fixed to a vertical flat wall can be employed for measuring height. The Stanley 'microtoise'[24] is a relatively new and low-cost apparatus in which the tape container is fixed to the wall 2 m above

[24] Stanley Tools, 600 Myrtle Street, New Britain, Connecticut 06050, USA.

the floor and the bar lowered down on to the subject's head. A direct height reading can be taken through the bar window. A refinement of this apparatus is the 'Nivotoise'[24] in which a heel rest and an upright support is included. The height attachment on certain weighing scales, such as the adult Detecto, is often used, but has the disadvantage that the head-piece is wobbly, narrow, and difficult to use accurately. The measuring scale should be 2 m (78 3/4 in) high and capable of measuring to the nearest 0.1 cm (1/8 in) in young children and 0.5 cm in adults.

Specialized manufactured instruments[25] are very accurate and convenient, but are prohibitively expensive for most purposes. They are indicated in special research projects when small differences in stature require measuring. For such purposes, stadiometers (board with a scale attached) or measuring tables with a digital read-out and counterbalanced movable vertical boards are available.[25] In some circumstances, *one* such apparatus may be made available to check the accuracy of less complex, low-cost measuring rods or length boards.

A growth screening chart[26] has been introduced in the UK to screen for abnormal height, especially on school entry (Aynsley-Green and Macfarlane 1983). The child stands against the upright chart and the height can fall into three categories — normal range, consider referral, and refer. The referral levels are both for children who are abnormally tall or short.

Technique After removing the shoes, the subject should stand up as straight as possible on a flat floor, or board, by the scale with feet together and with heels, buttocks, shoulders, and back of the head touching the upright. The feet should be bare, flat on the floor, and with the heels almost together. The legs should be straight and the shoulders relaxed. The head should be looking straight forward and held comfortably erect, with the lower border of the orbit in the same horizontal plane as the external auditory meatus (the 'Frankfort plane'). The arms should be hanging by the sides in a natural manner ('stand tall and look straight ahead').

The headpiece, which can be a metal bar or a wood block, is gently lowered, compressing the hair, and making contact with the top of the head. If a child has unusually thick hair, it should be taken into account. When an assistant is available, this person should place one hand against the child's knees to detect any flexion of the lower limbs and the other hand on the upper surfaces of his feet to detect any lifting of the heels from firm contact with the floor or platform. The eyes of the measurer should be as level as possible with the reading to avoid optical errors (parallax).

[25] Holtain Ltd., Brynberian, Bwynmych, Pembrokeshire, Wales (or) Pfister Import-Export Inc, 450 Barrell Avenue, Carlstadt, New Jersey 07072, USA.
[26] Castlemead Publications, Gascoyne Way, Castlemead, Hertford SG14 1LH, UK.

Weight-for-height

Weight-for-height has not often been assessed in child health programmes because of difficulties of measuring children's height, the need for two types of apparatus, the increased chance that an error might occur with two measurements, and problems with calculating weight as a percentage of the expected weight-for-height. To make it easier, the OXFAM Emergency Kit[27] contains a laminated plastic card giving the weight-for-height percentage for children of different weights and heights.

If children's ages are not known (or if children are seen infrequently), the weight-for-height chart (Nabarro and McNab 1980) may be used on its own to identify 'thin' or 'wasted' children who are in need of urgent help. Serially, changes in changes in weight-for-height can be monitored from month to month and can be recorded on a special chart.

This weight-for-height chart or 'Thinness Wall Chart' consists of a number of vertical columns printed on a large sheet (140 cm × 100 cm) of plastic-coated paper (Figs 2.16(a), (b)). Each column is marked with a different weight (5–25 kg) and has three coloured sections at its upper end.[28] The chart should be firmly fixed in an upright position, often against a wall. A health worker assessing the nutrition of a child, weighs the child and places him (her) standing, against the column marked with his weight. The colour at the top of the child's head indicates his weight-for-height. A red colour indicates the child whose weight is less than 80 per cent of the standard weight for his height. A narrow *portable* wooden weight-for-height board has been tried out in Africa (Campbell *et al.* 1985; Binkin *et al.* 1985; Cutting 1986); its practical use is being evaluated.

Problems can arise with the use of the 'Thinness Wall Chart' in that the highest red zone identifies tall (but thin) children. Careful training is needed to avoid confusion and to ensure correct usage by community health workers. Indeed, recent use of the chart in large-scale famine relief operations in the West Sudan revealed unexpected difficulties. However, these occurred because two charts were used with slightly different standards (Soeters 1986).

Another device was introduced by Franks and Cutting (1985, pers. commun.). This is a modified Salter scale. After the child's height has been measured, the weight-for-height 'category' — green, yellow, or red — can be read off directly.

[27] An OXFAM Emergency Kit contains a thinness chart, weighing scale, a height tape, and plastic card giving percentage weight-for-height (W/H). The W/H percentage can either be read off the card or directly viewed on the thinness chart. Available from OXFAM, Oxford, UK.

[28] The weight-for-height wall chart together with an instruction booklet and record cards are available from the Department of Nutrition, London School of Tropical Medicine and Hygiene, Keppel Street, London WCI 7HT, UK

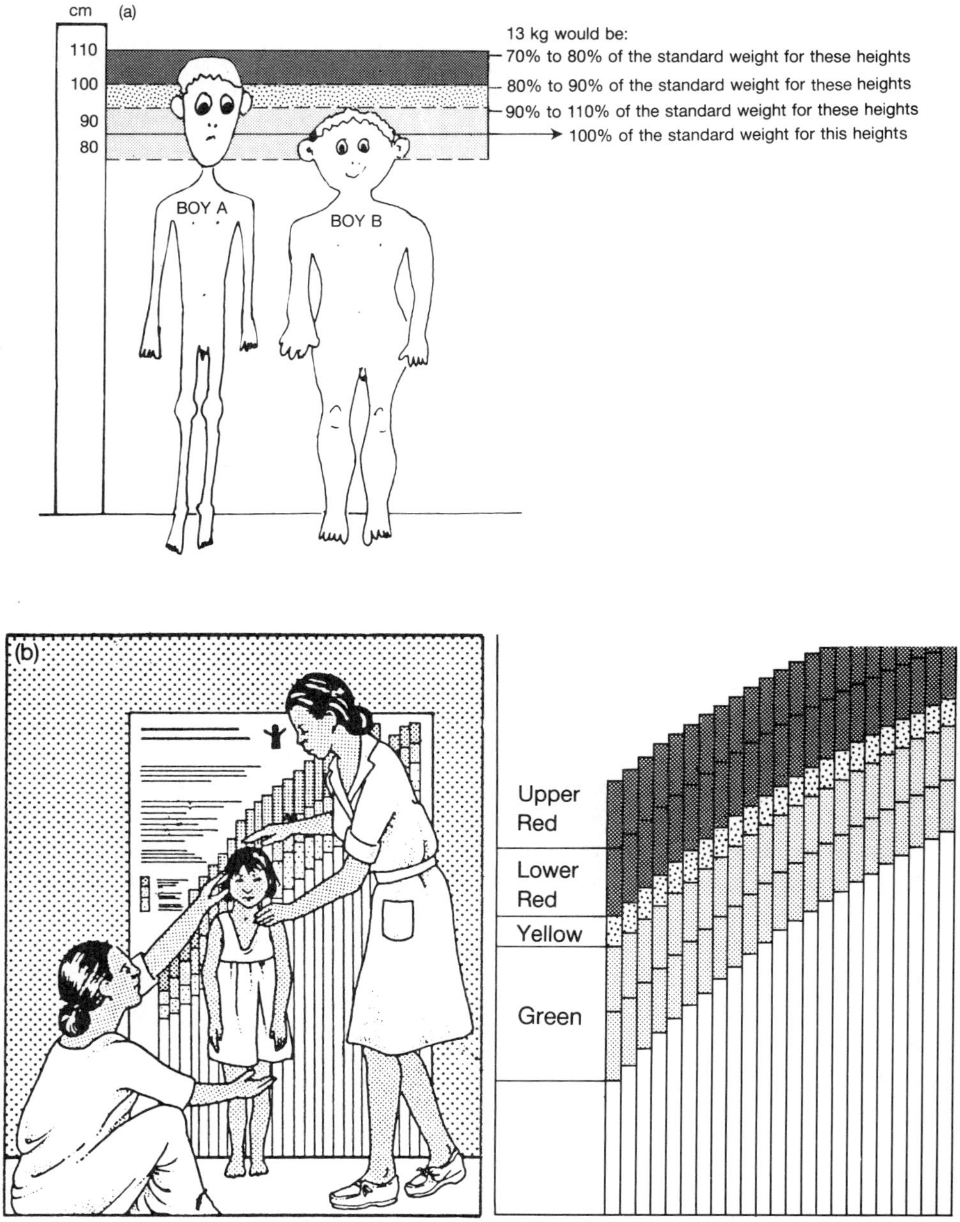

Fig. 2.16 (a) Weight-for-height or Thinness Wall Chart (Nabarro and McNab 1980). This illustration shows the different reading on the wall chart of two boys both weighing 13 kg. Boy A is thin, while boy B has a normal weight-for height. In the actual wall chart the top zone is red, the second from the top is yellow, and the bottom two zones are different shades of green. (b) Thinness weight-for-height wall chart (Nabarro and McNab 1980).

Length
In very young children, recumbent length (crown–heel length) has to be employed, as the measurement of standing height is either impossible or very inaccurate with an uncooperative child. It is usually measured with a length-board, often made of wood.

Recumbent length is usually considered necessary for children up to 2 or 3 years of age or until the child can stand unassisted, according to different authorities. Length can be more than standing height by as much as 2 cm (nearly 1 in), so that the procedure used has to be reported.

Equipment Very expensive, elegantly precise instruments are available, such as the Harpenden measuring table. Conversely, in paediatrics, the inexpensive table-top 'infantometer' (Model 1334)[29] (100 cm × 0.5 cm) has been widely employed, but is insufficiently accurate and needs a completely flat surface on which to be used. A low-cost durable, easily portable, commercially available length-board is a neglected piece of apparatus, needing an 'appropriate technology' (p. 361) approach.

Usually length-boards have to be made locally by carpenters. These have the advantage of being relatively inexpensive and can be adapted to the needs of the particular task. Plywood, pine, or similar locally available woods have been used satisfactorily. They need to be strong, smooth, and lightweight. A flat steel metric tape, or an old-style brass-hinged carpenter's rule can be used as the scale, and fitted on to (or let-into) the flat baseboard. Less expensively, a tape can be tacked on or fixed with a resin glue.

If a lightweight board is needed, because of transportability, it can be made of plastic (which greatly increases the cost), or a lattice-work of holes can be drilled through the wood on which the child lies. The wood should be varnished to prevent shrinkage, water-damage, or warping.

Several prototype boards, usually of wood, have been developed in recent years, although none as yet on a commercial basis. A folding model suitable for air transport has been widely used by the Caribbean Food and Nutrition Institute. In this, the wood is lightweight and the baseboard patterned with numerous 1 in (2.5 cm) holes to further reduce weight. The UCLA Nutrition Assessment Unit (1975–78) used a portable board for height and length measurement, in several African national nutrition surveys (Fig. 2.17). AHRTAG[30] and the Center for Disease Control[31] (Brink *et al.* 1977) have also developed a portable board for which plans are available (Fig. 2.18). The latter uses a hinge mechanism, so that the

[29] Grafco, Graham-Field Surgical Co, Inc, 415 Second Avenue, New Hyde Park, New York 11040, USA.
[30] AHRTAG, 83 Marleybone Road, London, WIM 3DE, UK.
[31] Center for Disease Control, Atlanta, Georgia 30333, USA.

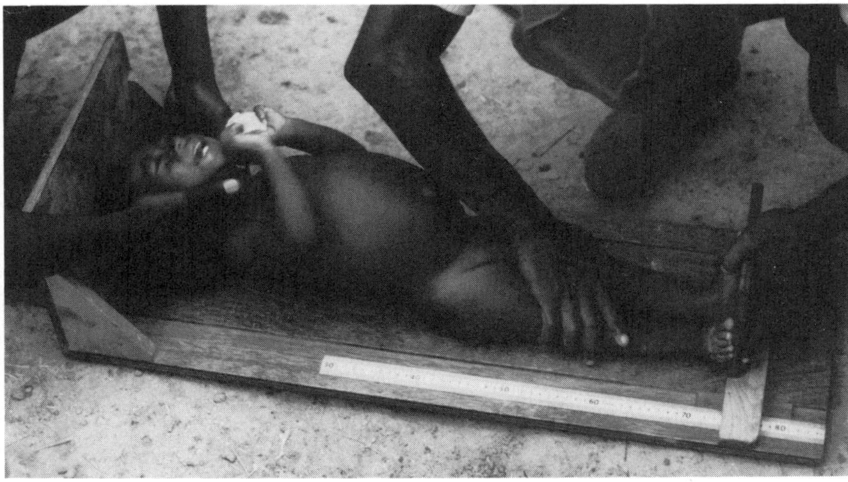

Fig. 2.17 Locally made wooden length-board (UCLA model). West African surveys.

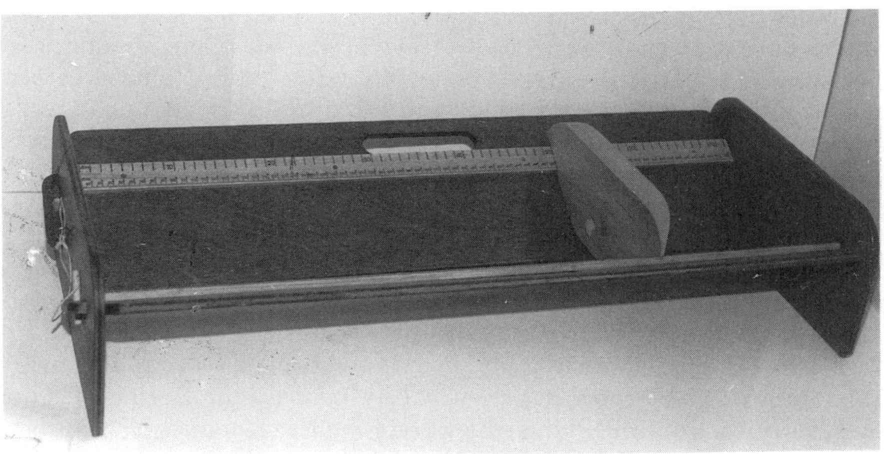

Fig. 2.18 AHRTAG wooden length-board.

headboard becomes the base of the instrument when it is used for the measurement of height.

Other designs are available — for example, from the Caribbean Food and Nutrition Institute, Jamaica, or as detailed in the recent publication by Shorr (1986).[32]

[32] Shorr Productions, 467 Prospect Street, Woonsocket, Rhode Island 02895, USA.

Technique

In the measurement of recumbent length, the infant is laid on the board which is itself on a flat surface. The head is positioned against the fixed headboard, with the eyes looking vertically. The legs are straightened and the knees (or, at least, one knee) are kept together and extended by gentle pressure applied by an assistant; the feet are upright at right angles. The upright sliding foot-piece ('cursor') is moved to obtain firm contact with the heels and the length is read to the nearest 0.1 cm. The mother should be present to calm the young child when length (or height) is measured.

The difficulties of using a length board with terrified struggling young children can be considerable, especially in rural survey work. Much practice, patience (in waiting for the right moment), and the assistance of two, or preferably three, people are required to make adequately accurate readings.

Breadth ('frame size')

In some reference data of weight for *adults*, such as the 1959 Metropolitan Life Insurance Tables, the figures given are sometimes divided into three 'body frames' — large, medium, and small — which are not defined.

Attempts to categorize breadth and frame size include radiographic measurements of bony chest breadth (Garn and Hawthorne 1984) and elbow breadth (Frisancho and Flagel 1983). The simplest method uses elbow breadth. From this measurement and the individual's height without shoes, body frame type for adults can be categorized, using the Lindner diagram (Lindner and Lindner 1985)[33] (Fig. 2.19). However, this procedure needs further testing in different ethnic groups with visibly different body proportions and physiques. (Also see: Addendum 1988.)

In practice, frame size is usually not considered and reference data are give for the 'medium' frame size.

Head circumference

The measurement of head circumference is a standard procedure in paediatric practice and is used to detect pathological conditions accompanied by a large head or one of increasing size (e.g. hydrocephalus), or too small a skull (e.g. microcephaly).

Head circumference is related mainly to brain size and — to a small extent — to the thickness of the scalp tissues and the skull. Brain size increases rapidly during the first year, in which head circumference normally reflects age rather than health or nutrition.

The head circumference was measured in the 1960s to detect a low (below 1:1) chest/head circumference ratio, considered to be suggestive of

[33] Cambridge Scientific Industries, P.O. Box 265, Cambridge, MD 21613, USA.

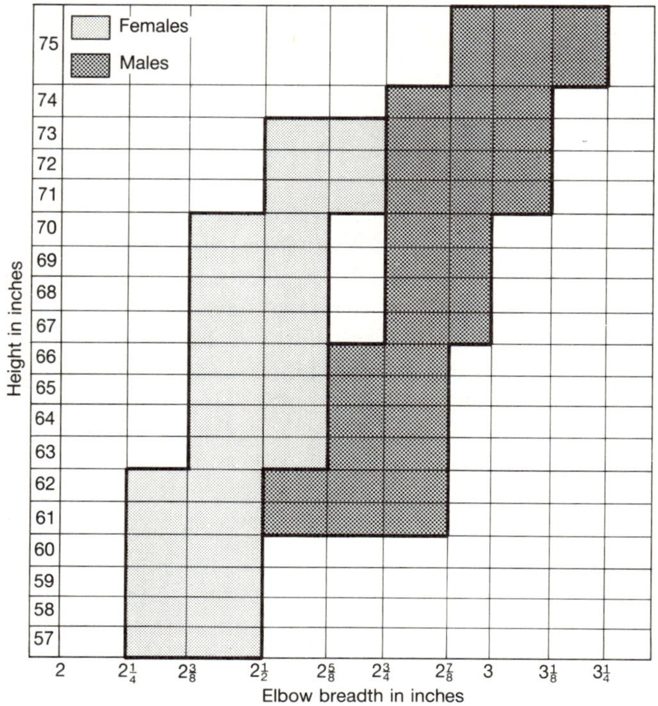

Fig. 2.19 Lindner diagram for estimating body frame size based on height and elbow breadth (Lindner and Lindner 1985). Medium frames for males and females, respectively are represented by the shaded areas. A measurement to the left of the shaded area indicates a small frame; a measurement to the right of the shaded area indicates a large frame.

less marked protein–energy malnutrition in young children in the second year of life. Recent work has shown this ratio to be unreliable (Martorell *et al.* 1975).

Recent investigations in the newborn have suggested that the mid-arm circumference/head circumference ratio (MAC:HC) might be used in assessing intrauterine growth (Sasanow *et al.* 1986). Further investigation is needed.

Equipment Measurements should be made with a narrow (less than 1 cm wide) flexible, non-stretch tape, made of steel or preferably fibre-glass. Cloth tapes should be avoided as they tend to stretch in use. If they have to be used, they should be checked frequently.

Technique The child's head should be steadied and the greatest circumference measured, by placing the tape firmly round the frontal bones just superior to the supraorbital ridges, passing it round the head at the same level on each side, and laying it over the maximum occipital prominence at the back. Measurements should be made to the nearest 0.1 cm.

Body composition

The brain, liver, heart, kidneys, and other internal organs together make up an appreciable part of the body weight, but are inaccessible for measurement in living individuals without ultrasophisticated apparatus. Muscle and fat constitute the soft tissues that vary most with protein depletion and excessive or deficient intakes of energy (calories or joules). Tissue anthropometry can be used to estimate *approximate* stores of both of these as part of the assessment of nutritional status.

Approximate amounts of subcutaneous fat and muscle are apparent on inspection. In adult males, the chest–abdomen: girth ratio can be used as a simple measure to confirm or screen for obesity.

Subcutaneous fat

Body composition studies, including information concerning the amount and distribution of fat, and hence of calorie reserves, can be carried out by various technically complicated methods, including: ultrasonics (Kuczmarski *et al.* 1987) (with a compact portable model available); densitometry (by water displacement in a densitometer, or underwater weighing); gaseous uptake of fat-soluble gases; isotope dilution techniques; radiological methods; total electrical body conduction (TOBEC) (bioelectrical impedance) (Lukanski 1987; Van Loan and Mayelin 1987; Malina 1987); and anthropometry (multiple fatfolds, using calipers). Whole-body chemical analysis at autopsy is the only direct method, but has rarely been carried out.

While techniques listed above can be important in detailed nutritional investigation in well-equipped research centres, only anthropometry using calipers is convenient and reasonably practicable in field circumstances as an indirect but objective indicator of complete body stores of fat. Even then, great care has to be taken with the technique employed and with the interpretation of results. However, scientific technological studies in specialized centres can be very valuable in validating the accuracy and significance of caliper measurements. It was found that the correlation between caliper measurements, radiological findings, and direct measurements made during surgery was good (Garn 1962). Investigations have shown a high correlation with ultrasonic and electrical conductivity measures of fatfold thickness (Van Loan and Mayelin 1987) as well as with total body fat. More recent studies have shown more difference between fatfold measurements and actual fat thickness. (Also see: Addendum 1988.)

Fat is most abundant subcutaneously, especially in children. However, considerable amounts also are present around the kidneys and heart, within the abdominal cavity (omental fat), and between muscles. Caliper measurements, therefore only give an estimate of superficial and accessible fat, as manifest by a *double* layer of skin and fat. This is usually called a 'skinfold.' However, as it is mostly fat and the caliper is concerned with measuring fat thickness, it seems more accurately descriptive to use the term 'fatfold'.

The fatfold measurement is of two layers of both fat and skin. Results are in millimetres, *not* in centimetres as is the arm circumference measurement (p. 91). As noted later (p. 101), the mid-arm fat *area* (p. 102) or *volume* (p. 102), can be roughly estimated from the triceps fatfold and the arm circumference measurements.

Equipment Various skinfold calipers have been devised, but experience suggests that the instrument used should have a standard contact surface or 'pinch' area (20–40 mm^2), should read through a range of 2–40 mm, with gradations of 1 mm (or less), and exert a constant pressure (10 g/mm^2) through the whole range of skinfold thicknesses at all distances of separation of the jaws. The caliper dial should be set to zero before each day's work, or allowance made for zero error by subtraction.

Although precision calipers are designed so that their jaws exert a constant tension, in practice, this has different results according to fatfold compressibility, which in turn varies with age, sex, hydration, and fatfold site. The subcutaneous fat in babies and young infants has been shown to be very compressible, while the obese appear to have decreased compressibility.

Precision calipers are expensive costing over US$100. Three models have been used in recent decades. The Lange[34] (Lange and Brozek 1961) remains the most popular in the USA (Fig. 2.20). In the UK, the Harpenden[35] (Edwards *et al.* 1955) has been largely superseded by the Holtain[36] (Tanner and Whitehouse 1978) (Fig. 2.21). (Also see: Addendum 1988.)

Small metal blocks are available from suppliers for standardization of the calipers, but do not duplicate fat compressibility. However, fatfold measurements differ somewhat with the type of caliper used. For this reason, a conversion factor has been suggested (Parizkova and Goldstein 1970), but rarely used.

[34] Lange Skinfold Calipers, Cambridge Scientific Industries, Inc, 101 Virginia Avenue, Cambridge, Maryland 21612, USA (approximately US$175).

[35] British Indicators Ltd, Acewood Way, St. Albans, Herts, England (or) Quinton Instruments Ltd, 2121 Terry Avenue, Seattle, Washington 98121, USA (approximately US$285).

[36] Holtain Ltd., Brynberian, Bwymmych, Pembrokeshire, Wales (or) Pfister Import–Export Co, 450 Parrell Avenue, Carlstadt, New Jersey 07072, USA (approximately US$211).

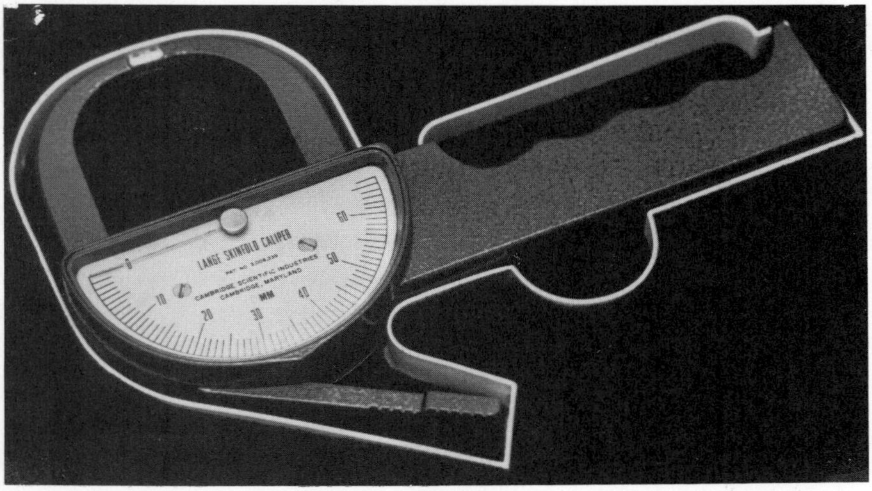

Fig. 2.20 Lange skinfold (fatfold) caliper.

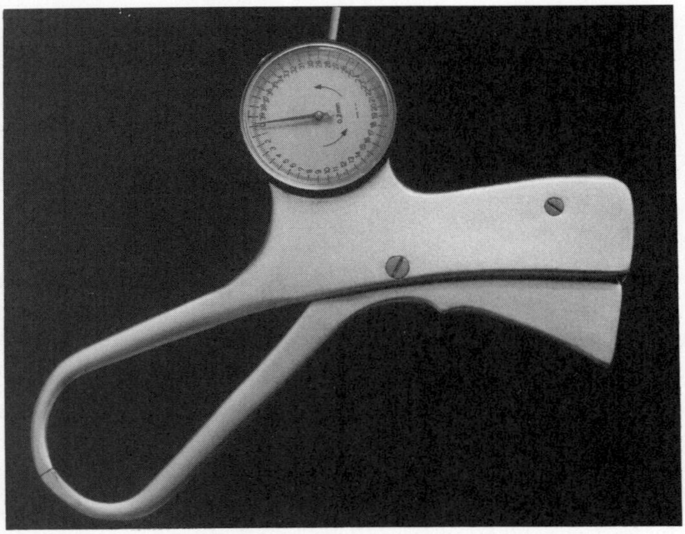

Fig. 2.21 Holtain skinfold (fatfold) caliper.

The critical limitation of these calipers, their considerable cost, is due, at least in part, to their metal construction and high standard of precision. However, this accuracy is often not matched by the results obtained in practice, because of observer error and because of differences in technique (e.g. the site, depth, and duration of application of the instrument at the selected skinfold area). Therefore, it makes sense to accept a little

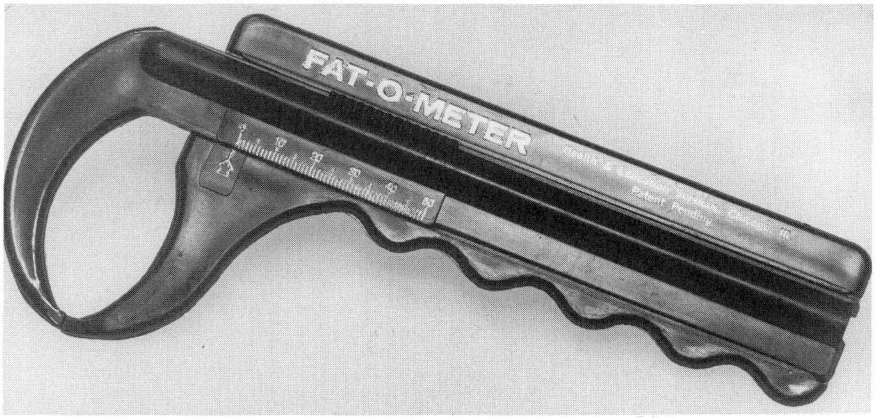

Fig. 2.22 Low-cost plastic fatfold calipers ('Fat-o-meter') (Garn 1983).

less precision, to overcome the cost problem, if reasonable accuracy is maintained.

In recent years, various inexpensive plastic calipers have been manufactured in response to the practice of self-assessment of fatness in the home, especially in the USA. These include the McGaw caliper[37] and the 'Fat-O-Meter'.[38]

Inspection shows such calipers to vary greatly, as regards tension applied and size of fatfold measured. Most, but not all, seem likely to be inaccurate, only giving gross estimates, and being unsuitable for measuring small changes.

McGaw and Lange calipers have been compared. The cheap plastic model gave results which were highly correlated with the Lange, but were consistently lower. Also, they could not measure fatfolds in the very obese as their highest reading was 40 mm (Burgert and Anderson 1979).

Another recent model in this low-cost field in the USA is the 'Fat-O-Meter', made of smooth injection-moulded black plastic and fitted with a protected steel spring to provide constant pressure along its 50 mm measurement capacity (Fig. 2.22). It is inexpensive (US$12.95), reasonably sturdy, and is calibrated from zero to 50 mm at 1 mm intervals. The jaw depth is 54 mm, the contact area about 20 mm, and the force exerted by the spring is about 0.5 kg (e.g. 25 g/mm^2) (Garn 1983).

In view of the current 10–20 times higher cost of the main scientific calipers, the more reliable plastic calipers need further trials in both clinical and survey circumstances.

[37] McGaw Laboratories, Irvine, California, USA.
[38] Health and Education Services, 80 Fairbanks, Addison, Illinois 60101, USA.

Techniques Fatfold calipers may be employed in communities in developing regions with more concern for depleted energy reserves. However, large numbers of measurements at different sites will usually neither be indicated nor feasible. Despite the fact that an increase or decrease of subcutaneous fat stores is not uniform all over the body, the essence of the problem is to select one or two easily accessible sites that may be expected to give an approximate practical indication of calorie reserves. For this purpose, both with poor calorie stores and in obesity, the triceps fatfold is the most practical measurement for all age-groups. This can be combined, if needed, with the subscapular fatfold as the preferred second site. Furthermore, especially in young children, the triceps fatfold is not only useful as an indication of energy (calorie) reserves, but enables the underlying mid-upper arm muscle circumference to be calculated (p. 102). The triceps fatfold also has the practical advantage of not altering substantially during the pre-school period, and so from 12 to 60 months it is relatively independent of precise age in well-nourished populations.

At all sites, a lengthwise fatfold is firmly grasped and slightly lifted up between finger and thumb of the left hand, care being taken not to include underlying muscle. This may be difficult to do in the obese. The calipers are applied about 1 cm below the operator's fingers at a depth about equal to the fatfold, while the fatfold is gently held throughout the measurement. Fatfold calipers are difficult to use, with considerable potential for error within, and particularly between observers. Three measurements should be made and the results averaged. Difficulties in obtaining accurate results can occur because of technical errors and increased compressibility in frank, or even subclinical, oedema, and the normal occurrence of softer fat in babies than in adults.

Triceps fatfold (upper arm, dorsal arm, arm fatfold) As the fat in this region is not uniform in thickness, the site needs to be carefully selected at a measured point half-way down the arm, between the tip of the acromial process of the scapula and the olecranon process of the ulna (Fig. 2.23). The left arm is usually measured by international agreement. However, some investigators use the right side. The midpoint can be marked with an appropriately coloured skin pencil. The measurement is made with the arm hanging relaxed at the side. The fatfold at the back of the upper arm parallel to the posterior long axis is picked up between the thumb and forefinger of the left hand, away from the underlying muscle, and measured at this point (Fig. 2.24). The triceps fatfold is easily accessible and no undressing is needed.

Subscapular fatfold (infrascapular, back fatfold) The subscapular fatfold is measured just below and laterally to the angle of the left scapula. The

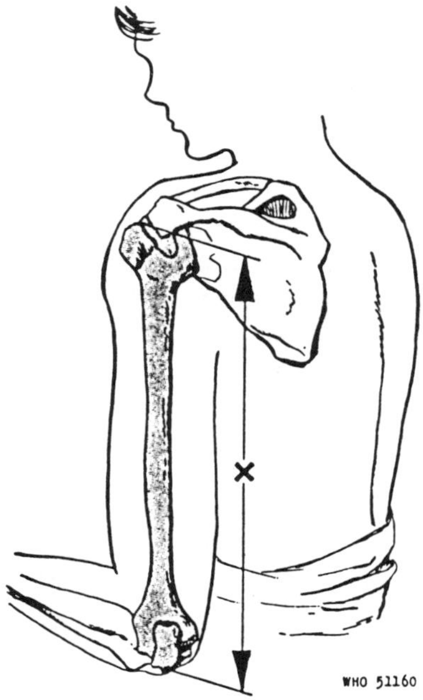

Fig. 2.23 Determination of the midpoint of the arm (half-way between the acromial process and the olecranon process). (Jelliffe 1966).

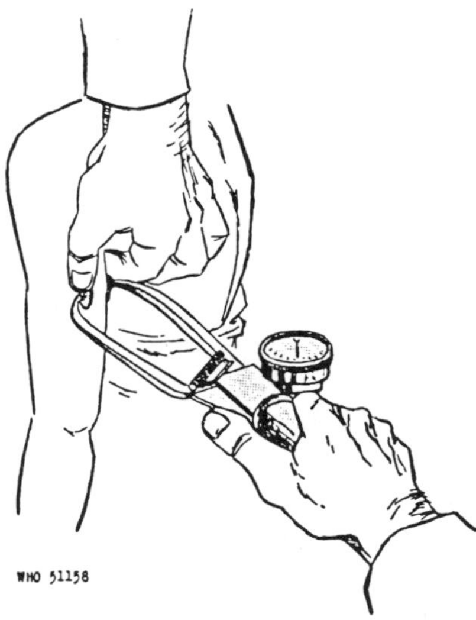

Fig. 2.24 Measurement of triceps fatfold with Harpenden calipers. (Jelliffe 1966).

fold should be in a line running at approximately 45 degrees to the spine, in the natural line of skin cleavage. It is often used as a secondary site for adults. It has the advantage of providing a uniform layer of subcutaneous fat, not requiring precise localization. It has the disadvantage of inaccessibility, needing partial undressing.

Combined fatfolds In the clinical assessment of obesity or fat stores formulae are available based on combined fatfolds from three or more different sites (Durnin and Rahaman 1967).

Arm circumference measurement

The arm circumference was first used in community nutritional assessment in a 1958 country-wide survey for protein–energy malnutrition in Haitian pre-school age children (Jelliffe and Jelliffe 1960). The reason for its selection was the obvious long recognized thinness of the limbs of malnourished individuals, noted, for example, in children in 1878 in Dibgy's *History of the Irish Famine*:

> The head looked unnaturally large by contrast with the emaciated trunk, the shoulder blades projecting as if they had been inserted by mistake in too small a carcass, the arms and legs shrivelled to the size of their bones, except at the knees which are swollen.

Based on these marked changes in severe protein–energy malnutrition, it was considered that the arm circumference would give an approximate composite picture of labile stores of energy (fat) and protein (muscle), and that the arm circumference would be diminished in lesser degrees of protein–energy malnutrition, reflecting *both* fat and muscle depletion. In obesity, by contrast, the arm circumference would be greater than normal, as a result of increased subcutaneous fat.

In almost 30 years since its introduction, much information has been collected on the value of this simple measurement from many workers from all over the world. Initially, this concentrated on young children (Jelliffe and Jelliffe 1969), but recent work has included consideration of the meaning of low- and high-arm circumference measurements in school children (p. 332), adults (p. 339), pregnant women (p. 227), and newborn babies (p. 245). The arm circumference measurement is often useful when screening for protein–energy malnutrition, and attempts are being made to use modified tapes for growth monitoring in circumstances where weighing and weight charts are not possible, for various reasons (Jelliffe and Jelliffe 1988*b*).

As a measurement it is relatively simple to take and can be done accurately, provided the tape is snuggly fitted and not squeezed too tight. A tape is very cheap and easily carried. It has special value when weighing scales and/or a length-board are not available, because of cost, convenience, and portability.

Two other limb measurements have been suggested — the circumference of the calf (Singh 1970), and of the thigh. The latter is larger and hence it is easier to appreciate smaller changes (Zeitlin 1979; Zeitlin *et al.* 1981) However, the arm circumference (and other measures derived from it) have been more widely employed, particularly because it is more accessible and usually requires no undressing.

Equipment Tape measures generally should not be wider than 12 mm nor thicker than 0.2 mm (Zerfas 1979). Metal and firm plastic tapes are more likely to retain a circular shape during measurement, while less rigid tapes tend to follow the actual surface of the arm. Cloth or paper tapes are not recommended, as they can stretch or tear. The readability of the numbers on commercial tapes varies greatly. The numbers should be clearly visible and understandable by the measurer. They are best printed along the long axis of the tape and not cross-wise, as the latter are more difficult to read. Currently, there appears to be a trend towards using tapes reading in *millimetres* — to avoid confusion with the decimal point.

Fibre-glass, plastic (or plastic-coated), or laminated tapes are suitable. Permanent creasing may occur with plastic tapes. Laminated tapes may adhere to the skin surfaces in humid conditions and should be smoothed during measurement.

An 'insertion tape' has been developed which has a window for reading the measurement, and a slot for stabilizing at one end (Zerfas 1975) (Fig. 2.25). As a further requirement, a Vernier scale can be built as in (Fig. 2.26). This can be more important when measuring a small arm circumference, as in the newborn (Ramachandran 1986), or when calculating muscle circumferences (p. 101).

Technique Measurements of the mid-upper arm circumference (sometimes abbreviated to MUAC) appear to be useful in practice, as the limb is roughly circular, heavily muscled, and is easily accessible, even with a young child sitting on the mother's lap in front of the examiner. Also, even in kwashiorkor the upper arm is not usually clinically oedematous, remaining obviously wasted and thin.

The arm circumference is measured to the nearest 0.1 cm with a flexible steel or vinyl-coated fibre-glass (or plastic) tape, which must be placed gently, but firmly, round the left limb to avoid compression of the soft tissues. Various tapes have been devised with attached springs to try to standardize measurement and avoid over-compression. Cost makes such tapes impractical in most circumstances and disproportionate to the extra accuracy. In newborn and young infants, it is difficult to measure the small circumference of the arm with a steel tape, and it is necessary to use a non-stretch fibre-glass tape.

By international agreement, the *left arm*, while hanging freely, is mea-

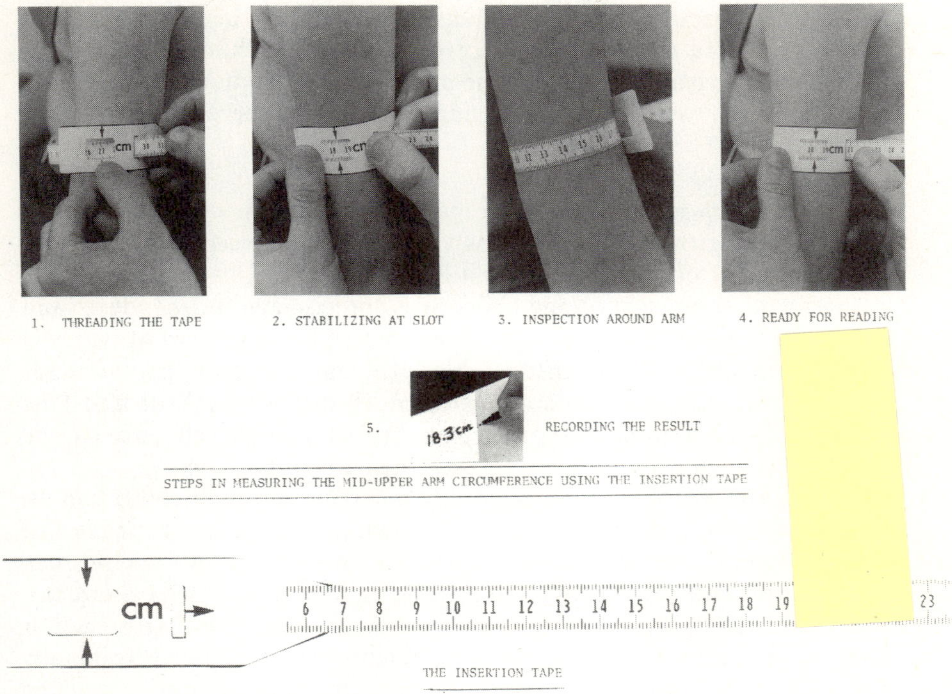

Fig. 2.25 Zerfas insertion tape.

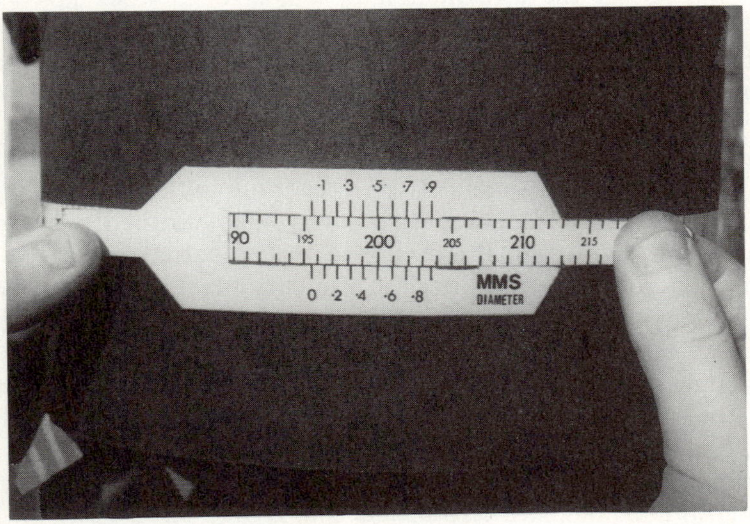

Fig. 2.26 Vernier scale addition to Zerfas insertion tape, enabling measurement of arm circumference to the nearest 0.1 mm.

sured to the nearest 0.1 cm at its midpoint, which has been identified for the triceps fatfold measurement. However, in young children in developing countries a visual estimate of the midpoint (or maximum site) is often made, especially when screening using a tricolour tape or similar device (p. 95).

Precise age-independent The average mid-upper arm circumference in well-nourished groups of children is very similar between 1 and 4 years (12–59 months) of age (Burgess and Burgess 1969). This means that the measurement in pre-school age children is 'precise-age independent' and can be used without knowledge of the exact age, the discovery of which is often a difficult or even insuperable problem in some communities (p. 318). Also, according to some workers (Fisher 1976; Yost and Pust 1987), the 7–12 months change is so slight that a single reference can be used for this period (with a lower cut-off point of 12.5 cm).

If the age is known, the appropriate reference level (p. 000) can be applied. However, if the age is not known precisely, an approximate single 'midpoint' reference level — often 16 cm — for 1–4 year olds can be used instead. Alternatively, some workers have used the arm circumference level compared with a less labile measure of bone growth. For example, the arm circumference for height was employed originally with the QUAC stick by Arnhold (1969) in Nigeria, and the head circumference has been used similarly (McLaren and Kanawati 1972). In both, the labile arm circumference (muscle and fat) is related to a less affected measurement of bone growth, which, in addition, does not decrease. Details for the construction of a QUAC stick are given by de Goyet *et al.* (1978). Usually, the arm circumference measurement by itself is preferred, and, in primary health care circumstances, the mid-point of the upper arm is not measured exactly, but estimated.

Simple screening devices Arm circumference measurements taken in community surveys are usually classified later into different levels, such as 'low', 'borderline', and 'normal', or 'very malnourished', 'moderately malnourished', and 'normal'. Owing to this, a variety of devices have been introduced which categorize the arm circumference of a young child directly as it is measured, based again on the knowledge that the circumference of the mid-upper arm changes little from 1 to 4 years, so that the instrument used can use a single midpoint 'reference'. Similar methods have been introduced to categorize pregnant women (p. 244) and newborns (p. 254).

Simple 'appropriate technology' (p. 361) methods for categorizing levels of low arm circumference also include the QUAC stick (Arnhold 1969) and the Bailey stick (1975), the Shakir string, or tape, or strip (Shakir and Morley 1974) (Fig. 2.27(a)), the *quipu* (Jelliffe and Jelliffe 1975), the 10

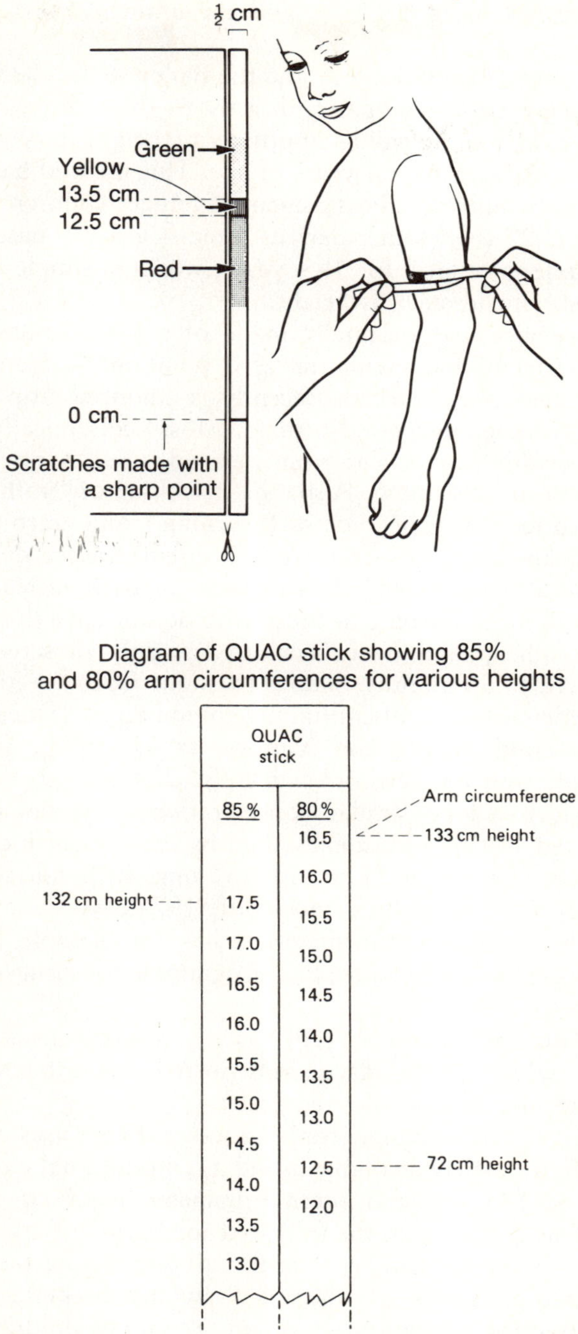

Fig. 2.27 (a) Shakir tape or strip. (b) Diagram and basic data of the QUAC stick. (Courtesy of de Ville de Goyet *et al.* 1978.)

anna bangle test (Laugesen 1975), and the anthrogauge (Zerfas *et al.* 1977).

The QUAC stick (Arnhold 1969) and the Bailey stick (1975) enable the arm circumference to be compared directly to the reference levels (and percentages below) for the child's approximate height (p. 000). They are more useful for children over 5 years of age. This method has been used, for example, in the nutritional assessment of refugee children (de Goyet *et al.* 1978) (Fig. 2.27 (b)). Other devices listed below are based on use of the midpoint reference level for 1–4 years, which is simple and requires no other measurement, such as height.

The Shakir device was originally made of a piece of string or cord about 12 in (30 cm) long with the zero point marked and with red, yellow, and green zones marked. Recently, a coloured strip of paper or plastic tape have been suggested instead. Most economically, a strip of 0.5–1 cm in width can be cut from cleaned, used X-ray film, which would otherwise be discarded. Also, this tricolour or 'traffic-light' tape can be coloured red ('danger'), yellow ('warning'), and green ('adequate'), with felt pens, and used to categorize arm circumference measurements. Different culturally significant colours may be used instead; the term 'traffic light' will mean nothing to those who do not have them. Such arm tapes are very cheap and have been used mainly in screening young children from 12 to 60 months. Similar tricolour tapes have been devised for school children (as part of continuing community self-measurement in the CHILD-to-child programme (Guthrie *et al.* 1978), for pregnant women (p. 244), and for newborn babies (p. 254).

The *quipu* is based on similar considerations. The name is derived from the knotted strings traditionally used by the ancient Incas to record historical events. It is about 12 in (30 cm) long, with coloured knots at 100, 80, and 60 per cent (Jelliffe and Jelliffe 1975), which can be used to classify pre-school children immediately. It has, for example, been used as a screening process in a graded feeding programme for refugee children in Africa.

Similarly, Korte and Lambert (1975, pers. commun.) have devised a MUAC meter, which gives danger levels (in red) for different ages, contrasted with normal ranges coloured green.

The so-called '10 *anna* bangle test' (Laugesen 1975) uses cheap plastic bangles, which are widely available in India, with internal circumferences of 12.6 cm, and 14.0 cm, and internal diameter of 4.0 cm and 4.5 cm, respectively. This is passed up the fully extended arm and over the elbow. If it passes up the upper arm easily without compressing the tissues, the test is considered positive — i.e. there is a low arm circumference. Ghosh *et al.* (1976) used the bangle test in Indian pre-school children and found it useful for detecting severe and moderate malnutrition. It seemed especially useful in the second and third year of life. They concluded that the bangle test was a simple screening procedure and that it took less than a minute to perform. A health auxiliary without much training of nutrition anthropometry could therefore screen children suffering from moderate to severe malnutrition and give them nutritional advice and supplementary food. In any natural disaster where large-scale malnutrition in young children occurs, resulting in an increased death rate, the bangle could be used as a quick screening test to plan feeding programmes. However, Shah and colleagues (1976), did not find the bangle test reliable in differentiating levels of nutrition.

A recent device is the plastic or cardboard 'anthrogauge' which has been designed to screen for both upper arm *diameter* and triceps fatfold (Zerfas *et al.* 1977) (Fig. 2.28(a)). Further field testing is required. Additional consideration of the practiced usefulness and limitation of these methods is given later.

As an ultimate in simplification Morley (1979) suggested that it is possible to train individuals to detect a low arm circumference in young children by palpation alone (Fig. 2.28(b)).

Several new arm tapes have appeared recently. These include four simplified tapes: (1) the TALC tape[39] in millimetres which can be used for measuring the arm circumference in young children or pregnant women, *or* the fundal height of the uterus in pregnancy (Fig. 2.29), and can be marked with yellow and red zones if need be for illiterate measurers; (2) the red–white newborn arm tape forming part of a 'birth coupon' in Guatemala for traditional birth attendants to identify low-birth-weight babies (Lechtig *et al.* 1983); (3) the four-colour arm tape (Zeitlin *et al.* 1982); and (4) a modified eight-colour zone tape for 'growth maintenance monitoring' by illiterate community health workers (Jelliffe and Jelliffe 1989*b*; see also: Addendum 1988, p. 000).

Two more complicated tapes are (1) the UNICEF Brazil tape which is intended for screening arm measurements in five age-groups (using both sides of the tape) (Fig. 2.30), and (2) the Echeverri tapes.

The Echeverri tapes include two tapes for *infants*. One for 0–3 months and another with two levels for 4–7 months and 8–11 months, respectively. Another tape devised by the same worker enables the measurer to record the result directly from the tape to an arm circumference growth chart and also indicates developmental milestones appropriate for different ages in the first 6 years of life. These may fit special needs in different places, but there is a risk that increasing refinement and complexity may limit practical usefulness, moving the technology back from 'appropriate' to 'inappropriate'.

Muscle mass

The mid-upper arm circumference can be an objective confirmation of the clinical observation of thinness or fatness. In young children in developing

[39] Obtainable from TALC, P.O. Box 49, St. Albans, England.

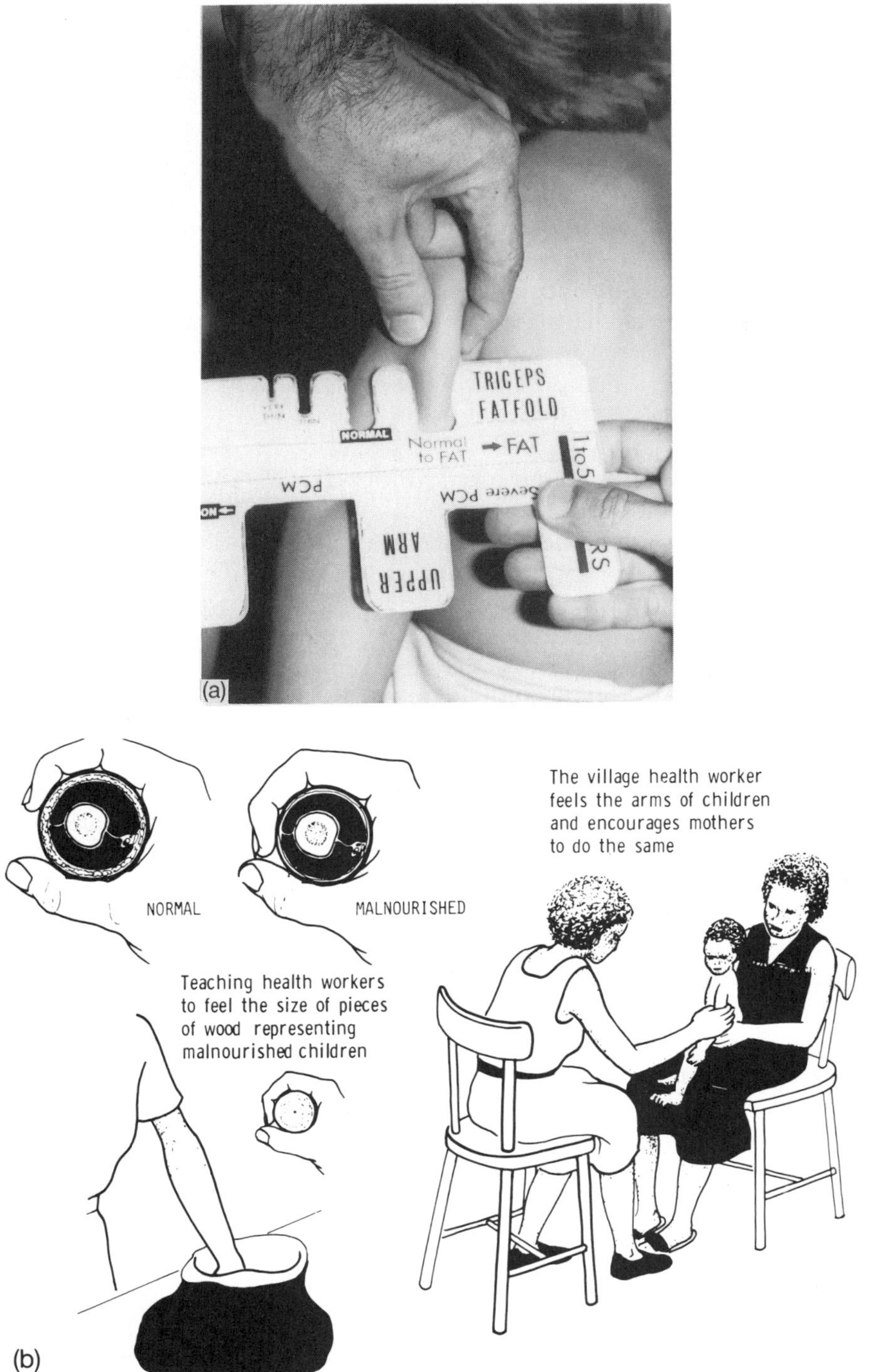

Fig. 2.28 (a) Anthrogauge for 'categorizing' triceps fatfolds and midarm diameter (Zerfas *et al.* 1982). (b) Training community health workers to detect 'low arm circumference' by palpation (feel) (Morley 1979).

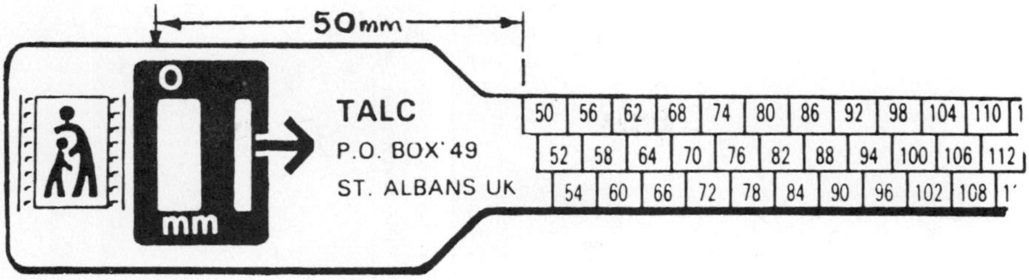

Fig. 2.29 TALC insertion tape using millimetres at 2 mm intervals for use in measuring arm circumference of a child or pregnant woman or fundal height in pregnancy (p. 246).

countries, who usually have little subcutaneous fat, it principally reflects muscle tissue. In adults in urbanized Western societies, the arm circumference is often related to subcutaneous fat.

Poor muscle development or muscle wasting are cardinal features of all forms of protein–energy malnutrition, especially in early childhood. This is also true in older children and adults, but usually to a less marked degree. Conversely, in older children and especially in adults, muscle mass in the arms is also related to the amount of exercise or work undertaken by these muscles. Extreme hypertrophy is seen classically in weight-lifters and 'body-builders'. In general, it is particularly important to measure the left or non-dominant arm in adults. From the opposite point of view, over-nourished, under-exercised, middle-aged adults can have a low muscle mass from disuse atrophy plus the decrease which seems a concomitant of ageing, even with a normal or increased arm circumference.

Muscular strength can be measured by dynamometry (p. 51), involving different body movements, and by estimating overall work productivity (p. 51). However, such measurements cannot be used in field circumstances, especially in young children.

Body composition, mainly muscle mass (or lean body mass), and body fat, may be assessed in various ways:

1. *Total.* Body radioactive potassium (as a measure of cellular mass, of which muscle is the principal component); chemical urinary analysis (for muscle break-down products, e.g. creatinine excretion); body analysis (at autopsy); electrical impedance (Cochrane *et al.* 1985; Klish *et al.* 1984; Lukaski 1987)
2. *Localized.* Soft-tissue radiology (of leg or arm); physical anthropometry (by measurement of a limb).

However, with the possible exception of timed, 24-hour urine samples for creatinine excretion (p. 495) and/or radiology in hospital circumstances, the most practical method is by direct anthropometry of a limb.

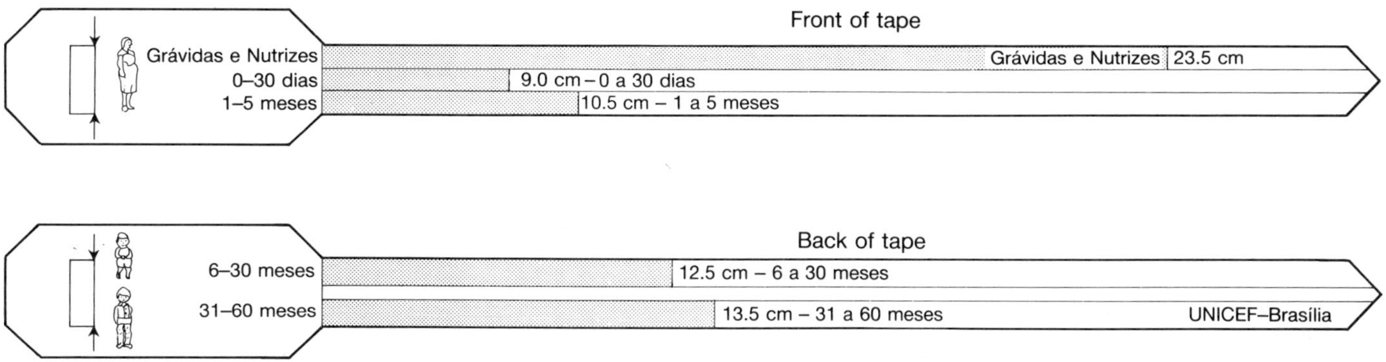

Fig. 2.30 UNICEF tapes (Brazil) with levels for five age-groups on one tape.

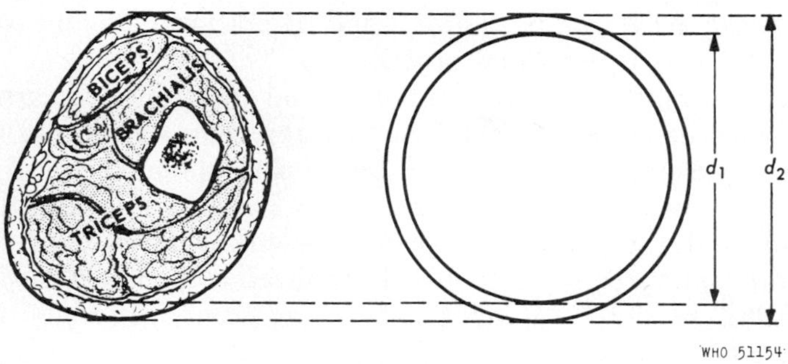

Measurements are made of arm circumference C_1 and triceps skin-fold S. Let d_1 = arm diameter and d_2 = muscle diameter. Then skin-fold $S = 2 \times$ subcutaneous fat $= d_1 - d_2$, and arm circumference $C_1 = \pi d_1$. Now, muscle circumference $C_2 = \pi d_2 = \pi [d_1 - (d_1 - d_2)] = \pi d_1 - \pi(d_1 - d_2)$. Hence, $C_2 = C_1 - \pi S$.

Fig. 2.31 Method of calculating approximate midarm muscle circumference (Jelliffe and Jelliffe 1960).

First, pre-school children in developing countries usually have little subcutaneous fat, so that low arm circumferences are mainly related to depleted muscle tissue. In children with severe protein–energy malnutrition, body muscle mass has been estimated by radioactive potassium assay to be only 42 per cent of normal, but returned to 92 per cent after treatment and recovery (Reeds *et al.* 1978).

More direct measurements of muscle can be made ('inner anthropometry'). For example, if the triceps fatfold (p. 85) and the arm circumference (p. 91) are both known, it is possible to calculate the inner 'circle', which is composed principally of muscle, with a small central core of bone, and with a relatively small area occupied by blood vessels, nerves, and fascia. It is usually assumed that the bone remains relatively constant in size, so that the calculated value is termed the 'midarm muscle circumference' (Jelliffe and Jelliffe 1960). Alternatively, it is possible to make allowance for the humerus by subtracting an approximate standard value according to the age of the subject, but usually this is not done. Alternatively, the IAD ('inner arm diameter'), composed principally of muscle and bone, has been used as a gauge of muscle tissue (McFie and Welbourn 1962). (Also see: Addendum 1988.)

The formula for the calculation of the midarm muscle circumference (Jelliffe and Jelliffe 1960) is (Fig. 2.31)

$$c_2 = c_1 - \pi s$$

where c_2 is muscle circumference, c_1 is arm circumference, and s is the triceps fatfold.

In this equation, the millimetre reading of the triceps fatfold needs altering to centimetres to conform to that of the arm measurement. It is sometimes suggested that both biceps and triceps fatfold be measured and averaged, but this is not usual practice.

In recent years, the arm circumference and sometimes the arm muscle circumference have been widely used as approximate indicators in the nutritional assessment of young children in developing countries (p. 294), and also for newborns (Gueri *et al.* 1977; Daza and Lechtig 1980) (p. 245), and adults (especially pregnant women) (Kusum Shah 1980) (p. 234), and hospitalized patients in industrialized countries (Blackburn and Harvey 1982 (p. 349)). Reference data for different age-groups are considered later (Appendix 9).

The arm-muscle circumference represents a practical, if approximate, measure of body muscle mass, and one that can be easily obtained. However, an apparent disadvantage is that it is a linear expression of a three-dimensional tissue, muscle, which should, ideally, be measured by weight or volume. However, this single measurement correlates well with more general manifestations of protein–energy malnutrition, despite the fact that it is an attempt to assess a body-wide tissue, which may perhaps be affected unequally in different muscle groups, by a measurement at a single site.

To allow the midarm measurements of arm circumference and triceps fatfold to give an estimate of arm muscle *area*, nomograms for children and adults have been prepared (Gurney and Jelliffe 1973) (Appendix 4). It was felt that these two-dimensional results might be more helpful in estimating reserves of *both* protein (muscle) and energy (fat). In a similar manner, Amador *et al.* (1981, 1983) have devised an 'energy/protein ratio' (E/PR) (p. 317). (Also see: Addendum 1988.)

Recently, it has been suggested that an approximation of the midarm muscle *volume* should be made (Jelliffe and Jelliffe 1979*b*). This has been based on the examination of X-ray pictures of the upper arm and on tests of surface anatomy, which suggest that a considerable proportion of total muscle bulk, mainly the belly of the biceps, is present for the middle one-fifth (20 per cent) of the length of the humerus. Midarm muscle volume can, then, be arbitrarily defined as midarm muscle area (derived from the available nomogram) (Gurney and Jelliffe 1973) (p. 000), multiplied by one-fifth of the length (cm) of the humerus, measured from the acromial process to olecranon tip, with the arm hanging loosely by the side (Jelliffe and Jelliffe 1979*b*).

$$\text{M vol (cm}^3) = \text{M area (cm}^2) \times \frac{\text{length of humerus (cm)}}{5}.$$

There is a considerable need to evaluate the relative usefulness and biological significance of the different arm measurements. In this respect laboratory tests at research centres (p. 50), including such techniques as soft-tissue radiography in the assessment of hospitalized patients in industrialized countries (p. 348), can be most helpful. (Also see: Addendum 1988.)

Standardization and quality control

The apparent simplicity of taking measurements is deceptive. Yet in field work in the past such procedures as weighing have been delegated to the most junior, poorly motivated, least well-trained member of the team, who may be left to work without adequate supervision and without regular checking of the apparatus used. The effects are particularly unfortunate, since the inaccurate results obtained are expressed numerically and, therefore, are too often viewed as scientifically precise and objective, capable of being analysed with statistical sophistication.

The time spent in obtaining a measurement is only a small fraction of the time required for subsequent calculations and interpretation, so that effort as well as time are wasted, if the original measurement is inaccurate.

The techniques employed, including such apparently simple and commonplace procedures as weighing, must be carefully carried out, standardized, thoroughly understood by all team members, and given adequate preliminary practical testing to ensure uniformity of results. Accuracy of both technique and equipment is especially needed with small children, especially when growth is being assessed by the measurement of small increments in uncooperative subjects. To ensure the accuracy, reliability, and comparability of results, standardization and quality control are needed for instruments and techniques.

Formal standardization exercises simply compare the results for the same measurements on the same individual (Zerfas 1986; WHO 1983*b*). For example, the result obtained by the 'supervisor' is subtracted from that by the trainee, on the assumption that the supervisor is competent. A single exercise should be performed for at least 10 children, initially. As an approximate guide, it is suggested that there should be no more than one difference *in any of the 10 measurements* greater than the following: 100 g (3 oz) for weight; 1 cm (½ in) for length or height; 0.5 cm (¼ in) for head or arm circumference; 2 mm for triceps fatfold. These figures apply with subjects up to 5 years of age. They may be altered according to the age of the child and the type of study required. During the actual survey, some form of field check should be made by the supervisor (p. 410).

Measurements poorly performed are usually not worth doing and the results can be dangerously misleading. Errors may be due to poor instruments or techniques, especially those of reading and recording. Common errors of measurement are listed (Table 2.16). A suggested anthropometry training schedule follows (Zerfas 1979):

Table 2.16 Common errors of measurement. (*Modified from Zerfas 1979*)

All measurements	Inadequate instrument Restless child (procedure should be postponed) Reading part of instrument not fixed when value taken Reading Recording errors
Length	Incorrect instrument for age Footwear or headwear not removed Head not in correct plane Head not firmly against fixed end of board Child not straight along board Body arched Knees bent Feet not vertical to movable board Board not firmly against heels
Height	Incorrect instrument for age Footwear or headwear not removed Feet not straight and together, nor flat on vertical platform or wall Knees bent Body arched or buttocks forward (body not straight) Shoulders not straight on board Head not in correct plane Headboard not firmly on crown of child's head
Weight	Room cold, no privacy Scale not calibrated to zero Child wearing unreasonable amount of clothing Child moving or anxious
Triceps fatfold	Wrong arm (should be left) Midarm point or posterior plane incorrectly measured or marked Arm not loose by side during measurement Examiner not comfortable nor level with child Finger-thumb pinch or caliper placement too deep (muscle) or too superficial (skin) Caliper jaws not at marked site Reading done too early, pinch not maintained, caliper handle not fully released One measurement made, rather than averaging three measurements
Arm circumference	Tape too thick, stretched or creased Wrong arm (should be left arm)

Table 2.16 (Continued)

Arm circumference (Continued)	Midarm point or posterior plane incorrectly measured or marked Arm not loosely hanging by side during measurement Examiner not comfortable nor level with child Tape around arm, not at midpoint; too tight (causing skin contour indentation), too loose (inadequately opposed)

1. Procedures and instruments demonstrated.
2. Instrument practice under supervision.
3. Trial practice review.
4. Standardization test.
5. Review and further practice under simulated field conditions.
6. Further standardization test if required.
7. Field trials under supervision.
8. Review.

Further consideration of training procedures is given later (p. 405).

Anthropometry: selection of measurements

Assignment of numbers (in measurement) nearly always functions as a communication, and unless the recipient knows the rules by which the sender has made that assignment, he will be unsure of its meaning.

J.L. Phillips (1971) Interpreting individual measures, In: *Statistical thinking.*

The central role of anthropometry in the nutritional assessment of protein–energy malnutrition and in obesity is clear and has been emphasized many times. However, the most effective use of anthropometry does not depend only on the use of appropriate instruments and careful, precise techniques. It also hinges on the choice of the most useful measurements for particular purposes in different age-groups and on selecting reference data (and abnormal levels or 'cut-off points' below and above) with which results can be compared (p. 122). Variation in any of these can give a very different picture of the nutritional situation both in individuals and communities. Considerable confusion and disagreement has arisen in recent years, often due to specialists in one field or one part of the world generalizing too widely from information of limited application. Clearly, an auxologist measuring detailed growth for research purposes will need different information and much more precise reference data than will a primary health care worker screening for persons with malnutrition requiring extra rations in a refugee camp.

Anthropometric indicators

A wide range of anthropometric measurements have been made in specialized auxological studies. However, as noted earlier (p. 66), for practical purposes, four basic measurements are commonly employed as anthropometric indicators — weight, height (length), arm circumference, and (much less frequently) triceps fatfold.

Anthropometric indices

These are essentially ratios of one measurement to another. They can have one or more of the following uses:

1. *Comparison of labile tissue (muscle, fat) with a less affected tissue (skeleton).*[40] Examples include weight-for-height, arm circumference for height (Arnhold 1969) (or for head circumference (McLaren and Kanawati 1972));
2. *Independence of knowledge of precise age.* Examples include the weight-for-height in young children, as judged by making two measurements or directly using a Thinness chart (Nabarro and McNab 1980), and the arm circumference in young children;
3. *Ratios of one-dimensional linear tissues with three-dimensional 'volume' tissues.* Weight is in one sense a reflection of body volume and density, so that it can be regarded as three-dimensional. By contrast, height (or length) is one-dimensional. Over the past century, numerous ratios have been developed based on attempts to make height dimensionally more comparable with weight. These include the original Quetelet Index (1836): W/H^2, now known as the 'body mass index' in adults; the Rohrer's Index ('ponderal index') (1921): W/H^3 in the newborn; and the Dugdale Index: $W/H^{1.6}$ (Dugdale 1971) in young children.

Differences between these 'power indices' is considered to reflect variation in body proportions in the newborn, young children, and adults, and to be least correlated with height (or length) at each age. However, they can represent confusing refinements, unlike the basic weight-for-height (W/H) which is understandable.

A large number of complex composite indices based on several anthropometric measurements, sometimes with clinical signs and/or biochemical tests, have been devised at various times. Some were in vogue prior to

[40] Currently rather crudely termed 'flesh–bone indices'.

World War II (Bigwood 1939) and were largely based on clinical judgement and anthropometric measurements. More recently, mathematically derived composite indices have been devised (Telwar 1975). None seem to have real practical value nor to have been adopted widely.

Considerations in selection

The selection of measurements (indicators) and their combination in various calculated ratios (indices) needs to take into account the following overlapping considerations:

1. *General purpose.* The general purpose and the degree of detail of an investigation will obviously influence the choice of measurements, including whether they are longitudinal or cross-sectional. In general, five main practical purposes can be identified: screening, assessment of nutritional status (of individuals or communities), monitoring, evaluation, and analytical epidemiological studies (including statistical investigation of causation) (Habicht *et al.* 1982).

Differences between longitudinal and cross-sectional studies can be illustrated by the following two examples. Serial weighing is an important method of assessment in pregnancy, while repeated height measurements are obviously not indicated. Cross-sectional surveys of young children in developing countries need to include both weight *and* height where possible — to differentiate 'stunted' and 'wasted', when ages are known (p. 312) and to give weight-for-height figures, when ages are not known (p. 80).

2. *Problem being investigated.* For example, obesity in adults is best detected by fatfold measurements — either the triceps alone or, if possible, combined with other sites (p. 342). Early protein–energy malnutrition in young children is best sought for by serial weighing and interpreting recordings of growth changes (p. 296).

3. *Age-group.* The significance of various measurements has to be known in different age-groups, as body proportions and growth rates vary. These will include: (1) the slower rate of increase in arm circumference in young children; (2) mathematical differences sometimes employed in expressing weight in relation to height (p. 106) in babies, in early childhood, and in adult life; and (3) the slow 'speed of change' in height in school children (until the pre-pubertal growth spurt).

4. *Biological significance.* An understanding of the biological significance of different measurements is needed (Table 2.17), in order to select those which give information needed for the particular study and to recognize their relative usefulness for assessment over shorter or longer periods of time ('speed of change').

For example, height gives a composite picture of growth up to the present. It does not decrease with recent acute malnutrition and increases

Table 2.17 Biological significance of basic four measurements and their potential speed of change in protein–energy malnutrition and obesity in a conceptual approach

	Biological significance	Potential speed of change in protein–energy malnutrition or obesity
Weight	Composite: lean body mass, fat, fluid	Very fast: increase or decrease
Height	Cumulative skeletal growth	Slow increase and no decrease (in children)
Arm circumference	Composite: muscle and fat (with relatively constant bone)	Fast decrease in protein–energy malnutrition Slow increase in obesity
Fatfold	Calorie stores	Slow decrease in protein–energy malnutrition Slow increase in obesity

slowly in children as they grow (apart from the rapid pre-pubertal height spurt). Height is, therefore, a useful indicator of the past and also can be used for comparison with more labile body tissues, such as muscle and fat (e.g. weight-for-height) ('flesh–bone indices'). However, because of its slow increase, height can only be used in the evaluation of a community nutrition programme for young children if measured over a considerable period, minimally 6 months, and preferably over some years. Also, height measurements of similar age-groups at intervals of years can demonstrate a positive or negative secular change (p. 59). The height of 7-year-old school-children has been suggested (p. 334).

Essentially, the potential speed of change of the four measurements gives insight into their usefulness. Those with the fastest potential for change give evidence of recent nutritional experience, including acute deficiency, and also can be useful in assessing the effectiveness of treatment of an individual or a community programme in a relatively short time. Those with a slow speed of change give evidence of past nutrition, including chronic malnutrition, and are most useful in assessment over a long period of time.

This also means that 'malnutrition rates' judged by abnormalities in one measurment are not the same as with another measurement. This often seems to cause concern when it is discovered, for example, that the percentage of children with low weight-for-height is different from those with a low arm circumference. In fact, arm circumference and weight-for-height do not measure *exactly* the same thing (Nichaman *et al* 1978;

Carter 1986), nor do the other measurements or indices commonly used. Similarly, obesity rates defined by increased weight-for-height do not give exactly the same findings as estimates based on fatfolds.

To clarify matters, sequential anthropometry may be employed, if time and other resources permit, going from simple single measurements giving limited information, to multiple measurements, which enable the situation to be defined more accurately. For example, in protein–energy malnutrition, anthropometry can be undertaken and interpreted in the following sequence: weight-for-age→height-for-age→weight-for-height→arm circumference→triceps fatfold→calculated arm muscle and fat estimations. Similarly in obesity, sequential anthropometry might be: weight-for-height→triceps fatfold→multiple fatfolds.

5. *Epidemiological significance*. The selection of anthropometric measurements also needs to be guided by two epidemiological concepts — their ability to detect the malnourished and to avoid including the non-malnourished (sensitivity versus specificity), and their relationship to functional outcome. Detailed consideration of epidemiological criteria in the selection of anthropometric field measurements has been given by Habicht *et al.* (1979).

In practice, consideration of the sensitivity and specificity of anthropometric measurements is complicated by the differing effects on body tissues of various forms of protein–energy malnutrition (and obesity) at various ages, and by the purpose of the investigation.

The functional outcome — that is the consequence as regards mortality, morbidity and ability to work and learn — is difficult to measure, but is increasingly recognized as being important in identifying measurements needed for different purposes, and the significance and definition of abnormal levels ('cut-off points') above or below them (p. 122). For example, a low weight-for-age and arm circumference have been shown to predict an increased risk of death in early childhood, but an essential question is at what level this occurs. Similar considerations apply to the long-term consequences of obesity in adults.

6. *Practicality*. In real life, selection of anthropometric measurements depends in considerable measure on various practical considerations, including *resources available* (funds, trained personnel, time, cultural acceptability), *availability of appropriate reference data* (p. 110), *parental knowledge of the age of young children* (p. 317), and *understandability of measurements* — to the measurers, when possible to those measured, and especially to those who need to act on the information obtained.

Conclusion

The question of which measurement is most useful depends on practical considerations, including its purpose and the resources available, more than anything else. Unfortunately, there often tend to be unnecessary schisms into different groups each of whom see one particular measurement as *the* measurement. This is not so.

For example, in a village survey weight alone *can* give a useful (but mixed) picture of the local situation, provided ages are known. Nevertheless, it is better if the *different* types of underweight children can be differentiated using the Waterlow classification (1973) (p. 312). This has, however, the disadvantages of having to take two measurements and of needing to know the children's ages. If the ages are *not* known, then the weight-for-height is very valuable. Once again, two measurements and two sets of apparatus increase the possibilities of error, unless the 'Thinness Wall Chart' is used (p. 80). The arm circumference measurement has its defects as well, but, with a tricolour arm band, screening can be rapidly undertaken by primary health care workers with little cost and with easily transportable and replaceable apparatus.

It is apparent, therefore, that the selection of anthropometric measurements needs to be guided by a variable blend of scientific and value judgements based on biological and epidemiological consideration and practical concerns, especially the purpose of the investigation and the resources available.

Anthropometry: selection of reference data

A universal external growth reference may seem to be a convenience, but experience shows that it invariably gets reified into some kind of absolute, ideal standard.

Goldstein and Tanner (1980)

Growth standards developed in industrialized countries are appropriate for measuring child growth in developing countries.

Graitcer and Genery (1981)

There is not sufficient evidence at present to justify the conclusion that one set of standards would represent the ideal growth of young children of all races.

Marshall (1981)

The question of what growth standards to use seem to me to have generated enormous quantities of rather useless discussion.

David Morley (1981)
(personal communication)

Table 2.18 Selection of anthropometric data: six principles

(1) All reference data are imperfect
(2) Practical usefulness (versus) comparability
(3) Relation to 'optimal health'
(4) Use most genetically appropriate
(5) Avoid unnecessary confusion with previously used data
(6) Recognize possibility of non-nutritional nationalistic misinterpretations

Anthropometry is the most widely used method of nutritional assessment both in more and less technically developed areas of the world. In all circumstances, results of body measurements of individuals or of communities ultimately have to be compared with some reference data[41], if conclusions are to be drawn, and deficient or excessive growth identified.

However, the selection of such anthropometric reference data has been the subject of much debate, disagreement, and confusion in recent years. This is indicated, for example, by the four quotations given above — all of which are partially true.

This dilemma has been due, in part, to the difficulty (or impossibility) of defining optimal growth and the different views held about the relative influences of genetic versus environmental factors, especially nutrition, on growth (Neumann 1979). This has perhaps been increased by the understandable attention focused on problems of protein–energy malnutrition in young children in Third World countries, and on the relative value of 'international standards' versus 'local standards' in assessment in this age-group.

Practical principles

It is suggested that the selection of reference data can be helped by bearing in mind six practical principles (Table 2.18).

(1) Appreciate that all anthropometric reference data are imperfect

Careful examination of sources of *all* anthropometric data indicate that *all* are imperfect; some more so than others. Flaws may be biological (e.g. genetically mixed population, or communities with widespread disease, or with nutritional disorders, including obesity), statistical (e.g. inadequate and/or biased sample), technical (e.g. measurements inaccurately taken), or a mixture of all or some of these.

The arbitrariness (yet practical utility) of earlier WHO-approved refer-

[41] An exception is the comparison of the same population (e.g. 7-year-old children) at intervals of some years to detect any secular trend in a community (Bengoa *et al.* 1959).

ence data were noted in 1966, 'because the figures for different age-groups and measurements have been collected by various investigators, using varying techniques in non-identical populations in different, recent decades' (Jelliffe 1966). However, more recent valuable and currently widely used reference data also show defects (Wrigley 1984). For example, the Metropolitan Life Insurance Society of Actuaries weight-for-height data (1959, 1981) are based on huge samples of over 4 million and try to relate to functional outcome (mortality and, hence, insurance risk). At the same time, they were taken from an economically biased group (who were able to afford insurance), with no attempt at controlling the quality of the measurements made (or testing weight scales) in individuals wearing light clothes and shoes (which were adjusted for), and with differentiation into three undefined frame sizes. As Ancel Keys *et al.* (1972) noted, the 1959 weight-for-height tables had serious limitations. The samples were 'clearly biased', the measurements 'crude', and the frame-size based on an 'actuary's imagination'. Also, some decades later, it has been pointed out that the tables prepared were incorrectly labelled, regarding clothing and shoes (Robinett-Weiss 1985).

With regard to young children, the valuable and much-used Harvard (Boston or Stuart) weight-and-height figures (Stuart and Stevenson 1975) have been criticized because of the small numbers of children included, the limited genetic representativeness, out-of-datedness (1930s), and unavailability of original raw data (from which weight-for-height, for example, can be derived statistically). Also, measurements of arm circumference and triceps fatfold were not included in anthropometry at that time.

Their successor, the NCHS (National Center for Health Statistics) data, were compiled from careful measurements of a large, randomly selected population, from birth to 18 years, from different economic and ethnic groups in the United States (Hamill *et al.* 1979). They include raw data for both sexes on weight, height, arm circumference, and fatfolds, from which statistically valid distributions and weight-for-height have been obtained. Nevertheless, despite their usefulness and advantages, the NCHS data have their limitations. They were compiled from two investigations in different decades — one longitudinal (0–3 years, Fels Research Institute)[42] and one cross-sectional (2–18 years, HANES — National Health Examination Survey), with overlap from 2–3 years. In the latter study, there was incomplete documentation on whether length or height was measured in children 2–3 years old. As is usually the case, no estimate of functional outcome — that is the consequences of different anthropometric levels as regards subsequent health and mortality — was

[42] Approximately 100 boys and 100 girls of 'above average' economic group followed longitudinally in Yellow Springs, Ohio from birth to 18 years (1942–62).

possible. Also, data were derived from some obese children (Gortmaker *et al.* 1987), adolescents, and adults, and potential anthropometric differences between the main genetic groups in the US may have been blurred by combining all the information obtained into one set of figures.

In fact, no anthropometric data are available for all four basic measurements from a single population for all age-groups. This is reflected in the reference data given in this publication (Appendix 9), which are not all from the same population, although most are from NCHS data.

In other words, all anthropometric data need to be recognized as approximate, but useful, yardsticks, and not as mathematical absolutes. This seems particularly difficult for Westernized scientific workers to appreciate. Once such data are calculated and expressed numerically, they tend to assume an unwarranted infallibility far removed from the inadequacies of their often unappreciated origins, which, in any case, are usually neither readily available nor read.

This lack of precision needs to be reflected in the labels used. The terms 'reference standards' or 'reference levels' cannot be recommended as they both seem to imply certain unwarranted ideal targets (Waterlow 1979). The less value-laden term 'reference data' appears preferable, as such figures need to be regarded as a frame of reference rather than a level of excellence. Care should also be taken with the use of such expressions as 'desirable', 'optimal', or 'ideal' rather than simply 'reference'.

Similar considerations need to be given to generic terms. For example, the label 'international' can be misinterpreted as being universally *optimal*, rather than being widely available and, thus, always useful for comparison between groups or countries. A less laudatory label may be more suitable, such as 'universally available reference data' (p. 116).

(2) Differentiate practical utility from comparability

Comparing body measurements with reference data has two main purposes: (1) *practical utility*: determining the prevalence of protein–energy malnutrition in a village, diagnosing obesity in an individual, screening for malnutrition in a Young Child Clinic, etc. — all obtained with a view to possible action; (2) *comparability*: determining the relative commonness of protein–energy malnutrition or obesity in different countries or regions at different times, by comparing results obtained using the same reference data, leading to information of scientific and public health significance, suggesting changing relative needs in different geographical areas.

If possible, it is preferable to obtain and present information which has *both* practical utility and comparability, especially for physiologically vulnerable groups — that is young children and pregnant women. However, local practical utility always needs to be the main concern.

(3) Relate reference data used to 'optimal health'

Anthropometric reference data used should, as far as possible, be those accompanied by the lowest mortality and morbidity rates (Goldstein and Tanner 1980), or, put less negatively, they should be those judged to be associated with 'optimal health'. The predictive value or functional significance of anthropometric reference data may be associated with increased as well as decreased values for anthropometric measurements. It can be immediate or long-term, and related to the risk of developing severe, clinically obvious malnutrition (such as protein–energy malnutrition or obesity) or non-nutritional diseases (such as infections in protein–energy malnutrition, and atherosclerosis or diabetes in obesity).

The determination of functional significance is, of course, very difficult to undertake in humans, because of their relatively long life span (paralleling that of the investigators and much longer than the length of time for which grants are awarded by research agencies). Also, numerous other factors influence health in each individual's 'life-flight'. However, this type of approach is by no means new; witness the approximate, but useful, 2.5 kg (5½ lb) low-birth-weight level introduced decades ago by WHO, partly because the figures were easy to remember but partly because it was related to neonatal mortality and immunity (Neumann 1984). More recently, Kusum Shah (1978) was able to define reference data for weight gain in pregnancy in rural Bombay by observing the predictive value of a birth weight of 2.8 kg or more. The functional significance approach has also been used in defining cut-off points or abnormal anthropometric levels above or below reference data in young children, and is discussed later (p. 124).

(4) Use most genetically appropriate reference data

In general, current evidence indicates that genetic influences on body size and proportions seem to increase in importance with age in different well-nourished ethnic groups (Eveleth and Tanner 1976). This means, in practice, that genetically-specific anthropometric reference data are more likely to be required for older children or adults than for pre-school children (1–4 years old) on whom the effects of environmental factors, especially nutrition, usually predominate (Habicht *et al.* 1974).

Most attention concerning genetic similarities in the two basic measurements, weight and height (length), has understandably been directed towards nutritionally vulnerable children in the 1–4 year age-group. Numerous studies indicate that growth during this period of life is comparable in most, but not all, ethnic groups (p. 117). For example, three tribes in Zaire showed quite different anthropometric measurements. This was felt to be partly genetic and partly due to differing ecologies and life styles (Manshande *et al.* 1985).

Genetic differences in fatfold thicknesses and distribution seem fairly

Table 2.19 Recently advocated and previously used internationally available reference data: selected examples

	Recent*	Previous*
Weights and heights for children	NCHS (Hamill *et al.* 1979)	Boston (Harvard) (Stuart and Meredith 1975)
Arm circumference for children	NCHS (1977)	Wolanski (1966, pers. commun.)
Weights and heights for adults	Frisancho (1984)	Metropolitan Life Insurance (1959)
Arm circumference for adults	Frisancho (1981)	Jelliffe (1966)

* Dates given refer to most recent publication, not to when the data were collected.

clearly documented (Harsha *et al.* 1980). In general, 'size' seems more influenced by nutrition and other environmental factors than 'shape' or body proportions.

The practical significance of this is the question of determining whether 'general reference data' can be used or whether 'local reference data' are needed.

(5) Avoid unnecessary confusion

With the recent involvement of more mathematically oriented workers, there has been an understandable tendency to introduce new reference data and cut-off points, based on real (or more usually marginal) statistical advantages (Table 2.19). Such changes need careful consideration as to whether the confusion produced by the displacement of well-established and familiar reference data by new, differently named data is worthwhile or not. When such change is widely regarded as helpful, then the new figures introduced should, if possible, be given with attention to overall comparability with both the previous reference data and, whenever feasible, the levels used as 'cut-off' points (e.g. percentages, centiles, standard deviations).

Such is the case with the NCHS reference data which have succeeded the Harvard data for young children (Appendix 9). From a practical point-of-view, they are reasonably close to each other and the British reference data (Tanner 1976).

(6) Recognize the possibility of non-nutritional nationalistic misinterpretations of reference data

Although not often stated, non-nutritional nationalistic and even political misinterpretations may sometimes occur, and these possibilities need to be borne in mind. Thus, advocacy to use reference data largely derived from populations of European ancestry for other genetic groups may be rightly or wrongly interpreted as reflecting an unintended ethnocentric anthropometric imperialism ('West is best') (McLaren 1987), or, alternatively, as suggesting racial superiority. Conversely, advising the use of local reference data, may also be criticized as stigmatizing the community as second-class world citizens and as missing the diagnosis of malnutrition in some under-sized individuals, especially children.

Types of reference data

Anthropometric reference data may be classified into two broad types: (1) internationally available; and (2) local.

(1) Internationally available reference data

The term 'internationally available reference data' is used here to apply to carefully collected measurements from a randomly selected population, which are widely available in the world's technical literature and, thus, may sometimes be used for purposes of international comparison. In fact, most such data have been collected from populations of predominantly European ancestry,[43] sometimes by cross-sectional studies, sometimes by longitudinal measurements, and sometimes by a combination of methods. For example, recent reference data on weights and heights of children include those from Switzerland (Heimendinger 1964), Sweden (Karlberg *et al.* 1968), the UK (Tanner 1976), and the USA (NCHS) (Hamill *et al.* 1979). Overall, such data show a general conformity in these genetically similar populations.

However, the term 'internationally available reference data' is meant to indicate availability and acceptance rather than implying an absolute, proven global standard of excellence and uniformity for all genetic groups, or that they should be used in all circumstances.

Various, more recent internationally available reference data have been presented in recent years as alternatives to those previously used (Table 2.19).

The comparative merits of older or more recently collected internationally available reference data need careful consideration — even in similar ethnic groups. Among dissimilar genetic populations, even greater care is needed.

Also, the relative usefulness of such data has to be considered for eight age-groups or physiological stages of life — pregnancy, newborn, infant, pre-school age child, school-age child, adolescent, adult (24–54 years),

[43] The NCHS data are from a national US sample, including African Americans and some Hispanic populations (Hamill *et al.* 1979).

and elderly in different groups (55–74 years and ⩾ 75 years). This is because genetic factors and cumulative nutritional influences appear to play increasing roles after early childhood. This means that 'internationally available reference levels' are often not genetically relevant for older children and adults, sometimes obtained from obese populations. Consideration of the appropriateness of internationally available and local reference data applies more to the most nutritionally vulnerable group — young children.

In view of this complexity, the availability, comparability, and utility of previous and current internationally available and local reference data are referred to separately in later sections dealing with nutritional assessment in different age-groups.

(2) Local reference data

In some parts of the world, local anthropometric reference data have been compiled, especially for young children, as it becomes apparent that the internationally available reference data are not appropriate to levels or even growth patterns in all genetic groups. This is the case, for example, in parts of Africa (Van Loon *et al.* 1986), New Delhi, India (Ghosh and Bhargaya 1985), Bangladesh (Brown *et al.* 1982), and Hong Kong (Davies and Leung 1985).

Local reference data may have been derived *either* from measurements of well-fed, medically and socially protected children of the élite — *(i) 'presumed optimal reference data'* — *or* from children attending Young Child Clinics (excluding those seriously ill with acute or chronic disease, including those with clinical malnutrition) — *(ii) 'practical interim reference data'*. As with all reference data, it is essential to know the source of such information, including the method of sampling the numbers involved, the definition of the population included, and the quality of the measurements and analyses made.

(i) Presumed optimal local reference data If local reference data do not exist, their preparation may be attempted. However, to undertake this scientifically is an expensive, time-consuming task involving the carefully controlled measurement of large numbers, ideally longitudinally (Goldstein 1978; Goldstein and Tanner 1980). At least 100 in each 3-month group of young children has been recommended. This type of investigation will focus on the privileged ('special group') — that is, those with higher income, better education, access to preventive and curative health services, and adequate home hygiene. By this means it is hoped to obtain what may be termed 'presumed optimal local reference data'. Such studies have been undertaken in some countries for some basic measurements — for example, in Guatemala (Johnson *et al.* 1984) and Nigeria (Janes *et al.* 1981).

Difficulties may occur in some countries in that this segment of the population may be genetically very or somewhat dissimilar to the majority of people in a country. There may not be sufficient numbers available. Also, such a population may be relatively obese, both children and adults, for cultural and/or nutritional reasons. The problem of definition is often most difficult, and likely to vary from country to country. Limited resources frequently are a major block to obtaining a statistically adequate sample.

Furthermore, in some communities or countries, the presumed optimal local reference data from the privileged section of the population may not be of much immediate value. This can lead to a practical dilemma, when the majority of the population, often young children, have measurements so far below these reference data that they cannot be used to differentiate those at greatest risk, with a view to taking appropriate action.

(ii) Practical interim local reference data Alternatively, local data may be prepared from measurements of presumed healthy individuals in the population by excluding those with obvious acute or chronic disease, including clinical malnutrition. Such data are obviously easier to obtain. For example, the median results from non-sick young children attending Under-Five Clinics can be used. Such reference data have, been developed in an area in Zaire (Manshande 1980) from records at Young Child Clinics.

The realistic utility of practical interim reference data is apparent in every-day work in health centres and clinics, as it 'relates to what currently holds true' (Pakrasi *et al.* 1986). In fact, it permits limited resources to be channelled to those found to be most at risk. Obvious and serious disadvantages are that growth retardation will be underdiagnosed (Gopalan 1984), with some poorly nourished children misrepresented as being 'well'. This not only gives a falsely optimistic picture, but may prevent specific action being taken for children in need and political recognition of the seriousness of the situation.

This means that if practical interim local reference data are used, their limitations have to be fully recognized. They need to be reviewed and updated at intervals of not more than 5–10 years. Also, those concerned with the overall surveillance of nutritional status in a community or country need to recognize the artificiality of such practical interim reference data — and the effect of their use on the local statistics. In fact, they represent 'targets for action' and not 'cut-off points for true prevalence rates' (Mora 1982). Unfortunately, they often become fixed as optimal' rather than 'interim'.

Genetically diverse communities Difficulties with preparing local reference data will obviously be greater in countries with several genetically very dissimilar groups. This is well-marked, for example, in Fiji with the completely different stature, physiques, and frame sizes of Melanesians and East Indians, originally from India. With such distinct genetic groups, different local reference data may need to be prepared.

Internationally available versus local reference data Comparison of internationally available and local reference data show them to have different advantages and disadvantages (Table 2.20). By definition, internationally available reference data are usually widely and easily available, and are often based on large sample sizes. They usually have raw data available for mathematically correct extrapolations (e.g. weight-for-height, standard deviations, etc.) and they permit international comparability of results. Older established data (e.g. the Harvard growth figures) are often familiar (i.e. well-known) to health personnel. However, both older and newer internationally available reference data may not be genetically appropriate for all communities.

Local reference data often have the opposite characteristics. First, they may not exist; second, they are usually difficult and costly to prepare in a statistically valid manner. Moreover, they may not permit ready international comparability. However, they are more likely to reflect local genetic influences on growth. It is essential to examine the source of such local reference data to see if they can be considered as 'presumed optimal' or as 'practical interim'.

Considerations in selecting reference data

Anthropometric reference data are used for two main purposes: (1) assessment of the commonness of protein–energy malnutrition or obesity in a community, ranging in size from a nation to a school, often by cross-sectional prevalence surveys (p. 356); and (2) diagnosis of individuals by single or serial measurements (as with growth charts) (p. 296).

The significance and value of the results will hinge on the accuracy of the equipment, the training of the investigators, and, in young children, on the ability to ascertain correct and verifiable ages.

In addition, selection of appropriate anthropometric reference data is critical for interpretation. The following sequence is suggested, on the assumption that 'internationally available reference data' are always actually or potentially obtainable for use in work in all countries. Enquiries need to be made in the particular country or region concerning the availability of 'presumed optimal', or 'practical interim reference data', or both.

If presumed optimal local reference data alone are available, they should be compared with internationally available figures. If they are similar, the internationally available reference data should be used to help

Table 2.20 General types of reference data: with special reference to the assessment of protein–energy malnutrition in young children

Type of reference data	Sources	Advantages	Disadvantages
Internationally available	Large-scale statistical sample, largely from populations of European ancestry	Raw data available for further analyses (e.g. weight-for-height, distribution) Data for commoner measurements available (e.g. weight, height, arm circumference, triceps fatfold) from same population International recognition by World Health Organization	Subject may be obese Results may not be relevant to all genetic groups Results may not be relevant to majority of population
Local			
Presumed optimal	Varied size samples of healthy, immunized children of well-to-do, with no acute or chronic illness from particular country or region	Usually genetically appropriate	Population difficult to define and to find in sufficient numbers Subjects may be obese. Data values may currently be too high for majority of population
Practical interim*	Varied size samples, usually apparently healthy children attending Young Child Clinic, without acute or chronic illness, or clinical malnutrition	Genetically appropriate Immediate practical use in suggesting children priority action	Population difficult to define in sufficient numbers Minimizes the amount of less severe protein–energy malnutrition present, so that some malnourished children not treated Self-selected population

* Sometimes an arbitrary level of 'internationally available' reference data (e.g. 80 per cent or −2 SD) is selected (see p. 124).

with comparability. If they differ markedly,[44] the local 'presumed optimal' reference data may be used, preferably expressed as a specified numerical level (usually a selected percentage) of the internationally available data for reports and comparability, by age-group. For example, in the recent past the Indian Academy of Paediatrics suggested that 80 per cent of the Harvard reference level of weight for age should be used as 'normal' — with lower limits being 70 and 60 per cent of the Harvard data.

If, as in many circumstances, only the international reference data are available, they should be compared with measurements from a *special group*[45] preferably comprising at least 200 apparently healthy, genetically homogeneous children who have been well-fed and protected from major infections, and who are not acutely or chronically ill (Zerfas *et al.* 1982). This 'special group' will be from the more educated, higher economic section of the population, often including the families of senior civil servants, university faculty, officers in the armed forces, etc. They will often, but not always, be living in more Westernized urban circumstances. The main difficulty with this approach is that the definition indicated is bound to be imprecise, as some of this group may be obese and/or may be genetically somewhat dissimilar from the general population.

If 'practical interim reference data' are available, these are usually lower than both the international and the uncollected presumed optimal for the community. They will be used mainly for guiding actions by health workers for priority children and not for survey work.

If both local types of reference data are present, results of surveys and similar investigations can be reported in relation to both internationally available and local levels.

Conclusions

The selection of anthropometric reference data is a key activity and yet remains complex and debatable. The choice of using 'internationally available', or 'presumed optimal local', or 'practical interim local' data depends on the circumstances. Some advantages and disadvantages are given in Table 2.20.

In all instances, especially in training and in survey reports, the source and type of reference data need to be clearly described and really understood by those using them. This is often not the case.

Reports can include comparison of the data used with the interna-

[44] Marked difference: local median approximately 1 SD (or more) from general reference data median.

[45] Preparation of statistically representative, local, presumed optimal reference data is preferable, but usually impractical.

tionally available reference data, if different and if felt to be desirable and useful.

'Internationally available reference data' should certainly be used when appropriate. This approach is neat, orderly, and uniform. However, humanity is diverse genetically, culturally, and ecologically. Comparability is an understandable and worthwhile goal, but is insignificant compared with practical utility in stimulating worthwhile action.

Anthropometry: selection of cut-off points

The issue is not whether we can draw a line. Any fool can draw a line and many do. The issue is to produce a reasonable criterion for drawing such a line which will look like a sober decision and not a matter of caprice.

E.A. Murphy (1976)
Defining the Normal

Nutritional assessment using any method, including anthropometry, presents no problem with extremes. It is easy to diagnose marasmus or gross obesity by visual anthropometry — that is, at a glance. However, it is much more difficult and important to decide upon and agree to cut-off points (or abnormal levels), below or above the reference data, which can be used to indicate less severe degrees of malnutrition.

In the past such cut-off points have often been derived from percentages of the reference,[46] leading to qualitative categorization into different nominal levels, such as 'malnourished' or 'not malnourished', or into ordinal levels, such as 'severe', 'moderate', and 'mild'. For example, the long-valued Gómez classification of weight-for-age in young children defines three degrees of malnutrition based on mortality in *hospitalized* young children in Mexico: $\leq$ 90–76 per cent, first degree; $\leq$ 75–61 per cent, second degree; and $\leq$ 60 per cent, third degree (Gómez *et al.* 1956). Conversely, obesity is often considered to be present (or likely) with a weight-for-height of 120 per cent or more of reference level.

Such types of mathematical categorization are simple, tidy, and easily understandable. However, such cut-off points neither take into account 'normal' distributions in a community (Gueri *et al.* 1980) nor the significance of selecting a particular point to be abnormal in terms of immediate or long-term consequences (functional outcome), as regards subsequent morbidity or mortality.

[46] See Appendix 4 for commoner epidemiological terms.

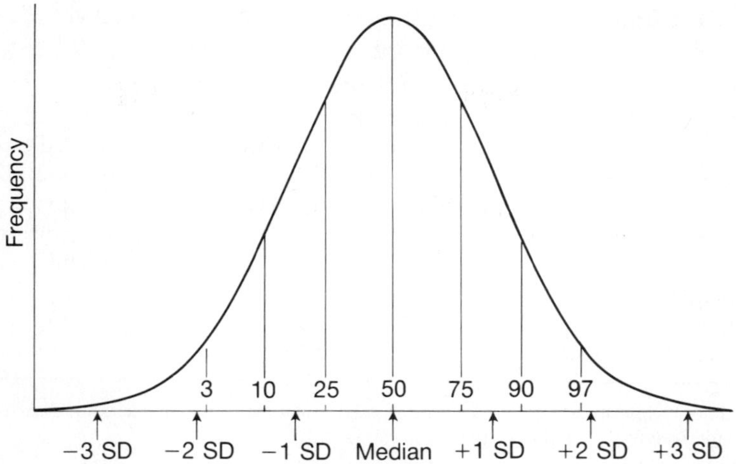

Fig. 2.32 'Normal' (Gaussian) distribution curve. Conventionally, individuals less than the third percentile or centile (approximately −2 SD) are regarded as probably abnormally low. In fact, by definition, three out of 100 of a normal or reference population will fall into this group. Numbers 3−97 are centiles.

Statistical distribution

Almost all anthropometric measurements have a 'normal' Gaussian distribution in an ethnically homogeneous population. In other words, some healthy, well-nourished adults will be smaller or taller than the average. However, the chances of their height being abnormal increases the further they are from the median. The most usual statistical limits of the 'normal' range are from +2 to −2 standard deviations (SD), or (approximately) from the 97th percentile (or centile) to the 3rd centile (Fig. 2.32).[47]

It follows, therefore, that individuals above or below reference levels may be classified statistically with regard to their distribution in relation to centiles or standard deviations from the median. For example, X per cent of a population may be below the 3rd centile (or − 2 SD) for weight-for-age, but may have Y percent of schoolchildren above the 97th centile (+ 2 SD) for height. This type of system, using + or − 2 SD has been recommended by WHO (Waterlow *et al.* 1977).

Recent emphasis on the statistical importance of expressing results in this way is correct and valid, yet can have the danger of being imperfectly understood by those with little statistical training. This seems likely to change slowly with increased emphasis on epidemiology and statistics in the curricula of medical and nursing students and other health workers.

[47] In some circumstances, as with paediatric measurements in the USA, the 95th and 5th centiles are used instead.

Table 2.21 Comparison of percentage below median (reference) corresponding *approximately* to third centile (−2 SD) and to 97th centile (+2 SD) in young children up to 60 months of age.

	97th centile (+2 SD) (per cent)	Median ('Reference') (per cent)	3rd centile (−2 SD) (per cent)
Weight/age*	120	100	80
Weight/height†	120	100	80
Height/age	110	100	90
Arm circumference/age	115	100	85

* *Severe* underweight for age: 60 per cent often used — simple to remember; long clinical use.
† *Severe* underweight for height: 70 per cent (−3SD).

From a practical point of view, it can be very helpful to see if and how easily understood mathematical percentage levels compare with centiles or standard deviations. For example, in young children the commonly used 80 per cent of weight-for-age equates *approximately* with the 3rd centile or −2 SD.[48]

However, different measurements have different 'normal' distributions. Weight in healthy, well-fed individuals varies more than height. Also, some normal distributions, such as fatfolds, are irregular (non-Gaussian or skewed). This means that abnormal percentage levels for various measurements differ from their approximation with standard deviations, centiles, or 'Z-scores'. Thus, − 2 SD for weight-for-age is roughly 80 per cent of the median, but for height is approximately 90 per cent of the median.

Very approximate comparisons between statistical and mathematical levels for commonly used measurements are given in Table 2.21, with special reference to young children with growth retardation caused by protein–energy malnutrition.

Functional outcome

In addition to knowledge of the distribution of an anthropometric measurement, it is important to try to recognize the meaning or significance of different levels in terms of function, and risk of illness and death.

[48] The often mystifying term 'Z-score' has been emphasized recently. It is merely a confusing statistical code term for the number of standard deviations below or above the reference (median). It has been referred to in the present publication as it is widely used in scientific assessment. It could more simply be termed 'Standard Deviation score'.

Although the concept of 'functional outcome' has been highlighted in the recent years, it actually has a long informal history. For example, the Gómez classification was initially devised because of the correlation of different 'degrees' of underweight with the mortality of *hospitalized* malnourished young children. Similarly, the original WHO low-birth-weight level of 2.5 kg (5½ lb) was selected mainly because of the higher mortality levels in neonates with weights below this level. Also, it must be emphasized that these figures were simple and easily remembered.

Unfortunately, functional outcome is not easy to measure — for practical reasons and because of the many and diverse influences which can affect individuals and communities. Also, the term 'functional outcome' can be viewed in various ways. It may, for example, refer to *more immediate effects*, such as the development of (and/or death from) severe clinical malnutrition or impaired immunocompetence (Neumann 1982) and particular infections (e.g. measles). It can also apply to *more long-term effects*, such as neurological development, ultimate growth, etc. in later life following malnutrition in young children, or atherosclerosis, diabetes, etc. in adults associated with or following obesity.

A limited number of field investigations have been reported concerning the functional outcome in young children in less technically developed countries. For example, in Bangladesh Chen *et al.* (1980), and in North India Kielman and McCord (1978) found the borderline — as regards risk of mortality — to be about 80 per cent (− 2 SD) of weight-for-age and weight-for-height.

Also, as noted earlier (p. 112), the Metropolitan Life Insurance weight-for-height reference data, and levels above and below, have been correlated with subsequent morbidity and mortality, especially cardiovascular disease and longevity. Other similar studies have been undertaken in adults.

Conclusion

The selection of the cut-off points indicating 'dangerous' abnormality above or below reference data has to be made based on a blend of knowledge of the statistical properties of 'normal' distributions, on the (usually) limited information on functional outcome, on clinical experience, on practical usefulness, and on understandability. None of these can give absolute truth; combined they can help to make an imperfect, but useful, selection possible. A guide to the thought processes which have often followed in the selection and labelling of cut-off points is given in the flow chart in Fig. 2.33. In practice, cut-off points may need to be modified for particular situations — for example, screening in a refugee camp for different levels of rations compared with a cross-sectional prevalence survey.

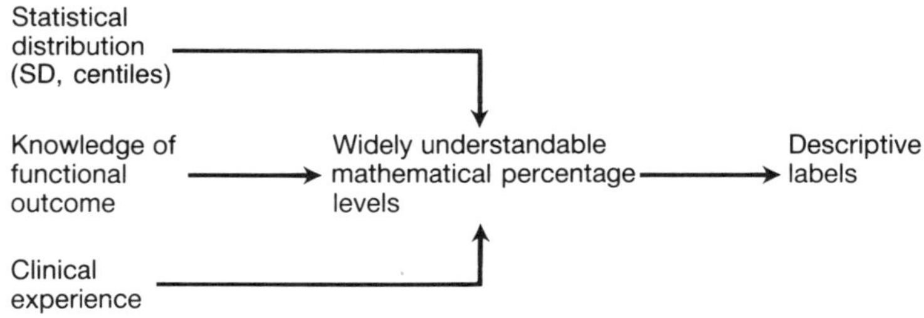

Fig. 2.33 Common considerations in defining and labelling cut-off points (or abnormal levels) in anthropometry: a flow chart. Modifications in selection of cut-off points may be required in different circumstances depending on practical needs (e.g. refugee camp versus routine survey). Descriptive labels include, for example, 'severe' (or) 'desnutrido' or stage III Gómez classification.

As with other aspects of reference data, detailed consideration is given in later sections to the definition, selection, and labelling of appropriate cut-off points for the different circumstances in various age-groups (p. 122). They need to be scientifically acceptable, of practical utility, and understandable to both measurers and recipients of reports. Definitions of levels used and how they have been selected need to be fully included in any reports.

Conclusions

> *Each of the above manoeuvres have something in common,* simplicity *(easy to administer by non-clinicians),* acceptability *(likely to lead to good cooperation),* cost, precision *(consistently reproducible in repeated trials),* accuracy, *(providing a true measurement of the attribute being sought),* sensitivity *(yielding a positive result in a high proportion of individuals with the disease or attribute being sought),* specificity *(yielding a negative result in a high proportion of those who are free of the disease or attribute under study), and* predictive value *(resulting in high proportions of diseased, and disease-free, individuals among those with positive, and negative, test results respectively). The importance of a given property may vary widely, depending upon whether one is screening, case-finding, diagnosing, or conducting a survey.*
>
> Sackett and Holland (1975)

As with all forms of nutritional assessment, a varying blend of methods should be used in direct assessment which are considered to be most useful in obtaining information for the particular situation as inexpen-

Table 2.22 Some characteristics of community nutritional assessment in less technically developed countries

Geared to inter-sectoral programme development for priority issues
Least expensive, limited resources
Avoid tests duplicating information
Use appropriate technology
Neutralize inaccuracies by combining methods ('triangulation', 'navigation')

sively and accurately as possible. Some characteristics are noted in Table 2.22.

It is useful if such data can permit comparability with results from elsewhere. However, the main purpose must never be lost sight of — to provide as rapidly, as economically, and as effectively as possible the most practical information for necessary action.

For individuals, such information should help to lead to early recognition and active preventive and/or curative measures. However, for *individuals* this is especially difficult as each person has an unique 'life-flight' (Trowell *et al.* 1954) and every individual is a package of variables impossible to duplicate (Tuchman 1982).

In communities, data should aim at assisting in developing inter-sectoral national policy and local activities, including feasible, economical methods for use in primary health care services.

3
Assessment from health statistics ('*indirect assessment*')

Introduction

Whatever was the father of a disease, an ill diet was the mother.

George Herbert (1660)

Malnutrition influences morbidity and mortality rates for various infections (such as tuberculosis), as well as maternal, young child, and perinatal mortality rates, life expectancy, and other health statistics as a result of the combined effects of inadequate nutrition and infections. A variety of vital and health statistics have, therefore, been considered as being *in part* (and in part only) indirect indicators of the nutritional status of the community.

Categories of information

Four categories of information can be considered: (1) age-specific mortality rates; (2) cause-specific morbidity and mortality rates; (3) health service statistics; and (4) nutritionally-relevant infection rates.

Practical problems

There are several obvious difficulties in using data of this sort in the 'indirect assessment' of the nutritional status of a community. First, there are the usual problems of collecting accurate data of this type anywhere in the world, especially in less technically developed regions. Before trying to obtain and analyse such data, it is necessary to ascertain not only their availability, but the probable degree of reliability. Neither will usually be great. Results will be related to the method of collection and its acceptability by the public, the percentage of deaths certified by doctors (occurring in hospital, autopsied, etc.), and the interest and concern of the particular government, institution, or agency. The situation varies greatly from one country to another. Sometimes deaths may be reported more regularly than births or vice versa, depending in part on local cultural concepts and social circumstances. For example, Akesode (1980) noted that, in Lagos, the total population is unknown and those living outside register births in the city because of the subsequent availability of better schooling.

In some areas, the numbers of deaths are recorded with comparative accuracy, although the stated causes of death may be inaccurate, or unavailable. Nevertheless, limited data may be found in government records, especially as only the *final* cause of death is recorded. They will usually be time-consuming to unearth and analyse. Officially compiled figures will be available, as in the WHO statistics annual report, from different countries. These can mainly be considered as approximate generalizations. They reflect all the inaccuracies mentioned and may also be influenced by indifference and/or political sensitivities (it is notable that the seventeenth century term for what is now called 'statistics' was 'political arithmetick').

Second, problems of interpretation are considerable in relation to many other concurrent factors interacting with nutritional status, such as a high incidence of infectious disease, overcrowding, and other conditions mainly related to socio-economic level.

For all their inaccuracies, selected vital and health statistics, analysed where possible according to region, season, sex, and age-group, can be potentially helpful. They can give approximate indirect insights into the nutritional situation in a community.

Age-specific mortality rates[49]

Some types of malnutrition have a particularly high incidence at certain ages, so that the mortality rates at these specific age-periods have been considered as indicators — or 'suggestors' — of the incidence of certain types of malnutrition.

2–5 month mortality rate

In areas where thiamine deficiency has been a potential danger, there is a relatively high mortality rate due to infantile beriberi between 2 and 5 months of age, compared with similar areas where dietary lack of thiamine is uncommon (Aykroyd and Krishnan 1941).

In view of the difficulty of assessing the incidence of infantile beriberi by other means, the 2–5 month mortality rate could be a valuable public health index. However, it will, of course, be imprecise, because other diseases, including pneumonia and diarrhoea, can be important causes of death in this age-range, although mortality is usually relatively low at this

[49] A World Bank publication entitled *World Atlas of the Child* (1979) was produced for the International Year of the Child, and contains valuable tables of infant and 1–4 year mortality rates for most parts of the world.

Table 3.1 Comparison of extreme levels of national, maternal, and child mortality rates*

	Highest levels (1)	Lowest levels (2)	Ratio of (1)/(2)
Perinatal mortality†	120	12–15	8–10
Infant mortality†	200	8–10	20–25
Childhood mortality‡	45	0.4–1	45–100
Maternal mortality§	1000	5–10	100–200

* WHO (Division of Family Health) 1980 estimates based on a variety of sources.
† Per 1000 live births.
‡ Per 1000 population.
§ Per 100 000 live births.

time in fully breastfed babies in traditional tropical circumstances, except where mothers are thiamine-deficient. Problems in obtaining data for such a narrow and precise age-range are very great.

Although the 2–5 month mortality rate is very frequently quoted, in retrospect, it has been a theoretical example, in practice. Furthermore, the dramatic decline in infantile beriberi in recent decades further decreases its usefulness.

1–4 year mortality rate[50]

While the infant mortality rate (IMR) has long been used as an indicator of the health of a community, it is now realized that, while the IMR in developing regions of the world may be 10 times as high as in industrialized countries in Europe and North America, the 1–4-year mortality rate may be 30 to 50 times as great. Relatively recent (1980) estimates contrast the situation in areas with the highest and lowest mortality rates in nutritionally vulnerable mothers and young children (Table 3.1).

This is because the so-called 'pre-school age' period, especially its earlier part, is often a time of combined nutritional, infective, and emotional stress. The high 1–4-year mortality rate is due to an accumulation of infections, parasitism, and malnutrition during this vulnerable period, which is normally characterized by rapid growth and, thus, high nutritional needs. The precise details of the responsible deficiency will vary from one area of the world to another, but in most less technically developed regions the principal condition is considered to be protein–energy malnutrition. However, recently, it has become recognized that

[50] The 1–4-year period includes children from 12 to 59 months (i.e. below their fifth birthday).

even 'moderate' degrees of vitamin A deficiency can greatly increase the death rate in this age-range (Leavell 1987). The significance of deficiency of other nutrients has almost certainly been underappreciated.

Estimation

In common with the collection of any such statistics, there is great difficulty in assessing the 1–4-year mortality rates. However, estimates may sometimes be attempted in the following ways:

1. *Analysis of birth and death records.* Records of births and deaths should be consulted, if possible. These may be kept by a local authority, such as a chief or mayor, or by a religious leader, such as the priest or a missionary. If these are complete and accurately kept, which is unusual, it may be possible to calculate the infant mortality rate and the 1–4-year mortality rate, and to enumerate the commoner causes of death in various age-groups. However, with precise ages not known, with no cultural incentive to register births and deaths, and with little likelihood of medical certification of the cause of death, it is unusual to obtain much useful information. Nevertheless, it may be worthwhile examining available records, and even incomplete or flawed information may be useful, provided interpretation takes such limitations into account. Sometimes, at least, it may be possible to note which causes of death are notified. However, these will give the final illness, which may be labelled symptomatically or by means of the vernacular name.

2. *Calculation from census figures.* This will be practicable only if a careful census has been repeated at intervals in an area. This is usually very difficult to do, for various reasons. These may include questionable accuracy in reporting ages of children, presence of illegal immigrants and abandoned 'street children', or concealment of children, if there is a strict governmental family planning programme.

3. *Questionnaire at village level* (Hill and Macrae 1985). A sample of mothers may be questioned carefully, by someone speaking the vernacular and preferably from the local community, on the number of children they have had, the number that have died, and the approximate ages at death, which may have to be expressed in general terms in descriptive age-groups such as 'still on breast', 'able to walk', 'circumcised', etc. The cause of death may also be sought and may be expressed symptomatically (e.g. 'diarrhoea', 'convulsions', 'voiceless crying' (infantile beriberi)) or as a syndrome recognized in the local culture (e.g. *obwosi* — one of the terms used for kwashiorkor by the Baganda people).

However, this type of enquiry is laborious and time-consuming, and may prove inaccurate. Where birth-rates are high and many children die, mothers often do not remember details exactly. In some areas, mothers can remember births and deaths well, but cannot relate them to a fixed time (Burgess *et al.* 1973). There may be local concepts that confuse such data as are obtained. Thus, an abortion, the placenta, or a miscarriage may be classified by local custom as a separate 'child', or it may be considered inauspicious to enumerate children, whether alive or dead. Some cultures do not include children unless they have survived for the first year of life.

Further attempts to obtain figures concerning family structure and particularly child mortality may be carried out by questionnaire and by observation in the course of rapid ecological visits (p. 224). The same difficulties arise as those connected with the questioning of mothers at a survey site. Moreover, in large extended polygamous families, or those with closely-knit clan ties, it may be difficult to sort out the relationships of children and adults, especially if it is customary for children to stay for prolonged periods with relatives. Also, in some groups, it may be considered incorrect behaviour for a woman not to acknowledge all the young children in her house as her own. Nevertheless, useful information has been obtained through this type of approach, as in Kenya, where Grounds (1964) calculated the infant and total child wastage rates, expressed per 1000 live births, for different regions of the country.

Expression of results

Mortality in early childhood can be expressed in various ways:

1. *Percentage of deaths of children below 5 years in relation to total death at all ages.* This can be calculated either from birth and death records or from census data. Figures in Western Europe and North America are below 10 per cent, but in some developing regions they may exceed 50 per cent. However, it is difficult to compare figures from more or less technically developed countries owing to their different population structures. Standardising for age would be useful, but is rarely practical.
2. *Annual 1–4-year deaths per 1000 of the 1–4-year population.* This method has the disadvantage that it is necessary not only to have a good registration of deaths but to know the size of the 1–4-year population in the area, which is difficult to estimate. Rates of 10 per 1000 or over indicate a high mortality in this group, suggestive of widespread protein–energy malnutrition. In some developing regions, this figure may reach 20 to 200 per 1000, whereas in Europe and North America the corresponding figures are usually 1 to 2 per 1000.
3. *Percentage of childhood deaths occurring in the 1–4-year period.* This information, with all the inaccuracies implicit in the method, can sometimes be sought by questioning the mothers about the number of their children who are alive or dead and the rough age (or stage of development) at which they died.

In rural Tanzania, Burgess *et al.* (1969) noted that the number of children stated by mothers to have died before their fifth birthday was compared: (1) to the total live births; and (2) to the total live births minus those still alive and under 5 years of age in other words subtracting those still at risk. The first method gives a figure which is falsely low as mothers with no surviving children under 5 years old were not included and some of the live children may still die before their fifth birthday. The second method gives a figure which is falsely high because the children 'alive' were born before the previous five years, whereas some of the dead children must have been born within this period. The final estimate for under-five mortality must be between these two extremes.

4. *Ratio of 1–4-year mortality rate to that of infants aged 1–12 months.* This method of expressing the 1–4-year mortality rate was suggested originally by Wills and Waterlow (1958), based on experience in Jamaica, as an index of protein–energy malnutrition of early childhood in the community. However, this depends on the assumption that complicating factors, such as infections and incomplete birth registration, are common to both age-groups, and that malnutrition affects the 1–4-year-olds most.

This is not always the case. In some areas, nutritional marasmus is the most common form of protein–energy malnutrition of early childhood and occurs mainly in the first year of life (e.g. Chile). In some more urbanized regions, the age-incidence of kwashiorkor itself decreases with the decline in breastfeeding, as, for example in Trinidad, where 20 years ago, the peak incidence of kwashiorkor (86 per cent) was between 5 and 7 months (Jelliffe *et al.* 1960). In both of these circumstances, the incidence of protein–energy malnutrition could be related to the infant mortality rate.

In many less technically developed countries the 1–4-year mortality is much influenced by malnutrition — the influence being greater than during infancy. This can be a useful index of malnutrition, although the impact of the recent EPI ('expanded immunization programme') will influence this through the prevention of such important contributory infections as measles and whooping cough. However, in whatever way the mortality rate is expressed, to be of value it must be interpreted in the light of: (1) knowledge of the local disease pattern in early childhood, and particularly of the age distribution of the different forms of protein–energy malnutrition and xerophthalmia (p. 265); (2) bacterial and parasitic infections in infancy and the 1–4-year period; and (3) an analysis of the ecological factors responsible for malnutrition in the particular region.

Second year mortality rate

As a refinement of this concept, mortality rates in early childhood ideally should be analysed in age-groups separated by one year only. This could then focus on the peak-age occurrence of malnutrition in the particular region, due to the cumulative burden of dietary inadequacy, infections, and (in some cultures) the psychological trauma of stopping breast-feeding. These would vary in different parts of the world, depending upon such factors as the age of 'weaning' and other infant feeding practices. However, as Gordon *et al.* (1967) emphasized, the 13–24 month (or 'second year') death rate yields more useful information in many countries, as this is the classical age-group principally afflicted with kwashiorkor and less severe protein–energy malnutrition, and the associated deficiencies of other nutrients that occur in affected children. This is the time when the child ('weanling') is experiencing the 'transitional' dietary period, when the main foods are likely to be largely carbohydrate pastes and gruels of low nutrient density, and when the child is between the breast-fed sufficiency of early infancy and the omnivorousness of later childhood. In view of the special dangers of the second year of life, an unsuccessful attempt at a specific term was made for the 2-year-old — the 'secotrant' (second year transitional) (Jelliffe 1969).

Ideally, mortality rates should be estimated for different *biological stages* of early human development — the 'exterogestate (or external) fetus', when the infant is exclusively (or predominantly) breastfed (Bostock 1962), and the 'transitional' (or weanling) — rather than by calendar age-groups. However, this is obviously impractical, as it would vary depending upon the feeding practices in the particular community.

Comparisons and changes

In countries where statistical data are available, presumed alterations in the diet of young children can be assessed, although other changes need consideration, such as a successful measles immunization programme. For example, Corteguera and Lopez (1977) analysed the 1–4-year mortality rates from many American countries. Between 1961 and 1972, this rate had fallen from 2.0 to 1.2 per 1000 per year in Cuba, and from 6.0 to 3.0 in Costa Rica.

Median mortality age

As another statistical indicator, Enderica (1974) has suggested the 'median mortality age', defined as the age in a country when 50 per cent of the mortality has occurred (Table 3.2). These figures vary dramatically from over 70 years to below 10 years and are felt to reflect the standard of living and economic level, including nutrition. However, as usual, the reliability of these figures is at most approximate.

Changing mortality rate by age-groups

In countries with sufficiently reliable statistics, changing mortality rates in different age-groups can be very informative. For example, in Costa Rica

Table 3.2 Median age of mortality in 15 countries. (*Modified from Enderica 1974*)

Country	Year	Median age of mortality (years)
Sweden	1968	74.8
Italy	1968	72.0
Australia	1969	70.4
Rumania	1969	67.5
Hong Kong	1969	60.8
Korea	1967	53.0
Ceylon	1968	47.7
Thailand	1969	39.4
Panama	1968	32.7
India	1964	27.7
Philippines	1967	18.6
Honduras	1968	16.4
Madagascar	1967	16.0
El Salvador	1969	9.2
Bolivia	1966	7.3

the 1–4-year mortality fell from 12.2 per cent of total deaths in 1965, to 10.0 per cent in 1970, to 4.7 per cent in 1975 (Mohrs 1978).

The general situation in one developing country was given by Hijazi (1977):

> In recent years there has been more attention to death rates by age groups. The mortality pattern in Jordan, as it is in most of the developing countries, reflects the socio-economic and health status in the country. The calculated infant mortality in this study (78.23 per 1000) is 4.4 times as great as it is in a country which is advanced; the 1–4 mortality rate 16 times greater. Another simple way of expressing this situation is that while in Sweden less than 5 per cent of the total deaths occur under age of 5 years, we have here a high percentage of children dying in infancy. Almost half of the deaths in the first year occur in the first month of life. It is known that where such a high mortality persists, it is obviously accompanied by a high morbidity. Together with a shortened lifespan and seriously reduced productivity, these factors have grave results on the physical, mental, and economic state of the country.

Cause-specific morbidity and mortality

Information concerning the incidence and mortality of certain forms of malnutrition may be available, if looked for. Data concerning the commonness and mortality rates of certain 'nutritionally relevant' diseases, mainly infections, may also be collectable.

Malnutrition

Once again, information specifically concerning protein–energy malnutrition and other identifiable forms of malnutrition should be sought.

Community Identification

The concept of 'lay reporting' (WHO 1978*b*) can be an essential part of continuing community self-assessment. It can include forms of malnutrition or infectious disease already well-known and with indigenous names. In different part of the world, these include kwashiorkor, (p. 276), night blindness (p. 52), Bitôt's spots (p. 475), whooping cough, and measles.

Cause-of-death-records

Where official records are reasonably accurate, the specific death rates due to malnutrition in 1–4-year-old children may be very useful. Results are best expressed per 100 000 population in this age-group.

In an attempt to draw attention to the problem and to differentiate it from other conditions, it has been suggested that kwashiorkor could be made a notifiable disease, in the same way as many specific infectious diseases. This never seems to have been put into practice.

However, the official notification of deaths in many countries provides a very distorted picture of the real problem, as a large proportion of deaths in children below 5 years is attributed to the final illness, such as diarrhoea, parasitism, pneumonia, or some infectious diseases, particularly measles and whooping cough. This can, for example, be seen in the otherwise excellent statistics from the National Children's Hospital, Costa Rica (Mohrs 1978). These demonstrate information on changes in pattern, such as a decreased mortality from diarrhoea, but children with malnutrition are not sufficiently disentangled from the often final cause of death, usually an infection.

Health service statistics

The prevalence of the major, clinically identifiable syndromes, such as kwashiorkor, nutritional marasmus, pellagra, keratomalacia, etc., will be noted in the course of community nutritional surveys (p. 362). However, a note also be made of the cases admitted from the same area to adjacent hospitals, and care taken to ensure that affected persons are not being overlooked or even hidden from the investigators.

Health centres

Useful, though biased, information concerning geographical distribution and seasonal incidence can be obtained by training staff, including paramedical personnel, to recognize kwashiorkor and marasmus at health centres and to record cases attending with these conditions (Burgess and Dean 1962). The bias is mainly because of the selective nature of the sample.

Diagnostic signs should be simple, clearly understood, and taught to personnel by means of practical demonstrations and photographs. They can also be illustrated by posters in clinics.

Kwashiorkor should be recorded for every young child with oedema, poor growth (low weight), and wasted muscles, and nutritional marasmus diagnosed by very low weight with marked wasting of muscles and subcutaneous fat, with no oedema. Results can be expressed as percentages of young children, probably in specified age-groups, often 1–4 years, attending the centre.

In well-organized clinics, the percentage of young children attending with 'inadequate weight gains' can be determined by examination of growth charts. Difficulties with analysing such records are considered later (p. 296).

Hospitals

Statistics from hospitals can be of some value, although they do not exactly reflect community conditions. Difficulties of interpretation may arise from the inadequacy of local transport and communications, the available bed space, the hospital's admission policy, the availability of other treatment facilities (such as nutrition rehabilitation units), the degree of trust of hospital staff, and indigenous beliefs concerning the cause of malnutrition and its treatment. However, a recent report from Zaire indicates the possible value of hospital admission data (Franklin *et al.* 1984). The hospital recorded an increase in children admitted with protein–energy malnutrition and linked it with rapidly rising food prices.

At present, hospital data often fail to furnish as much information as they could do, because malnutrition of early childhood, especially protein–energy malnutrition, is not identifiable in the disease classification used.

In addition, confusion may occur with regard to the diagnostic labelling of malnourished children who are also suffering from multiple infections. This was clearly shown in the classic 15-country inter-American investigation of the *causes* of mortality in childhood (Puffer and Serrano 1970). In this study, malnutrition was considered an 'underlying cause' when it was the direct cause of death, as evidenced by clinically severe protein–energy malnutrition or a weight less than 60 per cent of 'normal' for age. Malnutrition was considered as an 'associated cause' when it was felt to have influenced the course of the disease condition responsible for death, and with a weight of between 60 and 74 per cent of 'normal'. This study should be consulted for details. In general, it showed malnutrition to be widespread, yet especially under-appreciated as an 'associated cause' of death.

Whenever possible, hospital patients, including those coming to autopsy, should be labelled according to international classification (WHO 1977*a*). Clear-cut forms of malnutrition have specific numbers — vitamin D deficiency: 268; nutritional marasmus: 261; and iron deficiency anaemia: 280. Lesser degrees of protein–energy malnutrition are still given in relation to weight-for-age using the Gómez classification (p. 000) — moderate (60 to <75 per cent): 263.0; mild (75 to <90 per cent): 263.1. Possibly future editions of the WHO classification may revise the criteria to include weight-for-height. However, in practice even the recording of weight in hospitalized children will be helpful, especially in individuals with other primary diagnoses, but with 'associated malnutrition' in the form of moderate protein–energy malnutrition.

It is suggested that *all* cases of kwashiorkor, marasmus, other severe deficiency syndromes (e.g. rickets), and, if possible, moderate protein–energy malnutrition, should be recorded at hospitals, and that secondary conditioning factors should also be noted, especially associated, contributory infections (p. 355). Annual figures can best be reported as percentages of the total number of patients under a specified age admitted to the wards, often 5 years of age is suggested, but other ages may be more appropriate locally (e.g. 1–3 years). Similar records can be kept for out-patients. Care must be taken to avoid duplication of reporting if children with malnutrition are first seen in the out-patients' department and subsequently admitted. Figures should be separately summarized for infants and 1–4-year-old children, and, if age assessment has been sufficiently accurate, figures for the latter can be analysed in yearly age-intervals.

Hospital admissions with kwashiorkor and nutritional marasmus can also be used to supply information suggesting the seasonal incidence and the geographical distribution of these conditions in the surrounding area. Such information can play an important, although biased, part in national nutritional surveillance, especially through so-called 'sentinel hospitals', (which drain a known, constant population) (p. 359), or in the monitoring of the nutritional situation in a refugee camp.

The plotting of home-sites of affected children on superimposed transparent nylon-acetate maps may sometimes assist in the correlation with local ecological factors, including population distribution, urbanization, and staple food crop.

Children admitted to hospital with severe forms of protein–energy malnutrition or keratomalacia can yield valuable information on important local conditioning factors in the aetiology of these conditions, which can be helpful in planning appropriate preventive programmes (p. 355).

For this, detailed clinical histories concerning feeding practices, method of 'weaning' (separating) from the breast, and antecedent infections are needed. In addition, laboratory and other investigations, including a tuberculin test, a stool examination for helminth ova, a thick blood film for malarial parasites, etc., will have to be carried out. Such information may sometimes be available routinely, but this is often not so. More realistically, a group of children with malnutrition can be compared with those of a matched group of similar age and background admitted because of trauma, such as traffic accidents ('case control study', p. 508) (Waterston and Nhambe 1984).

Mortality figures for various hospitalized forms of malnutrition, such as beriberi or kwashiorkor, should be available, but, of course, these give no indication of mortality from these causes in the community. They are biased by the various factors common to all hospital data, and, especially, in the case of kwashiorkor, by the associated infections common to the region under study and by the effectiveness of the treatment employed.

In relation to the assessment of the prevalence of avitaminosis A, Oomen *et al.* (1964) suggested that the age-specific 1–4-year blindness rate may be related to past keratomalacia. This would be suggested by the presence of severe eye damage (leucomata, staphylomata, or phthisis bulbi) in older children or adults, dating from their early childhood.

Finally, where autopsies are obtainable, post-mortem evidence of protein–energy malnutrition and contributory conditioning diseases may be available.

Nutritionally relevant infections

Malnutrition is an important contributory cause of morbidity in such diseases as tropical ulcer, diarrhoeas of infectious origin, tuberculosis, measles, and whooping cough. Death certificates should include mention of severe malnutrition whenever it occurs, concurrently with the principal cause of death or primary disease. Conversely, diseases such as measles, whooping cough, etc., can be conditioning or contributory infections in the development of malnutrition.

Diarrhoea is one of the principal causes of death among young children in developing regions of the world. Its aetiology is often complicated and varies from region to region. However, interaction between alimentary infection (bacterial, viral and/or parasitic) and protein–energy malnutrition are probably the main causes. They often occur together and each can influence the other adversely ('weanling diarrhoea') (Gordon *et al.* 1963).

Therefore, in view of the relation between diarrhoea and malnutrition, and between these and the methods of infant feeding employed, statistics concerning the morbidity and mortality attributable to diarrhoea of early childhood may be further indirect evidence of malnutrition.

Measles is a world-wide disease. Unless effective widespread immunization has been carried out, the attack rate remains unchanged even in countries where mortality due to the condition is now very low. As there is apparently no evidence of variation in the virulence of the measles virus, the infection represents a uniform stress anywhere in the world.

Under this uniform stress, mortality rates and the severity of the disease seem to be related to the nutritional state of the group involved, although late attendance for treatment, availability of health services and their quality, associated parasitic infestations (including giardiasis) (Farthing *et al.* 1986) and a younger age incidence must also be taken into account. In a careful field study carried out over a 4-year period in rural Guatemala, the mortality was found to be 11.5 and 8.5 per cent in the first and second years of life, respectively (Gordon *et al.* 1967). In El Salvador, in 1959, the mortality rate was 105 times as high as in the USA (Scrimshaw 1964).

In some regions, measles is well recognized as a common precipitating factor in the aetiology of xerophthalmia (avitaminosis A) and kwashiorkor. Thus, in Western Nigeria, the hospital mortality rate was 25 per cent, and 13 per cent developed kwashiorkor (Morley 1962). A recent national survey of Cameroon found the mortality from measles in young children to parallel nutritional status — over 6 per cent in rural areas, 4 per cent in urban populations, and under 2 per cent in major cities (Zerfas *et al.* 1982).

Some infectious diseases with very striking and characteristic clinical features, especially measles and whooping cough, are easily recognizable conditions. The symptoms and signs are well-known to lay people and such infections often have specific local names, so that information can often be obtained by appropriate questioning, or as a continuing part of the community self-assessment. Attempts can therefore be made to collect data concerning mortality from measles and whooping cough in the community as a whole and in children admitted to hospital. Such data provides approximate information concerning the nutritional status of the young child population.

Conclusions

All the data mentioned are likely to be 'secondary' — that is, collected and/or compiled by someone other than the investigator, usually through government services. In Third World countries, distance, insufficiency of all resources, cultural anxieties, and lack of motivation or interest will mean that any such statistics should be recognized as being inaccurate.

However, when available, an attempt can be made to use such general and anonymously collected data cautiously as complementary information. This can be helpful in adding indirect evidence to the overall picture.

Sometimes, it may be possible to obtain information personally, if living and working in an area for a prolonged period, as occurs classically with anthropologists and missionaries with medical services. More reliable data on mortality and morbidity may be collectable from populations living in defined areas adjacent to health centres, or mortality rates from hospital attenders. Both have obvious biases. Last, with the development of a network of primary health care services important data may be collectable, certainly at a descriptive level, by village-level health workers, who have a detailed knowledge of events in the community.

4
Assessment of ecological variables I

The old ideas of simple causation are no more valid. In the first place, in actual existence, causation is always multiple. Still more basically, evolutionary and human processes are not based on cause and effect. They are all cybernetic, involving feedback, and their products are always simultaneously results and causes.

Julian Huxley (1964)
Essays of a humanist

Until relatively recently, we in the nutrition field had tended to stay within our discipline and generally only radicals claimed that poverty, land reform and work availability were more basic to the causation of hunger and malnutrition than the simple absence of nutrients. It is trite to say uneaten food has no nutritional value, but food that cannot be purchased is never consumed.

P.L. Pellett (1983) *Changing concepts in world malnutrition*

Introduction

Human malnutrition is always an ecological problem. It is the end-result of multiple overlapping and interacting factors in the community's ecology — that is its physical, biological, social, and cultural environments, including economic constraints and political priorities. The amount of various foods and nutrients available to persons of different age-groups will depend, among other things, upon such environmental conditions as climate, type of soil, agricultural practices, methods of food storage, transport, and marketing. It will also be related to a range of political and cultural factors, including the general economic level, governmental policy concerning an equitable distribution of resources (money, productive land) among the population, the educational level, and population changes, such as occur in urbanization and with an influx of refugees. Cultural influences including local cooking practices, meal patterns, and food classifications, and especially the distribution or restriction of more nutritious foods for vulnerable age-groups will be highly relevant.

The importance of contributory or conditioning infections in the production of malnutrition has become increasingly recognized in recent years. In particular, the synergistic influence of bacterial, viral, and parasi-

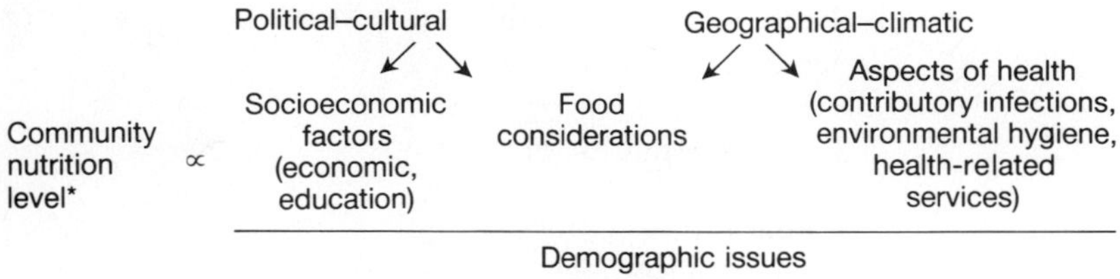

Fig. 4.1 Community nutrition level (CNL) 'equation'. *Especially vulnerable groups.

tic infections and nutritional status is now well recognized. This is especially so in relation to protein–energy malnutrition (p. 273) and vitamin A deficiency in early childhood (p. 265).

It is, therefore, important to try to identify the main causal factors responsible for malnutrition in a community or an individual, especially those amenable to practical action. These need to be differentiated as far as possible from coexisting, non-causal, associated factors, and given a priority rating as regards their importance and feasibility of amelioration. By this means, a locally appropriate preventive programme can be devised which is 'aimed at the vulnerable links in the chain of multiple causation' (Scrimshaw 1964). In current terminology, this is termed the 'risk factor' approach and is outlined later (p. 453).

In practice, at family, community and national levels, the CNL (community nutrition level) 'equation' (Fig. 4.1) (Jelliffe and Jelliffe 1978*a*) has been found to be a useful *general guide* to the main forces to be considered. (Table 4.1) This non-mathematical 'equation' suggests the information that needs to be collected, with special consideration being given to physiologically and culturally vulnerable groups in particular communities, usually young children and pregnant and lactating women and, increasingly, the elderly.

Preventive programmes aimed at eradicating or decreasing the incidence of malnutrition have to suit the particular area or community. Inadequate diets may be related to poverty or insufficient land, to overlarge, too closely spaced families, to lack of availability of foods, to inadequate knowledge of nutritional needs, to customs that limit the intake of available nutritious foods in locally vulnerable groups, or to any combination of these (and other) factors. Malnutrition in young children in less technically developed countries is rarely exclusively due to dietary inadequacy alone. For example, protein–energy malnutrition or vitamin A deficiency are often precipitated by, or made worse by, one or more infections. These include whooping cough, measles, or diarrhoea, or parasitic infestations, such as hookworm, malaria or giardiasis. Similarly, the psychological trauma of abrupt physical separation from the mother's

Table 4.1 Some ecological factors needing consideration

Socio-economic factors
Economics
Education
Food considerations
Availability
Accessibility
Preparation
Consumption
Utilization
Adequacy
Aspects of health
Contributory infections
Environmental sanitation
Health-related services
Demographic issues
Political priorities
Cultural factors
Geographical and climatic influences

breasts plays a part in some cultures during weaning (*sevrage*). A combination or sequence of infections and emotional trauma can often occur. In other circumstances, similar analyses can be made into the often complex aetiology of various types of malnutrition in the elderly (p. 354).

A rational preventive programme should be guided by a knowledge of the main causal factors considered to be of public health significance in the particular area that are most amenable to prevention by least-cost, practical methods that are considered locally feasible. Judgement of the factors that need priority attention is usually made by general overall considerations and knowledge of the local situation. Recently, epidemiological and management analyses have developed and are useful in combination with local knowledge. This means that, apart from other considerations, an immunization programme for young pre-school age children in some Third World countries may be planned, quite logically, partly for nutritional reasons.

At the same time, more fundamental issues ultimately at the root of malnutrition need to be recognized, such as high rates of urbanization, a very rapid increase in population, uncontrolled, unemployment, and in particular, an excessively inequitable distribution of income (and/or) productive land. While these are obviously not under the control of the nutritionist, awareness and advocacy may assist in effecting appropriate changes in national policy (Jelliffe and Jelliffe 1978*a*) (p. 449).

Investigations into ecological factors may also indicate the need for different programmes in various areas of a country or region. They can also assist in the definition of 'risk factors' (p. 453), which can enable public health workers and planners to identify those individuals, families, or communities in need of special care and supervision. Such information also assists in selecting essential topics and messages to be covered in nutrition education. In other words, programmes should try to focus on identifying 'preventable antecedents' and 'practicable changes' (Al-Dabbagh and Ebrahim 1984).

In collecting data concerning ecological factors, it is necessary to devise ways of recording information both qualitatively and preferably in a rough quantitative form using a numerical code — e.g. type of housing, degree of literacy, etc. These indicators have to be defined in ways which are relevant to local circumstances. They may, therefore, be difficult to compare from country to country. Highly sophisticated methods of data collection and analysis have been developed by social scientists, economists, and demographers in more technically developed circumstances. Interdisciplinary investigations of this sort, but on a more modest, realistic level, need to be developed collaboratively, when feasible, especially in judging priority needs in preventive programmes.

Also, in Third World circumstances, the range of information that can be included under the umbrella of 'ecological variables' can be very extensive, from prices of key staple foods, to income levels of the poorest segment of the population, to the availability and type of water supplies, to food habits of different cultural subgroups.

In all circumstances, only some of the relevant information can be collected, and, as usual, selection is always both an important and very difficult task. Decisions have to be made as to which data can be most easily and economically obtained, to yield useful, timely information as specifically as possible for programme managers, and to persuade policy-makers and planners. Quite often in the past, vast numbers of facts have been collected at considerable cost of money and effort but have never even been fully analysed, let alone used.

The range and detail of data to be collected depend on the purpose of the assessment, as do the methods employed. For example, in the special and extreme example of famines (p. 551), experience in agrarian cattle-keeping countries has shown that such crude indicators as the prices of the staple foods, and death rates of both humans and livestock give basic indications concerning the onset, location, and evolution of the disaster (Seaman and Holt 1975). This contrasts very greatly with the detail needed in an ecological assessment of the nutritional status of a technically advanced urban area, including the differentiation between 'causative' and 'associated' factors, and ranking of those considered causative.

Some of the main ecological factors that can play a part in causing malnutrition and which need to be borne in mind when devising preventive programmes can be considered under the following general, *artifically separated* headings as indicated in the community nutrition level equation: *socio-economic factors* (economics, education), *food considerations, aspects of health* (including contributory infections, environmental sanitation, health-related services), *population issues, political and cultural factors* and *geographical and climatic influences.*

These will be dealt with in sequence, except that *food considerations* will be considered last, as these are more often included in community nutritional investigations.

Methods of obtaining information

Information of varying degrees of usefulness and accuracy concerning ecological factors can be obtained in many ways, some of which may be more or less feasible in different circumstances. Some methods are detailed in this chapter, as they may be less familiar to health workers.

Information can be sought from individuals or mothers of children by carefully tested questionnaires. As noted earlier, complex and sophisticated methods of data collection, analysis, and interpretation may be available in areas with modern technological resources and sufficient funds. This is, however, usually not the case, so that the following is *mainly concerned with community studies, with limited resources, especially in technically less developed countries.*

Background data

Background data should always be sought. Library research, using books, journals, and other publications in medical, nutritional, anthropological, agricultural, economic, demographic, and other relevant fields, will be useful, if available.

Enquiries may be made from the various government departments whose officials and archives may be able to supply information ('archival data') — census figures, statistics, maps, national and regional food production systems, etc. The ministries, departments, or bureaux concerned with health, agriculture, education, economic development, etc. should be approached, if feasible. At the same time, the accuracy, often suspect, of such central information may vary and be difficult to check. In addition, it is rarely 'disaggregated' effectively — that is, broken down into geographical areas, economic levels, or age-groups of nutritional significance.

Discussion should be sought from nationals and foreigners who have had general or professional experience in the area. This may include administrators, physicians, nurses, anthropologists, and missionaries. In *all* cases, the possible bias and range of experience of the informant must be considered. For example, university students from overseas countries are often from the urban elite and have little personal experience of the living conditions of the rural or urban poor.

Further information and clarification of background data obtained will need to be sought in the field.

Field data

General observations Visual observations can be made in the field — for example, at an actual survey site when people have been assembled for examination. Staff should be encouraged to jot points down as observed (or shortly thereafter), and notebooks (or tape recorders) should be available for this purpose. In some surveys, co-ordination of these impressions can best be carried out by a team discussion each evening, and may suggest special features to be watched for on subsequent days.

As part of data collection, 'rapid ecological visits' should be made to gardens, kitchens, granaries, markets, village shops, and other places associated with food preparation and production, e.g. fish ponds, animal herds, etc. Whenever feasible, photographs should be taken to illustrate the real-life situation of the community investigated and used in reports, in slide presentations, and in subsequent training activities.

The type of information obtained — by means of observation, discussion, and enquiry — is mainly subjective and qualitative. Sometimes, it can be made more exact by the use of a suitable form, schedule, or check-list, giving the items to be noted on each visit. Sampling guidance will be helpful regarding the number of households, etc., to be visited, although in 'rapid ecological visits' it is usually only possible to obtain impressions of home-life. A social science research worker can be invaluable in advising on the preparation and testing of appropriate forms and questionnaires. A systematic approach to qualitative data collection was given by Scrimshaw and Hurtado (1987).

Although approximate and general, information obtained in the course of these rapid ecological visits is of considerable importance in that it provides a glimpse of local life and some of its food-related problems. In short cross-sectional surveys, if staff resources permit, one small mobile team can, with advantage, be made responsible for these activities. At the same time, it is desirable for *all* senior members of a survey team to take part in some ecological visits. Personal observation of the background and of general ways of life are essential, both for the subsequent interpretation of the survey findings and for making realistic suggestions in the eventual planning of preventive measures.

Home visits should always be carried out after obtaining permission, in a friendly, courteous, and diplomatic fashion, and should cause minimum disruption of domestic privacy. Survey personnel should be accompanied by a respected member of the community. The correct amount of time should be spent on greetings, which must be learned, and local etiquette should be most carefully followed. Appropriate culturally acceptable clothes should be worn. When feasible, it is sound policy, as well as humane, to be willing, in the course of the visit, to treat, advise, or, at least, be able to refer anyone who is really sick.

It is often unwise or impossible during these rapid visits to fill out a form within a household, since such action may be viewed suspiciously. The amount of practical information gathered from such home visits depends on the circumstances. Sometimes male visitors are disbarred by custom. Procedures must therefore be flexible to suit the probable reaction of the particular culture. In some circumstances, the head of the household should be interviewed alone; more usually several members of the family will be present, understandably curious as to what is happening. Minimally, only observation may be possible. If completing questionnaires in households is not acceptable, a small pocket notebook or tape recorder may be carried, and facts obtained entered briefly between visits to houses. To make this easier, the pages of the notebook can be prepared beforehand. The data so obtained can be transferred to the appropriate survey forms each evening, while the day's visits are still fresh in the observer's memory.

Information may also be sought from *local records*, if they exist, in churches, or town halls, or from *places where food is sold*, such as markets, street vendors, or village shops.

Clues to possible ecological variables responsible for malnutrition in the community can also be obtained by investigating the more obvious aetiological findings in malnourished persons (clinical case analysis or 'case control study'[51]) admitted to hospitals in the area, including their social, nutritional, and clinical histories, and laboratory investigations for contributory infections. However, this may not be possible because of shortage of staff, and because the notes on cases of malnutrition admitted to busy, understaffed wards often may contain inadequate information.

The gathering of accurate and detailed ecological information may be obtained by the use of appropriate *questionnaires*, preferably supplemented by investigations by specialist personnel, such as anthropologists, who may employ *specific techniques* (such as participant or close observation) These often require longer periods in the field for detailed study. Brief consideration of some of the main modern methods used in social science research is given later (p. 172).

Socio-economic factors

Human height becomes greater and growth takes place more rapidly, other things being equal, in proportion as the country

[51] See Appendix 4 for commoner epidemiological terms.

is richer, the comfort more general, houses, clothes, and nourishment better, and labour, fatigue, and privation during infancy and youth less; in other words, the circumstances accompanying poverty delay the age at which complete stature is reached and stunt adult height.

L.R. Villermé (1829)
Memoire sur la taille de l'homme en France

Many socio-economic factors are difficult to assess quantitatively, especially earnings and belongings, because people are understandably reluctant to reveal to strangers their income or other wealth, including land or livestock. In some circumstances it may be feared that these enquiries could lead to increased taxation, robbery, or, at least, hostile envy. Also, cultures differ in their display or concealment of relative affluence.

Ecological factors of relevance to nutritional status including those relating to economics and education, can include selected items from the list in Table 4.2. These can be determined for an individual, a family, or household, according to the local situation,[52] and the type of investigation.

The occupations of the 'head' of the household and other members of the family are likely to be relevant, although obviously needing review in the particular culture. Also, women employed out of the home may be a financial asset, but not necessarily of a nutritional benefit to young children (p. 200).

Attempts to assess social circumstances by tangible Western yardsticks, such as clothes or type of house, must be made cautiously as in some cultures these are of less importance. Wealth and status may be measured by the number of cattle (whether healthy and productive or not), or by gold ornaments owned by women, which will certainly not be displayed for the investigator. The local 'indicators' of wealth (or, conversely, 'poverty proxies')[51] must be known and, if readily identifiable by observation, carefully noted.

Some items selected from the foregoing points can be looked for during the rapid ecological visits; others require special questionnaires. In judging economic level, the structure and roofs of houses are often useful and easily observable without disturbing the community. These may include bamboo or mudbrick material, thatched or metal roof, etc. Other indicators or 'suggestors' include household furnishings and the type of water supply, which can range from natural (pond or stream) to man-made

[52] The publications by Yang (1971) and Schofield (1979) are of assistance in making selections. On a comparative national basis the UN has suggested an 18-point index of socio-economic variables.

Table 4.2 Some major ecological factors influencing nutritional status

1. **Occupation** — primary (e.g. farmer, fisherman, hired labourer, unemployed), secondary (e.g. home industry, seasonal employment).
2. **Tangible wealth** — land, number of livestock, boats, modern status symbols (e.g. sewing machine, bicycle, motor-scooter, radio).
3. **Family income** — wages and earnings (harvest/non-harvest), home industries, cash crops, non-cash income (e.g. foods grown foods, bartered), debts, intrafamilial distribution of goods or cash.
4. **Housing** — type, floor, roof, walls, lighting, ventilation, furniture, provision for sleeping, number of rooms, population per house, owned or rented.
5. **Kitchen** — building, location, stove, fuel, type and condition of cooking utensils, rubbish disposal.
6. **Budgeting** — expenditure on food, clothes, rent, fuel, light, education, transport, domestic services, charitable contributions, recreation (including tobacco and alcohol).
   Prices of foods — shops and markets, seasonal variation (with special reference to protein foods suitable for young children).
7. **Education** — literacy of men and women of parent and grandparent age-groups, presence of books and newspapers, children attending school (type of school, classes, examinations passed).
8. **Food storage** — size, contents, pest-proofing, refrigeration.
9. **Water supply** — source, distance from house, purity, approximate amount of water available per person and for livestock.
10. **Latrine** — type (if any) and condition (cleanliness, fly-proofing).
11. **Family details** — size, relationships, stability, intervals between children.
12. **Demography of community** — census data, including number, age, and sex distribution, geographical distribution, increase, migration (seasonal, illegal immigrants; refugees).

(roof-drainage to barrel or tank, or bore-hole and pump). The type of transport available may also be easily observable (buffalo cart, canoes or boats, bicycle, motorscooter, etc.). Other relatively expensive items, such as radios, may be noted during home visits.

The amount of land should be noted, when possible. However, this may be complicated and difficult practically. For example, a family may have multiple small cultivated plots in various places, and different parts of their land may or may not be suitable for the growing of different crops.

Approximate areas devoted to more nutritious plant foods, particularly legumes and ground-nuts, can be sometimes noted, and also the extent and type of cash crops grown, including the area under cultivation with cotton, coffee, tea, or cocoa, or the number of coconut palms.

The number of livestock and poultry can sometimes be estimated,

Table 4.3 Variables and scores employed in computing a socio-economic index in rural Guatemala *(Mata 1978)*

Land and animal resources		Housing material		Sanitary facilities		Education and cultural features*	
Land (cuerdas)		**Floor**		**Water supply**		**Literacy**	
10–98	3	Tile, cement	3	Home facility	3	Read, write	3
1–9	2	Earthen	1	Communal	1	Illiterate	1
None	1						
Livestock		**Walls**		**Faeces disposal**		**School, primary**	
Cattle and hogs	3	Adobe, cement	3	Toilet, latrine	3	> 3 grades	3
Hogs only	2	Stalk, bajareque	1	None	1	1–3 grades	2
None	1					None	1
Poultry		**Roof**		**Garbage disposal**		**Footwear**	
10–98	3	Metal	3	Fertilizer	3	Shoes	3
1–9	2	Tile	2	Buried, burned	2	Sandals	2
None	1	Straw, palm	1	Discarded	1	None	1

* These refer to the head of the family, usually the husband.

although this is usually not easy to do. Also, due account needs to be taken of the local cultural significance of various animals. These may be kept as symbols of wealth — for example, cattle among some African pastoralists — or as a source of food for the household (e.g. the buffalo for its milk in India), or as ritual celebration foods (e.g. pigs in the New Guinea Highlands), or as beasts of burden (e.g. the buffalo in Thailand), or as producers of saleable products (e.g. chickens for their eggs), or for a combination of these reasons.

In more technically developed countries, various indices of socio-economic status (SES) have been devised. Examples include the UK social classes, the socio-economic index of the US Bureau of the Census (1963), and the Warner ranking I–IV (Warner *et al.* 1960). Appropriate levels need to be defined for different cultures and circumstances in non-Westernized societies. For example, in rural Guatemala, Mata (1978) devised a socio-economic index based on scores from locally important items (Table 4.3). In more sophisticated communities, Belcher (1972) suggested a tentative cross-cultural scale, with 'scores' based on 14 categories, for measurement of 'level of living' (Table 4.4). All workers agree

Table 4.4 Preliminary cross-cultural scale for measuring level of living (used in rural Georgia, USA) *(Belcher 1972)*

		Score
Function 1.	**Shelter: construction of exterior walls**	
	Brick, concrete block masonry, painted frame	5
	Asbestos or asphalt siding	4
	Unpainted frame	3
	Scrap wood, Coca-cola signs	2
	Grass, leaves, none	1
Function 2.	**Shelter: construction of living room floor**	
	Finished hardwood, tile, terrazo	5
	Finished or painted softwood, bare concrete	4
	Unfinished hardwoods or softwood with tongue and groove	3
	Wood with cracks	2
	Earth	1
Function 3.	**Shelter: construction of roof**	
	Concrete, tile, good shingles	5
	Corrugated or sheet metal, warped shingles	4
	Roll roofing, thatch	3
	Straw, Coca-cola sign	2
	None, roof with large holes	1
Function 4.	**Storage of water**	
	Automatic: house piped	5
	Cistern	4
	Clay barrel designed solely for water storage	3
	Large clay jar	2
	Buckets, tin pails	1
Function 5.	**Transportation of water to home**	
	Automatic, faucet in home	5
	Hand pump, faucet in yard	4
	Bucket with pulley in yard	3
	Bucket from well or stream in own yard	2
	Carry over 100 yards	1
Function 6.	**Lighting**	
	Electric fixture, lamps	5
	Electric bare bulb	4
	Carbide or gasoline lantern	3
	Kerosene lamp	2
	Candle, open fireplace	1
Function 7.	**Preservation of perishable food**	
	Electric or gas refrigerator	5
	Ice box	4

Table 4.4 (Continued)

	Spring house, cellar	3
	Window box, clay jar	2
	None	1
Function 8.	**Eating: place settings of flatware**	
	Over two per person — (sets of knife, fork, and spoon)	5
	One to 1.9 per person	4
	One utensil or more per person, but less than one place setting person	3
	Partial for entire household — fewer utensils than people	2
	None — use hands	1
Function 9.	**Disposal of human wastes**	
	Flush toilets	5
	Modern pit toilet	4
	Privy	3
	Trench and stick in fence corner	2
	None	1
Function 10.	**Transportation**	
	Owned or leased automobile; in some situations, a motor boat or airplane	5
	Motorcycle or other small motorized vehicle	4
	Horse with wagon or buggy	3
	Bicycle, horse or mule	2
	Foot only, or public facilities	1
Function 11.	**Cooking food: equipment**	
	Electric or gas range	5
	Hot plate, kerosene or oil stove	4
	Manufactured wood stove	3
	Clay stove, mud table, hibachi	2
	Three rocks, bare ground	1
Function 12.	**Fuel for cooking**	
	Electricity or gas	5
	Oil	4
	Wood or charcoal	3
	Small sticks, scrap wood	2
	Weeds, leaves, dung	1
Function 13.	**Cleaning floors of home**	
	Vacuum cleaner	5
	Electric broom or sweeper	4
	Purchased dust mop and/or good grade broom	3

Table 4.4 (Continued)

	Native broom or mop	2
	None	1
Function 14.	**Washing dishes**	
	Automatic dishwasher	5
	Sink with drain	4
	Dishpan (no sink)	3
	Multipurpose pan: kettle or washpan	2
	Wash in stream or at pump	1

that such ratings need to be culturally specific, with functional equivalents related to local customs and styles of life. The method of deriving such scores must be clearly explained and justified.

Often a basic issue is defining locally meaningful 'poverty levels', both absolute and relative. Schuftan (1979) commented that the 'household purchasing power deficit' is one useful way to describe financial inability to purchase an adequate diet and to 'express malnutrition in economic terms'.

As noted (Table 4.2), the educational levels of the household members are relevant to nutritional status. This is partly because the level of education frequently parallels income. The significance of educational level is emphasized by the inclusion of literacy as one of the three items (combined with life expectancy at birth and infant mortality) in the PQLI (Physical Quality of Life Index) (Morris 1979). In particular, several recent investigations have emphasized the specially significant role of *maternal* education. This has been noted, for example, in parts of India, especially the State of Kerala (Gopalan 1984).

Education can be expressed as level of schooling achieved, and/or by some practical functional test of literacy (e.g. ability to sign name, read simple sentences), which can be defined locally in relation to international concepts.

Collection of information

Background data

Figures for national *per capita* income, sometimes broken down on a regional basis, and legal minimum wages may be available from the appropriate government departments and should be ascertained. This type of information is often not disaggregated to show distribution, especially the percentage below what is considered to be the local 'poverty level'. Also, it does not necessarily include the landless, nor those employed with wages below the legal minimum.

General field data

Approximate data can be collected by observation — for example, in the course of rapid ecological visits. More precisely, questionnaires may be employed, covering appropriate topics at least on a random population subsample.

Specific field data

Specific information on certain social data can be collected by special studies. However, overly long, complex questionnaires are rarely desirable. They often serve to fatigue and irritate both the investigator and the individuals being interviewed. In addition, limitation of funds can make the subsequent analysis of large amounts of data an impossibility.

Alternatively, recent investigations may have been carried out on these topics in the particular geographical area. Indeed, the selection of a region for a nutritional assessment study may be influenced by the availability of previously collected data (or actual ongoing studies). Sometimes, these can be usefully and economically incorporated ('piggy-backing'), or amalgamated. In particular, the availability of census data and an existing, appropriate statistical sampling frame may be of great assistance.

Discussion

As noted earlier, the selection of appropriate combinations of data to be collected varies greatly with needs and resources. For example, Graffar's classification has been widely used in Europe and elsewhere. It gives a score based on income, education, profession (employment), and housing (Graffar 1956). Numerous culturally modified variations of this type of coverage, together with family size, have been devised in many different parts of the world. When available, social and economic indicators used in Household Expenditure Studies in the country concerned should be considered both for guidance and consistency in reporting.

With present-day realization of the prime significance of maternal education and of adequate income and/or cultivable land, locally relevant, uncomplicated methods of assessment are priorities, including the most suitable 'economic level proxies' or visible indicators of income.

Various perspectives concerned with food availability need to be considered in interpreting the socio-economic significance of such information. Examples include, for example, the relationship of purchasing power to the price of major food items and their seasonal variation ('household purchasing power deficit' (Schuftan 1979)), and the cost–nutrient rating of different foods. These are detailed later (Appendix 5).

Aspects of health

Humanity has but these great enemies: fever, famine, and war.
Sir William Osler (1849–1919)

Three 'aspects of health' can influence nutritional status greatly: (1) contributory (or 'conditioning') infections; (2) environmental sanitation; and (3) the easy availability of relevant health-related services.

Contributory infections

The synergism between bacterial, viral, and parasitic infections and malnutrition has been recognized for many years (Scrimshaw *et al.* 1959, 1968; Cole and Pankin 1977).

'Opportunistic' infections occur more easily with more serious effects in the malnourished because of diminished immunocompetence and compromised barriers to infection. Conversely, malnutrition is precipitated by infections as a result of poor appetite, increased metabolic needs and nutrient losses, sometimes associated with vomiting and/or diarrhoea. In particular, the nutritional situation can often be made worse by treatment with prolonged dietary restriction, prescribed by either Western practitioners or traditional custom (Fig. 4.2).

Recent studies, notably the long-term field investigation carried out by Mata (1978*b*) in rural Guatemala, have re-emphasized the significance of a continuous succession of infections and of the 'dose' of infecting organisms, particularly diarrhoea-producing viruses and bacteria. In addition, the level of the 'worm burden' of intestinal parasites has to be considered in relation to the host's body size and nutrient needs.

Seasonal coincidence of outbreaks of infections and impaired nutritional status is well recognized in many places. For instance, malnutrition reached a peak in El Salvador in the early rainy season 2 months after the seasonal peak incidence of diarrhoea (Trowbridge and Newton 1979). Similarly, increased incidence of xerophthalmia has been noted following outbreaks of infections, especially measles, diarrhoea, and respiratory infections (IVACG 1982). Conversely, vitamin A supplements in deficient areas seem to reduce the mortality from measles (Barclay *et al.* 1987).

This means that programmes designed to improve the nutritional status of a community, especially of young children, have to give priority to the prevention and management of contributory or 'conditioning' infections (Mata 1978*b*).

Nutritionally relevant infections

Bacterial, viral, and parasitic infections considered most likely to be nutritionally relevant in the particular area need to be known. The list of

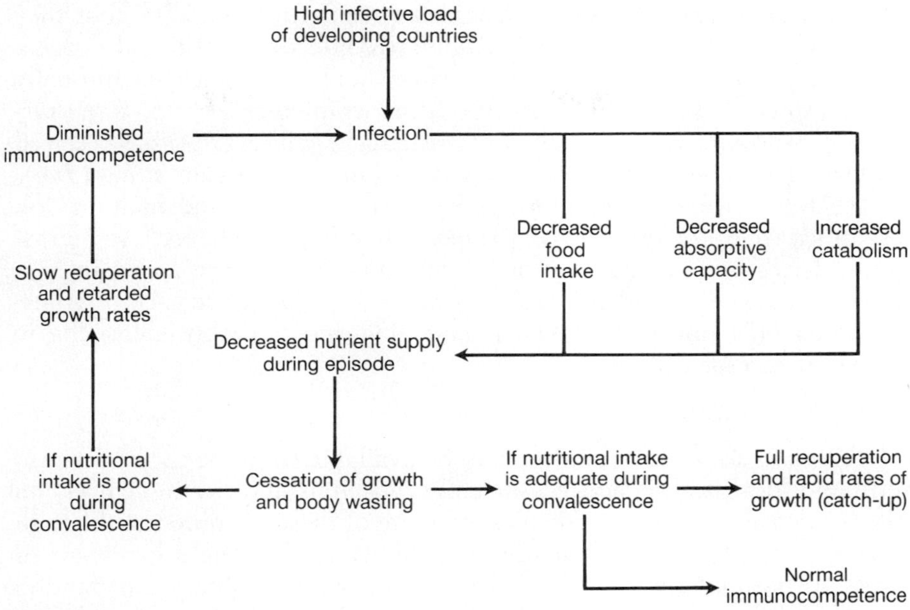

Fig. 4.2 Interaction between infection and nutritional status (Martorell 1982).

infections may include one, or usually more, of the following: *bacterial* — tuberculosis, whooping cough, pneumonia, diarrhoeal disease, including 'weanling diarrhoea', bacillary dysentery; *viral* — measles (Duggan and Milner 1986), rotavirus diarrhoea, HIV infection (AIDS); *parasitic* — malaria, intestinal parasites (giardiasis (Loewenson *et al.* 1986), amoebiasis, hookworm, roundworm, whipworm).

It may be noted that diarrhoea in early childhood is not a specific clinical or aetiological entity. For example, 'weanling diarrhoea' is a variable syndrome, usually resulting from combined bacterial and/or viral intestinal infection and malnutrition at the time when other foods, which are likely to be low in nutrients, bacteriologically contaminated, and indigestible, are given to the child in addition to breast milk. Its age-incidence varies with local infant feeding practices but is often between 6 and 18 months (Gordon *et al.* 1963). Recent work indicates that the *duration* of diarrhoea is particularly influenced by inadequate nutritional status (*Nutrition Reviews* 1985). However, any infection, even if clinically mild, adds slightly, but progressively, to the individual's nutritional burden, especially in already poorly nourished young children. Thus, in coastal New Guinea, even such a clinically uneventful condition as molluscum contagiosum has been shown to be an extremely widespread viral skin infection (Sturt *et al.* 1971). In fact, such skin infections as molluscum contagiosum, scabies, impetigo, and tropical ulcers can be considered not only as 'dermatological environmental sanitation markers', but they also from part of a community's cumulative infective-nutritional burden. Similarly, the significance of *heavy* worm burdens of such nutritionally underappreciated intestinal parasites as the whipworm (*Trichuris trichuris*) and the roundworm (*Ascaris lumbricoides*) (Jelliffe 1954) has received endorsement from several recent investigations (Stephenson *et al.* 1980).

The most clear-cut relationships between infections and malnutrition are in kwashiorkor (measles, diarrhoea, whooping cough, etc.), in marasmus (diarrhoea), in iron deficiency anaemia (hookworm), and in xerophthalmia (measles, diarrhoea) (pp. 270–3). The significance of transplacental HIV infection (AIDS) is emerging and probably increasing in some areas, especially in Africa.

Collection of information

Background data Information may be available from the medical literature and local health services, including hospitals and health centres, on the incidence (including epidemics) of some of these conditions. Although a biased sample, such information should always be sought by means of visits to hospitals, etc., when it may be possible to obtain information concerning attendances and admissions with malnutrition. In addition, the age-incidence of the possible conditioning infections can be noted, including diarrhoea in young children in order to estimate if 'weanling diarrhoea' is an important local entity (Gordon *et al.* 1963).

As noted earlier (p. 355), 'case analyses' can be undertaken on individuals, usually children, to attempt to identify the contributory infections, such as measles or roundworms, which commonly play a part in the aetiology of malnutrition. This is best undertaken epidemiologically as 'case control studies' in which non-malnourished children of similar background are compared.

General field data In field studies, three methods may be employed. First, inspection and observation will reveal such chronic infections as skin sepsis, scabies, conjunctivitis, trachoma, purulent otitis, leprosy, etc. The number (and percentage) of children with high fever has been used, employing a rapid-reading, low-cost, liquid crystal, re-usable skin thermometer.[53]

Second, questionnaires of varying degrees of complexity can be employed. These can be valuable, but their use is time-consuming. Prior definitions need to be agreed upon — for example, with diarrhoea.

[53] Available models, based on a liquid crystal principle (Lees *et al.* 1978), measure temperatures from 96–104°F (35.6–40°C) after being stuck to the skin for 15 seconds. The individual has to be out of sunlight. The 'EZ-TMP' model costs about US$2 from P.O. Box 1509, Dayton, Ohio 45401, USA.

Sometimes, questions concerning well-defined, clear-cut, much-feared diseases have specific (sometimes 'honorific') names in the local language (e.g. whooping cough, measles) and these may be usefully included. Most usually, such 'morbidity questionnaires' should focus on specific symptoms or signs which can identify or suggest syndromes and possible disease entities. The preparation of such questionnaires is much more difficult than often appreciated. Advice should be sought from social science research experts with practical knowledge of the local situation, when available. Questionnaires *always* need to be pre-tested in the population concerned, and should relate to recent events, such as these occurring during the previous week.

The pattern of therapeutic scarification can give guidance in some cultures. For example, a characteristic medicinal scar pattern beneath the left ribs of schoolchildren in a part of East Africa indicated clearly the commonness of *past* malarial splenomegaly.

Third, certain infections of a more chronic nature may be tested for, and may include:

1. *Intestinal helminths* — by examining stool samples taken in the field (by anal tube technique for young children[54]) and kept in preservative (e.g. 10 per cent formal solution, methiolate–iodine–formaldehyde, etc.) which can be examined later, on return to base, or in camp with a standard microscope or a battery-operated portable model (McArthur 1958);
2. *Malaria* — by clinical examination for an enlarged spleen and by a thick blood film, using carefully cleaned slides and stained with Giemsa or Field stains for malarial parasites;
3. *Tuberculosis* — by carrying out a tuberculin test with a Heaf gun or other apparatus. The main difficulty here is the need to read the result of the test at a subsequent attendance 2–3 days later, which is always difficult, and may be impossible, to organize. Furthermore, tuberculin sensitivity is diminished (anergy) by protein–energy malnutrition.

Conclusion

An obvious drawback is that, unless an epidemic is occurring at the time of a short-term field study, periodic or seasonal acute infections of nutritional consequence, such as measles, whooping cough, and infective diarrhoea, cannot be adequately assessed in prevalence studies. It may also be useful to obtain possibly biased information on the importance of

[54] An open-ended plastic or glass tube about 4 inches (10 cm) long and with an internal diameter of about 1/4 inch (0.6 cm) is used. The tube edges are rounded. The young child is positioned across his mother's lap and then the tube, lubricated with water, is gently inserted into the rectum. On removal, the faecal sample is pushed out of the tube with an applicator into the previously prepared screw-cap container of stool preservative.

these illnesses as contributory infections by investigating the aetiology of malnutrition from selected, adjacent hospital records ('case control studies'). The ability to document the occurrence of such illnesses is among the advantages of longitudinal studies (p. 367), and of collection of information by community health workers in primary health care services.

Environmental sanitation

At community level, numerous environmental factors have indirect nutritional effects, largely because of their influence on the spread of infections, which can contribute to the development of malnutrition. These have been included in an earlier list (Table 4.2) (p. 150). They especially should include information on the presence and use of latrines, rubbish disposal, water supply, and on over-crowding (with increased risks of contact and droplet spread of infections).

In particular, the significance of an adequate, reasonably clean water supply has been emphasized increasingly in relation to the prevention of skin infections, intestinal parasites, and especially diarrhoeal disease. For example, Tomkins and colleagues (1977) working in northern Nigeria have shown a rise in the prevalence of diarrhoeal disease at the end of the dry season, when water is in limited supply.

This has also been stressed by numerous books published on village water supplies (McJunkin 1982), by increasing use of oral rehydration, and by realization that an improved water supply can, in some areas, represent a priority method with long-term nutritional benefit as a preventor of diarrhoea.

Aspects of environmental sanitation can be categorized into various types and recorded in surveys. Recent concern and attention, on a worldwide basis, given to the role of the water supply in sanitation, cooking, and household irrigation has indicated that a functional classification scheme should include convenience (mainly nearness), quality, and minimal quantity (usually assumed to be 20–30 l/day per person). Basic information on various water supply systems in rural or urban areas can, therefore, be viewed in relation to health and nutrition, as well as reflecting economic status. The tremendous physical burden and time spent in carrying water from source to home also has obvious direct nutritional relevance to women and older girls who are responsible for this task in many cultures (p. 165).

Health-related services

In nutrition surveys, especially in technically less developed countries, information needs to be collected concerning existing health, educational, agricultural, and other extension and social services in the area. Programmes concerned with bettering the nutritional status of the community will almost always be in part related to the improvement of these services and in part channelled through them. In addition, information on community organization and the indigenous system of health beliefs and healing needs to be collected, at least in outline. Community involvement, understanding, and participation need to play a key role in nutritional assessment and in the subsequent development of programmes.

Health services

Some information should, if possible, be gathered on some of the following points, with special reference to their relevance to the local nutrition scene, and indeed, to see if their activities are contributing to, or hindering, the relief of malnutrition. A wide range is given below. Collection of information on many may be quite unrealistic. *A limited selection* of some items is usually possible.

General: number of hospitals and centres, location, and area served (related distances and transportation) ('drainage range'); number of beds (total, paediatric, maternity); records (especially information on individuals diagnosed as having malnutrition) (p. 356).

Admissions: number, age-groups, diagnoses, results of treatment (cured, improved, not improved, died, proportion of autopsies to deaths), mothers admitted with children, maternity admissions (rooming in), percentages of births to prenatal attendances.

Food services: meals provided and 'congruence' with nutrition education.

Out-patients: number, age-groups (including attendances at prenatal and Young Child Clinics), diagnoses (including malnutrition).

Follow-up system: home visiting.

Staff: doctors, medical assistants, nurses, and assistant nurses, midwives, and assistant midwives, community health workers, laboratory technicians, domestic staff; knowledge and attitude concerning nutrition.

Buildings: wards, out-patients, laboratory, offices, kitchens, accommodation for relatives.

Equipment: weighing machine, (type, whether checked) growth chart (type, understanding by health staff), transport, drugs, food supplements (including dried skimmed milk).

Training programmes (with special reference to nutrition): medical and other health professionals.

Community involvement: existence of primary health care services, community health workers and their general and nutritional activities.

Miscellaneous: immunization rate against contributory infections, methods of prevention and treatment of malnutrition (use of dried skimmed milk, and local food mixtures), procedures with dehydration (oral rehydration, early feeding), use of nutritional rehabilitation units, family planning programmes.

Indigenous health systems: types of practitioners and distribution, disease classification (including malnutrition), methods of prevention and treatment.

Educational influences

The following data are useful and locally priority items may be collectable.

School-age children: number, type, distribution, percentage in schools, training in nutrition (formal curriculum, school meals, school gardens).

Young people: clubs (Young Farmers, Scouts, etc.).

Adults: literacy (percentage, sex distribution), parent–teacher associations, clubs and mass organizations (community development, voluntary organizations, women's clubs, breastfeeding support groups, etc.).

Mass media: radio, press, television (content, advertising related to foods, nutrition education).

Agricultural services

Extension services: relevance to nutritional foods; cash crops (including easy, direct assistance to farmers with loans and locally preferable and improved seed); school gardens.

Collection of information

Background data These will be available, in varying degrees of completeness, complexity, and methods of collection, at the Ministries of Health, Agriculture, and Education and at the headquarters of other relevant agencies. These include Community Development, the Ministry of Information, Voluntary Organizations, and sources of information on major meteorlogical changes, especially rainfall.

General field data Concurrently with the gathering of data on conditioning infections from hospitals and health centres in the area, information concerning the medical, educational, agricultural community development, and other extension services should be noted. This can, for example, be obtained by questioning households regarding numbers of visits made to them and by discussion and informal observation.

Demographic

Each child brings his own supply of rice.

Traditional Korean proverb
(Robson and Wadsworth 1977)

Despite the traditional view expressed in this quotation, in the present-day world the level of nutrition in a community is often adversely related to the number of mouths to be fed. In fact, demographic issues (including the rate of increase, degree of urban migration, family (or household) size, and the closeness of child spacing) can be considered as a universal denominator for the rest of the 'community nutrition level' equation (p. 143).

Nevertheless, current investigations clearly indicate that present-day global food production is sufficient to feed the world's population. The main limiting factor, especially in poorer, less technically developed coutries is *lack of accessibility* of food, because of poverty or landlessness. At the same time increases in population size increase the numbers of mouths to feed.

The problem of lack of accessibility of sufficient food affects disadvantaged minorities world-wide. It particularly affects pre-industrial, largely tropical, resource-poor countries where food supplies are often already inadequate, often partly because of overemphasis on export cash crops and lack of land, sometimes associated with soil erosion, deforestation, and over-grazing. The situation has recently become further worsened in some countries, especially those lacking petroleum, minerals, and key foods, and/or with the general disruption of civil war or around disruption. This is because they become dependent on costly imported food and/or oil products to continue modernizing their agriculture via the 'green revolution' and the use of over-mechanized technology poorly adapted to the needs of the area. Fortunately, this may be beginning to change with major emphasis being given by many governments to self-sufficiency in the main *local* foods, using affordable 'appropriate technology' (p. 361). At the same time continuing very rapid population increase, especially in less technically developed countries, and world-wide ecological and climatic deterioration seem certain to pose huge problems in the future.

In addition, a tremendous population shift from the rural to the urban areas is now taking place all over the world including Third World countries. This is producing a different demographic situation with new problems related to the rapid change from rural to urban life-styles. Essentially, this represents a fundamental alteration from a subsistence, food-growing economy, with the support of a closely knit pattern of relatives and kinship groups, to the often hostile world and cash economy of the city. In such urban circumstances, almost all food has to be purchased, for which the 'new townsmen' have little preparation, and the foods most available are often those which are cheapest and most easily transported and stored. The pattern of infant feeding has been particularly affected, with change from breastfeeding to bottle-feeding and a consequent increased incidence of the marasmus–diarrhoea syndrome and decrease in the biological child-spacing resulting from lactation amenorrhoea.

Data collection

Information concerning population issues of nutritional relevance includes family details and the demography of the community (Table 4.2, p. 150), especially the sample or cohort under investigation.[55] Appropriate items may be obtained in the course of some field studies, or from existing data in government records, especially from recent demographic surveys.

In addition, knowing attitudes towards fertility may be helpful, if obtainable or available. Frequently, as is well recognized, these attitudes may strongly favour a large family size. In long-standing traditional agricultural communities, these attitudes are related to increasing the family work force at little cost, as well as the other traditional reasons for desiring large numbers of children. This is suggested by the ancient Korean proverb given at the beginning of this section.

Political factors

I want there to be no peasant in my realm so poor that he will not have a chicken in his pot every Sunday.

Henry IV of France (1553–1610)

Politics and policies

Political decisions lie at the heart of most aspects of community nutrition, particularly concerning realistic and sincerely carried out economic, agricultural, and social policies. Basic concerns include the level of real attention given to a relatively equitable distribution of resources (income, land, services) within a population. They also encompass such indirect adjustment mechanisms as price subsidies for basic foods, encouragement of their production locally, decisions concerning family planning programmes, and actual emphasis given to the practical development of primary health care services, particularly including nutritional activities using appropriate technology (p. 361).

Political factors have a key role in many ways, whether at international, regional, or community levels. Modern nutritional success stories have occurred in previously relatively less technically developed countries with capitalist regimes, such as Costa Rica, Taiwan, South Korea, and Singapore, as well as in Communist countries, such as Cuba and China. However, many countries with multiple problems, such as lack of practical commitment for nutrition and health programmes, poor management

[55] See Appendix 4 for common epidemiological terms.

and communications, economic problems, and deficient funding (especially for recurrent expenditure) have made limited progress. Not infrequently, the ultimate 'patient' may be the government and its political and economic priorities, exacerbated by civil strife.

Over-complex programmes are often limited to short-term goals (including pilot projects receiving unrealistic support which cannot possibly be replicated on a large scale) and, therefore, can be major constraints in implementing more generalized nutrition policy effectively. Also, obviously, an unstable political situation, particularly civil unrest or war, has severe short- and long-term nutritional repercussions. The very large present-day world refugee situation emphasizes this.

The improvement of the nutritional standard of a nation depends more than anything else on the political will of the government — that is, its understanding, priorities, and determination, especially related to policies regarding national food production and reducing inequities in the distribution of resources.

Knowledge of the local administrative hierarchy and of governmental policy is needed, both as practised and as theoretically defined in any written or informal national plans.

Cultural influences

The wildest dreams of Kew are the facts of Katmandu,
And the crimes of Clapham chaste in Martaban.
Rudyard Kipling (1865–1936)

Knowledge of the local culture pattern is essential for the successful conduct of any field investigation, for an understanding of the local causes of malnutrition, and for the ultimate implementation of any programe aimed at improving the situation. Indeed, malnutrition may be primarily due to cultural practices, rather than to poverty or food shortage. However, in many circumstances, cultural factors play a lesser role than economics, especially in urban areas which have cash economies, unemployment and inflation.

Also, several recent detailed studies by anthropologists with long residence in communities show that there is often considerable difference between stated custom and actual practice. In other words, the adherence to a custom varied from strict observance to modifications based on 'rules to break rules' (Lederman 1986).

Ideally, knowledge of cultural factors should include an understanding of the history of the society and the present leadership structure, social hierarchies, kinship systems, religion (including attitudes toward life, death, and disease), and the cultural philosophy concerning life-goals and values. As much understanding as possible should be acquired, especially concerning certain aspects of the culture pattern that have a more direct bearing on the nutritional problems. Only these will be touched upon here.

Food attitudes

Usually, humans do not eat all the potentially edible materials available, except reluctantly in extreme famine circumstances. More often, the cultural pattern, learned from parents and others in the community by subconscious observation and by explicit instruction, classifies items as appropriate or inappropriate, as food or non-food.

The food classifications employed, which have no relation to scientific divisions (e.g. protein, vitamins, etc.), are often extremely complex, but appear natural, normal, and obviously correct for the particular community, whether in Africa or North America. The more important and commonly found classifications of nutritional importance include:

1. *Food and non-food* — those of the potentially edible local items that are viewed as food and those which are not eaten.
2. *Age-group, or sex-linked, foods* — items regarded as suitable, or forbidden, for various age-groups or sexes, in particular for young children or women, and during pregnancy, the puerperium or lactation.
3. *Special occasion foods* — items especially associated with culturally defined holidays or periods of rejoicing.
4. *Disease-linked foods* — items deemed to produce illness in some circumstances (e.g. eggs and fish are believed to cause intestinal worms if given to young children in Malaya), or items to be avoided in certain diseases (e.g. the restriction on 'hot' (*garam*) foods in illnesses of the same classification in India).
5. *Foods to be avoided in illness* — including general restriction or periods of starvation.
6. *Cultural 'super-foods'* — often the main staple (e.g. rice in much of South-East Asia, corn (maize) in Central America, and plantains for the Baganda of East Africa), having great historical, psychological, and emotional significance to the particular community and tending to dominate the local diet.
7. *Modern prestige foods* — relatively newly introduced foods, most often in towns, which may have become symbols of prestige and modern living (imitation of socio-economic 'superiors'; influence of advertising). They may include various forms of tinned milk, milk-carbohydrate powders, aerated bottled drinks, etc.

A consideration of food attitudes can also include domestic task analysis (p. 188), particularly methods of food preparation (e.g. cooking practices, types of pots, stove and fuel, domestic measures) and meal patterns, including times, usual dishes, family order of eating ('intrahousehold distribution') — especially restrictions for women), special dishes for children, way of taking food, (use of cutlery, chopsticks, fingers, etc.)

Disease causation[56]

Local concepts of the causation, cure, and prevention of disease are extremely important. Illnesses, especially diarrhoea, are often treated by dietary changes, mainly of a restrictive nature, as well as with herbals and appropriate magical ritual. Knowledge of the methods employed, particularly the dietary practices in common illnesses such as diarrhoea (Jelliffe *et al.* 1987), and the ideology of indigenous healers is also important.

The advanced, and therefore more obvious, syndromes of malnutrition are often recognized and classified by indigenous peoples. The terms used usually refer descriptively to some striking feature, or to the presumed cause. For example, in an Indonesian language, *sisikan* (fish scale) is the appropriate descriptive word for a Bitôt's spot (p. 266). The Luganda word *obwosi* (synonymous with kwashiorkor), means 'disease of the displaced child'. However, such vernacular terms for types of malnutrition usually are not related to the main dietary aetiology.

Child-rearing

The general pattern followed in rearing young children can be most relevant nutritionally, especially with regard to the following:

1. *Obstetrical practices* — pre-natal maternal diet, immediate procedure with placenta (e.g. draining of blood and effect on neonatal iron stores).

2. *Neonatal practices* — 'pre-lacteal' feeds (given to newborn babies before lactation is fully established), laxatives, discarding of colostrum.

3. *Breastfeeding* — numerous patterns of breastfeeding exist, a fact that is not often appreciated. There is a need for a clearer, more defined system of classification, including frequency during day and night, use of other feeds, and many other variables. The term 'breastfeeding' by itself is quite unsatisfactory and inadequately descriptive. Local 'management' practices, including when started, techniques of nipple preparation, in-

[56] Disease-linked food classifications are often related to local concepts of body physiology (Foster 1952), as, for example, the ancient Indian view that health or ill-health are related to the balance in the body of three *dosha* (humours) (Jelliffe 1957). The food habits of many cultures have been listed on microfiches in the HRAF (Human Relation Area Files), available at many universities, notably in the USA.

digenous tests of breast-milk, duration of exclusive, predominant or partial breastfeeding, number of feeds per day (including night feeds), mixed milk feeding, local galactogogues (foods, herbs, or procedures believed to increase milk production), diet of the mother (normal, restricted, increased), community influences on breastfeeding (p. 200), when stopped.

4. *Animal milk* — type, quantity, dilution, feeding method (e.g. cup and spoon, bottle, local feeding-vessel, etc.), milk preparations (e.g. yoghurt, cheese).

5. *Feeding orphans and twins* — wet nurse, induced lactation, artificial feeding and method.

6. *Supplementary foods* — age introduced,[57] type, quantity, method of cooking, preparing (including 'pre-chewing'), feeding (e.g. spoon, finger, tongue).

7. *Other nutrient-rich foods* (animal and vegetable) — age introduced, type, quantity, method of feeding.

8. *Method of (and reasons for) stopping breastfeeding* (weaning) — age, abrupt or gradual, sent away or not, child prepared or not, the use of deterrent substances on breast, 'compensation' or not, apparent reasons for weaning.

9. *Food preparations for children* — special foods and their preparation; if none, which adult foods used, recipes, number of meals daily, methods of child feeding, diet given during infections.

10. *Person responsible for feeding* — mother, grandmother, older sibling, etc.

11. *Attention to sex of child* (and other attributes) — preferential treatment of male (more commonly) or female children (Khosla 1980); any special practices for unusual children, including breech delivery, albinism, born with teeth, etc.

12. *Emotional support* — love and attention by mother or others verous parental neglect.

Especially important are the 'cultural blocks' which restrict or limit the use of available nutritious foods for young children or pregnant and lactating women (Jelliffe 1957) and the impact on food habits of advertising, especially via mass media, which is often a form of cultural manipulation.

Food production

Important aspects of the local culture pattern will be concerned with food production and will include customs relating to methods of cultivation,

[57] When possible, differentiation needs to be made between small amounts given early on as part of traditional practices or Western ideas, and the introduction of increasing quantities of weaning food.

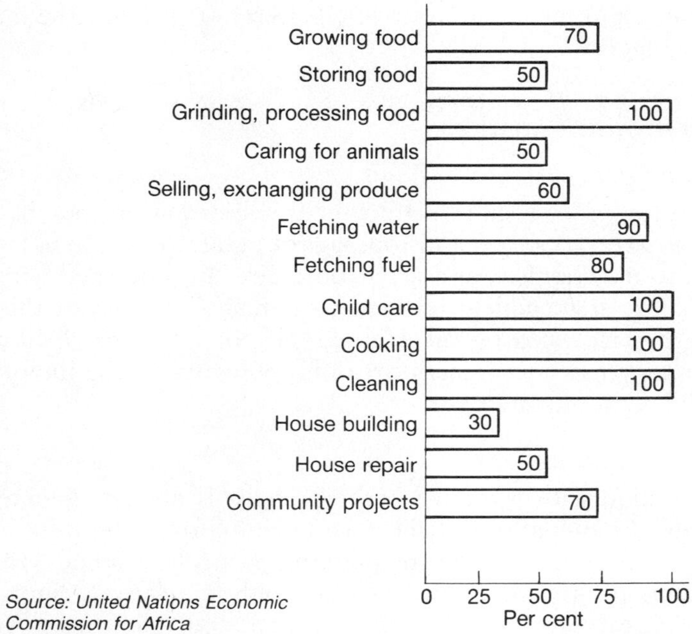

Fig. 4.3 Share of work performed by women in Africa. (Courtesy of Chandler 1985).

animal husbandry, and food storage (p. 165). Cultural influences can include the underappreciated, usually heavy work load undertaken by women (Chandler 1985) (Fig. 4.3).

Cross-cultural survey problems

Many problems may arise in survey work as a result of cross-cultural misunderstandings. The following difficulties, observed in various parts of the world, may make modification of the study design necessary:

1. *Local concepts of modesty.* These often limit the extent of the clinical assessment by restricting the examination of women to female team members. Likewise, people may be offended by the clothes or behaviour of the field investigators.

2. *Specimen collection.* This may be misunderstood and refused through fear that blood or urine may be used for magical purposes, or that its loss may weaken the donors, generally, or permanently weaken the arm from which blood was taken.

3. *Difficulties with names and numbers.* Problems can arise, for example, when the culture forbids that one's own name or that of one's

husband or child, or the number of children in the family, be mentioned before strangers.

Collection of information

Background data

Library research into cultural factors is important. It can be difficult because in some countries anthropological publications are not generally available to nutritionists, and are seldom directly concerned with aspects of the culture immediately relevant to nutrition. However, this is now changing as evidenced by the bibliography of Christine Wilson (1979) and a much greater awareness by anthropologists of the importance of food habits and nutrition.

General field data

If collaboration with a trained anthropologist is not possible, the nutritionist must be prepared to collect as much approximate information as possible concerning the culture pattern, particulary while visiting the homes. This is difficult to do, as often only a relatively short time is available. Great care must be taken to make only the most broad and tentative conclusions. Nevertheless, guided by such background information as is available, and by knowledge of the ways of 'parallel groups' with similar modes of life, a nutrition team can obtain at least limited insight into the local culture pattern, even in the course of rapid ecological visits, by means of such 'unobtrusive measures' (Webb *et al.* 1972) noted by intelligent, diplomatic observation. These 'unobtrusive measures' include the observation of physical evidence suggesting frequent or infrequent usages. In some cases, observation may be combined with interviews and the use of questionnaires, such as have been developed by Den Hartog (1977) and Scrimshaw and Hurtado (1987).

In relatively rapid prevalence studies, it is particularly valuable to have a daily meeting of all staff after the survey has been completed for the day, when impressions of the local way of life can be pooled and possible clues to relevant features of the culture pattern discussed. For example, it may be noticed that certain types of charms or amulets are commonly worn, or that certain medicinal scar patterns are frequent in some age-groups, or that differences of costume or physical adornment exist in different age-groups. Some clues are always to be found and can be followed up subsequently by further directed observation, and by discreet and friendly indirect enquiry at the survey site or in the homes.

Special field data

Detailed information can be best obtained by joint studies with a trained nutritional anthropologist. This field has emerged as a specialty in recent years. If obtainable, the results of intensive 'in-depth' investigations, such as can be obtained by participant observation, are of great value in community nutritional assessment. The use of 'life stories' or 'focus group interviews' can also be very helpful in eliciting attitudes towards foods (Manoff 1985; Griffiths 1987).

Occasionally, an anthropologist may already be working in the community to be investigated, in which case collaboration is indicated, if feasible and mutually agreeable. Alternatively, if there are several culturally and ecologically similar groups in an area, it may be possible to select one in which an anthropologist is already at work. If so, the ideal time for collaboration between nutritonist and anthropologist is in the second year or early in the third year of the latter's field study, by which time he or she will speak the vernacular fluently, be accepted by the community, and be deeply versed in many aspects of its culture. Furthermore, by that time, the anthropologist may be expected to welcome the further insight into the community being studied that can result from an investigation by a group with different perspectives, interests, technical knowledge and skill.

It may be found that the anthropologist has been concentrating principally on a particular aspect of the local culture pattern. For example, the main concern may be the clan system or kinship relations. However, at the same time a great deal of information useful to the nutrionist will have been accumulated, although sometimes the anthropologist may not appreciate its public health significance. Conversely, the subtleties of the causation of behaviour that so greatly influence nutrition may not be obvious to the non-anthropologist without explanation.

Nowadays, trained nutritional anthropologists are playing roles in teams concerned with nutritional assessment of communities. For example, their detailed ethnographic investigations, usually of a relatively small number of families, can complement very appropriately the results obtained on the prevalence of malnutrition in cross-sectional surveys.

Publications (Pelto and Pelto 1978; Jerome *et al.* 1980; Scrimshaw and Hurtado 1987) describe some current views on the range of techniques available to the nutritional anthropologist. These include participant observation, interviews with key informants, investigation of 'positive deviants',[58,59] unobtrusive observation (including child-following) (Wilson 1974), assessment for preferences ('hedonistic scale') (Peryam and Pilgrim 1975), the collection of life histories, activity analyses, structured interviews, and professional questionnaires, together with specialized

[58] 'Positive deviant' sampling involves identifying families *without* nutritional problems living in apparently similar circumstances to those having such problems and carrying out a small-scale comparative study of contrasting food habits and other ecological factors (Wishik and Van der Vynckt 1976; Zeitlin *et al.* 1987*a*).

[59] See Appendix 4 for common epidemiological terms.

methods based on ratings and rankings, semantic differential techniques, and projective methods, and the content and analysis of myths and folk tales. Pelto and Pelto (1980) also detail the use of modern technology, such as tape recorders, cameras, and video-recorders. Lozoff and Brittennham (1977) describe the use of portable field devices for the serial recording of community activities in the field ready for direct transcribing on to computer tape (Stephenson *et al.* 1975). With such devices, a continuous monitoring of family activities and energy usage, such as reported by Montgomery (1978) among the Machiguenga hunter–gatherers of South American rain forests (Table 4.5), becomes more feasible (although costly), as does the possibility of serially recording the dietary intake of young children. More often, records of activity have been timed by an observer (Acheson *et al.* 1980).

From another field altogether, the 'focus group interview' has been developed. Essentially, this comprises carefully guided informal discussion among a group of individuals concerned with the particular issue. With young child nutrition and feeding, this will usually be mothers. This technique is, of course, far from mathematically exact, but gives important qualitative guidance (Scrimshaw and Hurtado 1987). It is a major method in devising social marketing strategies (Manoff 1985; Griffiths 1987).

Geography and climate

> *The other races in Europe differ from one another, both as to stature and shape, owing to the changes of the seasons, which are very great and frequent, and because the heat is strong, the winters severe, and there are frequent rains, and again protracted droughts, and winds, from which many and diversified changes are induced.*
>
> Hippocrates (fl. 400 BC)
> *On Airs, Waters, and Places*

Many aspects of the environment, notably geography and climate, relate to nutritional status in numerous ways, most importantly via opportunities and potential for food production in general, and for certain types of food and cash crops in particular. Soil erosion may occur from overgrazing of herds or from attempted agriculture on the thin soil made available following the clearing of tropical forests. Annual cyclical changes in climate may lead to a yearly 'hungry (or lean) season', often before the harvest, with, for example, resulting lower birth weights (Bantje 1983). Drastic climatic changes, such as prolonged droughts or floods, remain major causes of widespread severe malnutrition or famine in less technically developed countries. This is illustrated, for example, by the

Table 4.5 Recorded activities among the Machiguenga hunter-gatherers of South America *(Montgomery 1978)*

Major activity* categories	Examples	Men				Women			
		Minutes	%	Calories/day	%	Minutes	%	Calories/day	%
Wild foods	Hunting, gathering	122	8.5	645	20.1	51	3.5	227	11.8
Garden labour	Garden activities	144	10.0	722	22.5	51	3.5	134	7.0
Food preparation	Cleaning, boiling, etc.	12	0.8	22	0.7	141	9.8	268	13.9
Eating	All, except in forest	71	4.9	135	4.2	55	3.8	71	3.7
Child care	Nursing, holding, etc.	1	0.1	2	0	69	4.8	96	5.0
Hygiene	Sweeping, laundry, bathing	20	1.4	47	1.5	35	2.4	88	4.6
Manufacture	Wood, cotton work, etc.	81	5.6	300	9.4	124	8.6	211	11.0
Visiting	Activities in others' houses	62	4.3	81	2.5	45	3.1	45	2.3
Idle/recreation	Playing, drinking, music	141	9.8	184	5.7	149	10.3	149	7.7
Other	Labour for trade goods, travel for trading, etc.	126	8.8	404	12.6	59	4.1	107	5.6
Daylight hours		780	54.2	2542	79.2	779	53.9	1396	72.6
Night hours		660	45.8	660	20.6	660	45.8	528	27.4
24-hour totals		1440	100.0	3202	99.8	1439	99.7	1924	100.0

* Results show a much greater share of the physical 'garden activities' (agricultural labour) borne by men than in many cultures.

severe, prolonged drought and civil war in sub-Saharan Africa in the 1980s, especially in Ethiopia and the Sudan, leading to widespread famine.

Other unique situations can affect communities living at high altitudes, in polar regions and in the tropics. An underappreciated human economic and nutritional dependence on the weather was highlighted recently by the severe effects of the 1982–83 'El Niño' ocean changes in the Pacific, and its impact on Peruvian anchovy fish shoals.

Although it has been appreciated for years that growth in children is usually greater in the warmer months of the year, the only nutritional syndromes specifically and directly related to climate seem to be rickets and osteomalacia. This is because biologically, human vitamin D requirements are mainly obtained as a result of irradiation of exposed skin to the ultraviolet rays in sunlight. Smaller contributions are obtained from the dietary intake, although this becomes more important in areas with less sunshine, extensive clothing, and/or customs which limit exposure for various reasons (p. 270). Seasonal influences also need consideration in nutritional assessment in many practical ways. These include accessibility of communities during the rains, the prevalence of some contributory infections (e.g. malaria, diarrhoea, etc.), and presence of the population at home or away (e.g. harvesting, school attendance, etc.).

Apart from the influence of topography and soil on agricultural productivity, the geography of an area, such as the existence of mountains, rivers, and deserts, influences the distribution of foods and the outreach of health and other services.

While detailed information may not be practicable, descriptions of general geographic and climatic factors need to be included as part of the overall picture in reports of all studies of community nutritional assessment.

5

Assessment of ecological variables II — Food considerations

General

Turning to contemporary human populations, we find an array of food habits running the gamut from almost total carnivory to almost total vegetarianism. Among South-East Asian agriculturists, meat, eggs, milk, and fish are only rarely consumed and even then only in miniscule quantities. Seemingly the list of foods and combinations of foods which can support human life is endless.

W.A. Stini (1980)
Human Adaptability to Nutritional Stress

Conflict over food is one of the oldest and most entrenched characteristics of human society. Yet is is often least visible. Sure enough, we see the battling moves and countermoves when there is, say, a food riot, or when a hunger march breaks the peace of a town. But in our normal day-to-day life the battling aspects of food entitlement are very much below the surface. Battles over food are persistently waged in widely different arenas, including (1) the market (2) political processes, and even (3) family relations.

Amantya Sen (1982) *Unequal Access to Food*

Assessment of the various links in the 'food chain' from agricultural production to consumption in the human diet (Fig. 4.4) can form an important aspect of the detailed analysis of the ecological factors responsible for the nutritional status of any community. The degree of detail with depend on need and resources available.

In some earlier public health investigations, 'food considerations' were sometimes given inadequate attention. This is partly because assessment by clinical signs, laboratory tests, and anthropometry were more familiar to often medically oriented staff, and because of the complexity of the food chain and the difficulties in carrying out quantitative studies.

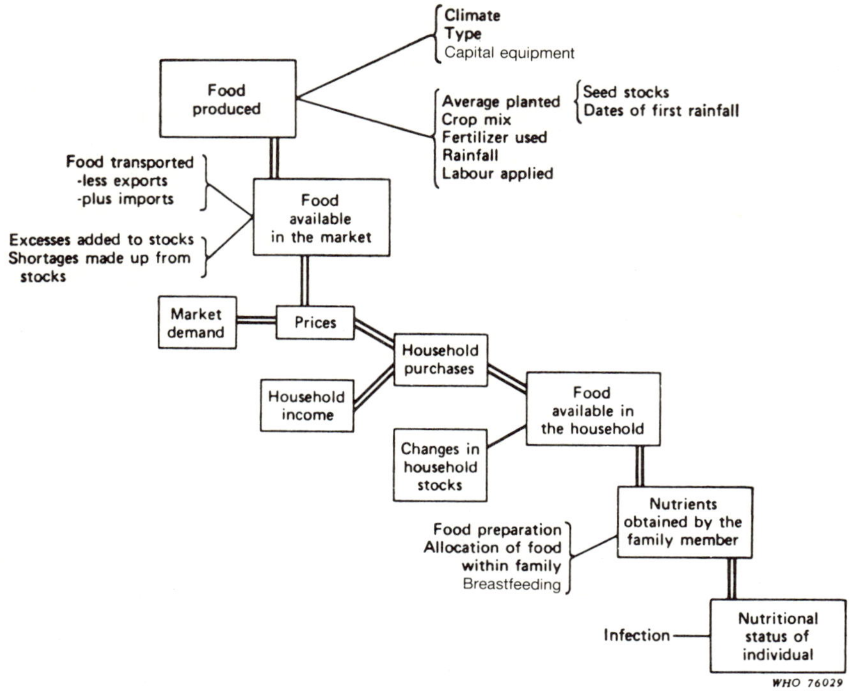

Fig. 4.4 Food chain from production to consumption (WHO 1976).

Many factors make up the food chain (Fig. 4.4), and these have also been described from a statistical viewpoint by Hay and Freeman (1978). Data on all or usually a selection of these can be collected as a part of nutritional assessment, depending upon resources of money, staff, and time; the acceptability and practicability of different methods; and the purpose or purposes of the investigation.

The reasons for such investigations may include, for example, one or more of the following: the identification of 'at risk' groups with dietary inadequacy (p. 453); the corroboration of clinical, anthropometric, or other findings; the recognition of changes in food habits over years; the suggestion of potentially remediable dietary practices (especially in infant feeding or excessive calorie intakes); and, on a national scale, changes in food prices relative to wages, and nutritionally illogical, costly import–export policies which often tend to benefit the well-to-do.

In-depth assessment of relevant factors affecting the food chain can best be based on the knowledge and skills of different available professionals, including, for example, agronomists, agricultural extension workers, veterinarians, home economists, anthropologists, and meteorologists. These types of specialized enquiry highlight the complex nature of community nutrition, and emphasize the need for appropriate interdisciplinary collaboration whenever possible. However, as always, careful consideration will be needed to select a limited number of feasible methods appropriate to the objectives of the investigation and the resources available.

In the present account, the following will be considered: *food availability, food accessibility, food preparation, food consumption, food utilization,* and *estimating nutritional adequacy.*

From a community or national point of view, this section is mainly concerned with less technically developed countries. Reviews of methods and results in industrialized countries have been given for Europe, North America, and Oceania (FAO 1977), France (Debry 1976), UK (Marr and Berry 1975), US (Beal 1967; Christakis 1973; Abraham *et al.* 1977; *Am. J. Clin. Nutr.* 1982), and West Germany (Haenel and Mohr 1974).

Disselduff *et al.* (1979) have described a method of assessing the intake of food additives. Recently, emphasis has been re-aroused concerning the often underappreciated widespread contamination of aflatoxin in many cereal grains and legumes, with a direct toxic ill-effect and a possible role in the aetiology of kwashiorkor (p. 276) (Hendrickse 1984). If this is of real significance, assessment of aflatoxin contamination may need to be considered with additional care in areas at risk.

Food availability

The availability of foods of different types depends on production, storage, preservation, distribution, marketing, and economic incentives. The data that are both collectable and valuable in nutritional assessment will depend on whether information is being sought from individuals or from families (or households or 'eating groups'), or from communities (e.g. villages), or from nations (either irregularly or as a part of continuing on-going nutritional surveillance) (p. 551), or from a combination of sources. Apart from important issues concerning cultural factors affecting the diet (p. 276), the two main considerations are usually actual physical availability, and 'accessibility' (mainly related to adequacy of family funds and/or land) (p. 185).

At the community or family level, many factors affect food availability including traditional and modern considerations:

1. *Family food supply:* home-produced, purchased, wild (collected, hunted, fished), obtained by barter; seasonal variation; cash crops; methods of storage (including loss to insects, rodents, etc.) and preservation (e.g. drying, salting, pickling); preparation and cooking (p. 188); intra-familial distribution (p. 165).
2. *Farming methods:* hoe, plough, mechanized; bush clearing, rotation;

double-cropping; irrigation; drainage; fertilization; insect and pest control; availability of extension services; modern versus technical methods.

3. *Land:* pattern of tenure, area per family, suitability (for different crops, pasture , infertile, etc.), actual utilization (especially staples, vegetable protein foods, cash crops); home gardens; number of agricultural workers (family, hired labourers).

4. *Livestock and fishing:* number of livestock (cattle, sheep etc.), milk production (yield, milk not used), fishing facilities (freshwater, ponds, sea; methods (e.g. nets, tackle, types of craft etc.); yields, including export items, such as shrimp, turtle, etc.

5. *Finance:* cost of key foods, cost/nutrient value of foods (p. 187); capital available, facilities for credit, purchasing power, stabilization of prices, co-operatives, indebtedness.

6. *Distribution:* communications (roads, transport); storage, preservation, and processing (home, industrial); marketing (local, regional, and world trade, prices and availability of foods).

Collection of information

Background data

In many countries, information on national food availability ('food balance sheets') is collected annually by governments. Since 1961, FAO has developed the Rome-based ICS ('Inter-linked Computer Storage and Processing System of Food and Agricultural Data'), which contains annually updated statistics on food and agriculture from more than 162 countries (FAO 1977).

Food balance sheets Health workers are often not aware of food balance sheets. These are estimates showing the total quantity of different foods or categories of food produced in a country during a specified period, usually a year, to which are added the total quantities of imported foods. Adjustments are made for any change in stocks which have occurred during the full reference period (Table 4.6). Deductions are made from this total amount of food for quantities of food exported, used for seed, fed to livestock, used in industry, other non-food uses, and general food losses incurred during storage and transportation. The figures obtained represent food available for consumption on a national basis.

From figures concerning the amounts of different foods available and population data, the theoretical *per capita* availability of each food can be obtained. These can then be converted into nutrients (e.g. protein, calories, fat, etc.) by using the appropriate conversion factors for each food.

National food availability can be estimated from food balance sheets. These have various obvious limitations and advantages, which have been fully described by FAO (1977). However, a general familiarity with their

Table 4.6 Sample Food Balance Sheet for Tonga. For larger countries, units are often in 10 000 metric tons (*FAO 1984*)

STANDARDIZED FOOD BALANCE SHEET
Tonga
Average 1979–81
units = 1 Metric ton

Population 97000

Imformation available as of 29 June 1983

	Production	Imports	Stock changes	Exports	Processed trade (E-I)	Domestic supply	Domestic utilization: Feed	Seed	Manufacture: Food use	Manufacture: Non-food use	Waste	Food	Per caput supply: Kilo-grams/Year	Per day: Grams	Calo-ries nos	Protein grams	Fat grams
Grand total															3200	67.3	105.8
Vegetable products															2660	37.4	61.4
Animal products															540	30.0	44.4
Grand total exc alcohol															3181	67.1	105.8
Cereals													55.6	152.3	422	12.0	1.5
Wheat		5	−178		−5164	5347					263	5085	52.5	143.9	393	11.3	1.4
Paddy rice					−112	112					2	109	1.1	3.1	9	0.2	
Maize					−1	1						1					
Prepared cereals nes		187				187						187	1.9	5.3	20	0.5	
Roots and tubers													508.7	1393.7	1361	13.0	4.1
Cassava	12823				2407	10416	1282				1282	7851	80.8	221.4	212	1.3	0.6
Sweet potatoes	79633					79633	26188				11945	41500	427.9	1172.3	1149	11.7	3.5
Sugars and honey													16.5	45.2	160		
Raw sugar		1540	36		−9	1513						1513	15.6	42.7	152		
Sugar confectionery		63				63						63	0.6	1.8	5		
Sugar and syrups nes		11				11						11	0.1	0.3	1		
Honey	16					16						16	0.2	0.5	1		
Nuts and oilseeds													94.8	259.6	375	7.8	31.2

Table 4.6 (Continued)

Groundnuts in shell	1387			3		1384	110			42	1233	12.7	34.8	124	5.3	10.2
Coconuts	99000		9511	358	31691	57440		46484	2994		7962	82.1	224.9	251	2.5	21.0
Vegetables												53.9	147.8	36	2.2	0.4
Tomatoes	1200			55		1145				120	1025	10.6	29.0	6	0.3	0.1
Fresh vegetables nes	4520	83		56		4547				460	4087	42.2	115.5	25	1.6	0.2
Dried vegetables nes		86				86					86	0.9	2.4	4	0.3	
Vegetables temp preserve		31				31					31	0.3	0.9	1		
Fruit												80.3	219.9	69	1.1	1.4
Bananas	2714			2406		308				83	225	2.3	6.4	4	0.1	
Oranges	2500	6				2506				125	2381	24.6	67.3	17	0.3	0.1
Lemons and limes	2500					2500					2500	25.8	70.6	16	0.4	0.8
Fresh tropical fruit nes	1797			39		1758				90	1668	17.2	47.1	19	0.2	0.3
Fresh fruit nes	1000	71		127		944				54	890	9.2	25.1	11	0.1	0.1
Prepared fruit nes		120				120					120	1.2	3.4	1		
Meat and offals												49.5	135.6	350	17.3	30.6
Beef and veal	186	130			−51	367					368	3.8	10.4	23	1.4	1.9
Edible offals of cattle	33					33					33	0.3	0.9	1	0.2	
Mutton and Lamb		2189				2189					2189	22.6	61.9	149	7.4	13.1
Goat meat	41					41					41	0.4	1.2	2	0.2	0.1
Pigmeat	1301	1			−10	1312					1312	13.5	37.1	133	4.1	12.7
Edible offals of pigs	87					87					87	0.9	2.4	3	0.4	0.1
Chicken meat	179	39				218					218	2.2	6.1	7	0.8	0.5
Meat nes					−534	534					534	5.5	15.0	31	2.6	2.2
Meat, dried, nes		12				12					12	0.1	0.3	1	0.2	
Hen eggs	349	2				351	11			18	322	3.3	9.1	13	1.0	0.9

Fish and seafood										36.0	98.7	75	10.2	3.4
Pelagic fish					−1480	1480			1480	15.4	42.3	39	4.4	2.2
Mabine fish nes	1995					1995			1995	20.6	56.4	36	5.8	1.2
Milk										12.7	34.6	27	1.3	1.4
Whole cow milk	268				−952	1220		5	1215	12.6	34.4	25	1.1	1.2
Whole cow milk cheese		17				17			17	0.2	0.5	2	0.1	0.1
Oils and fats										11.7	32.2	262	0.2	29.5
Vegetable oils and fats										8.2	22.5	189		21.4
Coconut oil	4529			3481		1048	474		573	5.9	16.2	143		16.2
Vegetable oils nes		8				8			8	0.1	0.2	2		0.2
Margarine, shortening		207	−10			217			217	2.2	6.1	44		5.0
Animal oils and fats										3.5	9.6	73	0.1	8.1
Cattle fat	7					7			7	0.1	0.2	2		0.2
Pig fat	130	1				131			131	1.4	3.7	30	0.1	3.3
Butter of cow milk		202				202			202	2.1	5.7	41		4.6
Spices	342	12		47		307		11	297	3.1	8.4	28	0.9	1.3
Stimulants										0.4	1.0	3	0.1	0.2
Green coffee		3				3			3		0.1			
Cocoa beans					−4	4			4		0.1			
Chocolate products nes		19				19			19	0.2	0.5	3		0.2
Tea		11				11			11	0.1	0.3			
Alcoholic beverages										14.0	38.4	19	0.2	
Beer of barley		1305				1305			1305	13.5	36.9	16	0.2	
Distilled alcohol		36				36			36	0.4	1.0	3		

fomat, usefulness, and limitations, needs to be included in the training of all working in community nutrition.

Food balance sheets have the following uses:

1. Trends may be identified in the consumption of foods among a specific population if maintenance of the food balance sheet data is possible over a period of years. Corrective measures may be suggested, especially if large-scale food shortages occur (Manetsch 1979).

2. Evaluation of the availability of food and agricultural production in the country can be made, including any undesirable reduction in *range* of foods available (Dewey 1978; Doughty 1979).

3. A country can assess degrees of self-reliance in terms of food supply or dependence on large amount of imported foods (which may entail difficulties with balance of payments and foreign debts).

4. The amount of food which could be consumed by humans, but is being diverted to the feeding of livestock, can be assessed, and this may promote reconsideration of policy.

5. Available figures on *per capita* food supply are of primary importance in making projections at governmental level for future food demands and economic policies, based on currently available data.

As with the collection of statistics in most fields, the data in food balance sheets are limited and approximate in many ways. In particular, they are usually 'aggregated data' combining information from different regions, age-groups, cultures, or socio-economic strata. Also, seasonal availability of foods in not indicated. The added data obtained from food consumption surveys can sometimes help fill gaps in information from food balance sheets.

The accuracy of food balance sheets has also been questioned and can only be approximate at best. It will depend very much on problems with collecting information, especially from subsistence farmers, and the geographical and demographic coverage of the information obtained. More recently, food balance sheets have sometimes been prepared as averages for 3–year periods. Both external and internal checks are made to validate results. Many difficulties are involved in the preparation of food balance sheets. For example, it is not possible to list all potentially edible items, including non-cultivated plant foods which are consumed in some parts of the world. Problems may occur when alcohol is not included. Also, the significance of human milk in national food balance sheets is often not considered and difficulties with doing so are unresolvable in relation to different forms of breastfeeding and volumes of milk consumed (Jelliffe and Jelliffe 1989*a*).

In summary, despite these limitations, the use of national food balance sheets can often usefully form part of investigations to assess the overall picture of the nutritional status of populations, and trends towards (or away from) national 'food security'. Results obtained can help to confirm, complement, or to bring an additional perspective to data obtained from clinical, anthropometric, and biochemical examinations, and from other methods.

Repeated food balance sheets also can give rough guidance concerning improvement or deterioration of national and world food supplies over time. For example, this is indicated in the FAO publicaton entitled *The fifth world food survey* (1981–83) (FAO 1986).

In some technically more developed countries, including the USA, a variety of information can be obtained on the international use and distribution of foods by market data and trends in purchasing of 'commodity groups' (Schwicker 1982), and by 'total food disappearance' and household consumption studies (Nesheim 1982).

Recent investigations have further emphasized the great significance in developing countries of post-harvest grain losses (including legumes), especially those caused by insects, micro-organisms, fungi, rodents, and birds. Methods of assessment of post-harvest losses have been given (Harris and Lindblad 1977). From this, it is apparent that detailed studies are difficult, complex, and likely to vary (especially with climatic conditions). They have to be undertaken by experts in different fields. This information is plainly very important, but can, at best, be undertaken with precision only in some selected areas.

According to Schofield (1979), food balance sheets can also be employed at the village level, in the unusual event that reasonably complete data on food production, crop sales, food exports, imports, and food wastage (seed and animal food) can be made available from the village. Taking all these losses into account, the total food supply and therefore the *per capita* availability of food can be measured and its nutrient content calculated. These data can then be compared with the calculated requirements or standard recommended allowances to give a measure of dietary adequacy. However, such analyses are based on village productivity data which cannot easily take into account food obtained outside the village, such as items purchased or food donations or school meals. Also, they do not measure the seasonal availability of foods or the distribution of subsistence crops within the village, between households, and between household members. This method does not provide any reliable indication of the number of people actually suffering from malnutrition and, at best, only allows rough comparisons of food availability between villages. In any case, it is very rare for this type of information to be available, unless a specialized agronomic study has been undertaken.

Attention has recently been directed to early warning systems for large-scale food crises (Currey 1984), including the potential value of satellite photographs. These can form a part of 'nutritional surveillance' (p. 374) and have been used in the recurrent Sahelian droughts of the late 1980s.

Specific survey data

In many field investigations, the collection of detailed information concerning the production of food and its availability to families may not be possible, as it calls for a lengthy and specialized investigation by agricultural nutritionists. Such studies are not normally possible in the course of most field surveys.

However, observations can sometimes be made by listing important vegetables and fruits in family gardens. Ideally, these should be particularly concerned with locally adapted plants that are nutritionally important in the particular area as 'natural vitamin–mineral supplements' with the customary staple. These include dark-green leafy vegetables and orange-coloured fruits and vegetables. They should also look particularly at 'low-effort' plants that are easy to cultivate, and 'three-dimensional' use of space in gardens (ground crops–bushes–trees). Important items in a home garden may include, for example, tropical spinach (*Amaranthus* spp.), (and other often under-used dark-green leafy vegetables), pigeon peas (*Cajanus cajan*), and papaya (or other tree crops). Details concerning the relatively speedy collection of information can form part of 'rapid rural appraisal' (p. 366).

Somewhat more detailed small-scale studies of food production and other ecological factors may be practicable for a limited sample of homesteads, as shown by early surveys carried out in Nigeria (Collis *et al.* 1962*a*, *b*) and in various Caribbean islands (PanAmerican Health Organization 1972). In such studies, at least one investigator ought to spend time in making a detailed study of a randomly selected sample of households. Where there is a considerable seasonal variation, as is usually the case, it is preferable to repeat the investigation at appropriate times within the year. Frequently, such quick investigations of traditional 'home gardens' can indicate under-used, easy-to-cultivate, 'low-effort' plant crops to be encouraged.

Other difficulties in estimating local food production and usage are due to different societies with varied mixes of foods grown, bartered, purchased, or obtained wild (caught, hunted, picked).

General survey data

In the course of rapid ecological visits to cultivation sites and markets, some outline information can be obtained concerning food production and availability. The approximate areas under cultivation with different types of crops (especially more nutritious plant foods and cash crops), the number of livestock (including small animals, such as ducks, rabbits, or guinea pigs), and methods of agriculture can be noted.

In the event that an agriculturalist is not available in a field investigation, any details of local methods of food production, preservation, and storage that cannot be understood should be noted, for discussion with such experts later. Similarly, if any food plants, cultivated or wild, cannot be recognized, the complete plant (i.e. leaves, fruit, etc.) can be collected, together with a record of the indigenous name, for identification later.

Visits to 'retail outlets', such as markets, stores (if such exist), small village shops, and (often neglected) street vendors (Cohen 1986) can be valuable since the range, cost, and possible dietary significance of nutritious and non-nutritious items available, including aerated (carbonated) drinks and infant formulas, can be seen. This also permits cost–nutrient data (p. 515) to be calculated. Information concerning the local system of credit can sometimes be collected, at least in general terms.

Shops at which local measures are purchased by housewives should also be included as part of the learning experience of field workers. Knowledge of the different sizes of spoons used locally, types of cooking pots, and measures is essential. From the visits to shops and markets, information will be acquired regarding types of units of weight and volume used in the country (i.e. kilograms, pounds; litres, pints, 'packets' of coffee beans, spoonfuls of so-called 'tonic powders', etc.). The unit cost of loaves of breads, of bean cakes, sweet biscuits, etc. may give those involved in a food consumption survey some indication of nutritional value of these commodities. (Also see: Addendum 1988.)

In some circumstances, additional qualitative information may be collected. For example, in rural Zaire, Brown and Brown (1979) undertook 'basket surveys' (inspections of the baskets of women who were leaving the market), as well as 'market surveys' (visits to markets through whole annual cycle) and home visits.

Food accessibility

It is insufficiently emphasized, although obvious, that foods may be available in adequate (or more than sufficient) amounts in a family, community, nation, or the world and yet not be accessible to all the population. As an extreme example, numerous famines have been recorded in which the overall supply of foods was adequate, but many starved. Inaccessibility of available foods is most usually 'man-made', and can occur in various political systems, as has become apparent in recent decades in Ethiopia, and among the 'homeless' in cities in the USA and Europe.

Geographical food accessibility (p. 174) can be influenced by *technical considerations*, such as the availability of methods of preservation and transport, and intra-familial accessibility by *cultural restrictions* (p. 166) affecting some groups or particular family members. However, more than anything else food accessibility depends on what is termed '*resource allocation*' by economists — that is income and/or arable land and/or social support programmes, such as rationing, governmental subsidizing of major food items ('fair price shops'), food stamps, etc. Poverty and/or ownership of inadequate amounts of land are usually major causes of malnutrition, especially in less technically developed countries.

The economic or other accessibility of different foods, especially key items such as the staple, the main legume, and cooking oil, can sometimes be estimated from national figures of income disaggregated to show its distribution and the percentage below the locally defined 'poverty level'. The cost of a basic diet needs to be calculated and the percentage of the family income of the poor needed to purchase adequate nutrients, especially calories, from foods which are traditionally the mainstay of the local diet. Attention has to be given to expenditure on 'recreational' items (e.g. alcohol, tea, aerated drinks, etc.), which can be considerable, and to the economic and nutritional significance of any social support systems that may be available, including rationing or subsidized prices of basic foods, food stamps, etc.

In rural areas, income is also important, but food accessibility usually needs to be considered principally in relation to land available together with labour and 'inputs' (seed, water, fertilizer) to produce sufficient food for the family.

Another technique of practical assistance in devising relevant nutrition education is to calculate the cost–nutrient value of local foods. In this, the cost is calculated of a specified amount of a particular nutrient in foods available. This approach can be illustrated by a cost–nutrient listing for 20 g protein and 1000 calories (usually stated as requirements for a 1-year-old child), based on a study in the late-1960s in the Caribbean (Table 4.7) (McKigney 1968). More recently, Gurney and Jutsum (1981) devised nutrient–cost nomograms for both energy (calories) and protein, based on cost of purchase and nutritional composition (Appendix 5). This procedure can be undertaken for any nutrient, especially those considered to be deficient in a particular area. This may include, for example, consideration of carotene (vitamin A precursor) or iron.

Another technique pioneered by the CFNI (Caribbean Food and Nutrition Institute) is the N-CURT ('Nutrient-Cost Users Reference Tables'). This is issued as a booklet for use by nutritionists and is up-dated several times a year. In it, the commoner foods used in the English-speaking Caribbean are listed, with major 'nutrients' (calories, protein, fat, and various vitamins and minerals) given *for different costs* (US dollars per lb). As prices fluctuate, nutritionists can compare the relative *cost* of particular nutrients in different foods at the time. This enables suggestions to be made as to the 'best buy' nutritionally.

Table 4.7 Cost–nutrient table, showing average cost of some available foods in the West Indies as sources of protein and calories (*McKigney 1968*). (Cost in East Caribbean dollars: EC$.)

Cost per 1000 calories	Food	Cost per 20 gm protein
0.22	Pulses	0.05
0.10	Cornmeal	0.08
1.20	Salt fish	0.10
0.13	Rice	0.12
0.60	Sardines	0.18
0.55	Fresh milk	0.20
0.60	Fresh beef, goat, mutton, cheddar cheese	0.20
1.80	Fresh fish	0.20
0.25	Bread	0.20
1.10	Chicken necks and backs	0.20
1.20	Corned beef	0.20
0.47	Peanut butter	0.22
0.55	Dry whole milk	0.23
0.25	Sweetened condensed milk	0.23
0.55	Evaporated milk	0.25
0.90	Minced (ground) beef	0.25
0.25	Ground provisions (root crops)	0.28
0.40	Fresh pork	0.28
2.20	Broiler meat	0.35
0.60	Irish potatoes	0.40
1.10	Frankfurters, sausages	0.40
1.60	Fresh eggs	0.40
0.80	Milk-based, cereal-based, infant foods	0.51
0.80	'Health promoting' foods	0.56
0.29	Plantain, green bananas, Ripe bananas	0.59
4.87	Infant Foods — strained meats	0.69
4.58	Infant foods — strained vegetables and meat	2.08
0.55	Arrowroot	13.00
0.09	Sugar	Infinity
0.15	Margarine, cooking oil	Infinity
0.80	Glucose	Infinity

Food preparation

A most important, but often neglected, aspect of nutritional assessment is concerned with methods of food preparation, including their effects on nutrients.

These methods can usually only be reported on in general, especially

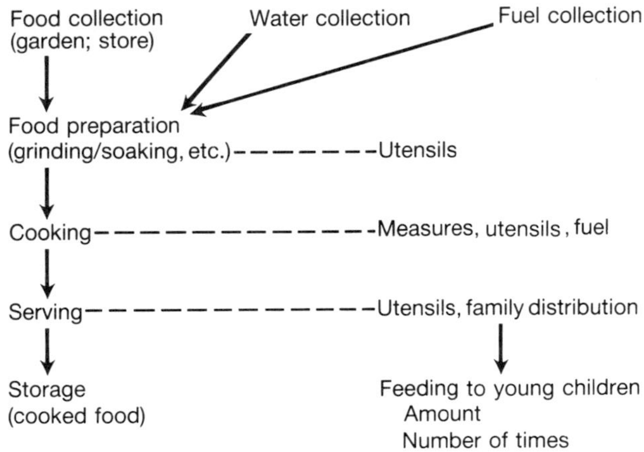

Fig. 4.5 Task analysis: some aspects needing consideration in the preparation of homemade weaning food mixtures (Jelliffe and Jelliffe 1983).

concerning the actual cooking process. Ideally, 'task analysis' can be undertaken (as described below), at least with a small number of food preparers, almost always women.

Task analysis (Fig. 4.5).

This consists of a 'time and motion study' of activities undertaken in the process of food preparation, especially cooking, but also pounding, grinding, soaking, milling, serving, feeding, and storing of cooked foods. Such analyses of existing 'culinary technology' need to consider probable effects on the availability of nutrients and the risks of introducing intestinal infections. In addition, they need to note time, cost (money, fuel, water, etc.), physical labour, utensils, and methods customarily used for preparation, serving, feeding of adults and children, order of feeding, storage, and re-use. Information can be obtained from several sources near the house as well as the kitchen (Fig. 4.6).

This type of task analysis is not generally undertaken in a planned manner, nor will this often be possible. However, a general 'focus group discussion' with the women concerned and unobtrusive observation of a 'cycle' of food preparation can be helpful. More detailed information can be obtained in careful studies of a sample of mothers by observation of the whole process as indicated in the flow sequence shown in Fig. 4.6, obtained from various sources of information in addition to the kitchen.

The results of task analyses may suggest whether advice on available foods given in current nutrition education fits into actual practices. More particularly, it may indicate if specific appropriate technology (p. 361),

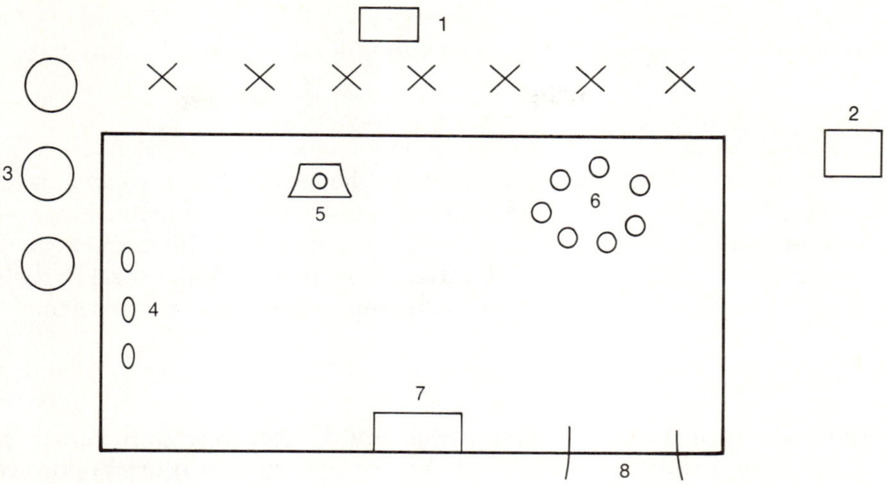

Fig. 4.6 Household nutrition: appropriate technology and sources of information. (1) Three-dimensional multipurpose garden (including compost); (2) water (collection, source); (3) crop storage; (4) food preservation and preparation; (5) cooking (energy source); (6) serving; (7) storage (cooked foods); (8) home visit (nutritional assessment, treatment, advice, referral).

within cultural, economic, and physical restraints, can be suggested to improve the nutritional value of local food, reduce risks of intestinal infection from food contamination, decrease cost of fuel used, and minimize the mother's time and labour in food preparation.

Food consumption: general

It is important to have as much detailed knowledge as possible concerning the foods actually eaten in the community, through food consumption (dietary intake studies). This information is needed for assessing nutritional status and for suggesting dietary causes that may be amenable to correction. Indeed, some form of basic dietary assessment should be included in most investigations of the nutritional status of individuals and communities. However, collecting meaningful, detailed information on dietary consumption can be extremely difficult and time-consuming. Compromises need to be made, using a method, or combination of methods, which ideally should be 'reproducible, objective, unbiased and economical in time and personnel ... with procedures standardized (as far as possible) to permit comparability between population groups' (Hankin 1982). The validity, reliability, and reproducibility of methods need constant consideration, or quite unwarranted conclusions may be drawn (Appendix 4).

Information is needed on different aspects of the background that influences family eating patterns, including food cycles and eating habits.

Food cycles

The seasonal production of crops affect the types of foods available at different times of the year. This often means that, when practicable, food consumption studies should be repeated at appropriate times in the agricultural cycle. Other sources of variation include periodic market days, and religious and other holidays, including 'weekends' or equivalents.

Eating habits

Some aspects of the cultural determinants of the diet were given earlier (p. 165). The main dietary pattern in the community will often be known already, but changing habits need to be investigated. For the poor, recent urbanization can mean that the accustomed range of foods are no longer available. In sophisticated Westernized circumstances, the possible influence of alternative dietary practices needs to be borne in mind, including, for example, faddist and slimming diets.

At the domestic level, knowledge of usual recipes and details of methods of cooking are important. Knowledge of the customary meal patterns is needed, as these may differ greatly in different cultures as regards timing and 'heaviness' (e.g. snack or main meal). This information should also include which household or family members eat together or alone and in what sequence; the eating utensils employed; and whether separate servings are given to each individual or a shared pot or dish is the usual pattern. The last mentioned practice may mean that the weakest, smallest, and least dexterous members are able to obtain little food and/or less choice of ingredients, especially if these are in the form of an often nutritious sauce eaten with the staple. The general distribution of food within the family and among the upper socio-economic groups surveyed needs recognition in general terms, as does the distribution of foods to servants and employees in households. The overall pattern of dishes served during weekends or on feast days should be known, as well as the potential for dietary restriction or change in feeding pattern during days or periods of fasting, such as Ramadan.

Methods

Various methods of estimating food intake in individuals or households have been employed in many parts of the world. One important bibliography and summary showing the countries covered from 1965 to 1970, the main methods used, and how the results are expressed was

Table 4.8 Some commonly used methods of estimating food consumption or dietary intake in more and less sophisticated communities. (*For recent bibliography: Krantzler* et al. *1982*b)

	Recording	Observing and measuring	Questioning
More sophisticated communities	Food diary by subjects	Home weighing by subjects	Self-administered standardized questionnaire (administered over 3–6 months)
		Home inventory measurement	
			Telephone dietary recall (usually 24 hours)
			Telephone dietary recall (plus portion size used)
			Food frequency recall
Less sophisticated communities		Weighing by investigators (+/− observation of distribution at meals in household measures)	24-hour dietary recall
			24-hour recall (plus estimated portion size)
			Group interviews

published by FAO (1980). Krantzler *et al.* (1982*b*) collected a more recent annotated bibliography. Such studies are often easier to conduct in some less technically developed countries because of the limited range of food consumed and cooking methods used.

The methods selected should, as always, take into account the available resources (funds, manpower, training facilities, transport) and needs as regards the purpose of the investigation (e.g. the hypothesis being tested), the group to which directed (e.g. young children, elderly, whole families, frequency of guests, etc.), and the characteristics of the population (e.g. separateness of dwellings, literacy, social organization, and co-operation). There are three main practical ways in which food intake can be measured: (1) *recording;* (2) *observing and measuring;* and (3) *questioning* (Table 4.8).

In addition, *chemical analysis of actual diets* can play a role under special circumstances. In this method, aliquot portions of all meals are removed and their nutrient content analysed (Alleyne *et al.* 1977). This approach is precise, but is too costly, complicated, and impractical, except in special research circumstances. These can include small-scale analyses of mixtures used for children during the weaning or transitional period (6 months to 2 years), or in special investigations of individuals in metabolic wards. However, even these analyses give no indication of the bioavailability of nutrients from the food mixtures after their ingestion.

Difficulties in assessing the exact composition of a meal by chemical analysis are considerable, especially if the item is a composite cooked dish. Often, standard recipes for dishes do not exist and a better meal than usual may be prepared. Some workers have suggested that, if an accuracy greater than 20 per cent were required, the uncooked ingredients should be weighed prior to the cooking of the dish. However, the housewife understandably may object to the repeated presence of strangers interrupting her cooking arrangements. The use of a replicated meal which duplicates as far as possible the household fare can be made and anaylsed, as well as the plate waste from the dish prepared by the housewife. A reliable laboratory is needed in which the chemical analysis of the different nutrients can be made with accuracy. This is very rarely available in less technically developed countries, although the possibility of freeze-drying representative, weighed samples and air-freighting them to appropriate laboratories may sometimes be feasible for research purposes.

At a more practical level, the *composition of basic cooked foods* widely eaten in a particular country (e.g. boiled yam, *tortillas*, corn meal porridge, etc.) and of common food mixtures prepared with a 'common recipe' need to be known and analysis of their nutrient content may be possible without too great expense ('nutrient data bank'). (Also see Addendum 1988.)

Commonly used practical methods (Table 4.8) The most commonly used practical methods are either 'recollective' — that is, relying on what people *say* concerning their diet (e.g. recording and questioning), with obvious opportunities for error and for over- or under-statement — and/or what investigators *see* (e.g. observing and measuring food preparation). Various methods can be used in each of these methods. Selection will depend on such issues as *the purpose of the investigation* (e.g. screening for malnutrition, assessing average food intake, determining the intake of key foods, identification of high-risk groups, etc.), *the age-groups concerned* (e.g. families, infants, elderly), *the nutritional focus* (e.g. general dietary adequacy; specific locally significant nutrients, such as beta-carotene, sodium or sugar (for dental caries)[60]; *other items*, such as fibre, environmental pollutants, goitrogens, aflatoxin, etc.), and the *local situation* (e.g. degree of literacy and motivation, availability of a telephone, etc.).

[60] A 'sucrose questionnaire' can include liquid, solid, and 'sticky' items in studies concerned with dental caries.

Examples of the use of different methods for different purposes in different circumstances, range from the assessment of dietary intake of cereal by 24-hour recall as an overall measure of calorie sufficiency by the National Institute of Nutrition in India, contrasted with detailed opportunities for the comparison of dietary recall, weighing, and diet analyses in an isolated Antarctic base (Acheson *et al.* 1980).

Whatever method, or preferably combination of methods, are selected, appropriate forms need to be prepared. Pre-testing is always required in the particular community being investigated.

Recording

In this method, the daily household consumption of different foods is recorded in a diary. This technique has been used mainly in industrialized countries, with literate, motivated, nutrition-conscious housewives or other individuals. In developing countries, it has been employed occasionally, since the very limited numbers of foods have made record-keeping easier. However, illiteracy and understandable lack of motivation and time usually make the method impractical.

Observing and measuring

The precise weighing method measures the amount of foods (both raw and cooked) consumed daily and at each meal, usually by a whole family, taking into account food wasted in preparation and leftovers. This method may be employed over a varying number of days — 7-, 4-, and (most usually) 3-day time periods being common.

Accurate weighing is carried out by specially tained staff, preferably with dietetic skills and/or knowledge of nutrition, who visit households and record the quantities of all foods eaten during a set period, preferably of 7 days' duration, but usually for 3 days. Foods are weighed and measured in the raw state. If possible and if methods of cooking are fairly standard, cooked food portions can also be weighed. At the same time, details of the family composition and other domestic information may be collected, including some aspects of task analysis (p. 188), as well as the cost and source of different foods.

Obviously, the longer the period of investigation the better. Cost, practicality, and exhaustion of both observer and observed usually limits this to, at most, a 1-week cycle, including the weekend (or equivalent), and usually only 3 days can be covered. In Fiji, Lucas (1978) included Sunday and two other randomly selected days. Repeated observation perods are ideal, if, as is often the case, marked seasonal differences occur.

While this is a most exact method in theory, certain difficulties are inherent in this type of investigation. Human problems are especially relevant, including establishing friendly rapport, and trying to ensure that the diet is typical and unmodified during the survey period. Practical problems are considerable, such as the estimation of wastage, refuse, and foods borrowed or lent, alteration of foods produced by cooking, use of local domestic units of weight and volume, the need to record some foods descriptively rather than by weight (including alcohol intake), and assessment of food eaten away from home (one or more meals, snacks, or collected items, such as wild berries, etc.). Probably the most common disadvantage of this method is the possibility that the diet may be consciously or subconsciously altered, for better or worse, during the period of intensive investigation.

Organizational and administrative considerations with staff may be a major key to success or failure, particularly questions of training and sustaining morale and motivation. As Alleyne *et al.* (1977) noted

> Sufficient staff must be employed and trained to carry out observations in the subjects' homes continuously throughout the day to deal with both regular and irregular mealtimes; it may not be possible for an observer to cover more than one family unit at a time. Each evaluation must be continued for at least a week to make sure of a reasonable representative sample. The qualities needed in staff selected for such a task are exacting; they must be capable of working accurately and conscientiously on a routine task for long periods but, above all, they must have the type of personality which enables them to integrate into the normal life of many different types of people. These qualities have been emphasized because they have been too little appreciated in the past.

The precise weighing method is time-consuming, difficult, and physically and emotionally exhausting. The survey worker has to keep all the records as she (or he) has to be present when all meals are prepared and preferably also when they are served. It is only possible to investigate very few families at a time. The number will depend on the distances between households, and on meal patterns, but usually cannot be more than three. Usually, this means that investigators have to be at household sites very early in the morning and remain on-duty until the evening.

However, these intensive periods of home-visiting also permit much other valuable information to be gathered unobtrusively, partly by questioning and partly by observation. Food preparation and task anaylsis (p. 188) (including methods of cooking, storage, the number of meals daily, and the common dishes that are taken), food purchasing, local household economies, agricultural practices, and social patterns can be observed, discussed, and recorded at the time or soon after leaving the home.

Training

General comments on training are given later (p. 405). However, the specialized nature of the precise weighing method makes particularly necessary specific training, based on carefully considered definition of the tasks and subtasks to be undertaken (Jelliffe and Jelliffe 1989*b*). The length and level of the training must vary with different circumstances, but, above all else, it should be practical. This should include an overall motivation and enthusiastic understanding of the purpose of the investigation and its practical relevance to improving the level of nutrition of the community, as well as an awareness of the difficulties which face workers in frequent daily communication with very busy, sometimes suspicious or apprehensive households.

Practical handling of foods, including weighing, measuring, and recording results on appropriate forms (p. 402), in similar conditions to the village or slum home is essential, as is a knowledge of local units of weight and volume, and the need to record some foods in units of different sizes (e.g. eggs, bananas, *tortillas*, etc.).

Part of the practical training will consist in the use of the weighing scales which are to be employed, together with exercises in 'quality control' (p. 410). Trainees need considerable continuing supervision in their use, as well as in the packing of the scales and the daily checking of the apparatus. Reh (1962) advised the use of two types of scales — those for foods weighing up to 1 kg and those for measuring foods up to 5 to 10 kg. The brand often depends on availability and cost.

The balance type of weighing scale with a hanging pan, may cause difficulties in handling, especially on windy days. Dietary balances with a wide base and a saucer in which to place the foods may be more acceptable to some workers. For example, the Salter 33D[61] dietary balance graduated to 500 g (by 5 g intervals) has been widely used. It has a saucer diameter of 17.8 cm, a net weight of 0.64 kg, and a height of 15 cm.

Selection of trainees If available, it is usually preferable to employ females who are experienced in cooking in similar circumstances. Preferably, they should have some knowledge of nutrition, but this is often not possible. The personality of the trainees is an important factor in their acceptance within households. They should have a pleasant disposition, as well as the ability, tact, diplomacy, and compassion to deal with human situations, and they should have the physical endurance to be able to work under field conditions. Trainees should be mature, as they usually command more respect from heads of households, and, if possible, should be relatively well-educated, so they can deal with the complexity of the social interactions involved, and the use of scales, and recording results correctly. However, locally recruited workers from the village or neighbourhood may not always be acceptable to families who feel that confidentiality of their personal lives may be violated (Reh 1962). Nevetheless, in small communities, especially among the poor, personal life-styles and habits may already be generally known to neighbours.

[61] George Salter and Co. Ltd, Weighing Machine Division. 31–33 Holborn, London, WCI.

Supervision of such field staff by experienced personnel is very important, and frequent checks of weighing results and calculations and discussions in the evenings regarding difficulties encountered can be valuable in ensuring accurate results, and in the difficult task of stimulating continuing high levels of commitment.

Other approaches In more sophisticated circumstances, subjects themselves may undertake home weighing (Graham 1980). The home inventory method has also been used, but apparently less in recent years. In this method, the amount of different food items in a household is listed by the investigator and householder, before and after a specified number of days. Together with information on items purchased during this period, utilization of different foods can be calculated.

Questioning

Various types of questioning ('recollective') techniques are available (Table 4.8), the most commonly used and most realistically practicable remains the '24-hour recall'. This method has been most widely used, especially for young children in less technically developed countries when a mother is asked to name the foods eaten by her infant or weanling during the previous day. This descriptive procedure is rapid, inexpensive, and tends to be easier and more representative in developing countries where the range of items consumed is usually relatively limited. It can still have problems with memory, maternal motivation, or communication (e.g. language misundertstandings). Last, the method only supplies *qualitative* data, unless attempts are made to estimate amounts eaten.

Longer periods of recall (3–7 days) have been attempted occasionally. However, it is generally agreed that many dietary details will not be remembered for such periods of time and the 24-hour recall method is most widely used by experienced investigators (Flores and Sogondares 1976).

Food frequency In enquiring into the frequency of use of different foods, it may be sufficient to concentrate entirely on certain foods considered to be particularly nutritionally significant in relation to known or probable nutrient deficiencies in the locality — the more important food or 'protective food' recall (Hunt *et al.* 1983). For example, specific, locally important carotene foods could be enquired for in areas where xerophthalmia is a problem, and sucrose-containing items if caries is a main consideration. In addition, Jenkins and Guthrie (1984) developed the idea of 'index nutrients' in the 'typical American diet'. These are iron, calcium, and vitamins A and B6. According to this procedure and in this particular society, if the RDAs (p. 520) are satisfied for these nutrients, then others will be taken care of. Obviously, different 'index nutrients' will be needed in societies with quite different dietary patterns.

Various foods may be inadvertently not included or overlooked in dietary surveys. For example, in adults, alcoholic beverages, in children, out-of-home snacks or sweets (candies), and in infants, breast milk.

As with any procedure to assess dietary intake, the enquirer needs to be on the alert for, and discourage, responses which may be given either to conform to the investigator's presumed views or to make the situation seem better (or worse) than is the case. Pre-testing and checking during a study are both most important. Usually, it is best to ask questions courteously and rapidly, but out of earshot of waiting mothers or others.

As with all field procedures, prior pre-testing should be accompanied by a small-scale pilot study and reinforced by checking during the study.

Semi-quantitative 24-hour recall The recall method can usefully be made semi-quantitative by incorporating questions concerning the *amount of foods taken*, based on known standardized local household measures (with specimen spoons, cups, etc. available) and/or on real or model portions eaten (small, medium, large) (again with examples for mothers to observe for comparison). This also requires a knowledge of the nutritional composition of household measures (e.g. spoon size, etc.) of the main foods and mixtures eaten. Details regarding use of this method for investigating the diets of young children are given later.

In less technically developed societies, the anthropological and marketing technique of the 'focus group interview' is used. With this method, informed guided interactive discussion with mothers can give useful qualitative information, and insight, and leads regarding food habits and their causation.

An 'interactive dietary assessment method' was introduced by Zeitlin *et al.* (1984). This is initiated by the preparation of a locally adapted form. This requires the following steps:

1. An inventory of foods commonly eaten in the project area;
2. An inventory of household utensils, meal patterns, serving and eating practices: decisions concerning reference utensils and documentation of their household availability;
3. Decisions concerning reference serving sizes and visual aids to illustrate these serving sizes;
4. Computation of nutrient content of the reference serving size of each food category;
5. Decisions concerning permissible clustering of foods of similar usage and nutrient content (e.g. green leafy vegetables);
6. Translation of computations in graphic representation (box size for calories and symbols for protein and vitamin A); design of instrument;
7. Selection of reference values for measuring adequacy.

Examples of items included in Bangladesh were the size and volume of commonly used kitchen utensils, brass spoons, enamel soup plates, and mollusc shells (about 5 ml). The nutrient content of reference servings of cooked dishes were determined by pre-weighing the raw ingredients, cooking in the usual manner, and defining an average serving of the cooked preparation. Similarly, the average size and weight of pieces of some vegetables were determined. 'Permissible clustering' of foods of similar usage and nutrient content was undertaken. The record form enabled the dietary intake to be noted not only as items of food, but also with the calories consumed recorded by pencil in an appropriate box per serving of each food. Total calories can then be measured on the form using an ordinary tape measure. Similarly, simplifications were made for reporting protein and vitamin A intakes.

This method was pioneered in Indonesia and Bangladesh. After the preparations indicated, the dietary practices of a family are observed as unobtrusively as possibly for an entire day, recording quantities served and eaten. The following day a different interviewer administers the 24-hour recall form for the same mother.

This method needs further trial. It needs care and time in preparation, but combines observation and recall, with reasonably accurate estimates of nutrient intakes, recorded with a tape measure in the field. Details of this ingenious procedure should be consulted (Zeitlin *et al.* 1984).

Other techniques based on questioning In more sophisticated circumstances, other techniques may be employed based on questioning individuals on their own or their families' diets. These include self-administered standard questionnaires, food frequency recall for longer periods, and telephone dietary recall (plus portion sizes used, as indicated by sending illustrations to subjects beforehand).

Comparisons Numerous studies have been undertaken attempting to compare methods of estimating food consumption, especially in young children. These have to take into account relative costs and the degree of detail of information required. In general, the 24-hour dietary recall is preferred, especially in less developed countries, *when large numbers are examined as in community studies*. However, whenever possible, an attempt needs to be made to collect some quantitative information.

Food consumption by special groups: the hospitalized and young children

Innumerable different special groups may need to be investigated, based for example, on age (e.g. the elderly), or cultural community (e.g.

gatherer–hunters; slum-dwellers; culturally underprivileged members of low castes in India), or by institution (e.g. schools, prisons), etc. All have their particular difficulties and special considerations.

Two particular groups will be singled out for particular attention — *the hospitalized* (all over the world) and *young children* (especially in less technically developed countries).

The hospitalized

Both in resource-poor countries or in large highly technological medical centres in industrialized countries, inadequate attention has been given to nutritional assessment of hospitalized individuals. This now seems to be changing (p. 348), but the need for practical methods to measure *dietary intake* is only beginning to be given some recognition. The role of nutrition in treatment has been and often continues to be very much underappreciated. Nurses, for example, are often not so much concerned with the food intake of their patients, as with more technological aspects of treatment, such as medicines and intravenous drips. An over-emphasis on the valuable technique of parenteral nutrition also may distract attention from the need for continuing measurement of the nutritional adequacy of patients' diets, both prior to admission and while in hospital. This is often overshadowed by biochemical and anthropometric measures of nutritional status.

Various experimental programmes have developed in some industrialized countries. In Denmark, Hessov (1978) calculated nutrient intakes in hospitalized patients, using a computer-based program based on Danish food composition tables and meal patterns. He analysed the foods actually eaten (and plate waste) noted by patients, relatives, and nurses. Although seemingly obvious, this represents a significant advance.

Young children

The dietary intake of young children is especially difficult to measure. This is particularly so in the important first 2 years of life, when the volume and composition of breast milk taken are very hard to estimate, as discussed later (p. 200), and when the quantity, type, and even consistency of other foods taken fluctuate irregularly during the 'weaning' or accustoming process. In addition, the dietary intake by the mother during pregnancy and lactation should, if possible, also be known. The infant's needs are partially taken care of by fetal stores, while the composition and the output of breast milk are related in some measure to the mother's diet, especially if this becomes *severely* limited in calories (Jelliffe and Jelliffe 1988*a*). Some details of perinatal care are also relevant, especially whether the cord is cut immediately or if additional iron supplies are permitted via 'placental transfusion'.

If some form of household dietary assessment has been undertaken (e.g. by the weighing method), then the question of determining the proportional allocation to different family members is particularly difficult with regard to young children whose appetite and intake are slowly increasing, but vary from day to day.

The diet in early childhood can be considered in two interrelated, overlapping aspects — *breastfeeding* and *semisolids* ('weaning foods').

Breastfeeding

The pattern of breastfeeding can be investigated at many levels of simplicity or sophistication. Problems of 'labelling' and verification in assessing types of breastfeeing in communities (complete, partial, mixed, etc.) have been discussed in detail (Baer and Winikoff 1981), and are much more difficult to define, corroborate, and agree upon than usually appreciated.

Retrospective or 'recollective' enquiries concerning the length of breastfeeding of older children are usually unreliable. Current information can be obtained as to whether babies are being breastfed or not, although mothers' concern with giving the 'correct' answer needs to be borne in mind. Moreover, without qualification or verification, this information is of very limited value, as 'breastfeeding' is a variable procedure. It can range from an occasional feed to many 'sucklings' throughout the 24 hours. To obtain meaningful information, it is necessary to try to ascertain the number of times the child is nursed, the range of timing of feeds (e.g. during the day and/or night, and the use of other foods) etc. This is often very difficult. The type of information varies from many traditional village societies, where 'biological breastfeeding' — that is, on-demand throughout the 24 hours, with the mother nursing the baby without conscious effort, or recollection of having done so, to early 'mixed milk feeding' and introduction of semisolids.

Such questionnaires become of greater relevance in cultures where breastfeeding is traditionally accompanied by other foods from the early months, or in communities tending to follow an old-style Westernized pattern of several feeds during the day, with bottle-feeds ('mixed milk feeding') and the introduction of semisolids in the early or later months of infancy. The last situation is more usual in urban areas, but is extending into rural communities in some countries.

As well known, the volume of breast milk secreted or ingested is very difficult to measure, even under ideal conditions. Two practical methods have been commonly used for many years — test-feeding (test-weighing) and expression.

In test-feeding, the child is weighed before and after a feed. This shows only the amount of milk taken rather than the amount secreted. If the child is at home and if (as is usually the case in developing countries) permissive breastfeeding is being practised, this presupposes a continuous surveillance in the home, theoretically through the full 24 hours. As a practical compromise, estimates have been made in Burma for 12 hours, and the result multiplied by two (Oo and Naing 1982). However, this approach is not useful in communities where the babies usually sleep apart from their mothers at night, as in the USA (De Carvalho and Pittard 1982). Also, because of the often small quantities taken at irregular intervals, an accurate, expensive weighing machine is needed and continuous close contact between investigator and mother concerned. Wherever carried out, but especially with a set feeding schedule in hospital, inhibition of the emotionally labile let-down reflex may occur as a result of the mother's anxiety. This is so even with well-motivated volunteer mothers.

Second, a period can be allocated when the breast-milk can be expressed manually or with mechanical or electric breastpump by the investigator or mother at 3–4 hour intervals from one or both breasts, measured, and then fed to the child, preferably with a cup and spoon. It may be more convenient to do this at a nearby health centre or hospital, in which case the mother may require compensation for her trouble. Considerable interference with the let-down (milk ejection) and prolactin reflexes is almost certain to occur, and the method cannot be recommended.

Both methods are difficult and likely to be inaccurate (Jelliffe and Jelliffe 1989*a*). This is especially so when the amount of milk obtained during an actual feeding is so much related to the baby's contribution in sucking stimulus and in inducing a full 'let-down reflex'. Also, the amount of milk received by the baby decreases gradually as other foods are introduced.

Two novel approaches have been introduced. In one of these, Lucas and colleagues (1979) developed an apparatus with a special nipple shield, into which a microminiaturized ultrasonic flowmeter was incorporated, which measured milk flow and, when needed, took samples at intervals during a single nursing. This apparatus is still at the experimental stage. It may be of value as a research tool for checking the validity of simpler methods, but the shield would seem automatically to interfere with normal mother–baby interaction. Second, Coward *et al.* (1979) developed a dilution method in which a calculated dose of non-radioactive heavy water (deuterium) is given to the nursing infant or, in a recent modification, to the mother. This needs further testing (see Addendum 1988).

The adequacy of breastfeeding is usually gauged ultimately by growth of the baby, mainly assessed by weight gain (Jelliffe and Jelliffe 1989*a*). However, recent studies indicate it is more difficult to evaluate, especially in the first 6 months of life, than previously realized, because of the use of inappropriate growth curves as reference levels, based on out-of-date data from infants bottle-fed with high-solute formula and receiving semisolid

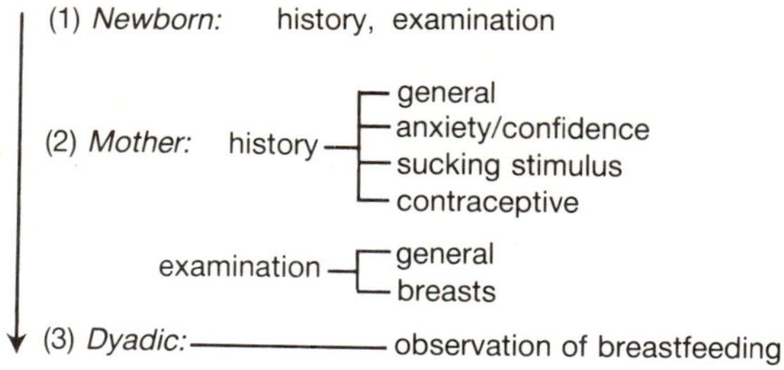

Fig. 4.7 Management diagnosis of reported inadequate breastfeeding (Jelliffe and Jelliffe 1978).

foods early (e.g. in the first weeks or months of life) (p. 110). *Stated inadequacy* of breast milk production by mothers needs to be verified practically by observation during actual nursing, by test-weighing, and by reviewing the babies' growth *and general appearance*. If breast milk is considered to be inadequate in volume, investigation is needed into: (1) practices which may be affecting the management of breastfeeding (Fig. 4.7) and possibly interfering with, or causing difficulties with, the maternal reflexes (dysreflexia) and leading to practical side-effects (e.g. sore nipples, engorgement), as well as into (2) the health and nutrition of the mother.

Conversely, details of artificial feeding with animal milk, formula or other liquid breast-milk substitute need to be collected, when relevant and feasible, either when they are the sole source of milk or as part of 'mixed milk feeding'. These can include the type of feed (species of animal milk, brand of formula), their preparation (dilution, addition of sugar), the number of feedings (and timing), and the method of administration (bottle: type, number, technique for cleaning; cup and spoon, etc.). At the same time, information can be obtained on the cost of formula compared with family income — that is, what percentage of a family budget will be needed to bottle-feed the infant adequately at his particular age. Also, facts concerning other prerequisites for safe bottle-feeding need to be collected, including number and type of bottles and teats, the available water supply, kitchen cleanliness, food storage, and the fuel situation (p. 188). Sometimes clues concerning the use of formula (and other foods) may be given by the presence of discarded cans ('garbageology') (Rathje and Harrison 1978), or their widespread use for other purposes, such as for food containers or cooking pots.

Many recent investigations concerning breastfeeding have been seriously flawed. Breastfeeding has been judged solely by response to a question, without clarification as to number of times or of the simultaneous use of bottle feeds, and without visual verification of the baby being breastfed.

Most accounts have been qualitative — a 24-hour recall (with or without questioning of mothers concerning details), or field observation of feeding practices (often including whether the mother breastfeeds the child at the investigator's suggestion), or unobtrusive observation of the local scene in the course of rapid ecological visits to homes, kitchen, gardens, markets, etc.

With present-day concern about promoting breastfeeding by community or national programmes, studies on infant-feeding practices will often extend to analyses or factors for individuals or communities that tend to make breastfeeding easier or more difficult (Jelliffe and Jelliffe 1989*a*) (Table 4.9). These include particularly support and encouragement, and *practical* information on management.

Semisolids (complementary foods)

Information with regard to the small, varying, and usually increasing amounts of food given to young children is not easy to obtain, especially in poorer homes in developing countries — particularly quantitative data.

As noted earlier, a special problem with regard to the measurement of dietary intake in this age-group is that infant feeding is, or should be, a progressive process, with breast milk being supplemented and eventually replaced by other foods. It is quite different from the relatively static and often montonous (though seasonally variable) diet of the average adult in less technically developed countries. To achieve accurate results, longitudinal studies by direct observation are required on a number of children. This is not often possible.

Nevetheless, it is useful to obtain an approximate outline of practices in the early years, including the number of daily meals and the preparation, or lack of preparation, of special dishes for young children, particularly for use during the dangerous transitional or weaning period.

Questioning of the mother as to the foods eaten by her child on the previous day (24-hour recall) can give useful qualitative information, if a sufficiently large group of women is sampled. This may be undertaken by asking the mother to say spontaneously what her child ate the day before. In some studies, she has also been asked if the child was well and if he seemed to eat with usual appetite.

Following the main 24-hour recall enquiry, it is desirable, if possible, to question the mother specifically concerning a list of foods (especially available nutritionally important foods, including breast milk) drawn up from a knowledge of the local feeding pattern. Such questions should be neutral and non-leading. This two-stage approach will help to check the initial enquiry.

Attempts at roughly estimating the amount of various foods eaten include methods to obtain information on the number of times items are eaten daily, or on the size of portions, times/day, and hence an approximate measure of total intake (Table 4.10) (Flores and Sogondares 1976).

Table 4.9 Type of data that can be collected in a community analysis of common factors influencing breastfeeding: Listing is not all inclusive and has to be used selectively *(Jelliffe and Jelliffe 1988*b)

Pattern of infant feeding	
Maternal diet:	pregnancy, puerperium, and lactation (especially cultural food restrictions)
Breastfeeding:	when commenced; use of colostrum; prelacteal feeds; frequency (including night feeds); scheduled or not; customs interfering with lactation (traditional or modern)
Artificial feeds:	what, cost dilution, method (bottle, cup)
Introduction of semisolids; use of pacifiers (dummies):	when, how, what
Removal from breast (*sevrage*):	when, how, compensatory actions
Community influences	
(1) **Health services**	
Prenatal care:	information on breastfeeding management; dietary advice
Puerperal care:	supervision of breastfeeding; out-dated hospital practices interfering with lactation reflex; routine inhibition of lactation (e.g. oestrogens); rooming in; cutting umbilical cord (at once or delayed)
Premature unit:	use of breast milk (especially colostrum); breast milk bank; mother–baby contact; nearby accommodation for mothers; traditional cultural practices
Children's ward:	opportunity for breastfeeding; admission of mothers; hospital policy on formula, purchasing, and distribution
Health centres:	supplementary food distribution policy
Health education:	formal and informal; 'ill-health education' (advertising; etc.)
Family planning services:	methods advised (in relation to lactation)
Staff training:	curriculum content (nutrition, infant feeding, psychophysiology, modern knowledge of properties of human versus cow's milk, practical management in theory and practice; relationships with food industry; knowledge of the WHO/UNICEF Code of Marketing of Breastmilk Substitutes)
(2) **Food industry**	
Advertising (shops, press, radio, television):	coverage (time, space); motivation; relevance (income, domestic hygiene, present infant-feeding practices)

Table 4.9 (Continued)

Promotion (via health services:	direct (posters, calendars, brochures; free samples; professional journals) indirect (funding of meetings, hospitality, prizes, research)
(3) **Role of women**	
Working women:	percentage working for wage out of home; types of jobs; facilities for breastfeeding; cost-benefit to family
Voluntary groups (concerned with breastfeeding):	name, size, activities, and methods of breastfeeding mothers' support groups
Legislation:	maternity protection laws (with special reference to lactation)
Attitudes to breasts and breastfeeding:	information from women, husbands, young girls, grandmothers, and health workers; status, modernness, acceptability in public

Table 4.10 List of foods and units used in Central American dietary intake studies *(Flores and Sogandares 1976)*

Foods	Unit
Cereal: cooked	spoonfuls
Cereal: pre-cooked	spoonfuls
Corn cakes (tortillas)	unit
Bread (or salt crackers)	unit
Bread in slices	slices
Sweet biscuits	unit
Rice	spoonfuls
Spaghetti (or macaroni)	spoonfuls
Sugar	spoonfuls
Carbonated beverages	ounces
Fats	spoonfuls
Total intake	
% of adequacy	

Also, the consistency of foods given to young children can be estimated in some circumstances. This can often be of great importance in relation to nutrient density, especially calories, in gruels or porridges.

A simplified, rapid technique for use in a dietary enquiry was suggested by Blankhart (1965) for field work, both at survey sites and in home

Table 4.11 Foods taken each week in a Sierra Leone village *(Blankhart 1965)*

Type of meal	Average number of times different foods taken per week at following ages (number of children studied)		
	7–12 months (12 children)	13–18 months (15 children)	19–24 months (11 children)
Breast-milk	21	10	2
Rice	6	13	14
Cassava and *foo-foo* pap	6	3	1
Sweet potato		⅓	½
Custard or cornflour	4	2	
Leafy vegetables	1	12	10
Bananas		2	1½
Oranges		1	1½
Tomatoes			
Milk	13	1½	½
Egg	½		
Fresh fish			
Dried fish		5	5
Oil			

visits. In this, the mother is first asked to say spontaneously what foods the child is eating currently. Following this, directed by initial findings, she is questioned as to how many times a day each item is being eaten. The information obtained is recorded as given by the mother (e.g. rice, twice a day, etc.). When the mother has given her spontaneous answers, questions are put systematically on the intake of other foods, and, in the event of an affirmative answer, on the number of times daily. This questioning was done quickly, as, according to Blankhart (1965), too much interrogation and cross-checking defeated their purpose and left both the mother and the interviewer confused. The information may be entered on double foolscap lined sheets, on which columns are ruled for each of the local foods likely to be used for young children. The frequency of use of different foods can be calculated and expressed as the number of times they have been eaten per week per child (Table 4.11).

In view of common food restrictions during often almost continous infections, it may be useful to obtain information by direct questioning concerning foods avoided or used during infectious diseases, especially diarrhoea (Jelliffe *et al.* 1987).

Under special circumstances, detailed studies of the consumption of specific food items by families can be enumerated. Studies by an anthropologist resident in a village would enable a ranking of foods by the number of days on which they were eaten per month or even per year to be drawn up.

A rough indication of the nutritional blend or mix of the foods given to young children during weaning has been suggested. De Wijer (1977) advises initial questioning of the mother concerning the staple, then nutritionally complementary legumes, and then animal products and dark-green leafy vegetables.

As noted earlier, the 24-hour recall method can be elaborated to give an approximate account of quantities eaten using domestic measures. This approach has been used in particular in Central America by Flores and Sogondares (1976), who suggested the drawing up of a list of more commonly eaten foods and defined domestic units which are employed (e.g. spoonful, slices, locally, 'standard size' *tortillas*, etc.) (Table 4.12). Such lists will obviously vary greatly with local utensils and dietary patterns, and have to be based on some type of 'standard' recipes.

In this system, it is also necessary to know the nutrient content of cooked items commonly consumed as prepared with usual recipes and dilutions. Flores and Sogondares (1976) compiled a 'compressed' food composition table for ready use with widely available domestic measures of commonly used cooked foods (Table 4.12), so that the main nutrients in the diet can be easily calculated, added together for daily intake, and compared with the RDAs (p. 520). The whole process greatly simplifies matters.

Even in the absence of quantitative information, a useful qualitative general pattern of infant feeding can be obtained from 24-hour dietary recall data from a community. This can be expressed numerically, but can sometimes have more impact if presented visually in a frequency graph. This is shown for the combined results from some West Indian studies (Fig. 4.8) (Gurney 1971). Essentially, this graph shows which foods are being under-used or used too late for young children, and, therefore, suggests topics to be emphasized in nutrition education. These can include breast milk, dark-green leafy vegetables (as sources of minerals and vitamins), or oil (as a source of compact calories).

Zerfas *et al.* (1982) introduced the useful concept of the 'child–family deficit' with regard to a certain major food (Fig. 4.9). Thus, if 24-hour recall information is available for *both* the family and the young child of 6–11 months (or 12–23 months), the two percentages of use of selected foods can be usefully contrasted, and again give direction to nutrition education designed to promote the use of available foods consumed by adults in the diets of young children.

Longitudinal data is rarely available and extraordinarily difficult to obtain in view of the varying food intake from day to day in young

Table 4.12 Blank model food composition table for selected nutrients for common foods ready to be eaten-and household measures used in dietary intake studies in children in Central America (*Flores and Sogondares 1976*)

Food	Measure	Net weight g	Calories	Protein g	Retinol mcg
Cow's milk:					
fluid — whole	1 cup				
powdered — whole	1 spoonful				
Cheese — soft	1 ounce				
Egg	1 unit				
Chicken (white meat)	1 ounce				
Beef, only meat	1 ounce				
Beef, liver	1 ounce				
Beans, all kinds	2 spoonfuls cooked				
Lentil	2 spoonfuls cooked				
Chard	4 leaves				
Squash, mature	1 ounce				
Tomato	1 unit				
Apple	1 unit				
Orange juice	1 glass				
Papaya	1 slice				
Banana	1 unit				
Plantain	1 slice				
Sweet potato	1 ounce				
Potato	1 unit				
Rice	2 spoonfuls cooked				
Oatmeal	1 spoonful				
Sweet bread	1 unit of 1 ¢				
Bread (French)	1 unit of 2 × 5 ¢				
Bread in slices, white	1 slice				
Spaghetti, macaroni	2 spoonfuls cooked				
Corn cake (tortilla) (white corn)	1 unit				
Sugar	1 spoonful				
Margarine	½ ounce				
Incaparina	for 1 cup				

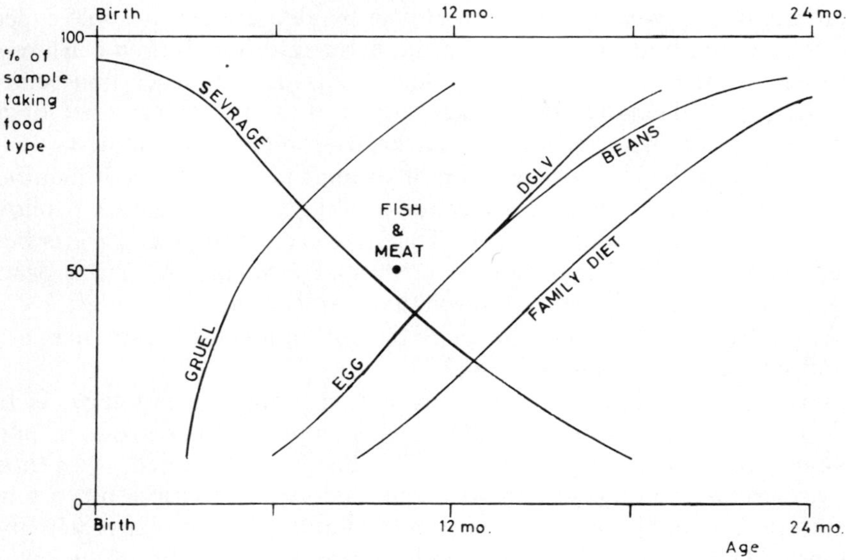

Fig. 4.8 Qualitative pattern of infant feeding obtained by questionnaires in some West Indian islands and graphed to show ages at which different foods are introduced into the diet (Gurney 1971).

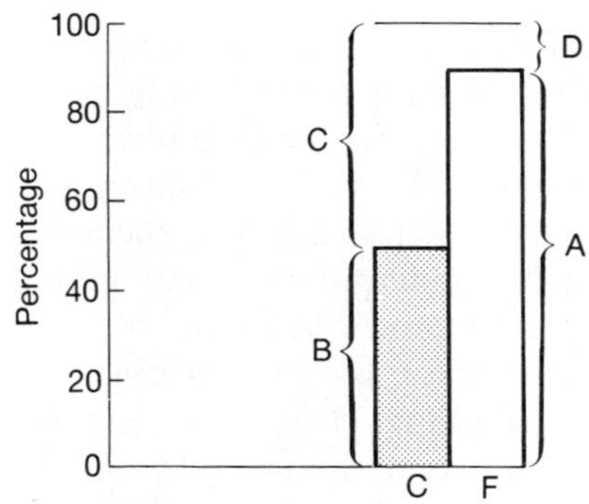

Fig. 4.9 Child–family food difference for one 'category' (oils). A, Percentage of families eating any oil (90 per cent; food available); B, percentage of children eating any oil (50 per cent); C = A − B, percentage of children not eating oil when available to family (40 per cent; child–family food difference or underusage); D, percentage of families not eating oil (10 per cent; food unavailable). C, Child; *F*, family. (Zerfas *et al.* 1982.)

children in the weaning period. However, two suggestions have been made recently, both of which need the more traditional, time-consuming approach of the orthodox anthropologist. That is they depend on being a familiar, trusted resident or frequent visitor in the village for a prolonged period. One of these techniques has been termed 'child-following' and, indeed, means the close observation of young children and recording their dietary intake throughout the day for a period of several days ('follow-behind technique') (Wilson 1974). This time-consuming method has been used successfully by the author in a Malaysian village. A similar procedure can be used following the technique of Zeitlin *et al.* (1984).

A system of observing the activities of hunter-gatherers has been mentioned earlier (Table 4.5) (p. 173).

A comparable technique, using expensive modern technology, is the SSR system (Stephenson *et al.* 1975). This employs a suitcase-sized portable electronic recording apparatus. This has been described as an 'open format event-recording system with computerized transcription'. In practical terms, it enables an observer to record multiple, cumulative activities by individuals in the community under observation, so that these can be available for instant analysis later. The SSR system has been used by Lozoff and Brittenham (1977) in collecting and analysing information on the activities of members of the !Kung gatherer-hunters of the Kalahari.

Characteristics of foods used in weaning

In addition to culturally-defined attitudes to foods preferred, accepted, or proscribed for children during the weaning period (p. 165) and the dietary and nutrient intake of young children (discussed in preceding pages), other characteristics should be reviewed and investigated, at least by observation. These characteristics will include probable *digestibility* (including, for example, undermilled cereal grain; ill-cooked legumes; irritant spices), *cleanliness* (and likelihood of bacterial contamination), evidence of *'calorie compactness' (or density)* (e.g. addition of oil, fat, increasing thickness, or malting) (Mellander and Svanberg 1984), *'origin'* (e.g. specially prepared for weaning or used from family pot or meal), and *task analysis* (p. 188) of the steps employed in their preparation.

Reporting results

As with all methods, detailed descriptions of the techniques used in assessment of food consumption need to be agreed upon, followed, and described in written reports. All have flaws, imperfections, and advantages.

In addition, careful and precise definitions should be used for aspects of infant feeding investigated, as these are often ambiguously labelled (e.g. 'weaning', complementary and supplementary feeds, mixed milk feeds, partial breastfeeding, etc.), which can have different meanings to different workers.

Finally, it is apparent, as noted by Beaton *et al.* (1983): 'There is no 'ideal' dietary method. There may be preferred methods for particular purposes'.

Food use within the body

This part of the food chain is often under-emphasized and, indeed, is very difficult to measure. It includes digestion, absorption and ultimately use of nutrients by the body. Two complex variables need consideration — physiological and pathological.

Physiological

At least three factors influence food use within the body, including digestion and absorption (bioavailability). First, the *mixture of foods* within the intestine may promote or interfere with absorption. As is well-known, vitamin C-containing foods assist in the absorption of iron; phytate-containing foods (such as lightly milled wheat flour) can diminish calcium and zinc uptake. Inherent enhanced bioavailability is particularly important in breast milk, from which zinc and iron are absorbed in greater amounts than the relatively low concentrations would suggest. In other words, it is not only the foods eaten which influence use, but the effects of the different nutrients consumed in combination with one another.

Second, the *physiological stage of life* can be relevant. For example, in pregnancy, various nutrients, such as iron, are better absorbed (p. 227). Also, recent work makes it clear that in both pregnancy and lactation metabolism can become adjusted, in ways as yet unknown, to lower intakes of calories, protein, and other nutrients than previously calculated theoretically (p. 229). Likewise, physiological variation and adaptation can obviously occur in young infants. Various studies have shown normal growth in breastfed young infants of comparable age consuming volumes of milk varying by two- to threefold (Underwood and Hofvander 1984), partly related to different levels of activity.

In the elderly, diminished absorption often occurs, while some of the medicinal drugs likely to be taken for common chronic illnesses can also limit or further interfere with the use of some nutrients.

Third, *genetic influences* affect food and nutrient use in individuals (p. 56). Some genetic factors which limit food use within the body are already known. The most recognized is lactose intolerance after early childhood due to an apparently genetically reduced intestinal lactase production. This limits the ability of large populations — for example, in Eastern Asia — to consume animal milk. The probability of such essentially varied metabolic mechanisms occurring seems to be endorsed by studies in pharmaco-anthropology, which show varying responses to certain drugs in genetically different ethnic groups.

In addition it seems highly probable that genetic differences occur in communities long adapted to particular diets, often restricted in range of foods and nutrients. A much quoted example is in the New Guinea Highlands where the diet, until recently, consisted predominantly of sweet potatoes. Another culture among whom metabolic adaptations may have occurred are Arctic-dwelling Lapps, whose intake of ascorbic acid is mainly seasonal — that is, in the brief spring and summer. How widespread other genetic variations and adaptations are appears little known — for example, modified calcium metabolism in non-milk drinking cultures.

Pathological

As emphasized throughout, in less technically developed countries, pathological limitation of food and nutrient use within the body is very often most important in causing malnutrition. This can occur from the cumulative effects of often continuous bacterial, viral, and parasitic infections (p. 139), and malabsorption from damage to the intestinal wall by repeated bouts of infective diarrhoea and/or by protein-energy malnutrition (p. 139), often exacerbated by dietary restriction in traditional or Western medical treatment.

The effects of such conditions can usually only be surmised based on available knowledge of the extent and severity of the infections limiting utilization. Detailed metabolic studies are needed to determine the commonness of malabsorption in any particular community and this is usually not feasible. Certainly, additional nutrients may be needed for the majority of young children in many tropical, less technically developed countries, since these children are not sufficiently protected from ever-present infections.

In all parts of the world, especially in technically more developed countries, food and nutrient use in the elderly needs much more consideration. Changes occur as a part of the physiological and pathological diminished metabolic functioning, including absorption, that accompanies the process of ageing.

In a more restricted sense, the effect of other pathological conditions may need consideration, particularly, for example, in hospitalized persons. Such conditions include the consequences of chronic alcoholism and cancer 'cachexia'.

Estimating nutritional adequacy

The adequacy of the diet of the individual or the community under investigation depends ultimately on whether sufficient nutrients can be made available at cellular level to maintain health and, in childhood and pregnancy, to sustain growth and development.

Numerous difficulties occur in making such calculations,[62] as will those already outlined concerning assessment of food intake (p. 198). Others include the possible nutritional ill-effects of various infections (p. 156) or malabsorption, the alterations that can result from different forms of cooking, and, very fundamentally, the fact that the absorption and utilization of nutrients (bioavailability) vary with the food mixtures actually present in the alimentary canal. These and other already mentioned practical sources of potential error indicate the need for considerable caution in interpretation.

Analysis of the results of detailed household food consumption surveys, usually with information obtained by weighing can be undertaken in five steps:

1. Conversion of weights and volumes into standard metric measures (if necessary);
2. Calculation of total household nutrient intake;
3. Calculation of total household nutrient needs;
4. Comparison of family intake with family nutrient needs;
5. Comparison of individual intakes with nutrient needs.

This analysis has for many years been undertaken laboriously by hand. Recent studies have increasingly employed electronic data-processing, using programmable calculators or computers.

Conversion into standard metric measures of weight

Initially the data collected on the weight and volume of foods consumed have to be converted into uniform metric units (if this is not already the case).

Calculation of total household nutrient intake

The total daily nutrient intake for the household (or family) needs to be made using the most relevant food composition tables for the particular area (p. 516). Some tables give information concerning cooked foods; some give conversion factors or coefficients to use with local measures of weight or volume. Computerized data on food composition may be available to aid calculations. If costs of foods and incomes are known, results may be correlated with purchasing power in different socio-economic strata.

[62] Detailed considerations for more technically developed countries have been reviewed recently in a volume edited by Simopoulos (1987).

Food composition tables

These are not uniform, but usually show average values for foods AP[63] ('as purchased') or as EP ('edible portion') for energy, moisture, protein, carbohydrate, calcium, iron, retinol, thiamine, riboflavin, niacin, ascorbic acid, fibre, ash, etc. Some modern food tables have special lists for nutrients more recently recognized as important (e.g. cholesterol, amino acids, fatty acids, trace elements). Occasionally, tables may have some composition values for madeup, cooked, or processed food mixtures, notably the US Department of Agriculture publication (USDA 1975*a*). When fortification or enrichment is practised by government regulation, these added nutrients need noting. (Also see: Addendum 1988.)

Usually composition tables are given for 100 g (3½ oz) portions (Table 4.13). In some areas, the nutrient content of long-established units of weight, such as pounds (lb), or commonly used units (i.e. slices of bread) (Table 4.14) may also be given for practical purposes.

Numerous food composition tables are available in different parts of the world (Appendix 6). These tables usually list names of foods both in the local languages and in English, together with the scientific botanical term.

Lists of foods used in different parts of the world have been compiled for some regions — e.g. for Africa (Jardin 1967) and Far East Asia (Wu Leung *et al.* 1972). These can be important as they contain food items not consumed elsewhere, and for which no composition data are available. In the latter case, analyses of similar species may have to be used instead (e.g. with species of *Amaranthus* or other dark-green leafy vegetables).

Recently, an international system and network has developed under the aegis of the United Nations University (UNU) to try to co-ordinate analyses of foods and the dissemination of information (Rand 1985)[64] This has begun to stimulate the analysis of foods in different parts of the world. A new publication — the *Journal of Food Composition and Analysis* — is forthcoming.

Food composition tables usually list foods grouped under certain conventional specific headings — such as cereals and derivatives, starches and starchy roots, dry leguminous seeds, oily seeds, nuts and coconuts, sugars, syrups and sweet goods, milk and milk products (e.g. cheese), fats and oils, meats and derivatives, fish and crustaceans, eggs (from different birds), vegetables (identified by different types), fruits — and a section in which miscellaneous items are covered.

Difficulties in the interpretation of the food-composition tables arise

[63] Raw and unprepared, including peel, seeds, and all inedible parts, subsequently discarded during preparation.
[64] INFOODS, c/o Department of Nutrition, MIT, Cambridge, Massachusetts.

Table 4.13 Page from food composition table: standard format showing nutrients per 100 g. (3½ oz) *(Caribbean Food and Nutrition Institute 1974)*

PULSES, NUTS AND OIL SEEDS		Composition of foods, in 100 g edible portion													
Item number	Food and description	Water (g)	Energy (kcal)	Protein (g)	Fat (g)	Carbo-hydrate (Total) (g)	Fibre (g)	Calcium (mg)	Iron (mg)	Vitamin A R.E.	Thiamin (mg)	Riboflavin (mg)	Niacin (mg)	Vitamin C (mg)	Refuse as purchased (%)
	BEANS														
	Broad bean (*Vicia faba*)														
0401	Whole seeds, dry	12.6	339	24.0	2.2	58.2	5.9	77	6.3	10	0.53	0.30	2.5	6	0
0402	Flour	11.1	343	24.4	1.8	59.7	3.4	66		5	0.42	0.28	2.7	4	0
	Butter bean, Indian, Banner bean, bonavist (*Lablab purpureus*)														
0403	Whole seeds, dry	13.1	334	22.1	1.0	61.2	7.9	46	7.3	—	0.44	0.12	1.5	—	0
	Horse bean, Jack bean (*Canavalia ensifermis*)														
0404	Whole seeds, dry	12.0	331	25.4	1.3	57.1	4.9	96	(4.9)	5	0.46	0.15	2.1	—	0
	Lima bean, Sugar bean, White bean (*Phaseolus lunatus*)														
	Whole seeds, dry														
0405	With skin	12.0	336	20.7	1.2	62.7	4.9	113	4.8	∅	0.34	0.21	2.2	0	—
0406	Without skin	12.0	337	21.6	1.4	61.6	1.0	38	5.2	0	0.55	0.21	2.2	0	—
	Green, immature														
0407	Fresh, raw	67.5	123	8.4	0.5	22.1	1.8	52	2.8	30	0.24	0.12	1.4	29	60-pods
0408	Canned, solids, liquids	80.8	71	4.1	0.3	13.4	1.3	26	2.4	20	0.04	0.04	0.5	7	0
0409	Frozen, cooked, boiled, drained	73.5	99	6.0	0.1	19.1	1.6	20	1.7	25	0.07	0.05	1.0	17	0
	Mung been (*Phaseolus aureus, P. mungo*)														

Table 4.13 (Continued)

PULSES, NUTS AND OIL SEEDS — Composition of foods, in 100 g edible portion

Item number	Food and description	Water (g)	Energy (kcal)	Protein (g)	Fat (g)	Carbo-hydrate (Total) (g)	Fibre (g)	Calcium (mg)	Iron (mg)	Vitamin A R.E.	Thiamin (mg)	Riboflavin (mg)	Niacin (mg)	Vitamin C (mg)	Refuse as purchased (%)
0410	Whole seeds, dry	11.0	340	23.9	1.3	58.3	(4.9)	145	7.8	30	0.56	0.17	2.0	5	0
	Sprout-see Item 0508														
	Red peas, kidney bean (*Phaseolus vulgaris*)														
0411	Whole seeds, dry	12.0	337	22.0	1.6	60.8	4.3	86	7.6	Ø	0.54	0.19	2.1	3	0
	Immature–apply Item 0407														
	Blackeye peas, cowpea (*Vigna unguiculata*)														
0412	Whole seeds, dry	10.6	341	24.1	1.2	60.7	4.9	77	7.2	5	0.87	0.23	1.9	3	0
0413	Immature pods	85.3	47	3.6	0.3	10.0	1.8	45	1.2	55	0.13	0.10	1.0	22	8-trimmings
	Chickpea (*Cicer arietinum*)														
0414	Whole seeds, dry	11.5	364	18.2	6.2	61.1	3.4	134	7.3	5	0.46	0.16	1.7	1	—

Table 4.14 Page from food composition table in common household units (e.g., loaves, slices, crumbs). The nutrients content is given in columns to the right as with standard tables. (*US Department of Agriculture 1975b*)

Fresh:		
Loaf, net wt., 24 oz. (1 lb. 8 oz.); approx. 24 regular slices (item 467b) or 28 thin slices (sandwich type) (item 467c).	1 loaf	--------------------
Slice:		
Regular, 4⅜ in. wide, 4 in. high, 9/16 in. thick; 1/24 of loaf.	1 slice	--------------------
Thin (sandwich type), 4 in. wide, 3⅞ in. high, ½ in. thick; 1/28 of loaf.	1 slice	--------------------
Loaf, net wt., 16 oz. (1 lb.); approx. 18 regular slices (item 467e; or 22 thin slices (item 467f).	1 loaf or 1 lb	----------
Slice:		
Regular, 4 in. wide, 4¼ in. high, 9/16 in. thick; 1/18 of loaf.	1 slice	--------------------
Thin, 4 in. wide, 4 in. high, 7/16 in. thick; 1/22 of loaf.	1 slice	--------------------
Cubes ---	1 cup	--------------------
Crumbs ---	1 cup	--------------------
Toasted slices:		
From 1½-lb. loaf:		
Yield from loaf --	24 regular or 28 thin slices.	
Slice, regular --	1 slice	--------------------
Slice, thin (sandwich type) -------------------------	1 slice	--------------------
From 1-lb. loaf:		
Yield from loaf --	18 regular or 22 thin slices.	
Slice, regular ---	1 slice	--------------------
Slice, thin (sandwich type) ----------------------------	1 slice	--------------------
Pound --	1 lb	----------------------
White bread, unenriched, firm-crumb type (made by conventional method):[84 85]		
Fresh:		
Loaf, net wt., 32 oz. (2 lb.); approx. 34 thin slice (item 469b).	1 loaf or 2 lb	----------
Slice, 3⅝ in. wide, 4¼ in. high, 7/16 in. thick; 1/34 of loaf.	1 slice	--------------------
Loaf, net wt., 16 oz. (1 lb.); approx. 20 thin slices (item 469d).	1 loaf or 1 lb	----------
Slice, 3¾ in. 4 in. high, 7/16 in. thick; 1/20 of loaf.	1 slice	--------------------
Cubes ---	1 cup	--------------------
Crumbs ---	1 cup	--------------------

Table 4.14 (Continued)

Toasted slices:	
From 2-lb. loaf:	
Yield from loaf	34 slices
Slice	1 slice
From 1-lb. loaf:	
Yield from loaf	20 slices
Slice	1 slice
Whole-wheat bread, firm-crumb type:[5 34 85]	
Fresh:	
Loaf, net wt., 16 oz. (1 lb.); rounded top, approx. 18 slices; flat top or sandwich style, approx. 20 slices.	1 loaf or 1 lb
Slice, rounded top, 4 in. wide, 4 in. high, 7/16 in. thick; 1/18 of loaf.	1 slice
Slice, flat top or sandwich style, 3 7/8 in. wide, 3 5/8 in. high, 7/16 in. thick; 1/20 of loaf.	1 slice
Toasted slices:	
Yield from 1-lb. loaf	18 or 20 slices
Piece, rounded top	1 slice
Piece, flat top or sandwich style	1 slice
Pound	1 lb
Whole-wheat bread, soft-crumb type:[5 84 85]	

from variations in techniques of food analysis, probable regional differences in composition of foods, the frequent non-inclusion of foods of local importance (alcohol, breast milk, wild berries, etc.), and confusion because of a lack of standardized terminology (Polacchi 1986). Also, all analyses are averages, sometimes based on a surprisingly small original number of estimations made on food samples collected without statistical consideration. Finally, results of small analyses are often copied from one food composition table to another. As with all facets of nutritional assessment, food composition data should 'only be used with caution' (Polacchi 1985).

Food composition tables for the country or region are to be preferred, as they will probably list many indigenous items. These include, for example, different types of dark-green leafy vegetables. There is a great need for a better knowledge of food composition using modern techniques from samples grown or reared in different ecologies and from different strains. Unfortunately, the expense of undertaking such activities may be limiting, except perhaps at regional centres or institutes concerned with research on certain crops (e.g. rice, tropical vegetables, etc.) (Appendix 7). It is hoped that the UNU 'INFOODS' programme may help (Rand 1985). In this scheme, collaborative studies of food composition are developed world-wide, including foods in particular regions (e.g. ASIA FOODS, EURO FOODS, etc.).

Calculation of total household nutrient needs

The total household nutrient needs can be estimated from a knowledge of the family composition (e.g. numbers; sexes; age-groups; levels of activity; physical condition, such as pregnancy or illness) and the recommended dietary allowance (RDA) (or recommended dietary intake) (RDI) for each individual. (The latter — RDI — seems gradually to be becoming the preferred term.)

Comparison of family intake with family nutrient needs

Obviously, the family nutrient intake gives no information on the adequacy or otherwise for individual family members, as it is very difficult (and usually quite impossible) to gauge the distribution within the family, especially amounts eaten by young children.

If the total family nutrient intake is known, the intake for individual members can be estimated *per capita* by dividing the total by numbers of family members of all ages. This is an absurd and invalid calculation as families vary in composition and no differentiation is made between the intakes and needs of adult males, pregnant women, and young children. This arbitrary decision takes no account of differences in dietary practices, cultural attitudes, and nutrient needs in different family members.

In some studies, attempts have been made to rate family members according to sex and age-group, using a family 'coefficient'. For example, the Oxford scale assumes an adult male to consume 1, while an adult woman consumes 0.8 and a 'child' 0.5. Such assumptions have little relevance to reality (Gopalan 1987).

The intrafamilial distribution of foods and hence of nutrients can best be undertaken by *meal-time observation*. This is very difficult to do for practical reasons and because of cultural sensitivities. The oberver must know the nutrient content of servings and household measures (e.g. spoons) of *cooked* foods and dishes.

For young children, the best combination of methods can often be a large sample for 24-dietary recall (with follow-up check using major locally significant foods) (p. 191), with a subsample using the semi-quantitative method of Flores and Sogondares (1976) and with a smaller subsample with the detailed information obtained by the 'child-following' method of Wilson (1964) or the 'interactive dietary assessment method' of Zeitlin *et al.* (1984) (p. 197). More usually, only 24-dietary recalls are feasible.

Nutrient needs

After measuring and calculating food consumption, ultimately the nutritional adequacy of a diet has to be compared with reference levels. These are frequently termed 'recommended dietary allowances' (RDA). In some parts of the world, 'recommended dietary intakes' (RDI) is the preferred name, as it is felt to be less 'paternalistic' and authoritative (Truswell 1983).

Tables of RDAs are available from numerous countries and from WHO/FAO (1974, quoted in Davidson *et al.* 1979). Recently, IUNS has reviewed compilations from 41 countries (Truswell 1983) and found considerable variation in suggested nutrient allowances and in age-categories considered.

The situation is particularly difficult with breastfed infants, in view of problems with assessing breast milk intake, variable composition in normal women, etc. (p. 260) (Jelliffe and Jelliffe 1989*a*; Fomon 1985). Also, because of the very different composition of breast milk, other mammal milks, and cow's milk-based formulas, in some countries, different RDAs are given for bottle or breastfed babies, as is, indeed, appropriate. For example, in Bulgaria, 3.0 g/kg of protein is suggested for the bottle-fed and 1.9 g/kg for the breastfed (Truswell 1983).

Definitions of the coverage and purpose of RDA also varies, but in the USA, for example, they refer to the 'daily requirements that healthy populations should consume over a period of time' (US National Academy of Sciences 1980). In other words, RDAs represent intakes sufficient for most of the healthy population (about 97 per cent) and thus more than usually needed by many individuals. Recent controversy in the US illustrates the difficulties inherent in this estimation (Herbert 1987*a*, *b*, *c*; Olson 1987*a*, *b*; Olson and Hodges 1987).

RDAs are categorized for both sexes, for various different age-groups, for pregnancy and lactation, and sometimes for different kinds of physical work. National data may sometimes be used. If not, allowances defined by WHO/FAO may be recommended for work in technically less developed countries (WHO 1985*b*). Sometimes, it may be feasible to express national data (when available) as percentage of WHO/FAO figures. This can help in comparability between countries.

At one time, caloric intake was corrected for environmental temperature, according to age, sex, and body size. Recent studies suggest that such categories are not based on actual evidence and are not recommended (WHO 1985*b*). Requirements for thiamine and niacin are related directly to calorie requirements (0.5 mg thiamine and 5.0 mg niacin per 1000 cal). Energy requirements are often expressed as an average for the population under survey assuming moderate activity. The UNU, WHO, and FAO have reviewed evidence concerning energy and protein needs (Torún *et al.* 1981; WHO 1985*b*) and made considerable modifications. Difficulties relating to compensating for infections and parasites are very great.

RDAs have usually been calculated on the basis of a certain physique ('reference man or woman', etc.) and on assumptions concerning the level of activity. Appropriate local nutrient requirements may need to be calculated in light of knowledge of body size, levels of activity, etc. In some regions, such adjusted values are already available, as in India and the Caribbean.

More recently, suggestions have been made that nutrients may more appropriately be related to the basal metabolic rate (BMR) (Weisell and Francois 1982). For example, individuals with energy intakes which fall below 1.2 times the BMR energy are considered to be malnourished. This concept is experimental and needs further investigation. It is much too complex for general use and seems more likely to generate confusion than clarity.

Questions of actual bioavailability depend on food *mixtures* consumed and on the potential impact of malabsorption and of infections, especially involving the intestines — all of which are common in various combinations in Third World countries, especially in children. Also, possible genetic variation in nutrient requirements needs to be borne in mind both in individuals and in different ethnic groups. All these variations and uncertainties obviously mean that much caution and flexibility are needed in interpretation of less marked findings, especially in individuals.

Cut-off points

Data collected needs to be analysed according to socio-economic level, ethnic group, etc. and the RDA tables used in analysis need to be identified. If the food consumption of the group or household or individual falls below the RDA for one or more nutrients, this finding should not be expressed in terms of degrees of 'undernutrition' or 'malnutrition', or 'overnutrition'. The report should state the difference between the observed consumption and the allowances as a percentage of the latter. Alternatively, the 'cut-off point' for inadequate intake can be taken as −2 SD or the 3rd percentile of the reference levels. However, this is really based on unproven assumptions concerning the range of distribution of needs for different nutrients in normal subjects. Last, on an arbitrary basis, various convenient cut-off points have been suggested (e.g. high 1½ times the RDA, medium 1⅓–1⅔ RDA, and low ⅔ RDA or below) (Stuff *et al.* 1982).

Attempting to solve this dilemma, some countries are considering establishing different levels of nutrient intake for various purposes. Thus, in Australia, a lower *diagnostic level* of intake has been suggested as a *physiological minimum*, and as a higher *recommended dietary intake* (RDI) for safe dietary planning (Truswell 1983). If this type of more complicated approach becomes widely used, results may be presented in relation to the different 'diagnostic levels'. Until such time, results are probably best presented for group or community studies as percentages of the RDA, with an accompanying explanation of the definition of the RDA. For individuals, a more cautious approach is indicated and a figure of two-thirds of the RDA can be used. Although imprecise, this seems an understandable diagnostic level with which results can be compared.

Unfortunately, as the RDAs are expressed numerically, they have an aura of scientific accuracy which is quite unwarranted in light of their derivation. It is obvious that there are numerous problems and uncertainties at every stage of the sequence leading to estimates of nutritional dietary adequacy in communities, households or individuals. Also, examples of apparent adaptation to lower intakes abound (Whitehead 1986).

Severe deficiencies will be detectable, but, as with all forms of nutritional assessment, great caution is needed to interpret lesser degrees. As repeatedly stressed for all methods of assessment, information on dietary intake needs to be combined with other types of information to give a useful general picture.

Conclusions

> *Epidemiological research consists in large part of sorting through tangles of associations between personal characteristics, environmental circumstances, and disease processes, searching for those biologically significant linkages that might be manipulated to prevent disease. Since everything is related to everything else, the search is often tedious.*
> *The tedium could be relieved substantially if we lived in a deterministic world and one in which the things we are measuring would stand still. However our world is probabilistic and all variables vary.*
>
> Reuel Stallones (1982)

This review of methods of assessment of ecological variables, including both causes and associated conditions, reveals that there are considerably more difficulties, complexities, ambiguities, and variations than often appreciated, especially when numerical results are the outcome. In turn, this leads to the need to select methods carefully to obtain the maximum amount of useful information (so as to avoid making scientific-sounding conclusions based on flimsy facts), at the least cost (time, money, and staff). It also again emphasizes the importance of combining methods to try to validate and corroborate results.

As with other aspects of nutritional assessment, any analysis of ecological variables in any form of community or individual nutritional assessment will vary greatly in complexity, depending upon the type and number of staff, the time available, and the purpose of the investigation.

Collecting as much information as possible is useful to give a complete picture of the existing situation and to suggest methods of improvement. Nevertheless, the amount and complexity of such information that theoretically could be collected can be inhibiting and even counterproductive. However, even rapid screening surveys, which record basic anthropometry and a limited number of clinical signs, can also incorporate some information on dietary intake and observation of a small number of selected local ecological variables in the course of a field survey (Table 4.15). Results can sometimes indicate the possible practical priorities for more detailed studies.

In many small-scale surveys conducted in technically less developed countries, both the size and training of the personnel and time available will be very limited. However, even in such circumstances, it may be possible for a sample of homesteads to be investigated in more detail. If even this is not feasible, qualitative information on major ecological factors can be obtained roughly during the actual survey by unobtrusive observation. Items that can be noted in practice will include only some of those in the lists given earlier in each section and in Table 4.15. Those chosen for inclusion in any particular field study will depend on various local circumstances and on probable relevance to nutrition and ease of identification in the course of rapid ecological visits. As noted earlier (p. 142), the risk of such an approach is that incorrect impressions may be obtained. Considerable caution must be exercised before making such generalizations sound like statistically verified facts. This means that reports of such investigations must give details of the methods used.

It follows, therefore, that all attempts at the assessment of the nutritional status of communities whenever possible should be multidisciplinary in scope (Gopalan 1987), as soon as such activities move from the basic enumeration and categorization of malnutrition into consideration of ecological variables. This is especially the case when trying to differentiate between ecological variables that are 'associated' with malnutrition and those which are judged to be 'causative'.

In less technically developed countries and from an immediate practical point of view, minimal attention to probable causes of malnutrition often should give priority to the assessment of: (1) relevant resources available to the less privileged portion of the population (e.g. adequacy of income and land related to needs of basic foods for families, especially for

Table 4.15 Guide list of selected features sometimes identifiable during rapid visits: intended to be used selectively

Home	
Family size	Number, relationships, ages, sex, interval between children
Occupations	Primary, secondary
Education	Adult literacy, presence of books and newspapers, children at school
House	Type and construction (roof, walls, floor), number of rooms
Economic	Furniture, clothes, radio, transport (bicycle, wagon, motor scooter, car)
Kitchen	Stove, fuel, cooking utensils, dishes in preparation
Feeding pattern	Meals seen, foods not used, breastfeeding, modern 'prestige' foods
Food storage	Size, types, contents, pest-proofing
Water supply	Type, distance, purity
Latrine	Type, state
Cultivation site	
Land	Area, use with different crops (including cash crops)
Farming methods	Tilling procedure, irrigation, fertilizer, reaping, drying
Livestock and fishing	Number of beasts and poultry, fish pond
Markets and shops	
Food and weaning equipment	Availability and prices of foods (especially protein foods for children), advertising, availability of bottles and nipples

pregnant women and vulnerable young children, with special emphasis on the main staple and legume, local vegetable oil, and breast milk); (2) the commonness of more important preventable contributory (conditioning) infections; and (3) qualitative (or preferably semi-quantitiative) assessment of the dietary intake in pregnancy and the first 2 years of life, especially breastfeeding and the use of available local foods during the weaning period, in both rural and urban areas.

Ultimately, there remain three difficult problems: (1) how to select the ecological variables to be included; (2) how to differentiate the 'causative' from the 'associative' factors identified; and (3) how to decide which causative factors are most significant. For these purposes, general judgement and observation can be assisted by sophisticated epidemiological computations, such as multiple regression analysis[65] and calculation of attributable risk[65], etc. In particular, it is often possible to select from general observational 'risk factors' (International Union of Nutritional Sciences 1977) those which are more important in the particular community ('attributable risk') (Backett *et al.* 1984). Further details are given later (pp. 452–6).

Such analyses can help in trying to decide on priorities in programmes, although in fact, non-mathematical considerations, such as feasibility, cost, acceptability, population concern, and politics, influence decisions more than numerical calculations.

[65] See Appendix 4 for explanation of common epidemiological terms.

6

Interpretation in different age-groups

The infant, mewling and puking in his nurses's arms ... the justice in fair round belly with good capon lined ... the sixth stage, the lean and slippered pantaloon...

Excised from Shakespeare's *As you like it.*

Introduction

Each stage of human life has different nutritional considerations. The preferred methods for assessment vary with the age-groups that are the main concern of the investigation. Different stages of the life-cycle have special physiological nutritional needs (p. 226), susceptibility to infections (p. 139), and cultural benefits or hazards (p. 165). The risk of different forms of malnutrition varies in different age-groups, and, as has been noted elsewhere (p. 14), even certain clinical signs suggestive of nutritional deficiency can be age-specific (p. 226). In addition, the anthropometric effects of protein–energy malnutrition in rapidly growing young children plainly will be different from those in an adult for whom physiological growth has ceased.

Although assessment of nutritional status may be undertaken to include all age-groups in a community, differences in nutritional problems and manifestations make it useful to consider the following categories: *materno-fetal nutrition, infant nutrition, nutrition of young children, nutrition of schoolage children and adolescents,* and *adult nutrition.*

Materno-fetal nutrition

We are what our mothers ate.

D. Oberleas *et al.* (1972)

A moderately-small toll on the nutritional economy of the mother for much of gestation, provision of adequate nutrients to support growth of the conceptus is clearly more complex and involves considerable adaptive responses on the part of the mother throughout gestation.

J. Bassett (1986)

Both these quotations are partially true. Because of this special complexity, in recent years much increased attention has been focused on materno–fetal nutrition, both from a scientific and a practical point-of-view. Indeed, the dyadic nature of the nutrition of the pregnant and lactating woman and the fetus *in utero*, the extero-gestate (or external) fetus (birth to 6–9 months) and the transitional or weanling (6–9 months to 2–3 years) has received wider recognition (Jelliffe and Jelliffe 1989*a*). Biologically, these stages form a continuum with maternal nutrition needing consideration in relation to transplacental fetal nutrition (p. 245), to breastfeeding the young infant (p. 260), to the care and feeding of the transitional or weanling (p. 262), and to the mother's own survival and health, with their obvious influence on her offspring. The present section is concerned with the assessment of nutritional status in pregnancy and in the newborn, as a reflection of fetal nutrition.

Maternal nutrition

Reproductive burden

Pregnant women are a nutritionally vulnerable group, especially in poor socio-economic circumstances anywhere in the world, notably in technically less developed regions (Liljestrand 1985). This becomes particularly so in extreme situations, as in famines or among refugees.

Nutritional needs are especially difficult to measure as assessment has to take into account the metabolism of two individuals, one of whom — the fetus — is inaccessible, without the use of highly technological procedures. The situation is further complicated by the nutrients required for the development of the placenta, uterus, and amniotic fluid, and by the difficult-to-analyse roles of maternal and placental hormones in inducing physiological adaptive changes in the mother during pregnancy, such as increased iron absorption and haemodilution.

Estimated recommended dietary allowances (RDAs) are often thought to be considerable. (US National Research Council 1980). For example, dietary requirements of iron and folic acid have been calculated to increase about sixfold. The significance of adequate calories has become increasingly emphasized.

On the other hand, many field studies indicate that physiological and cultural adaptations must occur commonly as adequate pregnancy outcomes occur with very much lower nutrient intakes than often recommended (Adair and Pollitt 1983; Kusin and Jansen 1986.)

Energy expenditure will be particularly high in some traditional cultures, where women may be responsible (sometimes throughout pregnancy) for much heavy, physical work often carried out with inefficient, clumsy tools. Cultivation, carrying the food to market, collecting water and wood, and pounding or hand-milling foods, as well as cooking for the family and carrying young children are commonly women's tasks.

However, in some communities — for example, in a part of New Guinea — pregnant women limit their activities somewhat as a physiol-

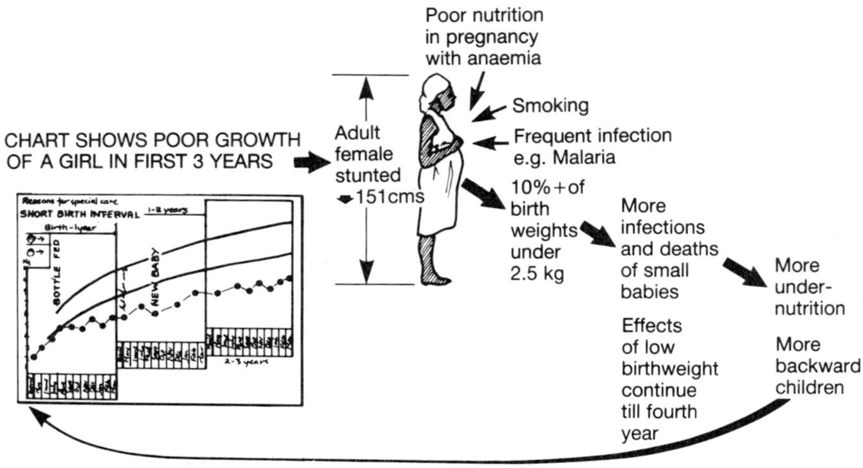

Fig. 5.1 Cycle of malnutrition: a common sequence in females in less technically developed countries. (Courtesy of Professor David Morley.)

ogical adjustment, often with cultural sanction (Greenfield and Clark 1974).

Nutritional stress can be aggravated by restrictive food customs which often are directed at women, especially during pregnancy and the puerperium. For example, in some East African communities women have been prohibited from eating chicken, eggs, mutton, and certain types of fish, which are the main local sources of animal protein (Jelliffe and Bennett 1962). A wide variety of other practices is found in different parts of the world. A relevant example is the custom of giving a very high salt intake in pregnancy among the Hausa of Northern Nigeria (Ebrahim 1982). In traditional cultures, it is rather unusual for any dietary improvement to be made during pregnancy, more often general or specific food restrictions are found.

An increased or improved diet can be given during the puerperium, as in some Chinese communities, or indirectly assisted by a culturally defined period of rest and seclusion after delivery. However, sometimes such cultural restrictions exist, but may not affect the dietary intake much. The *quantitative* effect of such restrictions needs considering and these may vary considerably with the strictness with which they are followed. Also, the diet may be restricted only for a short period after delivery.

In some areas, females may be in an almost constant state of nutritional stress from their own childhood up to the time of marriage and childbearing (often before their own growth has ceased). Continuous reproductive cycles can follow which may result in premature death in their thirties (Fig. 5.1; Table 5.1). The whole of adult life may be continuously reproductive, as a succession of pregnancies and so-called 'prolonged' lactations follow one another without pause. In some cultures, particu-

Table 5.1 Some possible effects on fetus and/or mother of *severe* inadequate maternal nutrition in pregnancy — more marked with repeated reproductive cycles

Maternal	
'Maternal depletion syndromes'	Protein–energy* malnutrition Specific nutrients (iron and/or folic acid anaemia, goitre, beriberi)
Maternal death	Anaemia and haemorrhage (iron deficiency)
Suboptimal lactation	Volume of breast milk limited Specific nutrients in breast milk limited (vitamin A, etc.)
Materno-fetal	
Stillbirths and abortions	
Fetal	
Low birth weight	Defective immunocompetence (susceptibility to infections) Possible growth retardation, especially in 'chronic' fetal malnutrition Possible impairment of mental ability
Suboptimal neonatal stores	

* Calories (energy) the most important deficiency.

larly in urban circumstances, the socio-economic and nutritional consequences of early teenage pregnancies are made worse by illegitimacy, with lack of social acceptance and support. This is increasingly the case in Westernized societies, such as the USA, but also seems to be a world-wide phenomenon.

In traditional cultures, early marriage and child-bearing are usual. For example, in a study in Hyderabad, the *average* maternal age for a first child was 16.2 years (Ebrahim 1982). Following this, repeated reproductive cycles of pregnancy and lactation can become a cumulative nutritional drain, leading to various forms of 'maternal depletion syndrome' (Jelliffe and Maddocks 1964). Probably the most common is protein–energy malnutrition. This is usually insidious, undramatic, and may only be revealed by decreasing body weight and subcutaneous fat with succeeding pregnancies. In extreme circumstances, oedema of nutritional origin can develop (Bailey 1962), and rarely adult kwashiorkor. However, for reasons as yet little understood, adaptive physiological processes obviously occur in pregnant women in some circumstances lessening the need for additional nutrients, including calories (Adair and Pollitt 1983; Kusin and Jansen 1986). The pre-pregnancy nutritional status of the mother seems critical, as does her 'life style'.

Specific maternal depletion syndromes involving particular nutrients can also occur, often becoming more marked with recurring pregnancies. These vary in different parts of the world depending on locally prevalent nutritional deficiencies. They can include osteomalacia, iron deficiency (or megaloblastic) anaemias, and iodine deficiency goitre.

In recent years, the opposite situation — obesity in pregnancy — has become recognized as a problem in Westernized well-to-do circumstances. Severe obesity in pregnancy can pose obstetrical difficulties during delivery. In addition, there may be an increased perinatal mortality rate, and prevalence of high-birth-weight babies, usually defined as 4000 g or over, with possible relationship to obesity in later childhood (Mcharen 1987) Also, the question of weight gain and dietary intake in already obese women is currently debated in clinical practice, since it is important to supply nutrients for pregnancy without increasing the individual's obesity. Probably the ideal would be a diet containing the additional nutrients required for pregnancy, especially minerals and vitamins, but with some limitation of calorie intake, given mainly in the form of carbohydrate foods. The remainder of the calories could be supplied from the mother's surplus fat stores.

With regard to the effects of lesser degrees of maternal malnutrition, problems of comparison and interpretation depend on the levels and forms of undernutrition under consideration in pregnancy and on whether the prior nutritional situation in the community was relatively 'adequate'. Contrasting situations exist as, for example, with the relatively short, but severe, food shortage in Holland in World War II, and chronically and continuously markedly inadequate, nutritional status, as in many less technically developed countries.

In some Western countries, especially the USA, 'obstetrical fashion' in previous decades advised dietary restriction in pregnancy and a limitation of weight gain to 7 kg in the belief that this would decrease the likelihood of pre-eclampsia and produce a smaller baby and an easier delivery. In the past 10 years or more, this dogma has been completely reversed (Pitkin *et al.* 1972; Jacobson 1983). Instead, a generous diet is now advocated, with a suggested weight gain of 10–12 kg and with the recognition of increased subcutaneous fat as a physiological reserve, especially for lactation.

Effects

The effects of maternal malnutrition in pregnancy on both the mother and her offspring depend on its severity, the nutrients involved, the woman's previous nutritional status, and the degree of maternal adaption.

As expected, the consequences on the mother and fetus are more marked with severe degrees of combined present and past malnutrition. In famines, especially in previously poorly-fed communities, amenorrhoea and loss of libido cause declining birth rates. There are also high maternal, perinatal, and infant mortalities. The last is partly related to the ultimate lactation failure seen in starving breastfeeding mothers. At the other end of the nutritional spectrum, in the UK, Edwards and colleagues (1979) have shown that women whose pre-pregnancy weight for height was 10 per cent or more below 'standard' had a higher than usual rate of low-birth-weight babies with poor growth in early infancy, and maternal anaemia. The effects of possible 'marginal' sublinical deficiencies of trace minerals remains uncertain (Hurley 1980).

Methods of assessment

The assessment of the nutritional status of pregnant women has an important place in public health activities because of their nutritional vulnerability. Also, at least some pregnant women are accessible at prenatal clinics, which are popular in many parts of the world. Sometimes, pregnant women can be an approximately indicative group for some wider community problems, such as iodine deficiency presenting as goitre. Maternal malnutrition has consequences not only for the mother, but for the health, nutrition (especially avoidance of low birth weight) (p. 245), and survival of her baby. Monitoring of mothers in pregnancy will enable nutrition-related 'at risk' indicators (p. 453) to be defined for the particular region, including those suggesting a high risk of a subsequent low-birth-weight newborn.

To obtain a valid picture of maternal nutrition in the community, appropriate sampling methods (p. 205) need to be undertaken. Often, biased studies have been carried out on limited samples of such women who are attending prenatal clinics. This remains a worthwhile approach, provided its probable lack of representativeness is recognized and noted in any reports.

While serial, longitudinal observations during the course of pregnancy are ideal, anthropometric measurements and other examinations in the early weeks can give an approximate idea of the mother's background nutritional stauts. If only a single examination is feasible, about the sixth month of pregnancy may be the best time to detect, prevent, and correct nutritional deficiencies.

Direct assessment

Clinical signs

Different signs may have a special importance in particular regions, depending upon the local nutritional problems. These may include angular cheilosis, conjunctival pallor, goitre, the bone pains of osteomalacia (especially severe and persistent low back pain), and suggestive signs of beriberi. Pre-tibial oedema can be due to various causes. Uncommonly, it can be nutritionally relevant in some areas where severe protein–energy malnutrition is common in pregnancy (Bailey 1962), notably in famines. Other more common obstetrical causes of oedema, need to be excluded such as toxaemia. Signs or measurements of pelvic narrowing or distortion may indicate past rickets or protein–energy malnutrition in early childhood. They can have direct bearing on the risk of obstructed labour and potential for neonatal injury.

Biochemical tests

Apart from difficulties with all biochemical tests (p. 31), the nutritional problems of local importance will determine the nature and utility of the tests given priority. For example, studies in Saudi Arabia have suggested that there is a high prevalence of marginal vitamin D deficiency in pregnant women (Serenius *et al.* 1984). Special reference data are required for pregnant women, such as those suggested by the US National Academy of Sciences (1980).

Haematological investigations

Haemoglobin concentrations are of great practical value in the nutritional assessment of pregnant women. This is especially so in regions where maternal deaths occur in pregnancy from anaemia alone, especially when compounded with even slightly increased blood-loss during delivery. The commonness of anaemia in pregnancy as a public health problem was shown by Petros-Barvazian and Behar (1978) who estimated that in numerous developing countries 30–40 per cent of women may have haemoglobin concentrations below 10 g/d in the third trimester of pregnancy. More up-to-date information from most countries has been given by Royston (1982), confirming its widespread prevalence.

Ideally, haemoglobin estimations should be made serially during pregnancy — for example, at each attendance at a prenatal clinic. However, regular or frequent attendances may be unusual, and the best single time for a haemoglobin estimation in relation to possibility of treatment and avoidance of later complications is at about the sixth month of pregnancy.

Appropriate technology As noted earlier, the question of an appropriate, low-cost apparatus for measuring haemoglobin concentrations has not been solved as yet, and is a major priority for 'appropriate technology' (p. 43). At community levels, screening with such simple devices as the anaemia recognition card (p. 25) (Ghosh and Mohan 1978) or the three band 'anaemiometer' (Shah 1980), may be helpful to community

Table 5.2 Critical levels for key haematological investigations in adult women. (*Modified from WHO 1972*b)*

Determination	Level
Haemoglobin	
Pregnant	< 11 g/dl
Non-pregnant	< 12 g/dl
Haematocrit	
Pregnant	< 33%
Non-pregnant	< 36%
Serum iron	< 50 μg%
Percentage saturation	< 15
Serum folate	< 3 ng/ml
Serum vitamin B_{12}	< 80 pg/ml

* Serum ferritin levels have been used more recent to estimate body iron stores (p. 500).

health workers in identifying more serious degrees of conjuctival and mucosal pallor.

The interpretation of haemoglobin levels in pregnancy must take into account the normal physiological fall in level of about 2 g/dl due to haemodilution. This 'pseudo-anaemia' is associated with a decreased haematocrit reading, but no hypochromia. Also, Micozzi (1978) has drawn attention to the need to view haemoglobin levels in pregnancy in relation to their 'functional significance' and even possible genetic, ethnic variations. In a study in the Philippines,, he reported that a pregnancy haemoglobin of 10–11 g/dl seemed to have no measurable ill-effect on subsequent maternal or neonatal health.

Nutritional anaemia in pregnancy remains a common and serious public health problem in less developed countries and the literature has been reviewed by Royston (1982). It is usually caused by iron deficiency, but may be megaloblastic, owing to an inadequate intake of folic acid and/or vitamin B_{12}. Anaemia due to combined iron and folic acid deficiency can occur. With regard to iron deficiency, Simmons and colleague (1982) have shown that the degree of anaemia correlates with the risks of fetal and maternal mortalities in the Caribbean. Based on large-scale studies, they suggest the following labels < 8g 'severe' and < 9 g 'moderate' anaemia Different levels may used to be used elsewhere in the world for practical management.

Critical levels for key haematological investigations are given in Table 5.2. More detailed tests related to the cause of anaemia will be needed in different regions (p. 500) including stool examinations for hookworm ova, thick blood fims for malarial parasites, etc. In hyperendemic areas, malaria is especially important, as immunity declines during pregnancy, especially in primiparae.

Anthropometry

This remains the main approach to the assessment of nutritional status in pregnancy, and can be considered in two ways: (1) *background anthropometry*; and (2) *changes during pregnancy*.

Background anthropometry

Prior to or during the first 1–3 months of pregnancy, before the onset of rapid fetal growth, weight-for-height ratios of 10 per cent or more *below* locally used reference level or 20 per cent *above* have been suggested as rough indicators of under- or over-nutrition.

With all genetic provisos recognized, maternal height is both a gauge of *past* nutritional state in particular, with correlation with pelvic bony growth in earlier life, and present size. The main problem in the possibility of obstructed labour.

Body fat stores can roughly be gauged by measuring the triceps fatfold (p. 89). At a more sophisticated, but still approximate level, it is possible to estimate total energy reserves and percentage of body weight composed of fat by various formulae combining fatfold measurements from several sites. The triceps, biceps, subscapular, and supra-iliac measurements have been recommended by Durnin and Rahaman (1967) (p. 91), based on results obtained from a sample of Scottish women. This combination may not be optimal in other ethnic groups or ages.

Other approaches could be by measuring the arm circumference and triceps fatfold and estimating the arm muscle circumference (p. 101), the arm fat and muscle areas (p. 102), or the arm muscle or fat volumes (p. 102). Additional ways of comparing energy and protein reserves have been described elsewhere, including the adiposomuscular ratio (Bray 1978) (p. 342) or the *E/P* (energy–protein) ratio (Amador *et al.* 1981).

For village workers, simple screening measurements may be devised. A height stick (Fig. 5.3) and arm band can be useful. 'Cut-off' levels will have to be appropriate for the local situation. For example, in some communities, a height below 150 cm (5 ft) and an arm circumference below 23 cm may be useful for basic screening of high-risk mothers. As a very simple form of 'appropriate technology' (p. 361), a bar or rod can be positioned across the door of the clinic at the local 'at risk' height (Everett 1978) (Fig. 5.2). Other practical methods may be useful for illiterate TBA (traditional birth attendants) (Fig. 5.3).

In Guatemala, simplified arm tapes have been employed for both pregnant women and newborn babies. These have only two colours — white: normal, red: abnormally low (Lechtig *et al.* 1983).

Basically, three simple anthropometric measurements can be used to

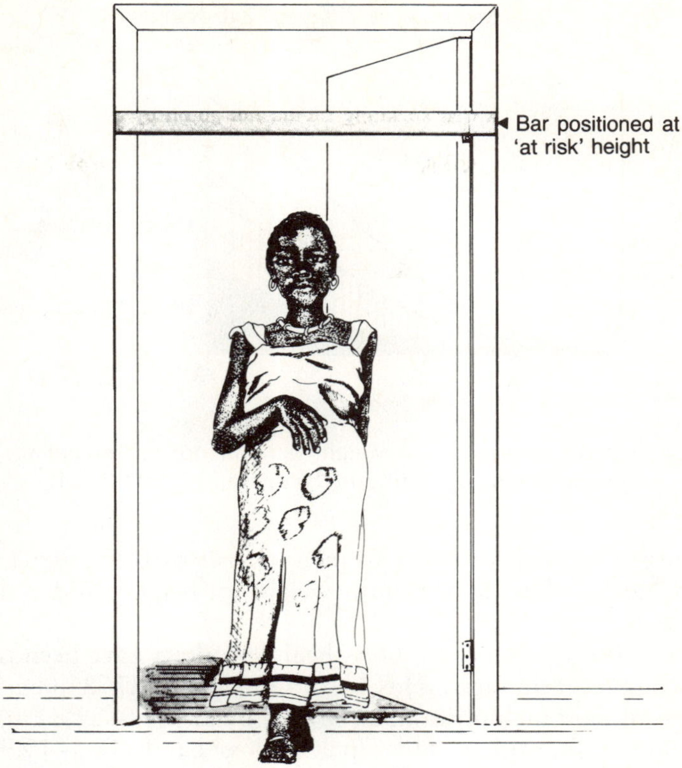

Fig. 5.2 Bar across door of clinic to detect small stature (Everett 1984).

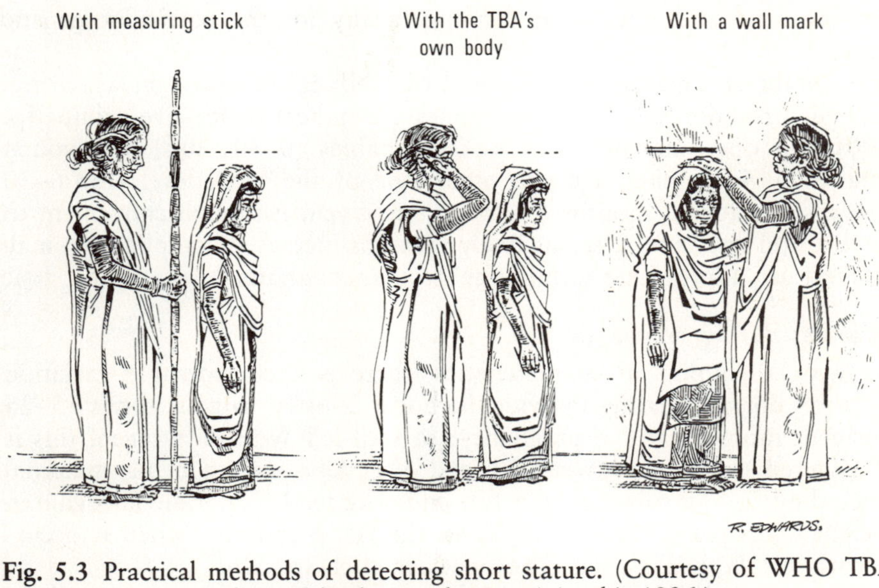

Fig. 5.3 Practical methods of detecting short stature. (Courtesy of WHO TBA (traditional birth attendant) training kit 1986.)

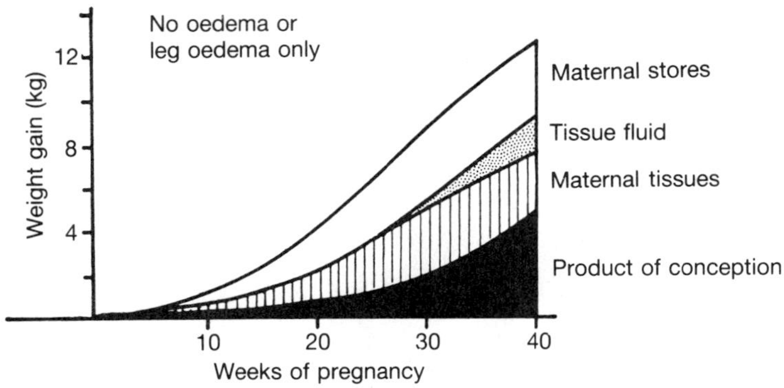

Fig. 5.4 Estimated components of weight gain in normal pregnancy: Scottish women in UK. (Courtesy of Hytten and Leitch 1971.)

identify probably malnourished women at risk of delivering low-birth-weight babies — low height, low weight-for-height, and a low arm circumference.

In parts of rural India, community health workers have been trained to use a 'tricoloured arm tape'. This has a red band (22.7–25.0cm) indicating normal-to-mild malnutrition, an orange band (20.0–22.6 cm) indicating moderate malnutrition, and a pale yellow band (18.5–19.9 cm) indicating severe malnutrition. The choice of colours can sometimes be culturally significant. In India, red is auspicious and 'healthy', and yellow is associated with sickness. The most useful measurements for the different zones on the tapes need defining locally for the particular genetic group.

A combined tape has been devised by UNICEF in Brazil on which red (danger or abnormal) and white zones are indicative for five groups (p. 100). On one side, pregnant women, babies (0–30 days) and young infants (1–5 months). On the other side of the tape, levels for 6–30 months and for 31 months to 6 years are given. Although convenient to have all on one tape, it seems likely that this increased complication may convert an 'appropriate technology' to inappropriate.

Changes during pregnancy

As with all biological characteristics, there is a considerable variation between normal healthy individuals, but it is usual to gain about 15–25 per cent more weight in pregnancy. In well-fed Western women, this is considered to range between 11 and 12.5 kg — 6 kg being maternal (including 3–4 kg subcutaneous fat) and 5 kg fetal (Fig. 5.4). This gain in weight takes place almost entirely in the last 6 months, when it occurs linearly at about 350–400 g per week in such women.

Weight gain in pregnancy has three phases: first trimester — very slight

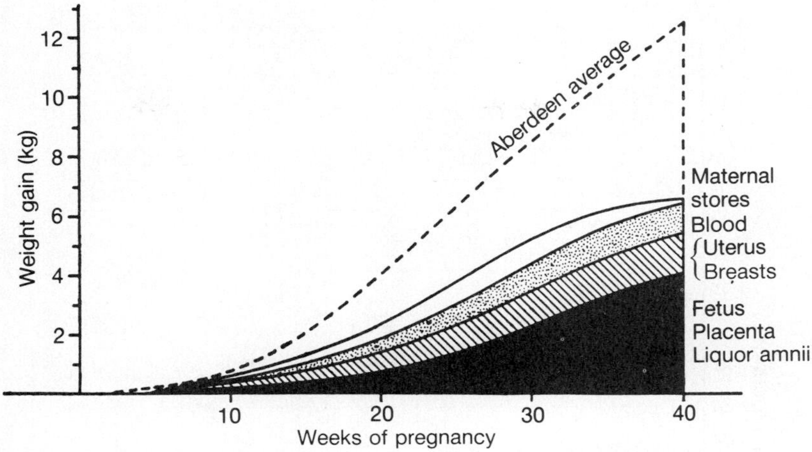

Fig. 5.5 Estimated components of weight gain in poor Indian women. (Courtesy of Venkatachalam *et al.* 1960.)

gain; second trimester — considerable linear increase involving maternal tissues and stores; third trimester — continuing considerable linear increase due to growth of the fetus, placenta, and aminotic fluid, together with the continuing laying down of maternal tissue and stores.

Recent work has shown a hormonally regulated biphasic metabolic activity with both fat and protein. In both cases, during the first part of the cycle in early pregnancy there is an increase in protein storage and in fat deposition. In the latter part of pregnancy when fetal growth is extremely rapid, these stores can be mobilized (Willocks 1977). The subcutaneous fat also acts as a bank of calories and fatty acids for subsequent breastfeeding (Jelliffe and Jelliffe 1989*a*).

By contrast, poorly nourished pregnant women show much lower weight gains. For example, Gebre-Medhin and Falk (1980) reported that privileged Ethiopian women gained an average of 10.6 kg in pregnancy, while non-privileged mothers of the same genetic group showed an average weight gain of only 6 kg. Differences in total gain and possible components were shown in southern India 20 years ago (Fig. 5.5) (Venkatachalam *et al.* 1960). However, the mother's pre-pregnancy size and physique have to be the practical basis for judging weight gain. In general, *percentage* weight gain (15–25 per cent) is more logical, with limits of locally desirable weight gains (in kg) needing to be estimated for the particular community, as judged by an adequate birth weight.

Growth charts Serial weight measurements in pregnancy can provide useful approximate insights into probable fetal growth and maternal nutritional status.

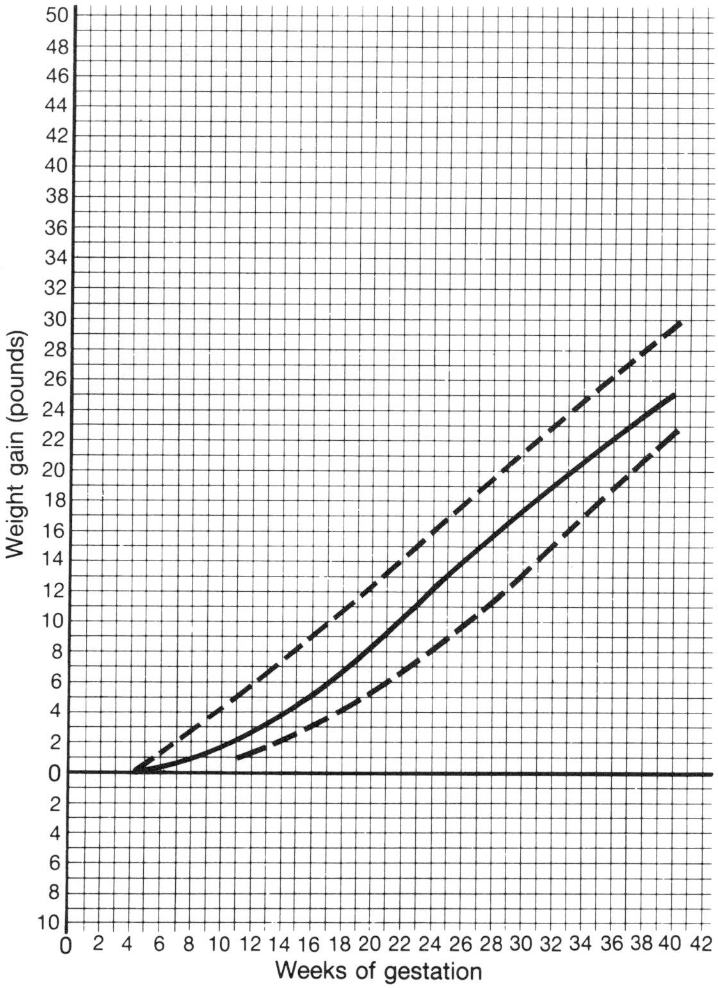

Fig. 5.6 Curve for the assessment of weight gain during pregnancy (Butman 1982).

Various pregnancy growth charts have been devised in the past. These include the US National Academy of Sciences (1970) chart in the USA, based on a total weight gain of 10.9 kg (24 lb), subsequently modified by Butman (1982) (Fig. 5.6). In Scotland, Thompson (1965) developed a chart (Fig. 5.7) based on a total weight gain of 12.5 kg (27.5 lb) and a rate of gain of about 0.45 kg (1 lb) per week in the second half of pregnancy. The 'norms' are shown as a series of parallel lines, and the actual weights at each attendance are recorded directly against the appropriate week of gestation. A patient who is gaining weight more

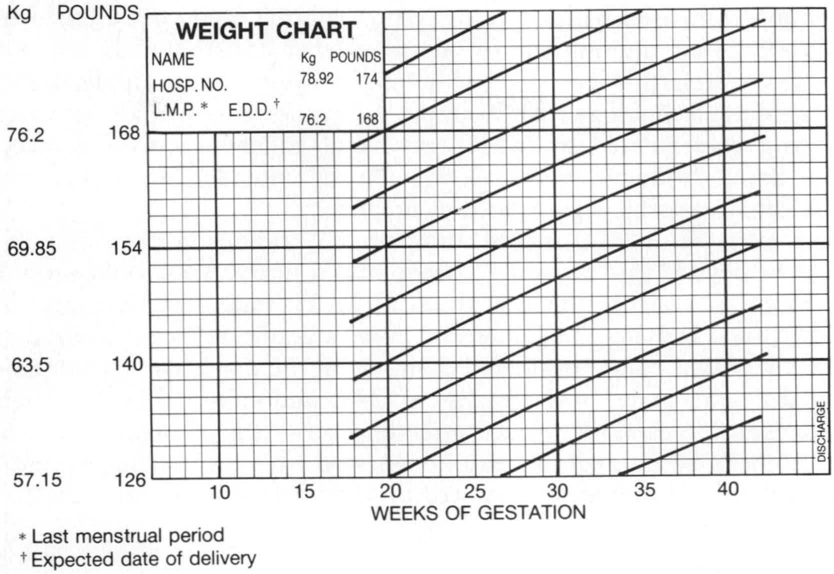

Fig. 5.7 Thompson pregnancy weight chart (Thompson 1965). See text for details.

slowly than the standard will show a trend downwards across the parallels, while one who is gaining weight faster than the standard will show a trend upwards.

Rosso (1985) described a new chart to monitor weight gain in pregnancy. This is based on a 'modified table of weight for average frame size'. It appears to be too complex for use in most Third World countries.

Particularly in less technically developed countries, problems often exist because the date of the last menstrual period will not be known, use of a Western-type calendar may not be part of the local culture, and the woman's pre-gravid weight will not be known. By contrast, in some cultures, the occasion of the most recent menstrual period will be known exactly according to the lunar or local calendar (e.g. Hindu), because it is a time of ritual impurity requiring seclusion and ceremonial cleansing. Last, a reasonable or optimal weight gain in smaller mothers is difficult to be certain about and needs investigation regarding the local situation and practical outcomes, especially the relationship to 'adequate' birth weights, maternal health, and ease of delivery.

Compared with very large amounts of work on growth charts for young children (p. 296), the creation and testing of appropriately adapted weight charts for pregnant women seems to have been neglected until recently. This is partly because of the difficulties mentioned, partly because nutritional problems of pregnancy have often been given inadequate attention compared with those of young children, and partly because of only occasional, intermittent, or late attendance at prenatal clinics. In the last few years, this has become a major area for the application of 'appropriate technology'. For example, a large long-term study in currently being co-ordinated by WHO in several countries into a prototype home-based mother's record (WHO 1985*d*), intended to include many variables of possible significance in pregnancy.

For example, a local modification of the Thompson chart (Fig. 5.7) could be devised in a particular developing country. This could show (1) the mothers' weights (on the abscissa) appropriate for the range seen locally, and (2) the parallel lines drawn with gradients based on total and monthly weight gains considered desirable in the particular communities, judged by 'adequate' birth weights (p. 245) and maternal health. Such a chart might be used for women attending very early in pregnancy, when the mother's gestational age can be assessed by obstetrical signs and/or the date of her last period estimated by local calendar on the occasion of the first weighing.

This concept has been improved on by Husaini *et al.* (1986) in Indonesia (Fig. 5.8) in a chart based on local weight gains, adequate birth weight, and various maternal heights. If the exact week of pregnancy is not known and cannot be plotted precisely, the weight gain should still parallel appropriate lines for the woman's height. However, this seems likely to be too complex for use, except in main centres.

Another approach has been pioneered in India by Kusum Shah (1978) in the form of a 'surveillance card for married women'. This is used by community health workers, who weigh all children under 6 years *and* all married women monthly during home-visiting. In addition, women's heights are recorded on the first visit. This information is recorded on the pre-pregnancy part of the self-retained card (Fig. 5.9), together with information concerning menstruation, family planning, and lactation, using symbols or locally understandable illustrations to record events. When a period is missed, the next page of the card is used, covering weight gain in pregnancy (Fig. 5.10). As with the 'Road-to-Health' growth charts for young children (p. 298), the purpose is to record a satisfactory curve rather than precise comparison with specific levels. Two lines are present on the cards. The upper line represents the mean weights of Aberdeen women who had a satisfactory weight gain in pregnancy and whose babies had a mean birth weight of 3.3. kg. The lower line represented weight changes of Indian women in the Project area in Kasa, rural Bombay State, who had delivered babies weighing 2.8 kg or more. A curve between these two lines and paralleling them was the aim. The card has a fold-out section allowing for records of four pregnancies in all.

This type of functional approach needs trying out in other parts of the world. It could sometimes fit into the possible range of tasks of primary

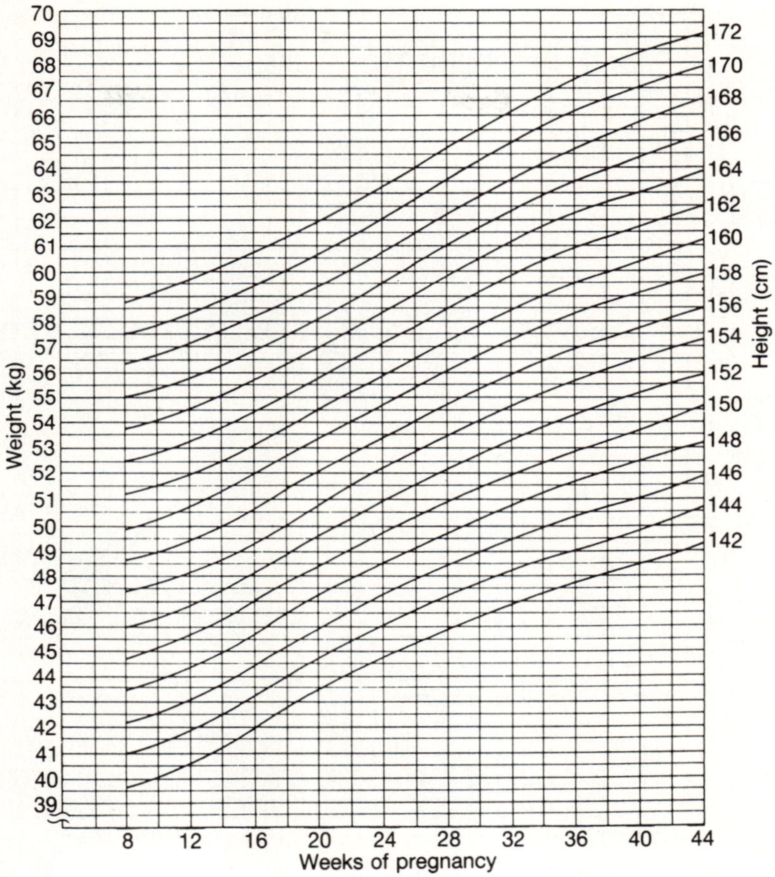

Fig. 5.8 Husaini chart for weight gain in pregnancy for women of different heights (Husaini *et al.* 1986).

care workers in the community. The use of home-based mothers' records is being tried out by WHO in various countries. However, practical and logistical difficulties, such as the feasibility of serial weighing of all fertile non-pregnant women and accurate early reporting of the last menstrual period will limit this approach to communities where pregnancy is unusual in unmarried women, such as India.

Percentage weight gain Well-fed, healthy women in Europe and North America usually gain about 15–25 per cent of their pre-gravid weights. In the United States, an inadequate weight gain has been defined as 1 kg or less per month in the last two-thirds of pregnancy (Pitkin *et al.* 1972).

In poorly fed communities, it is common for percentage weight gains

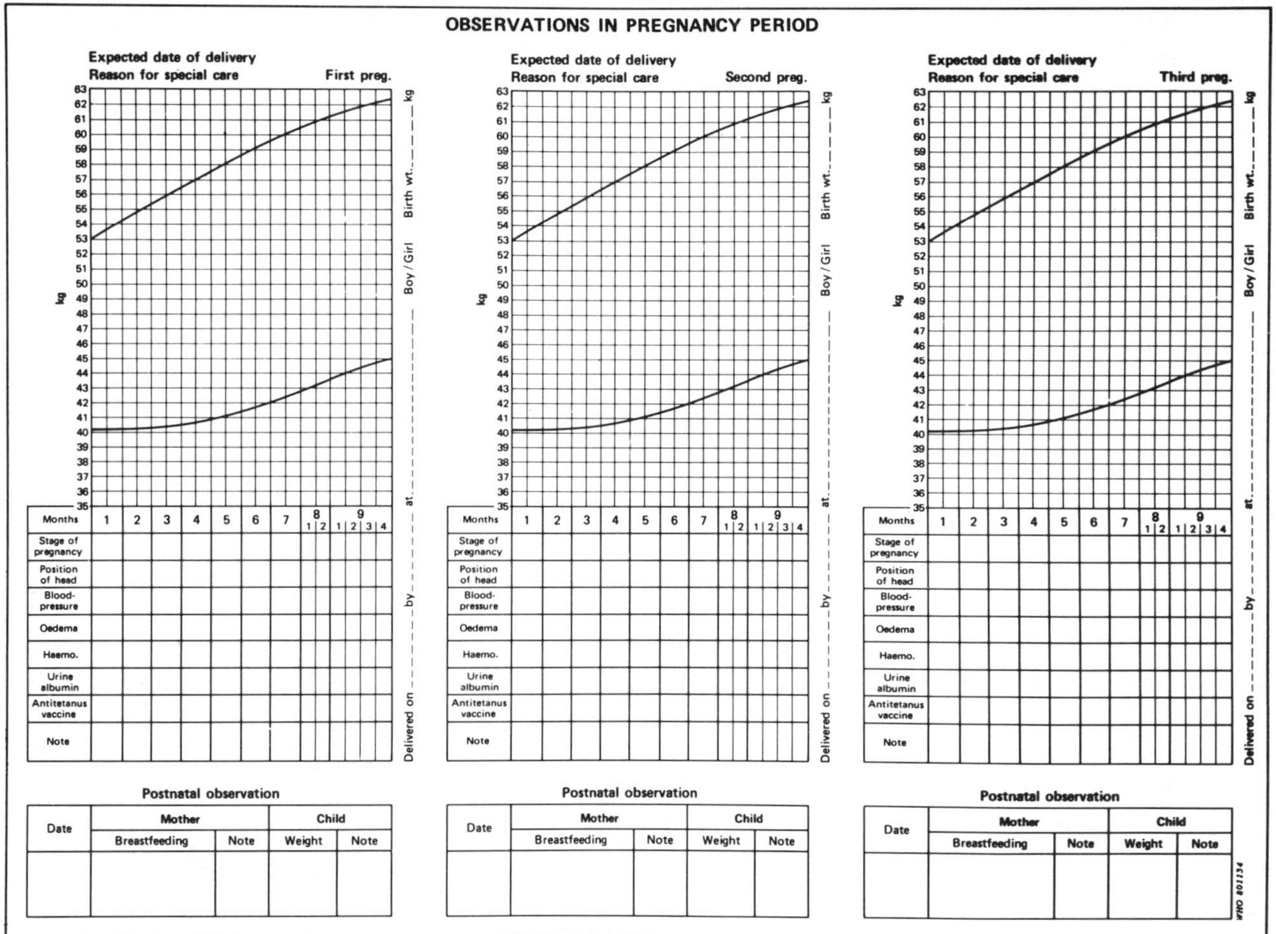

Fig. 5.10 Surveillance card for married women in rural India: pregnancy section (Kusum Shah 1978).

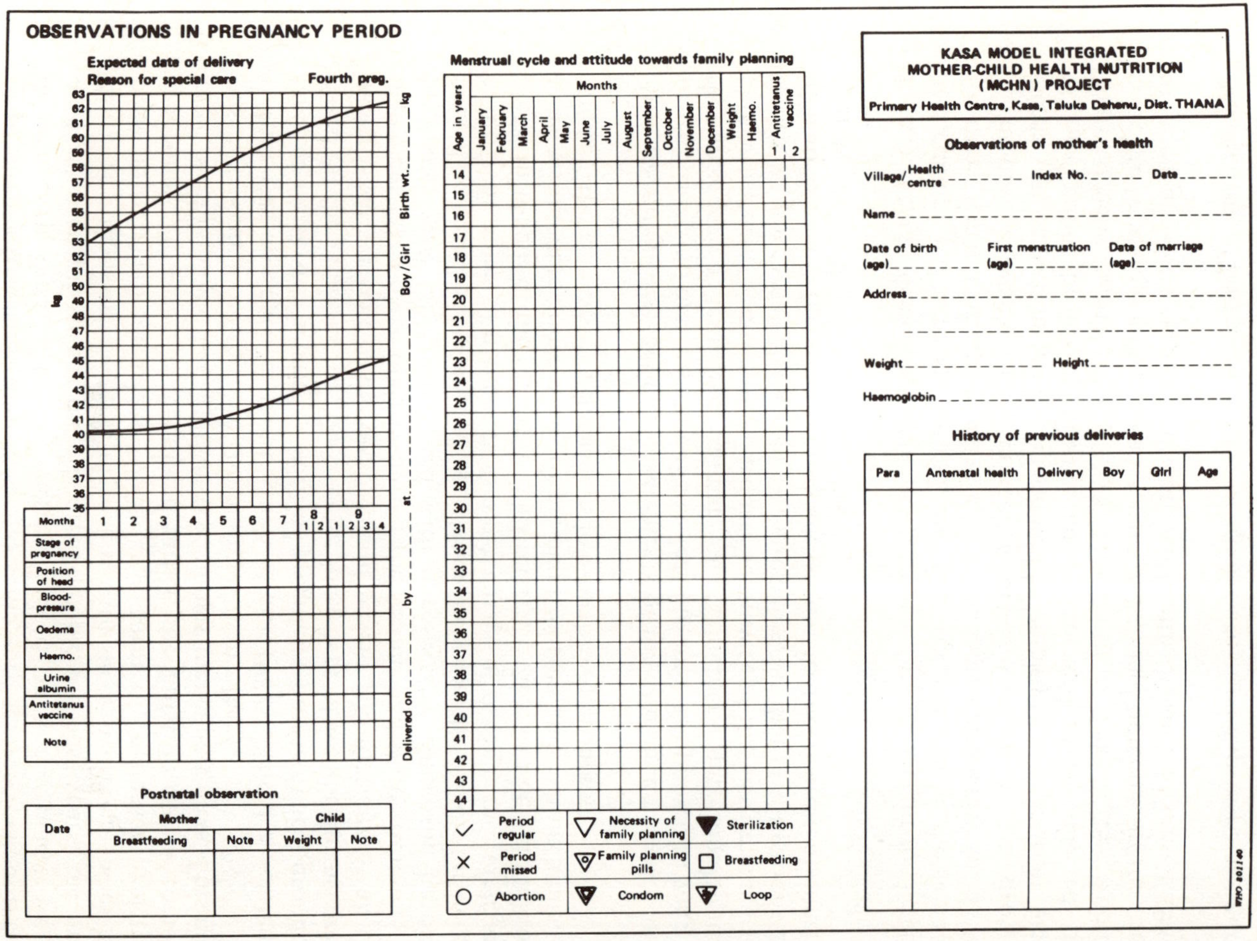

Fig. 5.9 Surveillance card for married women in rural India: pre-pregnancy section (Kusum Shah 1978).

in pregnancy to be less than this, and some very severely malnourished women even show a *loss* of weight. Indeed, in a few places where accurate prenatal weight records are available for past years, the incidence of progressive decrease in weight with successive pregnancies has been noted (Venkatachalam 1962), as a form of 'maternal depletion syndrome'. However, as mentioned earlier, the situation can be complicated by physiological adaptation to seemingly inadequate diets. This may possibly occur more in some communities than others.

With this approach in mind, Gueri *et al.* (1982) devised a reference table of weight-for-height by week of pregnancy on theoretical grounds, based on the premises that the average increment of weight during pregnancy is 20 per cent of the pre-pregnant weight and that almost all the increment takes place linearly during the second and third trimesters of pregnancy. The table was tested with retrospective clinic and hospital data. The results show a good correlation between the weight-for-height at different stages of pregnancy as a percentage of the reference table and the birth weight of the offspring. This reference table can be a useful tool to assess the nutritional status of pregnant women and, within limits, to 'predict' the chances of delivering a low-birth-weight infant.

Arm measurements Serial measurements of the arm circumference and/or triceps fatfold may occasionally be feasible, and, as opposed to weight, they may give a 'fetus-free' estimate of the mother's nutritional status. Difficulties arise because of inadequate sensitivity of the instruments used to detect rather small changes in measurements. Further investigations are indicated, as by the use of tapes measuring to the nearest millimetre (Zerfas, 1975; Ramachandran 1986).

Reference data Basic pre-pregnancy reference data for weight-for-height, arm circumference, triceps fatfold, and haemoglobin will be the same as for other females of reproductive age of the same community (p. 339).

The optimal weight gain is difficult to define. Current Western growth curves can be used as guides, but should be employed with caution. Data of *local* public health significance and value need to be collected and analysed when feasible (Shad 1978; Husaini *et al.* 1986). These should correlate weight gain in pregnancy with 'functional outcome' in the form of 'adequate' birth weight and maternal health (Kusin and Jansen 1986)

Presentation of findings Results of studies are often expressed as figures for mean weight gain (and distribution) compared with currently accepted Western levels. This does not seem to be realistic.

One more locally adapted method of expressing growth failure in pregnancy can be by the number of women with different levels of weight gain, particularly of less than 10 per cent between 'early pregnancy' and full-term. These can then be categorized as 10 per cent, < 10 to 5 per cent, < 5 per cent to no gain, and loss of weight. Again, the selection of such categorizations needs to be correlated with functional outcome, including 'adequate' birth weight of a viable baby capable of breastfeeding (p. 258) and maternal health.

Indirect assessment

For a number of complex reasons, maternal mortality and perinatal mortality rates are affected by the mother's socio-economic level (including her nutritional condition).

Relevant statistics should be collected, if feasible. However, this is rarely possible on a community basis, especially as the health of women is often much neglected. Sources of such data are usually the biased samples obtained from women attending prenatal clinics or admitted to hospital. Information should also be sought concerning women seen in wards and clinics with various forms of maternal malnutrition and relevant contributory infections (pp. 227, 348).

Assessment of ecological variables

In addition to the assessment of nutritional status of pregnancy, assessment of causative and/or associated ecological variables is also needed to permit the design of programmes appropriate for the needs of particular communities.

In addition to the assessment of availability and accessibility of key foods and in view of the special significance of the diet in pregnancy, a specifically designed questionnaire will be needed to investigate qualitative and/or semi-quantitative food consumption. Such a study should emphasize available nutritious foods that may be prohibited in pregnancy in the particular society (cultural blocks) (p. 168) and their quantitative significance. Particular attention needs to be paid to energy (calorie) intake in relation both to special needs in pregnancy and to physical work undertaken, and to available foods rich in nutrients known to be commonly deficient locally, such as riboflavin or vitamin A and to affect fetal growth (e.g. iron, zinc). In addition, nutritionally significant maternal infections need to be investigated when feasible, especially placental malaria (E.F.P. Jelliffe 1968*a*).

Fetal nutrition

The growth and nutrition of the human embryo and fetus are difficult to observe and measure directly. Intrauterine growth charts, such as the

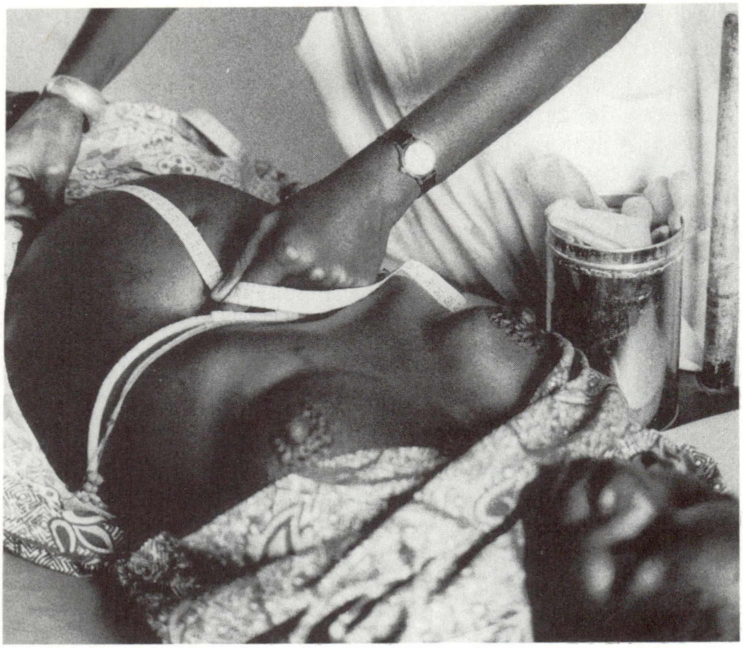

Fig. 5.11 Measuring height of fundus of uterus in pregnancy (Senegal). (Courtesy of UNICEF.)

classic ones compiled by Lubchenco *et al.* (1963), have been based mainly on the dimensions of live-born birth weight data at 24–42 weeks of gestation. More recently, ultrasound has been used for estimating various fetal measurements including the crown–rump length (Miller and Merritt 1979). Such sophisticated techniques have no direct practicality in technically less developed countries. However, they can be helpful in defining and validating simple anthropometric indicators, if carried out at national research centres.

Approximate direct estimation of fetal size has been advocated recently by measuring the height of the fundus of the uterus above the pubic symphysis (Fig. 5.11) (Belizan *et al.* 1978), as a result of studies in Argentina. Practical difficulties occur with taking such a measurement and with gauging the duration of pregnancy. A graph of symphysis–fundal height, showing the normal range of uterine height by week of gestation has been constructed by Everett (1978) (Fig. 5.12). Local adaptations will probably be required for different ethnic groups (Tjon A Ten *et al.* 1985). Garde (1986) has devised a composite score based on gains in fundal height, in abdominal girth, and in maternal weight during pregnancy. This will be too complicated for widespread use. Probably,

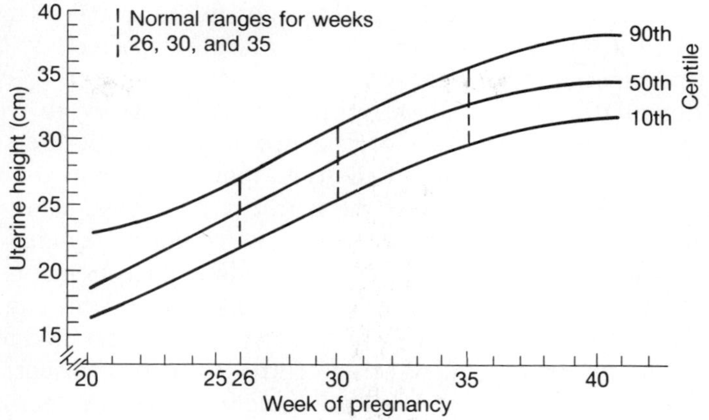

Fig. 5.12 Graph of symphysis–fundal height, showing normal ranges of uterine height in centimetres by week of gestation. (Courtesy of Everett 1984.)

fundal height has the most likelihood of giving useful information simply (Cnattingius *et al.* 1984).

Usually, prior fetal nutrition and growth has been judged at birth, mainly by anthropometry of the newborn, especially birth weight. However, cultural problems, particularly ritual puerperal seclusion, may make measurements difficult to undertake and almost always need to be made by female health workers.

Clinically, obvious vitamin and mineral deficiencies are rare in the neonate, although, with severe vitamin D deficiency in the mother, congenital rickets occurs very uncommonly. However, *latent* neonatal malnutrition is probably more common than appreciated in the form of low stores, such as hepatic iron or vitamin A. These can play a part in the subsequent causation of overt deficiency disease in the early years of childhood. This is indicated, for example, by marginal vitamin D deficiency suggested by biochemical tests in Saudi Arabian neonates (Serenius *et al.* 1984).

However, by far the most important consequence of materno–fetal malnutrition is low birth weight, which is now recognized as a very large public health problem. In fact, WHO has set ≥ 90 per cent of newborns with a birth weight of ≥ 2.5 kg as one of the 10 criteria to be aimed for in the struggle for 'Health for All' by the year 2000 (HFA 2000).

Low birth weight

Low-birth-weight babies are not a homogeneous group and very many complex, interacting factors may be involved (Kramer 1986). There are two main overlapping categories: the gestationally premature (or pre-term) born before term, and the underweight full-term baby ('small-for-dates', 'small-for-gestational-age', (SGA) or, most correctly, 'light-for-dates'). Combinations can also occur.

To differentiate between these groups, it is necessary to know the *gestational age*, from the date of the last menstrual period, and the *accurate weight of the neonate*. In addition, more detailed examination at birth can be undertaken to assess the maturity of babies, using physical and neurological tests (Ballard *et al.* 1979) or more detailed anthropometry suggesting fetal malnutrition, including measurements of arm muscle and fat (Brooke and Butters 1979) and weight-for-length. Such elaborate testing is not usually possible. However, such detailed investigations could be undertaken at research centres to help to disentangle the diagnosis of different types of low-birth-weight babies, and perhaps suggest uncomplicated methods to identify them.

'Light-for-dates' babies can be due to genetic factors, intrauterine growth retardation (from maternal malnutrition, some infections, and various forms of placental insufficiency), and possibly 'spatial constraints', with a mother whose height (and pelvic size) have been limited by malnutrition in her own childhood. As at any age, disentangling these and other variables can be difficult. Higher birth weights in well-nourished, upper socio-economic women from the same ethnic group suggest that intrauterine growth retardation (IUGR) is mainly responsible, rather than genetic influences. A similar conclusion can be reached by the well-documented lowering of birth weights in parts of Africa during the 'hungry season' prior to harvesting (Bantje 1982).

'Light-for-dates' babies due to intrauterine growth retardation also comprise at least two categories — delayed 'chronic' interference with growth throughout fetal life and diminished growth for a shorter period during later pregnancy. The end results may differ anthropometrically. The 'chronic' group approximate the 'stunted' young child's measurements (p. 312) that is a low weight and length. By contrast, the 'acute' group has a relatively normal length, but a decreased weight-for-length. The 'chronic' variety seem to show least ability for catch-up growth in infancy, even when well-fed (Villar *et al.* 1982), but the 'acute' group appear to have a higher mortality as neonates.

In general terms, it has been estimated that there are about 22 million low-birth-weight babies (2.5 kg) born annually. Of these the vast majority (20 million) occur in developing countries, where 80 per cent are 'small-for-dates' rather than pre-term.

Conversely, 'high-birth-weight babies' ($>$ 4.0 kg) can occur in large mothers, in diabetics, in some instances of prolonged pregnancy, and possibly in maternal over nutrition, with increased risks of dystocia and the need for Caesarian section. Because of this, emphasis is sometimes given to collecting birth-weight distribution showing both low and high

Table 5.3 Determinants of low birth weight in Latin America *(Lechtig* et al. *1977)*

Predominant	Of minor importance
Low socio-economic level	Altitude
Malnutrition	Toxaemia of pregnancy
Infection	Smoking habit
	Haemorrhage
	Repeated abortions
	Previous child with low birth weight
	Diabetes
	Cardiovascular disease
	Multiple pregnancy
	Hyperemesis
	Genetic factors
	Other

birth weights in the population as a whole, separated into upper and lower socio-economic groups. However, low birth weight remains overwhelmingly the major problem world-wide.

Many factors can be responsible independently, or often jointly, for the intrauterine growth retardation leading to 'small-for-dates', low-birth-weight babies (US Department of Health and Human Services 1986). These factors include *environmental* (altitude), *obstetrical* (pre-eclampsia, placental insufficiency), *biological* (parity, teenager, birth interval, multiple births)[66], *maternal malnutrition* (calories, zinc iron, iodine, folic acid (Morgan and Winick 1978)), *maternal infections* (placental malaria, chorio-amnionitis) (Tafari 1981)), *toxic* (smoking, alcohol, drug abuse), and *miscellaneous* (hypertension). Some determinants of low birth weight in Latin America have been listed by Lechtig *et al.* (1975) (Table 5.3).

Teenage or adolescent pregnancies are on the increase in many parts of the world, including the USA, with an increased risk of low birth weight from a varying blend of some of these causes. Interestingly, this trend is occurring also in some urban areas in less technically developed countries in almost all parts of the world. (Also see: Addendum 1988, p. 604).

Maternal infections appear to be especially important in less developed countries, but those mainly responsible are difficult to diagnose. However, in a special research project in Ethiopia, chorio-amnionitis due to a range of organisms was found commonly (Tafari 1981). Of particular importance in hyperendemic areas, placental malaria in symptomless women leads to lowering of birth weight by 240–300 g (average 263 g)

[66] *Twins:* Particularly common in some parts of Africa (Ransome-Kuti 1985).

(E.F.P. Jelliffe 1968*a*). This is especially significant with the resurgence of malaria in many parts of the world.

Maternal malnutrition is one of the most important contributing causes of 'light-for-dates' newborn. The fetus has long been considered a 'successful parasite', but it is only partially so. If maternal malnutrition reaches a critical level, there is a reduced transport of glucose and amino acids across the placenta, and, in severe cases, the placenta is smaller in size and weight than usual and has a diminished DNA content (Rosso 1980).

A suboptimal intake of energy (calories) compared with physical activity in pregnancy leads to a lowering of birth weight. This is less apparent in communities where the population was previously relatively 'adequately' nourished as in wartime Holland.

Most marked effects result, as might be expected, in women with very low pre-pregnancy weights and extremely inadequate dietary intakes during pregnancy. In South India, neonates with low birth weight, decreased length, and deficient fatfolds were born to mothers with poor diets and energy stores, as evidenced by maternal triceps fatfolds (Sibert *et al.* 1978). Also, in poorly-fed women in Guatemala, calorie supplementation of diets in pregnancy increased the babies' birth weights (Lechtig *et al.* 1975). Such supplementation can lead to an increase in birth weight from 100 to 300 g, depending on the amount of calories supplied.

Practical risk factors

Field investigations can have the valuable function of validating and/or identifying maternal (and family) 'risk factors' (pp. 452–6) for subsequent low birth weight. Thus, in Guatemala, a combination of anthropometric and social indicators has been suggested (Lechtig *et al.* 1983). Maternal height and head circumference, together with the quality of the home (as a proxy indicator of economic level) gave the best prediction of the risk of low birth weight. More recently, Lechtig (1987) suggested using several anthropometric measurements singly or in combination — arm circumference, weight-for-height, and percentage weight gain. (Also see: Addendum 1988.)

In Indonesia, Husaini *et al.* (1986) noted the following risk factors: maternal height < 140 cm, age ≥ 35 years, formal education ≤ 4 years primary school, interval between pregnancies ≤ 6 months, diastolic blood pressure about 90 mm Hg and haemoglobin < 8 g/dl.

Conversely, the question of the incidence and cause of 'overweight neonates' (4.0 kg) seems to be claiming more attention in some areas. Genetic factors may be more responsible in some groups — for example, in Samoans and in Raratongans. However, the possibility of maternal stature and high dietary intake of calories in pregnancy needs consideration.

Table 5.4 Percentage low-birth-weight infants and some health-related indicators for selected countries (*Petros-Barvazian and Behar 1978*)

Country	Infant mortality rate* (per 1000 live births)	Percentage of low-birth-weight infants	GNP US$ per capita	Physical quality of life index†
Sweden	11	3.16	3500	100
USA	17	7.39	5480	97
Cuba	29	9.44	650	86
Sri Lanka	45	19.00‡	130	83
Algeria	126	14.00	710	42
India	139	30.00	152	39

* Average figures from official existing statistics for latest available year.
† Physical quality of life index: life expectancy at 1 year of age/literacy rate/infant mortality rate.
‡ Estimated on data from the University unit in Colombo.

Special considerations

The incidence of low birth weight is closely related to socio-economic levels (Table 5.4). In Latin America in 1975, 1.5 million babies had a low birth weight (Lechtig *et al.* 1975). In most parts of the world, the birth weight in lower socio-economic groups is less than in the well-to-do groups of the same genetic stock (Table 5.5). This also applies in contrasting socio-economic extremes in industrialized circumstances. For example, Stanfield and Donnett (1978) found that 19.1 per cent low-birth-weight neonates occurred in a poor tenement area of Glasgow compared with 5.5 per cent in a wealthier area in the same city.

Low birth weight has considerable societal costs in the form of increased neonatal mortality and susceptibility to infection (due to diminished immunocompetence) (Neumann 1981) *and* possible subsequent growth retardation (Davies 1980) and likelihood of diminished mental ability (Willocks 1977). It also starts the child's 'life-flight' with subnormal stores of nutrients. Conversely, the incidence of low birth weight in a community or country can be one relatively accessible. Statistical indicator of the level of social development (Table 5.4.)

As with malnutrition in general, socio-economic factors play major causative roles, and, in turn, low birth weight is associated with many aspects of maternal and child health, and consequently has social and economic impacts. Secular trends in birth weight over periods of years have been suggested as one yardstick of national development and its influence on the population, particularly the health and nutrition of mothers (Sterky and Mellander 1978).

Table 5.5 Mean birth weights in different socio-economic groups *(Modified from Beaton and Bengoa 1976). (Sources given in original)*

Country or area	Population studied	Mean birth weight (kg)
India (Madras)	Prosperous	2.985
	Mostly poor	2.736
India (South)	Wealthy	3.182
	Poor	2.810
India (Bombay)	Upper class	3.247
	Upper middle class	2.945
	Lower middle class	2.796
	Lower class	2.578
India (Calcutta)	Paying patients	2.851
	Poor	2.656
Congo	Bantu	
	Very well nourished	3.026
	Well nourished	2.965
	Badly nourished	2.850
	Pygmies	2.635
Ghana (Accra)	Prosperous	3.188
	General population	2.879
Indonesia (Jogjakarta)	Javanese	
	Prosperous	3.022
	Poor	2.816

Methods of assessment

Difficulties include problems with birth weights being obtained from hospitals which do not reflect the general population, and the need for affordable portable scales for weighing newborns.

Anthropometry The most usual measurement is the birth weight which should be undertaken within an hour of birth on an accurate, frequently checked scale by a trained health worker who appreciates the need for care. Birth weights are often recorded by junior nurses with ill-checked scales, and sometimes with variations in techniques, such as taking the measurement with large artery forceps still clamped to the cord (Fig. 5.13). Also, babies delivered in maternity wards will be a biased sample in various ways, depending on local circumstances (e.g. more sophisticated parents, logistics, higher incidence of primiparae, etc.). In some countries, it has been suggested that birth weights could be incorporated on to birth certificates.

Recently, sufficiently accurate, light-weight, easily portable spring ba-

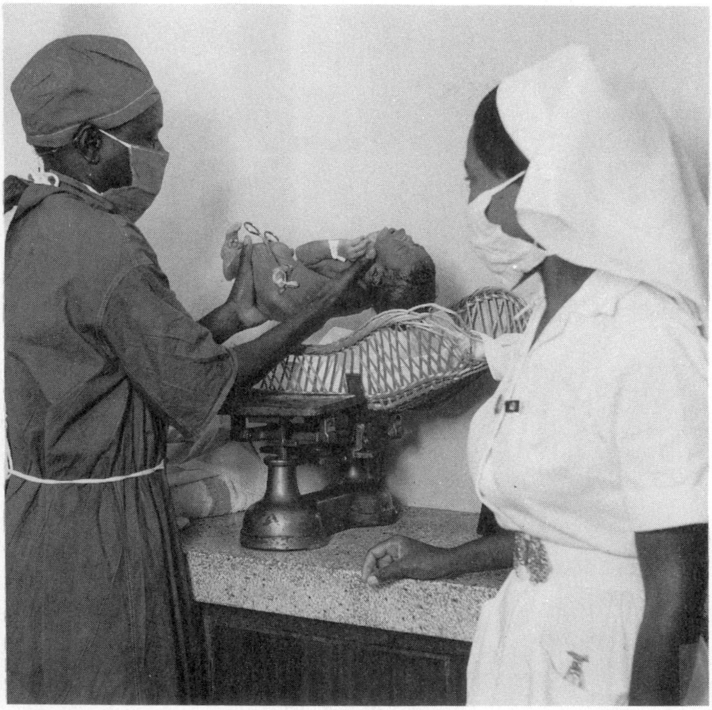

Fig. 5.13 Weighing newborn: showing inappropriate technique, with never checked scales and large metal forceps clamping umbilical cord.

lances have been introduced for use by community health workers, particularly traditional birth attendants (Fig. 5.14). These include: (1) the AHRTAG Baby Weigher; and (2) the Indonesian model spring scale (Alisjahbana *et al.* 1984) (Fig. 5.15) (both can be 'colour-coded' for categorizing birth weight when used by illiterate traditional midwives).

The PATHweigh newborn scale, manufactured in Malawi, only indicates babies above and below 2.5 kg, but costs only US$4 (1988). Another cheap locally available hanging spring scale, with a colour-coded strip pasted on, has been used in India (Kumar and Walia 1986) (Fig. 5.16). Both would seem sufficiently accurate for categorizing.

Light-for-dates babies usually appear thin for their length on inspection (Brooke 1980). This can be confirmed by measuring the length as well as the weight. As noted earlier (p. 81), length is not easy to obtain accurately and should be measured by two people. Other bony measurements which can be made by one person have been suggested as alternatives, including head circumference (Moskowitz *et al.* 1983), arm length (Brooke and Butters 1979), and foot length (Daga *et al.* 1987).

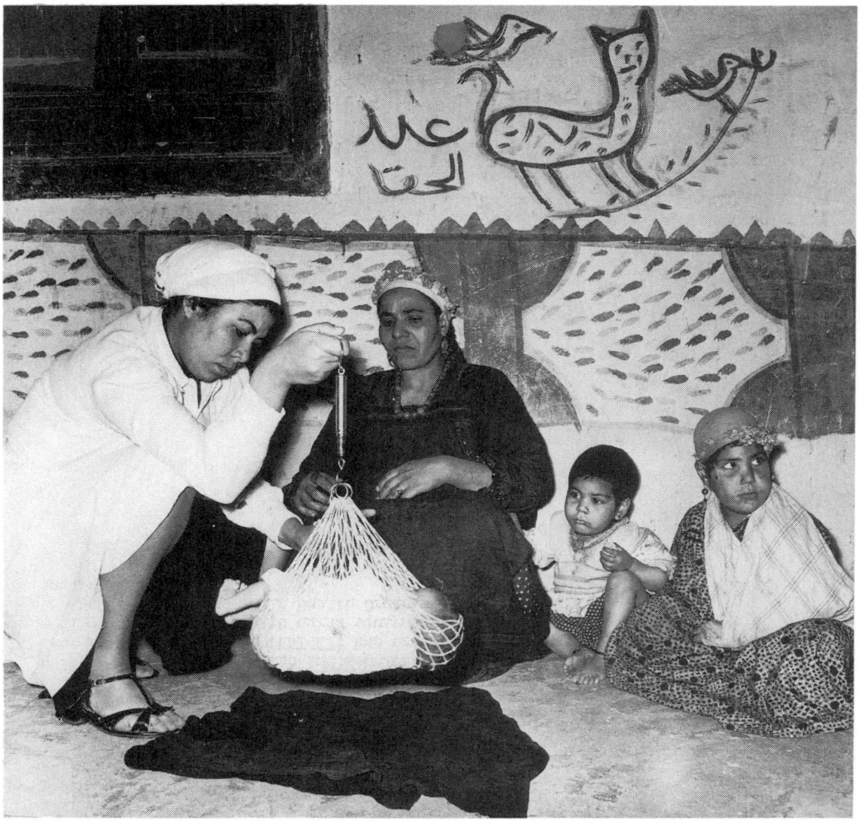

Fig. 5.14 Midwife weighing baby in the home during a postnatal visit (Egypt 1961). (Courtesy of UNICEF.)

Various different ratios of weight to height have been suggested as more correctly reflecting the body proportions of young babies. For the newborn, the:

$$\frac{\text{weight (g)}}{\text{length (cm)}^3} \times 100$$

(Rohrer's Index or the ponderal index) (Rohrer 1921) is still commonly used. This can be employed to categorize babies who are under- or over-weight for length. The following levels have been suggested: extremely overweight (obese) > 2.93, moderately obese > 2.85–2.93, moderately underweight (malnourished) 2.32–2.26, and severe malnutrition $<$ 2.26 (Miller and Merritt 1979) (Table 5.6).

Several workers have looked into the possibility of using other measurements that can be made with a tape measure, but which correlate

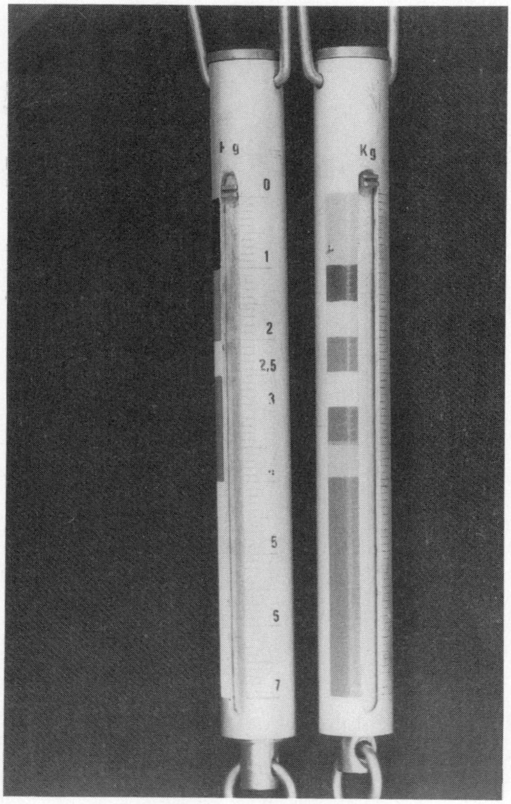

Fig. 5.15 Indonesian model spring scale for weighing newborn in the home with colour-coded model on right for illiterate midwife (Alisjahbana *et al.* 1984). Colour code is as follows. Black: less than 1000 g; red: 1000–2000 g, to be referred immediately; yellow: 2000–2500 g, may be cared for at home but with caution; green: 2500–4000 g, safe birth weight; white: more than 4000 g, care with caution.

with low body weight and with neonatal mortality. These could be used by village-level workers. Original studies in the Caribbean (Gueri *et al.* 1977), followed by work in Central America (Lechtig *et al.* 1983) investigated various surrogate measurements for birth weight. The arm circumference has been shown to be a simple, low-cost measurement which can be used to screen for low-birth-weight babies. A critical level of < 9 cm has been suggested in Guatemala, but needs verifying in different ethnic groups. In India, Bhargava *et al.* (1985) used 8.7 cm as the cut-off point for neonates in New Delhi, while 9.5 cm has been suggested in Burkina Faso (Sauerborn and Bouyain 1987).

Recent work in Guatemala showed neonates with arm circumferences

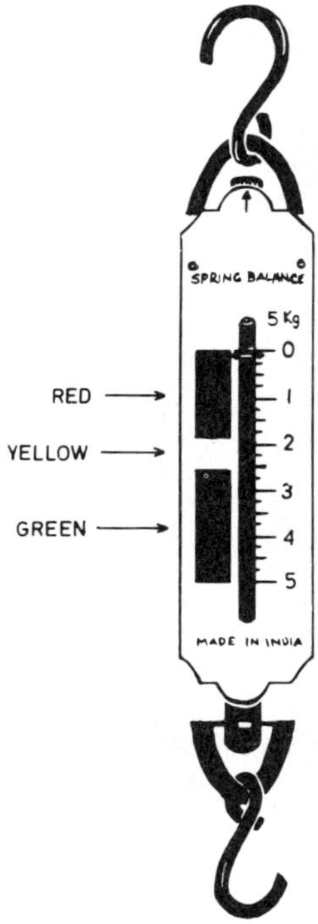

Fig. 5.16 Modified low-cost, colour-coded spring balance for use by traditional birth attendants in India (Kumar and Walia 1986).

Table 5.6 Suggested anthropometric indicators of underweight and overweight newborns: needing testing and possible modification in different ethnic groups. (*For details: see text*)

Measurements	Underweight	Overweight
Birth weight	< 2.5 kg	> 4.0 kg
Ponderal index		
($wt/lt^3 \times 100$)	Moderate: 2.32 (+0) 2.26	Moderate: 2.85 (+0) Obese 2.93
	Severe: < 2.26	Severe: > 2.93 Obese
Arm circumference	< 9 cm	Not known

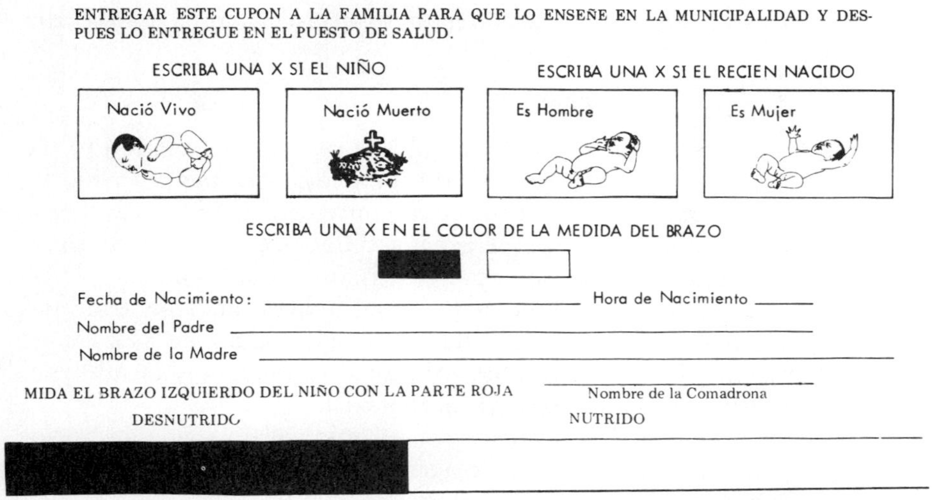

ENTREGAR ESTE CUPON A LA FAMILIA PARA QUE LO ENSEÑE EN LA MUNICIPALIDAD Y DESPUES LO ENTREGUE EN EL PUESTO DE SALUD.

ESCRIBA UNA X SI EL NIÑO

Nació Vivo

Nació Muerto

ESCRIBA UNA X SI EL RECIEN NACIDO

Es Hombre

Es Mujer

ESCRIBA UNA X EN EL COLOR DE LA MEDIDA DEL BRAZO

Fecha de Nacimiento: ______ Hora de Nacimiento ______

Nombre del Padre ______

Nombre de la Madre ______

MIDA EL BRAZO IZQUIERDO DEL NIÑO CON LA PARTE ROJA

Nombre de la Comadrona

DESNUTRIDO

NUTRIDO

Fig. 5.17 Certificate for use by illiterate or just literate midwife (SINAPS Programme, Central America). Suitable for recording: sex of child, born alive or dead, and undersized (as judged by arm circumference) (Lechtig *et al.* 1983). Black areas on the detachable tape in the illustration are actually red.

of < 9 cm to have a 10–17 time greater chance of dying in the first 2 weeks of life. The measurement was considered to have a high sensitivity (100 per cent) and specificity (De Vaquera *et al.* 1983). However, Ramachandran *et al.* (1978) point out that the small arm of a newborn is difficult to measure, and a Vernier tape has been suggested to improve the accuracy (Ramachandran 1986).

In the SINAPS Programme in Central America, midwives have been issued with a two-colour arm tape (red and white) for use with newborns. With the certificate supplied (Fig. 5.17), they can send in information concerning the sex of the baby, whether born alive or dead, and whether undersized (as judged by arm circumference) (Lechtig *et al.* 1983).

Ramji *et al.* (1986) suggested using the maximum thigh circumference (TC), as an alternative indicator of low birth weight. This is because the thigh is larger and relatively small changes can be noted more easily than with the arm. In New Delhi, they used a TC of 13.9 cm to detect infants of 2000 g, which they found to have a better predictive value than a mid-arm circumference of 8.0 cm.

A refinement of using the arm circumference alone has been suggested by Sasanow *et al.* (1986). This is the middle arm circumference/head circumference ratio (MAC/HC), which is considered as a useful method of assessing 'intrauterine growth and baby proportionality' at birth. Standard curves are available from these workers' paper. This may be useful in sophisticated hospital circumstances, but for general purposes the arm circumference alone is recommended.

Reporting results

The incidence of low birth weights should be reported in relation to the long-standing, widely recognized WHO level (2.5 kg) *and* to a locally constructed level appropriate for the community, which will have to bear in mind the possible influence of genetic differences, functional significance, and practical needs. For example, in Singapore, both the 'flesh–bone' ratios (such as the Rohrer or Ponderal indices) and the arm (and calf) circumferences were less in Indian neonates than in Chinese or Malay newborns (Bhan *et al.* 1985). The relative influences of maternal diet and genetic variation appeared undecided.

In an attempt to control for genetic causes of low birth weight, a 'socio-economic birth weight index' was suggested (Jelliffe and Jelliffe 1978*b*). This was defined as

$$\frac{\text{average birth weight of low socio-economic population}}{\text{average birth weight of upper socio-economic population}} \times 1000.$$

This approach is only valid when the community concerned is, in general, genetically uniform. Also, as always with such comparisons, problems may occur in defining the two groups. Generally well-nourished, genetically homogeneous communities with good prenatal services, as in Denmark, should have an index of 1000. In a study in an area in India, Prema (1978), reported results ranging from 872 to 885.

The functional outcome of low birth weight can be estimated at many different levels of complexity. At a detailed research level, different types of low-birth-weight baby can be investigated for immunocompetence and followed-up later to assess growth and mental development. For practical purposes, locally defined levels needing special care need defining. For example, in Cambridge, UK, studies have shown that 'small-for-dates' babies of 37 weeks gestation or more can be safely cared for without special precautions. In technically less developed countries, an immediate functional level of 'adequate' birth weight can be estimated mainly in relation to ability to suckle at the breast. For example, in the 1960s in Kampala, Uganda, an 'adequate' birth weight in relation to need for special care was considered to be 2.0 kg.

Conclusions

The use of largely anthropometric methods to assess materno–fetal malnutrition can be put to valuable practical use in surveys and in prenatal clinics. A range of appropriate technology suitable for use by community

Table 5.7 Summary of anthropometric assessment of the mother, fetus, and newborn: using appropriate technology

Measurements	Purpose
Mother	
Background anthropometry	
Early pregnancy	
Height: below local 'risk level'*	Future risk of low birth weight
Weight for height	
Arm circumference	
Changes during pregnancy	
Materno–fetal	
Pregnancy weight gain	Intrauterine growth retardation (IUGR)
Composite anthropometry (growth rate score)†	
Fundal height	
Newborn	
Weight: exact measurement	Low-birth-weight baby
: categorization	
Arm circumference (AC): exact measurement	
: categorization	
'Flesh–bone' ratios: AC/head circumference	Thin low-birth-weight baby — prolonged intrauterine malnutrition
: Weight/length (Rohrer's index: wt/ht^3)	

* High risk of obstructed labour.
† Combined scores for gains in maternal weight, fundal height, and abdominal girth (Garde 1986).

health workers have been described recently and are summarized in Table 5.7.

The identification of locally important indicators of high risk of maternal malnutrition or of low birth weight can be undertaken largely by community health workers. These results can assist in identifying 'risk factors' (p. 453). They can therefore indicate appropriate concerns for nutrition education and other practical prenatal activities, designed to improve the mother's health and nutrition and reduce the incidence of low-birth-weight babies. These activities can include the use of antimalarials or the issue of iron tablets or folic acid.

Nutrition in young children

In less technically developed regions of the world, malnutrition has its most serious impact on young children. They are at a stage of life when growth should be rapid and nutrient requirements are high. Unfortunately, inadequate diets are likely because of a variable combination of poverty, absence of suitable foods, lack of parental knowledge, and limiting cultural food beliefs ('cultural blocks') (Jelliffe and Bennett 1961). Malnourished young children also have diminished immunity (Neumann 1982) and continuous stress from bacterial, viral, and parasitic infections, sometimes associated with emotional trauma from abrupt separation from the breast.

Although there is no precise dividing-point, it has become customary to consider the malnutrition seen in young children in the two age-groups — infants and pre-school-age children (1–4 years). A more biological classification is that of Bostock (1962) — fetus, extero-gestate fetus (0–6 to 9 months), and transitional (or weanling) (6–9 months to 2–3 years). However, this is usually impossible to use in practice, because the last two stages vary in different cultures.

Infants

The nutritional status of children in the first year of life depends on the local methods of infant feeding and, through their fetal stores, on the maternal diet in pregnancy and on the mother's own previous and present nutritional status. However, the principal practical determinant in less technically developed countries is often whether the baby is breastfed, as is traditional, or whether, as is increasingly the case in urban areas, attempts are made to bottle-feed artificially, with cow's milk-based formulas or dilute animal milk or liquid gruels.

Breastfed infants

In well-nourished mothers with unimpaired maternal lactation reflexes, growth — as evidenced by weight-gain — is usually excellent for over 6 months (Ahn and MacLean 1980). In most traditional, less than well-fed societies, growth is well sustained in the first 4–6 months ('early infancy') (Venkatachalam 1975), as sufficient protein, calories, and vitamins are supplied by breast milk, exclusively or predominantly,[67] together with fetal stores. Also, protection against many infections, especially diarrhoea, is afforded by a wide range of anti-infective substances in breast milk (Jelliffe and Jelliffe 1989*a*). However, in some circumstances, breastfeeding by itself can be sufficient for a shorter period only. This may result from *severe* maternal ill-health (including *marked* malnutrition, anaemia, infections) and/or interference with the key prolactin and 'let-down' reflexes (dysreflexia) by new practices and/or life-styles, or, uncommonly, by some traditional customs (Jelliffe and Jelliffe 1989*a*), and with lack of knowledge of breastfeeding 'management' in recently urbarized mothers. It seems likely that dysreflexia is increasing, especially in urban areas.

Only three deficiency syndromes have been described commonly in 'early infancy' in breastfed babies, who are growing well in some parts of the world — infantile beriberi, deficiency of vitamin B_{12} or folate, and rickets. These syndromes occur only in areas where maternal intakes of thiamine, vitamin B_{12}, and vitamin D have been very low in previous years, including the current pregnancy and lactation, In the case of infantile rickets, mothers of affected babies also have had restricted exposure to sunlight for cultural reasons, sometimes from their own childhood. Endemic cretinism can also be observed in breastfed babies, due to fetal damage from iodine deficiency in pregnancy. Growth retardation and clinical signs of cretinism or mental deficiency from fetal brain development will be present (p. 272).

Generally, in traditional rural circumstances in developing tropical regions, infants in the second half of the first year of life will continue to be breastfed, usually with the addition of infrequent feedings with inadequate quantities of largely carbohydrate gruels or pastes. These are often insufficiently cooked, bulky, low in calories, protein, and other nutrients, and nutritionally dilute (with high water and fibre content.) In many parts of the world there is a trend towards the use of usually unnecessary complementary bottle feeds in the earlier months of life ('mixed milk feedings').

Severe malnutrition is usually not seen at this stage in infancy. However, avitaminosis A (as with keratomalacia in Indonesia) (p. 265), or early rickets (as in North Africa) (p. 270) may occur for dietary, social, and/or cultural reasons.

More commonly, the second 6 months of infancy — termed 'late infancy' by Venkatachalam (1975) — is characterized in many traditional societies by a slower weight gain, as shown by a somewhat flattened growth curve, and sometimes by a degree of iron deficiency anaemia. At this time, children are living, in part, on their fetal reserves and on stores laid down in early breastfeeding.

Artificially fed infants

At the present time, there is a world-wide trend towards urbanization. Among these new towns people, there is an increasing decline in breastfeeding because of the ill-effects of Westernized health services (notably unappreciative professionals without training in this field and inappropriate maternity units), the example of socio-economic 'superiors', the detrimental influence of over-advertised infant formulas, and, to a varying extent, the result of some mothers seeking paid employment out of the home in jobs where breastfeeding may not be feasible or culturally acceptable (Jelliffe and Jelliffe 1989*a*).

For the majority of families in less technically developed countries, artificial bottle-feeding is not practical — economically, educationally, or hygienically. Imported cow's milk-based formulas and other processed products designed for babies are too expensive for parents to be able to buy in adequate amounts, as are sufficient bottles and teats. Token, very weak concentrations of formula or milk are all that can be given. Mothers ordinarily have not had sufficient education to follow the necessary routine of preparation, dilution, and protection from contamination. Last, conditions in the home with regard to supplies of sufficient clean water and fuel, kitchen facilities, the means for storage protected from insects and dust, and difficulties with keeping feeding bottles clean make the preparation of uncontaminated bottle-feeds a virtual impossibility.

In these circumstances, the majority of non-breastfed infants reared artificially on the bottle receive very dilute, highly infected feeds, resulting in most cases in growth failure, if not marasmus. The children often die from associated or added infective diarrhoea.

In recent years, the prevalence of 'mixed milk' feeding has increased, especially in urbanized communities, where both human milk and bottle feeds are given. The consequences vary. Essentially, they are intermediate between the exclusively breastfed and the completely bottle-fed, but are likely to lead to the cessation of lactation and increased diarrhoea.

The type of resulting malnutrition depends on the artificial feeds the child has received. Most often, this will be over-diluted cow's milk-based formula, but thin gruels or locally available animal milk may be used. In any case, such feedings usually supply inadequate calories and protein. A disproportion betwen sugar (sucrose) calories and protein can be a particular issue, if diluted sweetened condensed milk is used. This is a practice which seems to be once again on the increase, probably because of the keeping quality of this high sugar product without refrigeration. Infective diarrhoea occurs frequently, and ultimately nutritional marasmus develops, so that the result has been termed the 'marasmus–diarrhoea syndrome'.

Such a decline in breastfeeding has wide effects on community nutrition, including an increased birth rate (because of shortened lactation amenorrhoea) and economic effects, as breast milk substitutes will need to be purchased (and often imported).

Pre-school age children (1–4 years)

This period of childhood, especially the second year of life, is notoriously fraught with risk. The young child is 'transitional' as regards diet, immunity to infections, and psychological dependence. This is a period of rapid growth with a high need for all nutrients, including calories, protein, vitamins (e.g A and D), and minerals, such as iron and zinc. It is a time when several meals a day are required and when foods should be easily masticable and digestible, and, in particular, should contain 'compact calories' capable of being accommodated in the small volume of the young child's stomach.

It is at this time also that the non-immune child comes in contact with a succession, or more often an accumulation, of bacterial, viral, and parasitic infections. Last, it is sometimes the occasion for the psychological trauma of 'weaning' (*sevrage*) that can occur in some cultures as a result of the sudden separation from the mother — after a prolonged period of continuous close contact and permissive breastfeeding throughout the 24 hours. For all of these reasons, this period of life is classically recognized as dangerous. It is the time when kwashiorkor, 'late onset' marasmus, and less severe forms of protein–energy malnutrition are seen most commonly in many parts of the world, particularly in traditional cultures.

Certain vitamin- and mineral-deficiency diseases occur with varying frequency in pre-school age children in different parts of the world. These include avitaminosis A (xerophthalmia), rickets, and iron deficiency anaemia. The incidence varies greatly from place to place, depending upon the local dietary, social, and other factors. Thus, rickets in sunnier parts of the world may be related to lack of actual exposure to readily available ultraviolet rays in sunlight due to overcrowding in urban dwellings, as in old-style walled cities or in slums, or to a deliberate sheltering of young children from the sun for various cultural reasons, such as trying to prevent them from acquiring a darker complexion or to escape the risk of the 'evil eye'.

Subsequent sections are concerned with methods of assessment appropriate for iron deficiency anaemia (p. 263), for avitaminosis A (xerophthalmia) (p. 265), iodine deficiency disorders (p. 272), rickets (p. 270), and especially with the complex and difficult questions concerned with the recognition, classification, and categorization of different forms and degrees of protein–energy malnutrition (p. 273).

Iron deficiency

Anaemia is extremely common in young children in many developing countries. It is often due to the cumulative effect of a number of concurrent factors, including nutritional deficiencies, bacterial and parasitic infections. Genetic abnormalities may play a part, including sickle-cell anaemia in children of African ancestry, or thalassaemia in other communities.

Iron needs are high in early childhood because of the rapid increases in the total number of red blood cells and in muscle mass which occur with normal development. Iron deficiency anaemia results when these needs are not met. This can result from one or usually more, of the following: *dietary inadequacy* (e.g. with delayed introduction of iron-rich foods, overemphasis on iron-poor cow's milk in some cultures); *loss* (*e.g.* infection with hookworm or bilharziasis); *suboptimal liver and bone marrow stores* (e.g. twins, prematures, babies of severely iron-deficient mothers); or *poor absorption* (resulting from malnutrition, together with limited bioavailability of iron in the foods consumed.) Recent work indicates increasingly that an adequate iron intake is needed for intellectual development (*Br. Med. J.* 1986), for satisfactory immunocompetence (Chandra and Scrimshaw 1980), or, indeed, for normal physical growth (Auckett *et al.* 1986). Current views of the impact of iron deficiency on growth, and impaired learning ability have been authoritatively summarized by Illingworth (1986).

Assessment in the community

Direct assessment

Haemoglobin estimations are the most useful screening test. Problems with low-cost haemoglobinometers of sufficient accuracy, reliability, and ruggedness have been discussed elsewhere (p. 43), as have the trials of such simple screening or categorizing methods as the anaemia recognition card (Ghosh *et al.* 1978) (p. 25), or the anaemiometer (Shah 1980).

Low haemoglobin concentrations may need further investigation to specify the *nutritional cause(s)* of the anaemia (e.g. iron, folate, vitamin B_{12}) (p. 264) and/or to ascertain *other causes* of anaemia (e.g. stools for hookworm ova, thick blood films for malaria, etc.) (p. 502). The serum ferritin is especially helpful in estimating iron stores (p. 502) in the absence of liver disease and infections.

Indirect assessment

The frequency of different forms of anaemia may be sought for from hospital data, particularly through enquiry at laboratories. Findings may be difficult to evaluate, as anaemia in young children in tropical regions is often due to several causes in combinations. Also, the necessary haematological laboratory facilities for ensuring accurate results and particularly to ensure correct aetiological diagnoses are not commonly available. As usual, the biased nature in hospital data needs to be taken into account (p. 355).

Assessment of ecological variables

Dietary studies are relevant, although it is difficult to accurately estimate the probable degree of absorption and bioavailability of iron present in a diet. Iron is also available from the water supply, from the soil — as with laterite dust — and from iron cooking pots.

Reference levels and reporting

Haemoglobin can be reported in various ways — as percentages below WHO reference levels (p. 48) or as percentages in different levels, which can be defined arbitrarily, or numerically, or in functional terms (p. 50). Adjustments need to be made in reference levels for populations living at high altitudes and perhaps for different ethnic groups, although this currently seems insignificant.

Avitaminosis A (xerophthalmia)[68]

Severe manifestations of retinol (vitamin A) deficiency have been recognized as widespread in young children in some developing countries for decades (McLaren 1963). Recently, increasing attention has shown xerophthalmia to be especially prevalent in some rice-eating areas of South Asia (such as Indonesia). It is also a problem of varying significance in parts of Africa, Latin America, the Caribbean, and the Eastern Mediterranean (Sommer 1978; Leavell 1987).

Aetiology

The most dangerous obvious manifestations of retinol deficiency (avitaminosis A) occur in the epithelium of the eye, collectively termed 'xerophthalmia' ('dry eye disease'). It is a condition almost exclusively affecting young children, and is associated with poverty, lack of education, and poor hygiene. Under such circumstances, children's diets are frequently restricted economically and/or culturally to exclude sources of retinol (vitamin A) (including animal milk) and to limit intakes of vitamin A precursor, carotene, present in darkgreen leafy vegetables, orange pigment fruits, and vegetables. In some communities, it may be related in part to too early a cessation of breastfeeding or to 'colostrum rejection' (cultural avoidance of vitamin A-rich colostrum). In urban areas, xerophthalmia can occur even among young infants, as a result of artificial feeding with vitamin A deficient skimmed milk, in powdered or condensed form. Poor storage may play a part, particularly in twins or premature infants, or with liver damage, as occurs in the fatty infiltration of kwashiorkor. Contributory infections, especially diarrhoeal disease and measles, may act at times as the final conditioning factor by limiting absorption, in-

[68] Detailed accounts of specialized surveys and other details concerning xerophthalmia are given by Sommer (1978, 1982).

Table 5.8 WHO Xerophthalmia classification: revised version (*Sommer* 1982b) (Illustrations in frontispiece)

XN	Night blindness
X1A	Conjunctival xerosis
X1B	Bitot's spots
X2	Corneal xerosis
X3A	Corneal ulceration/keratomalacia < ⅓ corneal surface
X3B	Corneal ulceration/keratomalacia ⩾ ⅓ corneal surface
XS	Corneal scar
XF	Xerophthalmic fundus

creasing metabolic needs, and directly by damaging the eyes, as in measles or in dehydration. Conversely, vitamin supplementation can decrease mortality from measles in areas where vitamin A deficiency is common Barclay *et al.* 1987).

Maternal nutrition can play a part in that neonatal liver stores can be less than normal if mothers are themselves retinol deficient in pregnancy. Also, vitamin A in breast milk can be somewhat diminished in women whose retinol stores are inadequate both in pregnancy and during lactation.

Studies in Indonesia have also suggested that children with mild vitamin A deficiency can show increased mortality (Sommer *et al.* 1983).

Assessment in the community

Under the guidance of WHO and the International Vitamin A Consultative Group (IVACG), the assessment of avitaminosis A in the community has become more systematic and clearly defined in recent years (Sommer 1978, 1982). In view of possible seasonal variations in incidence, due to dietary differences or patterns of contributory infections (such as measles or diarrhoea), it is important to obtain and evaluate information at representative periods during the annual cycle.

Direct assessment

The situation with regard to signs previously considered to be associated with vitamin A deficiency, such as xerosis of the skin and follicular hyperkeratosis (p. 483) has been reappraised in recent years. It is now recognized that they lack sufficiently clear association with avitaminosis A. Currently, only signs of xerophthalmia are sought for, and their description has been given elsewhere (p. 265). They can be best recorded following the WHO classification (Sommer 1982) (Table 5.8).

In evaluating these signs, four guidelines from the International Vitamin A Consultative Group (1975) need noting:

Table 5.9 Xerophthalmia: variation with age (*Sommer 1978*)

	Conjunctival (X1A, X1B)	Corneal (X2, X3)
Age (peak incidence)*	3–6 years	6 months–3 years
Protein–energy malnutrition	Usually mild	Usually severe
Precipitating illnesses: gastroenteritis, measles, respiratory tract infection	Uncommon	Common

* Either form of the disease can occur at any age. Most cases fall within the indicated range of peak incidence.

1. These signs are descriptive rather than diagnostic. All signs seen at the time of examination are recorded.
2. In general, a progression of severity is reflected in the classifications of primary signs.
3. The classification can be used both in field surveys and the routine recording of findings in patients in hospitals and clinics.
4. When tabulating the frequency of these signs each child should be included only once, under his or her most severe sign.

The relative age-specificity of corneal and conjunctival xerophthalmia needs emphasizing, as does the variation in detailed causation at different ages (Sommer 1978) (Table 5.9). Bitôt's spots, the most identifiable sign (Fig. 2.3), can be seen in older children and adults, but often seem then to be stigmata of vitamin A deficiency in the past (McLaren 1987).

Children with corneal scars (XS) or ocular destruction can be investigated further by means of a detailed history from a responsible, informed adult and a careful examination of the eye, preferably by a physician with opthalmoscopic experience. According to the International Vitamin A Consultative Group (1975), cases of vitamin A related corneal destruction should meet the following criteria: (1) clinical picture compatible with this diagnosis; (2) the absence of other forms of ocular disease that could have produced a similar picture (advanced trachoma, for example); (3) the lesions' appearance was unassociated with either trauma, gross purulence, or measles; and (4) historically, the child was at least 4 months old when the lesion first appeared.

Biochemical tests

Community nutritional assessment for xerophthalmia will always be mainly based on a search for 'suggestive' clinical signs, particularly Bitôt's spots (p. 23), although these mostly occur in older children after infancy.

Biochemical tests for serum vitamin A concentrations may be feasible and, can sometimes be helpful if 'abnormals' (e.g. with clinical signs) are contrasted with 'controls' (Sommer 1978). Alternatively or additionally, a subsample of all children examined may be tested biochemically, if facilities are available.

Serum vitamin A levels of 10 μg/dl or less are considered low, but allowance for decreased amounts of retinol-binding protein (RBP) should be considered in children with protein–energy malnutrition.

Biophysical method

Tests for night blindness — more correctly, dark adaptation, especially difficulty with seeing in a dim light — have usually been considered as only possible in co-operative older children or adults in carefully controlled laboratory circumstances (p. 31). The practical significance of night blindness has been re-emphasized, as it appears to be a relatively early feature of serious vitamin A deficiency (Sinha and Bang 1973). It can be recognized spontaneously by parents in areas where its occurrence is frequent and identified by specific words in the local language (Sommer *et al.* 1979).

The possibility of testing young children by games has been suggested, especially using older siblings as part of a CHILD-to-child Program. Two such games have been devised by the Institute of Child Health, London. They should be played at sunset at twilight, when it is beginning to get dark:

1. *Back-to-back*. Two siblings stand back-to-back, each holding a rock and a stick; each takes five steps and turns around; the older sibling holds up one of the items; the younger sibling must hold up the same object.
2. *Match the stick*. The older sibling has three sticks in his hand, one significantly shorter than the others; he takes 10 steps away from the smaller sibling, and places one of the sticks to his right, one to his left, and one directly in front of him; the smaller child must point to the shortest stick.

In very recent years the ocular cytology impression test (p. 53) has been developed, and appears to have promise as a practical, low-cost method for detecting pre-clinical vitamin A deficiency. (See also: Addendum 1988.)

Indirect assessment

Hospital figures, both in the children's and ophthalmic wards, may furnish useful statistics concerning admissions with keratomalacia. In the past, these have been underestimated because many orthodoxly trained paediatricians and ophthalmologists had little instruction in diagnosing the ocular manifestations of vitamin A deficiency.[69]

This may still be partially true. Sommer (1978) emphasized the value of examining children in communities or circumstances of 'special risk', such as slums, refugee camps, and paediatric infectious disease wards, and of 'chart reviews' and discussion with concerned health personnel. Keratomalacia is so frequently a disease of the toddler that 'weanling blindness' can be an age-specific epidemiological phenomenon. Local records giving the age-incidence of the onset of blindness, if available, may disclose suggestive data.

Assessment of ecological variables

Food consumption patterns (p. 187) These may play a special role in both mothers and their offspring. It is important to assess: (1) breast-feeding and weaning practices (including the use of retinol-rich colostrum); and (2) the degree of usage (or avoidance) of locally important retinol- and carotene-containing foods in pregnancy, lactation, and early childhood. In view of the importance of infections in triggering serious xerophthalmia, especially keratomalacia, assessment of the prevalence of contributory infections, especially measles and diarrhoea, should be included.

Cultural factors would seem to have an unique role in assessing xerophthalmia, because communities where severe vitamin deficiency has long been common may have specific indigenous names for night blindness and Bitôt's spots. In Indonesia, Sommer (1982) showed that a mother's recognition that her child has *buta ayam* (chicken's vision, referring to the inability of chickens to see well in poor light) correlates with low serum vitamin A levels. In such communities. 'a properly elicited history' of night blindness was a better index of early xerophthalmia than Bitôt's spots. The sequence used by Sommer (1982) consisted of questioning the mother about *buta ayam*, then enquiring from her about the child's ability to locate objects just after dusk or in a poorly lighted room. Last, the child's ability to recognized small toys at a distance of about 8–10 feet was tested just at sunset, when it was beginning to get dark.

Presentation of results and significance

Prevalence levels of xerophthalmia considered to represent a significant public health problem have been proposed to assist government adminis-

[69] Excellent slide sets with text appropriate for different levels of workers are available from Helen Keller International, 22 West 17th Street, New York, New York 10011. Current information on avitaminosis A is available in the Xerophthalmia Newsletter, c/o Nuffield Ophthalmology Institute, Oxford, UK.

Table 5.10 Criteria for assessing the public health significance of xerophthalmia and vitamin A deficiency, based on the prevalence among children less than six years of age in the community (1982 revision) *(Sommer 1982*b*)*

Criterion	Minimum prevalence (percentage)
Clinical	
Night blindness (XN)	1.0
Bitot's spots (XIB)	0.5
Corneal xerosis and/or ulceration, keratomalacia (X2, X3A, X3B)	0.01
Xerophthalmia-related corneal scars (XS)	0.05
Biochemical	
Serum retinol (vitamin A) less than 10 μg/dl	5.0

trators (Table 5.10). These apply only to children up to the age of 5-years in the area actually surveyed. The presence of one or more of the three *clinical* criteria at these levels should be considered as evidence of a significant xerophthalmia problem (International Vitamin A Consultative Group 1975; Sommer 1982).

The major social ill-consequence of xerophthalmia in an affected country is the number of children blinded annually. Methods of calculating 'blindness potential' have been given by Sommer (1982) in terms of numbers, social suffering, and national financial loss.

Rickets

Rickets is common in some tropical and sub-tropical countries, and has been considered to affect as many as 40 per cent or more of young children in some North African cities. It occurs where mothers, infants, and 'toddlers' received inadequate vitamin D, either as food or as supplement, and where they are not exposed to sunlight. The latter can occur because of crowded urban conditions or because infants are purposely kept indoors for various cultural reasons — for example, to keep the skin fair or to avoid the 'evil eye'. It is more frequently seen in crowded cities.

It more commonly affects pre-school age children, but can occur in 'younger infants' in the first 6 months of life (Borjesson and Hofvander 1970; Parent *et al.* 1987). Such early cases are undoubtedly related to poor fetal stores and lower concentrations in milk from mothers who are themselves vitamin D depleted, as a result of prolonged dietary lack and minimal exposure to sunlight for cultural reasons, such as the more restrictive forms of *purdah*.

Rickets is sometimes dismissed as an unimportant condition or a malady of the past. Neither is the case. The resulting bony abnormalities can lead to permanent deformities (e.g. stunting and unsightly bow-legs) and, especially important, contracted pelves in females with subsequent danger of a difficult 'obstructed' labour (dystocia). Rickets also has a direct effect on mortality in early childhood, as respiratory tract infections tend to be more severe. Geographically, rickets still remains a common public health problem in a number of countries, such as Ethiopia (Gebre-Medhin 1982) and Tunisia (Parent *et al.* 1987).

Assessment in the community

Direct assessment

Unfortunately, as with many conditions, serious cases are obvious clinically, radiologically, and biochemically, but children with less severe rickets are more difficult to diagnose with certainty. In fact, in view of the lack of specificity of many of the signs found in rickets, direct assessment is best based principally on the occurrence in young children of at least three signs (including epiphyseal enlargement or the wrist (p. 29), preferably supported by high serum alkaline phosphatase concentrations (> 20 Bodansky units/dl) and by radiological examination of the wrist in samples of those examined clinically, where facilities are available. This complete sequence is usually impractical. As a screening measure, one sign may be sought for to select children for further investigation. This is usually epiphyseal enlargement at the wrist (p. 29), but sometimes 'beading' of the ribs (p. 487) or craniotabes (p. 487) may be looked for. Actual measurement of the degree of epiphyseal enlargement at the wrist has been attempted without success.

Investigations by Hojer *et al.* (1977) re-affirmed that a raised serum alkaline phosphatase precedes clinical signs, even in marasmic children. Likewise, plasma vitamin D (25-hydroxycholecalciferol) estimations can be included in the rare situations where this is possible, as in Saudi Arabia in neonates and pregnant women (Serenins *et al.* 1985). In Manchester, UK, Grindulis *et al.* (1986) found biochemical rickets to be common in Asian toddlers, using levels of < 10 ng/ml as 'suboptimal' and < 5 ng/ml as deficient'.

Indirect assessment

Statistics of out-patient attendances and admissions of children with rickets may be useful, although the criteria employed for diagnosis need to be scrutinized.

Assessment of ecological factors

Dietary patterns and details of local cultural practices which exclude children and women from exposure of the skin to sunlight need to be investigated. The recognition of risk factors (pp. 452–6; see also Addendum 1988) is important in suggesting a specific preventive programme, including education concerning both diet and culturally acceptable exposure to sunshine.

Presentation of results

Basic positive results can best be presented as in a survey by Mankodi *et al.* (1974) of young children in urban Bombay and in villages nearby:

Clinical	**Urban** (per cent)	**Rural** (per cent)
(3 signs)	5.2	4.7
X-ray		
(wrist)	0.9	1.5

The serum alkaline phosphatase test was not considered to be useful as protein–energy malnutrition was common in the same children, possibly having a 'compensatory' lowering effect.

Additionally, the influence of causative factors, both dietary and cultural also need to be investigated, in order for realistic practical preventive programmes to be devised.

Iodine deficiency disorders

Recent evidence indicates a much wider spectrum of disorders resulting from severe iodine deficiency than previously realized (Hetzal 1986) (Table 5.11). This puts at risk more than 400 million people in Asia alone as well as millions in Africa and South America[70] These iodine deficiency disorders include *goitre* at all ages (especially in females); increased stillbirths; perinatal and infant mortality; *fetal effects*, presenting as endemie cretinism (Fig. 5.18) or as mental deficiency, often with deaf mutism, and spastic diplegia.

The social and economic impact of iodine deficiency is very great. Prevention is practicable through iodization of a commonly used food, usually salt, or by intramuscular injections of iodized oil. These measures can result in improved quality of life, and productivity, and increased educability of children and adults. In the meantime, diagnosis is mainly by clinical examination, with decreased urinary iodine as a biochemical test if laboratory facilities permit, which is very uncommon.

[70] The recent recognition of lodine deficiency disorders is reflected by the formation of the ICIDD (International Council for iodine Deficiency Disorders).

Table 5.11 Iodine deficiency disorders *(Hetzel 1986)*

Fetus	Abortions*	
	Stillbirths*	
	Congenital anomalies*	
	Increased perinatal mortality*	
	Increased infant mortality*	
	Neurological cretinism	Mental deficiency*
		Deaf mutism*
		Spastic diplegia*
		Squint*
	Myxoedematous cretinism	Dwarfism
		Mental deficiency*
	Psychomotor defects*	
	Fetal hypothyroidism	
Neonates	Neonatal hypothyroidism	
	Neonatal goitre	
Child and adolescent	Juvenile hypothyroidism	
	Goitre	
	Impaired mental function*	
	Retarded development*	
	Cretinism	Mental deficiency
		Dwarfism
	Myxoedematous	
	Neurological	
Adult	Goitre with its complications	
	Hypothyroidism	
	Impaired mental function*	

* Items indicated are non-specific and can be caused by many other pathological conditions.

Protein–energy malnutrition

From a practical point of view, the nutritional status of young children as regards protein and energy (kilocalories or joules) may be viewed as a gradient or downward slope running from 'normal', through moderately severe degrees of malnutrition, to severe syndromes, including kwashiorkor and nutritional marasmus (Jelliffe 1959).

Suggested terminology

The label 'protein–calorie malnutrition of early childhood' was suggested (Jelliffe 1959) as a generic term to cover the whole range of mild to

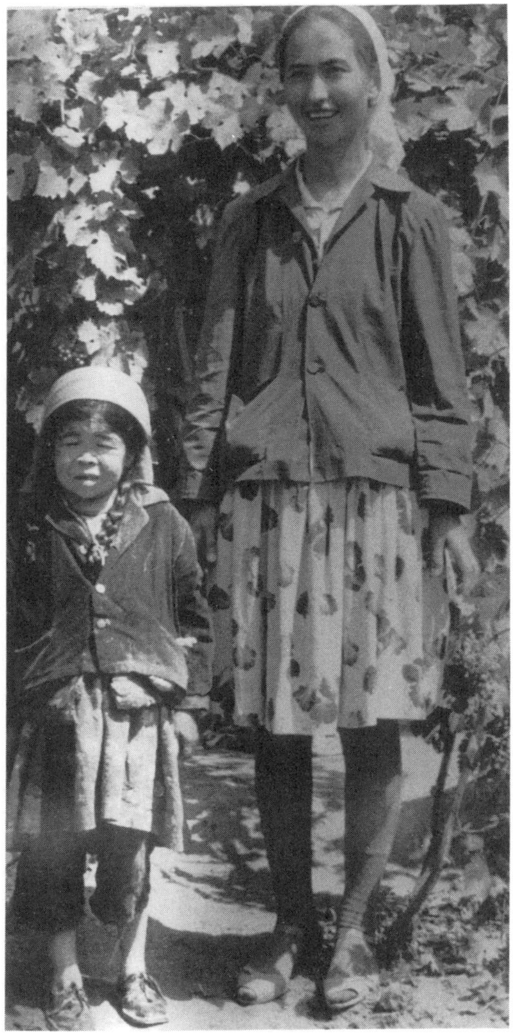

Fig. 5.18 Dwarfed cretin woman together with a 'barefoot doctor' of the same age from the Hetian District of Xinjiang, China. (Courtesy of Dr Ma Tai of Tianjin, China.) (From Hetzel 1986.)

severe, classifiable, and unclassifiable manifestations, including the two main severe clinical syndromes of kwashiorkor and nutritional marasmus.

The reasons that were advanced in favour of this term were:

1. It emphasized that kwashiorkor was *not* the only severe clinical end-result in young children. In an increasing number of countries nutritional marasmus has become the most common severe form, especially in

urban areas. Also, lesser manifestations of protein–calorie malnutrition are at all times far more frequent.

2. It stressed the need for consideration of calorie (energy) intakes as well as protein, not only in infant feeding in tropical regions, but in the treatment of all syndromes, including kwashiorkor.

3. All syndromes could be considered as related mainly to a diet low in protein, but with different levels of intake of calories in the form of largely carbohydrate foods.

4. The term 'early childhood' was considered appropriate, as the various syndromes occur most frequently from the early months of life up to late pre-school age, depending on local infant feeding practices.

The disadvantages of this overall label is that it neglects mention of 'contributory infections' (which are almost always present). These may be included in rather ill-defined 'noxious stimuli', as may the possible ill-effects of environmental toxins, especially aflatoxin, in some areas (Hendrickse 1984*b*). Also, it does not indicate that deficiencies of other nutrients are also certain to be present, such as folic acid, iron, etc., varying with the locality, and that some of these may also cause growth retardation (e.g. iodine, iron, and zinc).

However, work in recent decades has clearly indicated that calorie deficiency is the key, limiting nutrient in aetiology, prevention, and treatment. This is much more important than previously appreciated. Emphasis in feeding young children has moved to considerations of 'calorie density' or 'compact calories' (such as oil, fat, and sugar, and malted foods), as well as other nutrients, including protein. Also, it has become recognized that the main source of calories in many diets is also the principal source of protein. This applies, for example, with staple foods, such as wheat, rice, or corn (maize).

However, doubt has been cast on the view that varying proportions of calories to protein in dietary intakes are responsible for the very different clinical syndromes of kwashiorkor and marasmus (Alleyne *et al.* 1977). Nevertheless, this remains a useful practical working concept.

Prolonged detailed dietary histories for the weeks prior to the onset of severe syndromes are rarely obtainable in real-life studies. What is more, similar clinical pictures to kwashiorkor and marasmus have been produced by appropriate limited intakes of calories and protein in experimental animals. The difference in energy stores (subcutaneous fat) in marasmus compared with kwashiorkor is noteworthy. The greater dietary carbohydrate intake in kwashiorkor may also have metabolic effects leading to fatty infiltration of the liver, low serum albumin, and oedema. Increase in sodium retention may also play a part.

The term 'protein–energy malnutrition' has been adopted by WHO (Beaton and Bengoa 1976) and other international agencies, with the joule as the scientifically accepted international unit of *energy*. It seems unlikely that this seemingly logical change has helped clarify matters in practice. The word 'calorie' is part of everyday English in many countries. The use of the word 'energy' has a less obvious meaning, possibly referring to the activity level of the child. However, to conform with international opinion the term protein–energy malnutrition is used in the present publication. The two major, severe syndromes of protein–energy malnutrition are kwashiorkor and marasmus.

Kwashiorkor

Nomenclature

Williams (1933) introduced the socially descriptive West African word 'kwashiorkor'[71] to scientific medical literature. A variety of other terms have been used in the past for this dramatic, severe syndrome:

1. *Clinically descriptive: enfants rouges, culebrilla,*[72] *bouffisure d'Annam, syndrome depigmentation oedeme.*
2. *Pathologically descriptive:* fatty liver disease.
3. *Suggested nutritional aetiology: dystrofia pluricarencial, syndrome pluricarencial* (multiple-deficiency disease); *mehlnahrschaden* (flour malnutrition), nutritional oedema syndrome, malignant malnutrition.
4. *Vernacular name: obwosi*[73] (Luganda language).

Today, these terms are only of historical interest, since, by unofficial international agreement, the term kwashiorkor is currently used almost universally for this particular extreme form of protein–energy malnutrition of early childhood, even though there is disagreement about minimum diagnostic criteria.

Aetiology

Kwashiorkor can occur in infancy or in later childhood. It can develop, though rarely, in adults in famines, especially in women. However, in traditional circumstances, it usually has its maximum incidence in the second year of life, as this is when the main cumulative stresses of the 'weaning period' occur in many (but not all) cultures (Fig. 5.19). For example, in a classical analysis of 1141 cases by Trowell *et al.* (1954) in Uganda, 45 per cent were between 1 and 2 years of age, and 60 per cent between 1 and 3 years of age.

Kwashiorkor is never exclusively dietary in aetiology. Infective, psy-

[71] Meaning in the Ga language a disease occurring in a young child displaced from his mother's breast by a subsequent pregnancy.

[72] 'Snake skin', referring to the flaky-paint rash sometimes found.

[73] As with many vernacular names for the condition in African languages, *obwosi* has the same meaning as kwashiorkor ('sickness in the child displaced from the mother's breast').

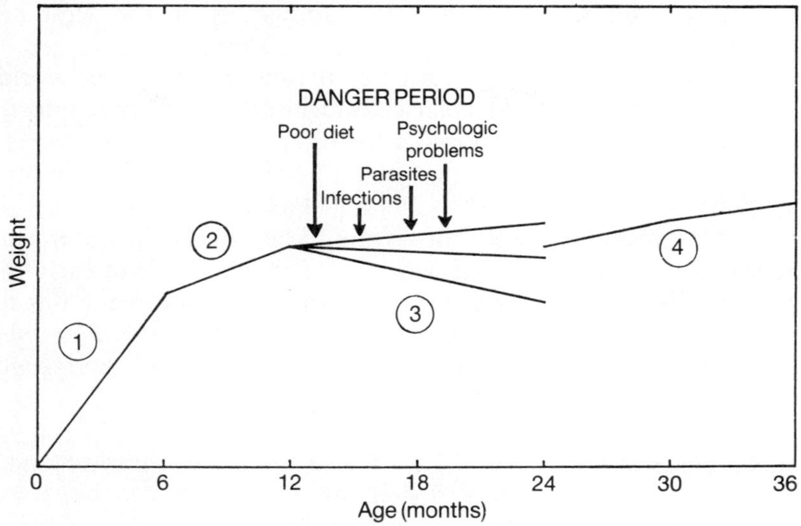

Fig. 5.19 Effect of cumulative stresses and danger period in second year of life on growth (weight gain) in many traditional communities.

chological, cultural, and other conditioning factors, either singly or in combination, are also operative. Nevertheless, for practical purposes the principal cause can still be considered to be a dietary deficiency and imbalance in early childhood — that is one which is low in protein, but which contains carbohydrate calories. A similar syndrome has been produced experimentally by feeding a low-protein, mainly carbohydrate diet to piglets (Platt 1958).

In the past, descriptions of the clinical features of kwashiorkor were confused by workers in one country or region who assumed that the clinical picture with which they were familiar was identical in detail to other parts of the world. Kwashiorkor can best be considered as a variable syndrome with certain constant features. Details of the clinical picture will vary with many factors, including: (1) the degree of deficiency and the amount and type of carbohydrate calories ingested; (2) the speed of onset; (3) the age at which the child is affected; (4) the duration; (5) conditioning factors, e.g. infections, psychological trauma; and (6) genetic characteristics (e.g. the normal colour of the skin and type of hair, etc.) in the particular community.

Thus, the infantile kwashiorkor seen in Trinidad 20 years ago had its peak incidence betwen 5 and 7 months of age, but the infants rarely showed hair changes and consistently had an enlarged liver (Jelliffe *et al.* 1960. This contrasted markedly with the classical tropical African textbook cases (Trowell *et al.* 1954). Similarly, obese, more 'chronic' variants of kwashiorkor have long been recognized in the West Indies ('sugar-babies') (Waterlow 1948; Jelliffe *et al.* 1954).

Despite these variations of detail in different parts of the world, it seems justifiable to divide the clinical features of kwashiorkor into three categories: constant; usual; and occasional.

Constant signs of kwashiorkor (Figs 5.20 (a), (b))

There are four constant features in kwashiorkor, which, though normally accompanied by other signs, can be regarded as diagnostic in early childhood, especially if found in regions where the conditions make this form of malnutrition likely to occur. There are *oedema, growth failure, muscle wasting* with *retention of some subcutaneous fat*, and *psychomotor change.*

Oedema Bilateral oedema is *the* cardinal sign of kwashiorkor and the syndrome should not be diagnosed in its absence. It can be detected initially in the pre-tibial region by the production of a definite pit as a result of *moderate* pressure for 3 seconds with a finger or thumb over the lower end of the tibia.

In tropical circumstances, bilateral oedema of the lower legs may also occur in hookworm disease, with severe anaemia, in beriberi, or in the nephrotic syndrome, when accompanied by heavy albuminuria. Particular difficulty may be encountered in some parts of the world with hookworm disease, as this parasitic infection can contribute to the development of kwashiorkor, as a result of protein loss in the blood ingested by the worms.

Growth retardation The growth retardation of kwashiorkor is much less strikingly obvious than in marasmus. The interpretation of weight in untreated kwashiorkor is complicated by the presence of oedema fluid. Also, so-called 'sugar baby' variants seen occasionally at one time in some parts of the world had a relatively thick layer of subcutaneous fat. The full degree of underweight only becomes revealed during successful treatment as the oedema disappears.

Muscle wasting and retention of some subcutaneous fat Muscle wasting is a constant feature of kwashiorkor, both clinically and at autopsy, and a reduction in the circumference of the upper arm and thin trapezius muscles are usually particularly evident. Often, affected children cannot hold up their heads because of such muscle wasting. It is much less obscured by oedema than the forearm or leg, although minimal oedema may occasionally be detectable, especially over the dependent triceps. However, even when none can be found, there is a further decrease in arm circumference when body oedema subsides, indicating the constant pre-

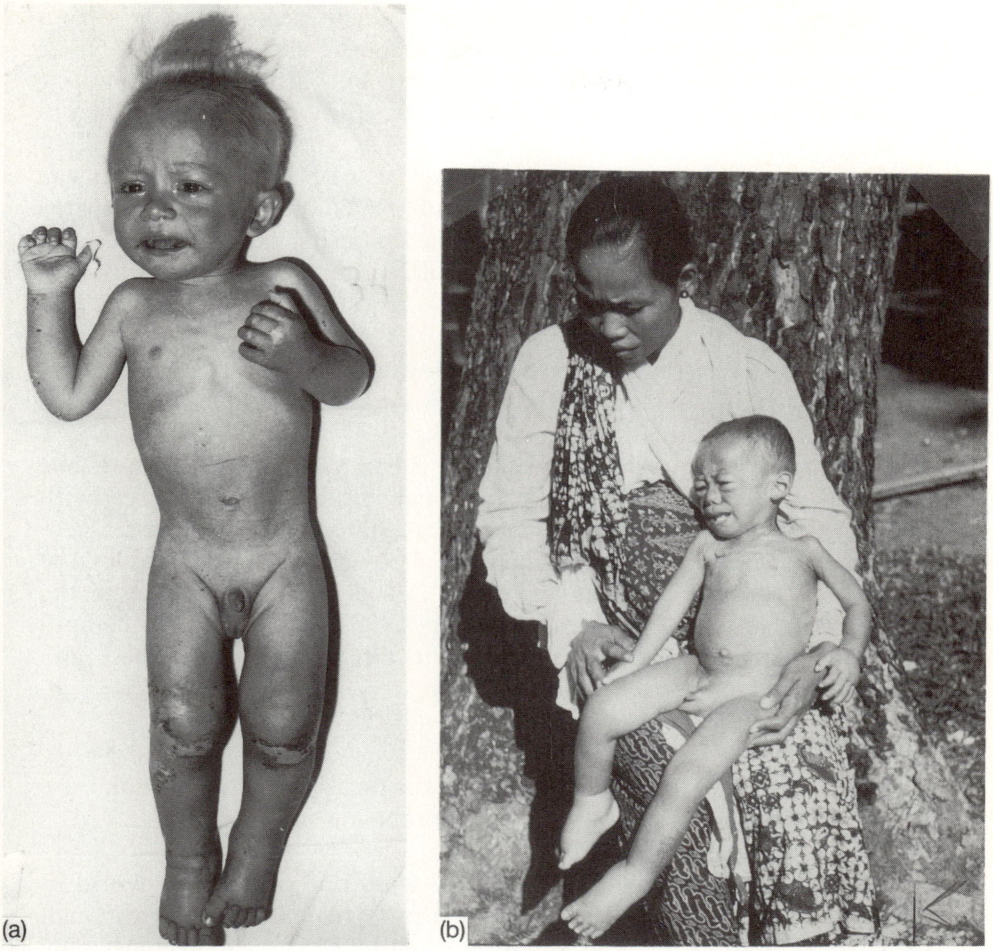

Fig. 5.20 Severe protein–energy malnutrition. (a) Kwashiorkor, showing oedema, misery, wasted muscles (with presence of subcutaneous fat), flaky paint rash, and hair changes. (Courtesy of INCAP, Guatemala City.) (b) Kwashiorkor showing marked oedema, misery, wasted muscles with some subcutaneous fat and with lightening of skin and hair (Indonesia). (Courtesy of the late Professor H.A.P.C. Oomen.)

sence of subclinical oedema and an increased water content of muscle and skin (Frenk *et al.* 1957). The midarm circumference has the advantage of being both simply measured and roughly circular. Its use in the assessment of lesser degrees of protein–energy malnutrition is considered in detail elsewhere (p. 307).

Clinical palpation suggests that a decreased limb circumference is principally due to muscle wasting, and this can be demonstrated both at autopsy and during life by surface measurements, and radiology. Muscle wasting and weakness can also be demonstrated functionally by testing the infant's ability to hold up his head when gently pulled from a lying to a sitting position.

In contrast with marasmus, a variable layer of subcutaneous fat can also be observed on both the body and the limbs. It can be palpated during clinical examination, and confirmed by using skinfold calipers. Its presence in part appears to reflect the child's calorie intake in the form of largely carbohydrate foods.

Psychomotor change The child with kwashiorkor is apathetic, miserable, inert, withdrawn, and anorexic. His motor development is retarded and has usually regressed in recent weeks.

The cause of this psychomotor change is complex. In some cultures the psychological trauma due to the maternal withdrawal associated with 'weaning' (*sevrage*) from the breast, sometimes including actual geographical separation from the mother, plays a part. The possibility of biochemical change affecting the brain is suggested by changes in the electroencephalogram (Nelson and Dean 1959), while physical components include a lowered basal metabolic rate, and the weakness and hypotonicity due to severe muscle wasting.

Usual signs of kwashiorkor

Certain signs, though not necessary for diagnosis, are common and are usually present either singly or in any combination:

Hair changes Although varying greatly from one part of the world to another, some degree of hair abnormality is usually found, although kwashiorkor can occur with wholly normal hair. The hair changes may comprise lightening in colour (dyspigmentation), straightness (if the normal hair is curly, as in African children), silkiness, and loosely attached roots, as shown by sparseness and 'easy pluckability' (p. 474).

Of the hair changes, dyspigmentation, if present, can be the most striking. A range of abnormally light hair colours can be found in kwashiorkor — light brown, reddish-brown, blonde, etc. It appears to occur most readily in African children. It is absent in cases of acute onset and, conversely, is most marked in chronic syndromes of gradual evolution, such as with some of the 'sugar baby' cases seen in the past in Jamaica. It is probably mainly related to interference with melanin formation due to inadequate supplies of sulphur-containing amino acids.

Dyspigmentation of the hair can occur from non-nutritional environmental and genetic causes. In some regions, it is commonly found in children without kwashiorkor. However, if genetic and environmental causes can be excluded, the correlation of dyspigmentation of the hair in pre-school age children with a community diet of largely carbohydrate, low-protein foods is suggested by several factors: (1) its absence in African children who are not protein-deficient (as among the Hadza hunters of Tanzania) (Jelliffe *et al.* 1962), as compared with the very high incidence among the children of the Baganda, whose diet is based on steamed plantain (Welbourn 1954); (2) its greatest occurrence at age 1–3 years, when, in most tropical regions, the child's diet is low in protein and high in carbohydrate calories; and (3) the fact that African children in the Congo with dyspigmentation of the hair have been shown to have a lower weight curve, especially in the second year of life, than children with normal black hair (André and Holemans 1955).

Diffuse depigmentation of the skin Skin depigmentation probably has the same causation as dyspigmented hair, and usually occurs at the same time of life. Light-coloured skin is a common feature of kwashiorkor, although with the genetic range of pigmentation found in many populations, it may be difficult to estimate with certainty. It is most easily seen in darker pigmented people, especially children of African descent, and, in the same way as dyspigmented hair, it is often most marked in chronic cases of gradual onset.

Moon-face The full, well-rounded, somewhat pendulous, and blubbery cheeks, known as moon-face, are often present in kwashiorkor. The pathogenesis of moon-face is uncertain. It occurs particularly in obese variants of kwashiorkor, and is presumably the result of increased fat locally, with possibly some degree of oedema. However, in addition to its probable relationship to the intake of carbohydrate calories, the effect of endocrine dysfunction also merits consideration, as the appearance can be similar to the Cushingoid face of pathological or steroid-induced hyperadrenalism.

Anaemia Again, this varies in commonness, and even more in precise causation from country to country. Various nutrient deficiencies may be responsible, including deficiencies of iron, folic acid, and protein. Anaemia is usually not severe unless infections or infestations, such as heavy hookworm burdens or malaria, are also present.

Occasional signs of kwashiorkor

The various signs that are occasinally present include the following.

Flaky-paint rash This well-known feature has been described elsewhere (p. 483) as occurring in advanced cases. It varies in commonness in different parts of the world. If present, it is diagnostic.

Hepatomegaly Although extreme fatty infiltration is a constant pathological finding, a considerably enlarged liver, sometimes extending down to the level of the umbilicus, is a pronounced feature of kwashiorkor only in certain parts of the world. In the past, this was the case in the West Indies (Waterlow 1948). From a world standpoint, hepatomegaly should be viewed as an occasional manifestation. In many rural tropical communities, the large livers found in late infancy and in the pre-school age-group are often associated with splenomegaly and are mainly the result of chronic malaria.

Other skin lesions Children with kwashiorkor may sometimes show indolent sores, fissures (as behind the ears), and a 'moist groin rash' (Trowell *et al.* 1954).

Associated vitamin deficiency A variety of signs possibly due to associated vitamin and/or mineral deficiencies may be found, including keratomalacia and angular stomatitis. Their commonness varies from one part of the world to another. They may appear during treatment, if the particular vitamin is not supplied as part of therapy.

Associated contributory conditions These may include chest signs of tuberculosis, severe anaemia in hookworm infection, and dehydration, from diarrhoea, even when peripheral oedema is present.

Marasmus

Nomenclature

The term at present used for this second severe syndrome of protein–energy malnutrition is imprecise, but clinically descriptive. It refers to a person, usually a young child, showing very severe wasting, principally due to a grossly inadequate diet. Older terms include athrepsia, decomposition, infantile atrophy, desnutrition, and inanition.

Aetiology

Marasmus is usually due to very severe under-nutrition — that is, a diet that is extremely low in both protein and calories — so-called 'balanced starvation'. While it can occur at all ages, including adulthood, it is seen most commonly in the first year of life ('early onset' or infantile marasmus) (Fig. 5.21). This is in contrast to kwashiorkor, which occurs mainly in the age-group 1–3 years. It occurs most frequently as a result of attempted artificial feeding with very dilute milk or formula, and is also often associated with infective diarrhoea and sometimes with tuberculosis. It can occur with very inadequate lactation, resulting from interference with the lactation reflexes (p. 260), with the use of high-dose

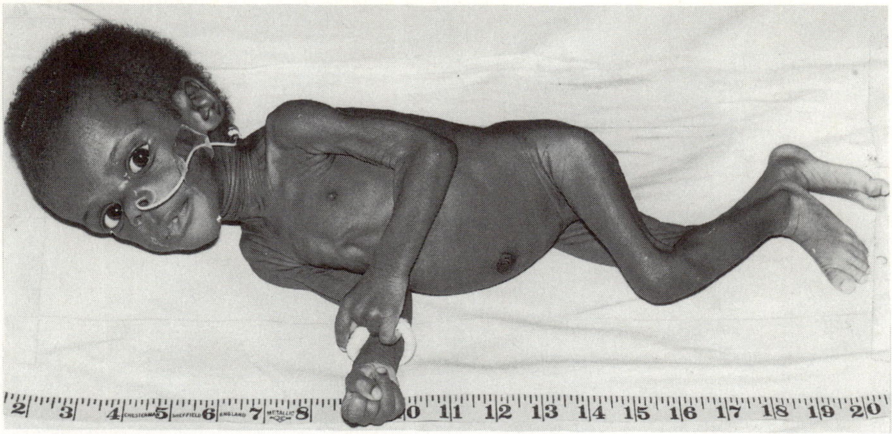

Fig. 5.21 Severe protein–energy malnutrition. Early onset (or infantile) marasmus, showing extreme wasting of muscle and fat (Kampala, Uganda).

oestrogen contraceptives, or more rarely from *severe* maternal malnutrition. 'Late onset' marasmus (Fig. 5.22) is a quite distinct syndrome occurring in the pre-school age period, often as a result of prolonged breastfeeding *not* supplemented with sufficient amounts of nutritious, calorie-rich foods — so-called 'breast starvation'. This very late introduction of semisolids may be for cultural reasons, as in parts of India and Burma, but seems to have been increased in recent years by rapidly rising food prices. Once again, a clinical picture similar to marasmus has been produced in piglets by feeding them a diet low in both protein and carbohydrate calories (Platt 1958).

The clinical signs of nutritional marasmus can be divided into two groups: constant and occasional.

Constant signs of nutritional marasmus

The two constant features of nutritional marasmus are severe growth retardation and marked wasting of muscle and of subcutaneous fat (Figs. 5.21 and 5.22).

Growth retardation This is extreme. Weight loss is much more marked than that of length. The child is usually below 60 per cent of the reference weight for age.

Wasting of muscle and of subcutaneous fat This can be detected by clinical inspection and by palpation. The arms look and feel very thin. The skin is loose, and measurements of the circumference and the skinfolds of the upper arm, and subsequent calculation of muscle circumfer-

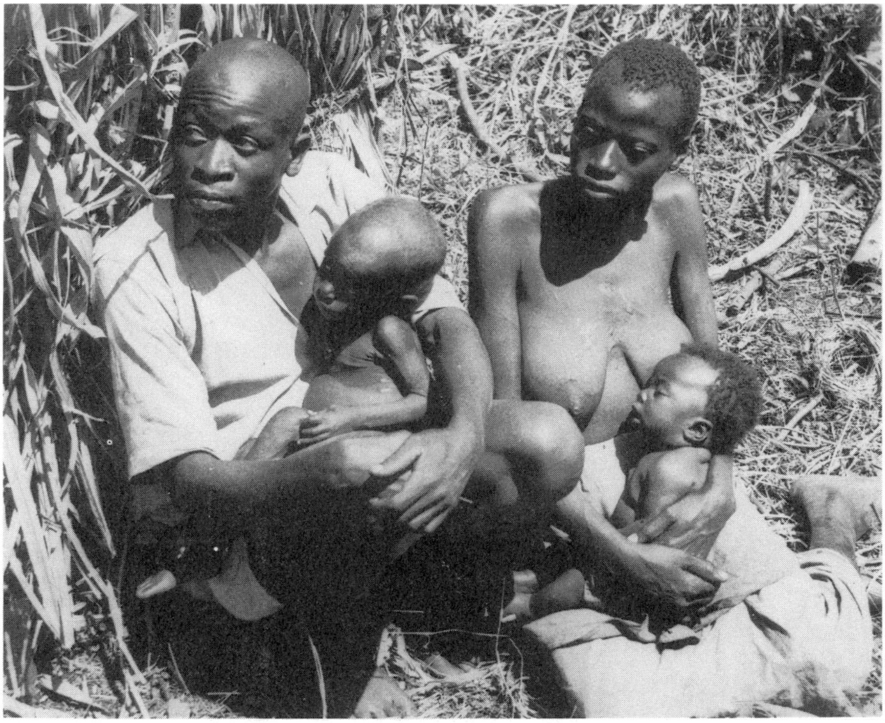

Fig. 5.22 Severe protein–energy malnutrition. 'Late onset' marasmus showing wasting of muscle and fat, in contrast with well-nourished 5-month-old breastfed baby. The mother shows signs of early 'maternal depletion' (diminished fat and muscle). The father is adequately nourished (rural Uganda).

ence are all very low (p. 51). Wasting is also clinically apparent in the wizened 'little old man' or 'monkey' face. This emphasizes the depletion of the buccal pad of fat, usually considered the last reserves to be metabolized.

Occasional signs of nutritional marasmus

Hair changes Minor abnormalities of the hair may be seen occasionally. These are never marked, although light-brown, somewhat sparse hair may be found. The conspicuously dyspigmented hair occurrng in many children with kwashiorkor never occurs.

Associated vitamin deficiency In particular, angular stomatitis and keratomalacia may be present.

Associated contributory infections These may include the dehydration resulting from infective diarrhoea, oral moniliasis (thrush), and chest

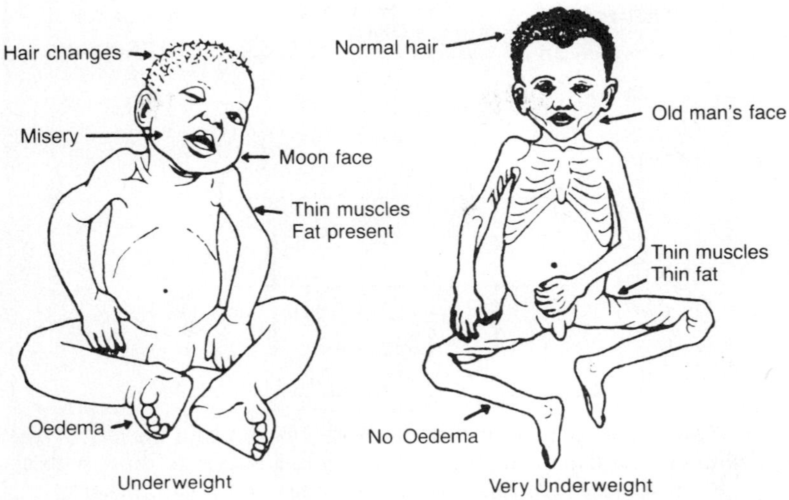

Fig. 5.23 Contrasting clinical signs in severe protein–energy malnutrition: (left) kwashiorkor and (right) marasmus.

signs due to tuberculosis. In contrast to kwashiorker, oedema is absent and the child seldom exhibits psychomotor change, such as apathy or anorexia.

The main features contrasting kwashiorkor and marasmus are given in Fig. 5.23.

Intermediate severe syndromes

The term 'protein–energy malnutrition of early childhood' has been used in an attempt to attach a tentative aetiologically helpful label to the group as a whole. Yet even with severe forms there will be frequent cases which are intermediate between the two clinical 'mountain peaks' of kwashiorkor and of nutritional marasmus, and in which categorization is debatable.

Less severe protein–energy malnutrition

Lesser degrees of protein–energy malnutrition have been labelled 'latent', 'hidden', 'marginal', or 'mild–moderate'. They are far more common than the advanced syndromes, as indicated conceptually in the protein–energy malnutrition icebergy (Fig. 5.24). In order to assess the full extent of the problem, less marked forms must also be enumerated in a nutritional assessment of the community (p. 297). It is suggested that the term 'moderately severe' be used for children with growth failure below the

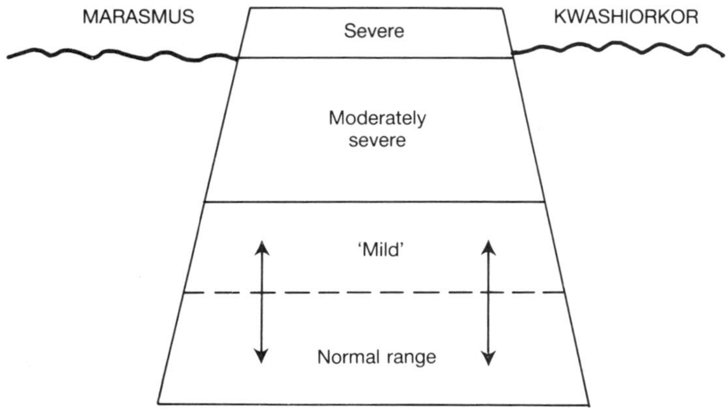

Fig. 5.24 Protein–energy malnutrition 'iceberg' emphasizing the large number of children with clinically inapparent malnutrition in addition to those with clinically obvious, severe forms (e.g. marasmus and kwashiorkor).

3rd centile of weight-for-age, using locally agreed upon reference data (p. 110).

The situation is complicated by the variability of the clinical picture. Difficulties include: (1) problems with objective definition and variability of most of the signs (p. 14); (2) the fact that a continuous gradient exists between the obvious severe case and the well-nourished, healthy child; and (3) children with less severe protein–energy malnutrition are not a homogeneous group, but need categorization into those acutely and chronically affected, as discussed later (p. 287) (Gurney *et al.* 1972, 1973; Waterlow 1972, 1973).

Classifications based on the percentage of weight-for-age percentage levels such as those of Gómez *et al.* (1956) and Jelliffe (1966) are still useful. Whenever possible, they need to be further differentiated by additional measurements (p. 312). However, all conclusions based on anthropometry should be corroborated from other sources of information, such as dietary intake.

Public health significance

In different forms and degrees of severity, protein–energy malnutrition is common in most less developed countries, and is the principal nutritional public health problem in the world. Thus, in very severe conditions in Haiti in 1960, it was found that 7 per cent of the 1–3-year-old children in representative villages of the country as a whole were suffering from kwashiorkor (Jelliffe and Jelliffe 1960). In Kampala, Uganda, 10 per cent of admissions to the childrens wards at Mulago Hospital demonstrated

Table 5.12 Range and median prevalence of protein–energy malnutrition in community surveys *(Beaton and Bengoa 1976)*

Area	No. of surveys	No. of children examined (thousands)	Severe forms		Moderate forms	
			Range (%)	Median (%)	Range (%)	Median (%)
Latin America	11	109	0.5–6.3	1.6	3.5–32.0	18.9
Africa	7	25	1.7–9.8	4.4	5.4–44.9	26.5
Asia	7	39	1.1–20.0	3.2	16.0–46.4	31.2
Total	25	173	0.5–20.0	2.6	3.5–46.4	18.9

Table 5.13 Total number of young children affected by protein–energy malnutrition *(Beaton and Bengoa 1976)*

Area	Population aged 0–5 years (millions)*	No. of children with protein–energy malnutrition (millions)		
		Severe	Moderate	Total
Latin America	46	0.7	8.8	9.5
Africa	61	2.7	16.3	19.0
Asia†	206	6.6	64.4	71.0
Total	314	10.0	89.5	99.5

* Averages for the years 1963–73.
† Excluding China and Japan.

this advanced syndrome (Musoke 1961), and more than 50 per cent of those attending local child-welfare clinics showed clinical and anthropometric evidence suggestive of lesser degrees of protein–energy malnutrition.

Beaton and Bengoa (1976) analysed results available from surveys in different continents (Table 5.12) and from these roughly estimated total numbers of affected young children (Table 5.13). Categorization into 'moderate' protein–energy malnutrition is based on the weight-for-age Gómez classification (p. 122), which does not differentiate the two main types of underweight children, as nowadays suggested (p. 312), nor are the methods used or samples included comparable from one country to another. However, an approximate world total of 10 million children with severe protein–energy malnutrition clearly indicates the very large magnitude of the problem (Beaton and Bengoa 1976; Keller and Fillmore 1983). More modern estimates of the main types of malnutrition in young children and mothers were given earlier (p. 2).

Protein–energy malnutrition syndromes have major public health significance as causes of death, both directly and as a result of increased susceptibility to infections. They also can have very large economic consequences to nations due to the cost of services needed for treatment. This may become less if primary health care services are developed to detect and manage early cases at the community level.

The later consequences of treated severe protein–energy malnutrition and of different forms of untreated 'moderately severe' protein–energy malnutrition (e.g. 'wasted', 'stunted', etc.) (p. 312) are imperfectly understood. The effects of different forms of moderate protein–energy malnutrition in late childhood and adult life are currently much under consideration in relation to their relative significance as regards more immediate or more long-term impact, and therefore, to their public health priority.

Historical considerations

As judged by the records of children attending clinics who subsequently develop kwashiorkor, and by the common flattening of weight curves in the second year of life in regions where kwashiorkor is widespread, the first clinical indication of protein–energy malnutrition appears to be growth failure, most usually recognized by inadequate weight gain following serial measurements. This is discussed in detail later in relation to the use of growth charts in young child clinics (p. 296).

In general terms, the clinical stereotype of moderately severe protein–energy malnutrition (Fig. 5.25) has been of an underweight disproportionate child, with a long-seeming body, thin limbs, a head that appears too large, and feet that seem unduly elongated. The buttocks may be flattened and the scapulae appear 'winged'. The chest appears to be small, especially in contrast with the abdomen, which may be somewhat distended because of thin abdominal muscles and a bulky, fermentable, largely carbohydrate diet. The child may also have a heavy burden of roundworms and enlargement of the liver and spleen, often due to malaria in hyperendemic areas. Other signs in the grouping suggestive of protein–energy malnutrition (p. 493) may be present in varying combinations. However, these are variable and subjective, especially in early cases.

In such children, the principal anthropometric abnormality has been a low weight for age, approximately paralleling the severity of the malnutrition. Despite early interference with bone metabolism, there is much less effect on linear growth, as indicated by measurement of body length. This is because bony growth, including length, has a much smaller range of normal variation. It is affected more by chronic deprivation (p. 312), and, unlike weight, it cannot *decrease* in malnutrition.

Historically, the characteristically lesser effect of malnutrition on

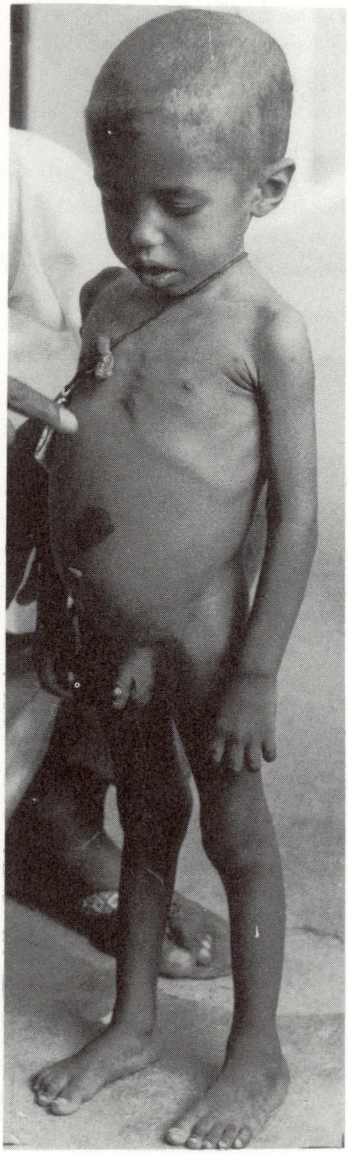

Fig. 5.25 Moderately severe protein–energy malnutrition in a pre-school age child, showing body disproportion (thin limbs, large-seeming head, small chest, elongated appearance of body and feet) (Mauritania). (Courtesy of UNICEF.)

skeletal growth has been recognized for many decades, with 'the body being elongated and the head large' (Jackson 1925). Similar results are also found in piglets experimentally subjected to severe undernourishment. They also develop heads that seem too large, legs that are too long, and bodies that are too small.

The head circumference is affected, though much less so than the weight, especially if malnutrition occurs in the second year of life. This is because 50 per cent of extra-uterine skull growth occurs in the first year of life. The apparent largeness of the head is due to the contrast between a relatively normal-sized skull with the thin limbs, and especially with the small chest, which is due in large part to wasted or poorly developed pectoral muscles, a finding which may be confirmed by a relatively small chest circumference.

In addition, earlier attempts to categorize lesser degrees of protein–energy malnutrition were confused by what was originally recognized as 'nutritional dwarfing' (Fig. 5.26), occurring in children with mild–moderate, prolonged malnutrition 'in as yet ill-defined circumstances', who were 'considerably underweight and undersized, while at the same time appearing to have relatively normal body proportions' (Jelliffe 1959). As Downs (1964) remarked children with nutritional dwarfing are light in weight, short in stature, with relatively normal body proportions, and subcutaneous fat appropriate to their weight; they are likely to be taken for healthy *younger* children. In the 1960s, this condition was only beginning to receive attention, but appeared to be not uncommon, as noted in Peru (Graham 1966) and among Arab refugee children in the Lebanon (Downs 1964).

Recent developments

In recent years, various changes have occurred, particularly in some parts of the world. In many 'dysurbanized' slum and shanty town areas in less developed countries, the onset of protein–energy malnutrition now occurs in younger children. This has lead to a rise in incidence of 'early onset' marasmus, often with infective diarrhoea, from changes from breastfeeding to inappropriate bottle-feeding, with over-dilute, contaminated formula, either alone or as a 'mixed milk feeding'. In addition, in some areas, markedly rising costs of basic foods are associated with an increased incidence of 'late onset' marasmus, in the 1–4 year olds.

In a small number of less technically developed countries, mortality in early childhood has been reported to have decreased in the last decade or so. In some instances, the vital statistics for such conclusions are unreliable or from limited populations. When correct, it has been suggested that this may be partly the result of improved basic treatment in primary health care services. However, according to Bengoa's 'surviving child'

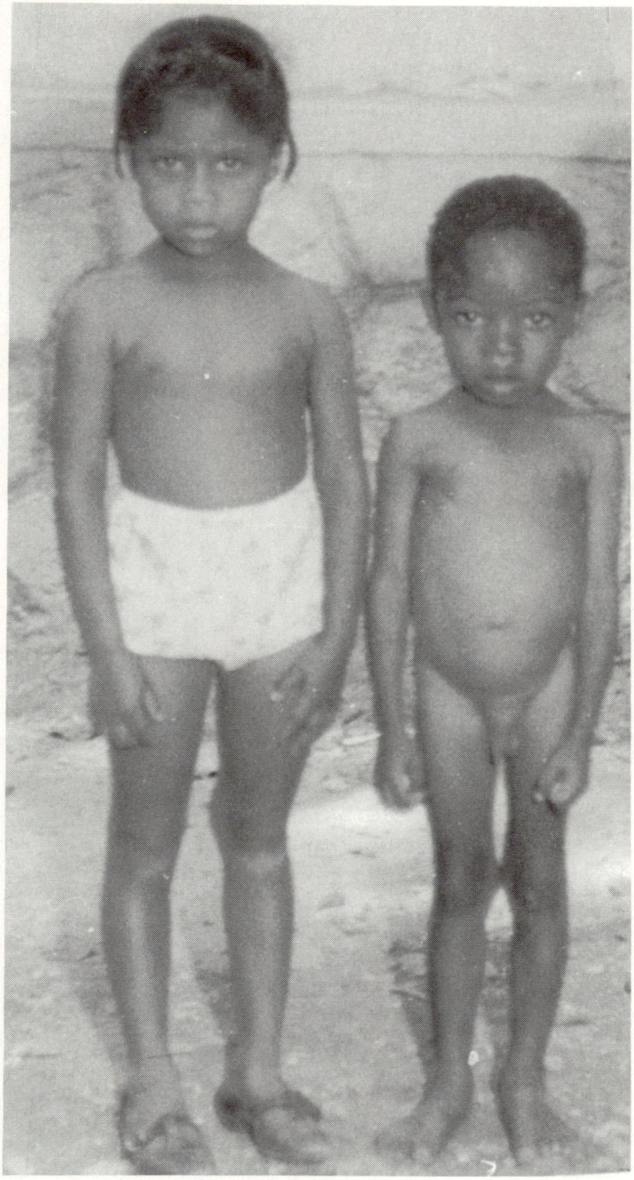

Fig. 5.26 Nutritional dwarfing or stunting in a young boy (right) in rural Jamaica with normal body proportions, compared with a girl of the same age.

hypothesis, such communities may be 'passing from an era of high child mortality' to 'an era blighted by increasing numbers of socially handicapped with chronic disability' (Bengoa 1970). However, in too many areas, young child mortality, considerably related to malnutrition, undoubtedly has increased as a result of economic problems, and man-made and/or natural disasters. This is exemplified by the large-scale refugee situations in Indo-China and in Ethiopia and the Sudan as a result of drought and civil war. During the past 10 years, the difference between two forms of moderately severe protein–energy malnutrition has been particularly emphasized by the work of Waterlow (1972, 1973). It is now agreed that the 'acute' condition (characterized by wasting or thinness) needs to be differentiated from the 'chronic' (stunting or dwarfing) (Fig. 5.26). Their anthropometric measurements and body proportions are dissimilar, their nutritional aetiology distinct, and their public health meaning as regards both prognosis and community programmes different. This important issue is discussed further in relation to interpretation according to the Waterlow classification (p. 312).

Obesity

All over the world in industrialized countries, obesity appears to have increased in recent decades, including infancy and the 'pre-school age-group. This is emphasized by a recent comparative study in the USA from 1963 to 1980 (Gortmaker *et al.* 1987), and by a British report on obesity in the young child (Poskitt 1986). It is also possible that overweight ('heavy-for-dates') newborns are occurring or being recognized more frequently (Sterky and Mellander 1978). The trend towards obesity involves the usually small percentage of children of the Westernized elite in many developing countries. While of varying and complex aetiology, the primary cause seems to be the 'caloric overdosage' that can occur more easily in infants who are bottle-fed (when the volume and concentration of the feeds are under the mother's control) and who usually also receive semisolid foods 'early', that is in the first 1–2 months of life.

Obesity in early childhood has certain inherent risks, including a greater likelihood of severe respiratory tract infection and skin disease. There is also the possibility of the mother continuing to overfeed because her baby is large. There often seems to be a link between excessive fatness in early childhood and obesity in later life, with all the known increased associated health hazards. However, the evidence is controversial and not as clear-cut as previously believed (Lloyd 1979). The connecting links may include early habituation to a large appetite, the general family dietary pattern, and an abnormal increase in the numbers of fat cells in obese infants, although recent studies have shown this last factor to be more difficult to prove than previously believed. Detailed consideration of obesity in early childhood is available elsewhere (Lloyd 1979).

Assessment

As with obesity at any age, the assessment is initiated by clinical inspection showing visibly obvious excess fatfolds, over-rounded limbs, and a corpulent abdomen, which can be recognized at a glance. Anthropometry is employed for objective diagnosis, with findings the opposite of those observed in protein–energy malnutrition. The weight-for-age is well above the 'normal' reference level — as is the weight-for-length (height), despite the fact that the stature of such children can also be somewhat increase. This is perhaps related in part to the high intake of protein, calcium, and other nutrients that accompany the excessive calories in the diet. The arm circumference will be above the 'normal'. Most significantly, the fat stores will be increased , as can be measured at standardized sites, usually the triceps fatfold.

In addition, more complex statistical analyses have been undertaken to develop 'obesity indices' for infants. For example, Crawford *et al.* (1974) suggested a composite index incorporating the weight gain since birth, the waist circumference, and the supra-iliac fatfold as being most appropriate for use in infancy, especially around 6 months of age. Like most more complex mathematical anthropometric formulas, these have little chance of effective use or adoption on a wide scale.

Simple, albeit approximate, measurements have to be the basis for assessment, especially for community investigations. For the individual child, borderline measurements on one occasion are more difficult to interpret, because of the normal range of variation. Serial weight measurements recorded on growth charts may be helpful (p. 296).

Reference data

This controversial subject is discussed elsewhere in general (p. 110). Difficulties include possible ethnic, genetic differences in fat patterning (Eveleth 1979) and uncertainty as to whether the 'reference data' collected in industrialized countries and in Westernized urban élite populations in developing countries in recent years represent truly optimal or overfat populations.

Reference data for weight, height (length), weight-for-height, arm circumference, and triceps fatfolds from NCHS surveys are given in tables in Appendix 9. Obesity is probable with a weight-for-height of $> +2$ SD ($\geq$ 120 per cent of reference level, especially if corroborated by clinical inspection. Obesity is confirmed by a high triceps fatfold (Appendix 9).

Nutritional assessment of protein–energy malnutrition and obesity

Direct assessment

Clinical signs (p. 493)

As noted earlier (p. 14), these are variable and subjective. The only sign which needs to be included routinely in survey work is bilateral oedema, which is the cardinal feature of kwashiorkor. However, it is often recommended that a small number of selected other signs (p. 493) be borne in mind, as they can give a general view of the clinical picture of protein–energy malnutrition, including kwashiorkor, in the particular region.

Biochemical tests (p. 38)

In general, these are not used much in less technically developed parts of the world because of practical difficulties, lack of laboratories, cost, and uncertainty of interpretation. Consideration of previous and current biochemical tests for protein–energy malnutrition are given elsewhere (p. 496).

Biophysical tests (p. 50)

The only test which has been used in field studies in some areas of the world is examination of the hair root morphology. Present views on this test are given earlier (p. 53).

Anthropometry

It has become clear that the field assessment of protein–energy malnutrition in young children will depend in practice mainly on anthropometry, both cross-sectional and preferably serial measurements, *together with* supportive information from other sources, especially dietary intake (p. 198). The numerous considerations concerning the special significance and value of anthropometry in children are given elsewhere (p. 68).

Assessment from health statistics

When reliable statistics are available (which is usually not the case in Third World countries), age-specific mortality rates (p. 129) can be helpful. This is especially so in the first or the second years of life, depending on local weaning practices. Consideration of other methods of indirect assessment is given elsewhere (p. 128).

Assessment of ecological variables

Evaluation of ecological variables (p. 142), such as socio-economic circumstances (p. 148), cultural practices (p. 164), contributory infections (p. 139), food considerations (p. 175), etc., need to be included, as far as practicable, in investigations into protein–energy malnutrition in individual children and in communities. It is only by so doing that locally important risk factors can be identified, and appropriate programmes devised to focus on the main preventable causes in the particular area. Qualitative and quantitative estimations of dietary intake are especially needed, although these pose special problems in this age-group (p. 199).

Commonly used anthropometric measurements

Widespread experience in many parts of the world indicates that four measurements are commonly used and are most useful in attempts to assess the prevalence or incidence of protein–energy malnutrition (or obesity) in young children. These are weight, height or stature (or length), arm circumference, and triceps fatfold. However, for practical reasons, particularly the high cost of fatfold calipers, the first three are most likely to be included — weight, height, and arm circumference.

The significance and limitations of these measurements as indicators of abnormal growth associated with malnutrition are considered below. This is followed by discussion concerning derived ratios, which can be obtained from the four determinations.

Weight

Single measurements

Weight has been used to classify malnourished or overnourished children for many years. The apparatus required is relatively simple and inexpensive. The significance of the procedure is recognized world-wide by health workers and the general population. It is still a useful guide to nutritional status, but with more limitations than previously recognized.

In particular, a single weight on one occasion only gives a composite measure of lean body mass (especially skeleton and musculature), internal organs, fat, and body water, together with some pathological conditions, such as oedema (or dehydration), marked enlargement of the liver or spleen, or even heavy burdens of roundworms. A low weight on one occasion in younger children especially may be related to birth weight or small maternal size.

A single weight measurement is a static estimate at one point in time of a dynamic process — growth. It can be affected by sudden temporary decreases due to dehydration or to a recent acute infection. At the same time, in young children, body weight remains a simple-to-obtain, approximate 'suggester' of malnutrition, reflecting particularly the depletion of the most nutritionally labile tissues — fat and muscle.

In an individual child, the interpretation of a single weight measurement must be made with caution, unless very high or low — in relation to the source of the 'reference data' with which it is compared (p. 119) and to the distribution of weight in any healthy, well-nourished community. In less technically developed countries, problems also commonly occur because of lack of knowledge of the exact age (p. 109), and because children who are underweight for age are not a uniform group. They may have arrived at similar malnourished conditions by past histories, as regards dietary inadequacy and infections (Gopalan 1987). What is more they include those who are 'wasted', 'stunted', and 'wasted and stunted' and who need differentiating for practical reasons (p. 312).

Repeated measurements

By contrast, serial measurements of body weight give a dynamic record of growth failure from protein–energy malnutrition and its associated infections and psychological stresses. The use of growth charts in clinics all over the world and in the community itself continues as a most important practical method of detecting children with early protein–energy malnutrition — and the same applies for obesity.

At more sophisticated levels, methods have been devised using recorded weight *gains* (De Winter 1977) or incremental growth velocity (Tanner *et al.* 1966) or 'catch-up' growth in successfully treated protein–energy malnutrition (Landman *et al.* 1979). Martorell and colleagues (1982) developed a weight chart for low-birth-weight children in the first 2 years of life. Results are based on current weight and weight gained over a specific time, and are categorized as 'insufficient', 'adequate', and 'excessive'. However, these more refined methods have little application in less technically developed countries, especially as such activities are usually carried out by community health workers with limited education and training.

Weight charts and growth monitoring

The use of a weight chart for monitoring growth, or its failure or excess, in young children is undoubtedly one of the most important practical techniques for nutritional monitoring introduced in recent years.[74]

For general purposes, some form of simplified weight chart — such as pioneered by David Morley (1963, 1968*b*) — has gradually been adopted

[74] Detailed discussion of some of the advances, controversies, and dilemmas are given in papers presented at the Second Consultation on Growth Monitoring, New Delhi (UNICEF 1986)

widely. If used correctly, this can be a dynamic and feasible method of monitoring nutrition and health in early childhood. It can also focus the attention of health staff on the prevention of malnutrition and, especially when kept by the mothers, it can serve both as an educational tool for parents and a permanent health record. Various other types of health information can be included, using the local language, pictures, or understandable symbols. These can comprise messages and information on infant feeding, spaces for recording of immunizations, use of antimalarials, family planning practices, and a list of risk factors for the particular area.

Weight charts of several types have been used with differing degrees of success by health auxiliaries in various countries. In Indonesia, mothers have successfully functioned as 'weight-watchers' — weighing their children and recording the results themselves (Rohde *et al.* 1975). This important approach needs further investigation, as its reported success in Java seems to be due in part to two traditional practices — the cultural habit of forming of women's (and other) mutual support 'clubs' and the widespread use of an accurate indigenous beam-balance scale in the village market. Varied results have been obtained from questioning and testing mothers' understanding of weight charts. For example, in Ghana and Lesotho often there has been little comprehension (Peilemeier 1985). This has also been the case in Papua-New Guinea (Forsyth 1984), Afghanistan (Grant and Stone 1986), and in different regions in India (Gopalan and Chatterjee 1985).

Whatever chart is used, the gain in weight, or failure to do so, is more impotant than the situation of the weight recording on the graph. The potential value of a growth chart was summarized by Morley and Woodland (1979):

> It provides a continous record of health. When a child is sick, there is valuable background information to help treatment. It is the basis for comprehensive health monitoring and care. It avoids the dangers of giving a single response to a specific need, without consideration of the total picture. It encourages positive action for all children. Promotion of adequate growth is a more useful target than prevention of malnutrition.
>
> The chart is of the greatest value in terms of preventive action as it makes serious disease or malnutrition easy to diagnose. The role of the weight chart is to identify the potential danger of malnutrition before management becomes too difficult at the primary health care level. The weight curve may identify trouble 6 months or even a year before the child has obvious signs of malnutrition. The opposite is also true. A child who is gaining weight regularly and whose curve is parallel with the curves on the chart will not develop malnutrition.

Types of weight charts

Three main types of weight chart are used: two-line, multi-line, and single-line.

'Road to Health' two-line chart This version has been advocated by Morley and by WHO (1978*a*) for young children. It is designed for use for both sexes and has only two reference lines on it. Various ways have been devised for selecting these two levels. The commonest is with (1) the 50th NCHS centile for boys as the upper line and 3rd centile for girls as the lower line (Morley and Woodland 1979). Other levels may be used in different countries. It is apparent that the *exact* levels are not of major significance *so long as the majority of the 'healthy' children of the community fall between the two*. The main purpose in using such growth charts is to see that the child is gaining weight regularly and that the growth curve or line is roughly parallel with and follow the curves on the chart (Morley and Woodland 1979).

The Morley 'Road-to-Health' chart uses the calendar system for recording the child's age and is designed to be kept by the mother. WHO (1978*a*) introduced a modification of this chart (Fig. 5.27). The chart spans from birth up to the fifth birthday, but in some countries it may be limited to the first 3 years and in others extended up to 7 years. Other information may be included, such as reasons for special care, family composition, infant feeding, immunization, family planning, etc. It is based on the need for least cost (but attractive) printing and the most 'user-effective' scales, very often of hanging spring type, such as the Salter model (p. 74).

If needed, the weight *levels* of young children attending a clinic can be measured, perhaps during a specified week, by using a plastic overlay showing lines with different levels placed on the 'Road-to-Health' chart, when mothers bring these to the clinic or weighing site.

Alternatively, the weights of children attending a clinic or in a community can be plotted during a particular period on a 'master chart' (Capone 1978)* (Fig. 5.28). In a few areas, duplicate or more elaborate charts may be retained at the clinic. This is so in some Caribbean countries.

Morley has argued strongly for standardized growth charts for use round the world, based on the 'Road-to-Health' model for the following reasons (Morley and Woodland 1979):

1. A standardized record can be based on experience gained in many countries. It can incorporate the best and most relevant experience and ideas.
2. Weight charts are not easy to understand and use. Training needs to be given to health workers with little formal education, and also to the community at large. This could be provided through schools in countries where governments realise the importance of growth in the first years. Thus the record needs to be simple to understand and use, and appropriate traning materials used need to be

* Catholic Relief Services, Nairobi, Kenya.

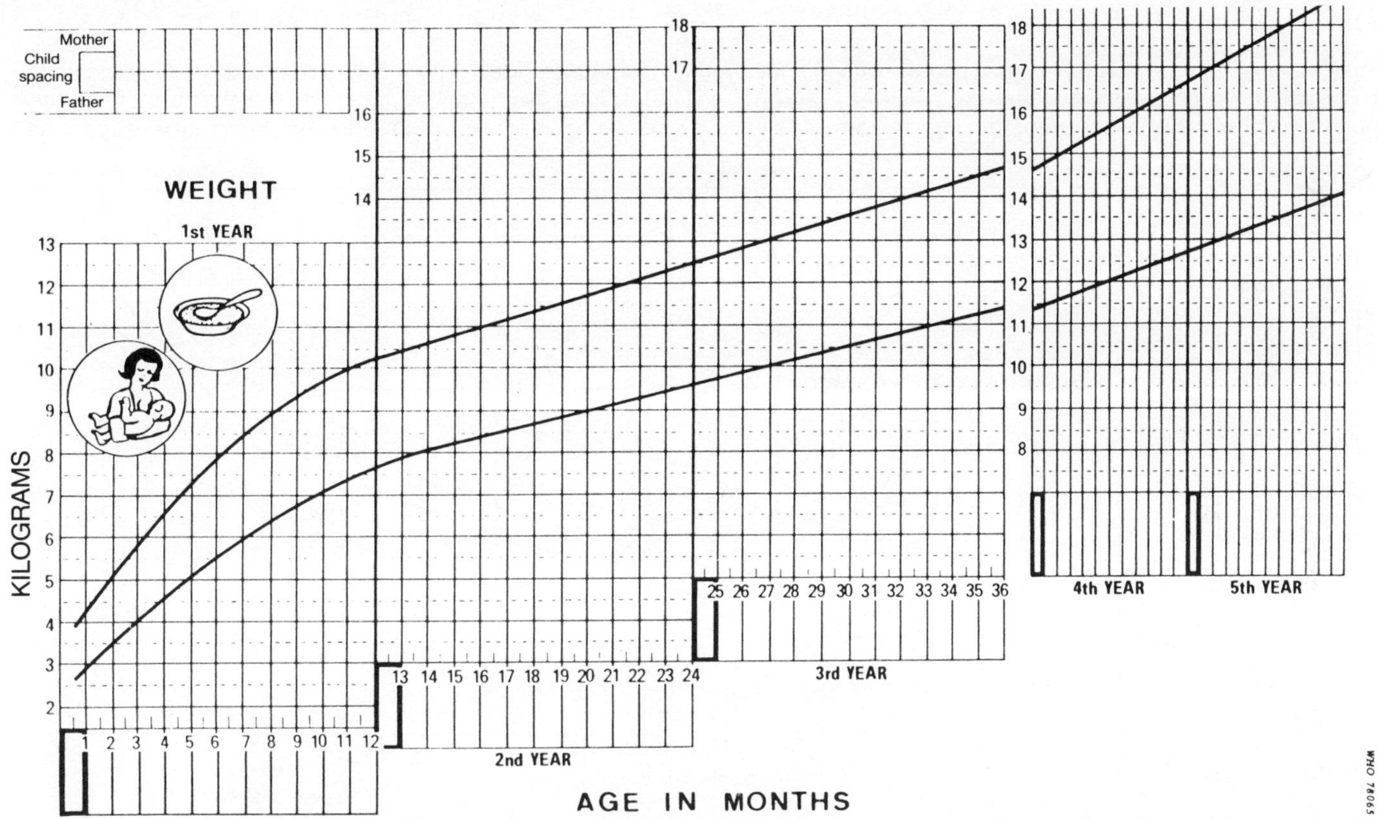

Fig. 5.27 Two-line growth chart for retention by mother (WHO 1978*a*). Home-based weight chart. Sexes are combined with two reference lines: 50th centile for boys and 3rd centile for girls (NCHS data: see Appendix 9.) Appendix 9.

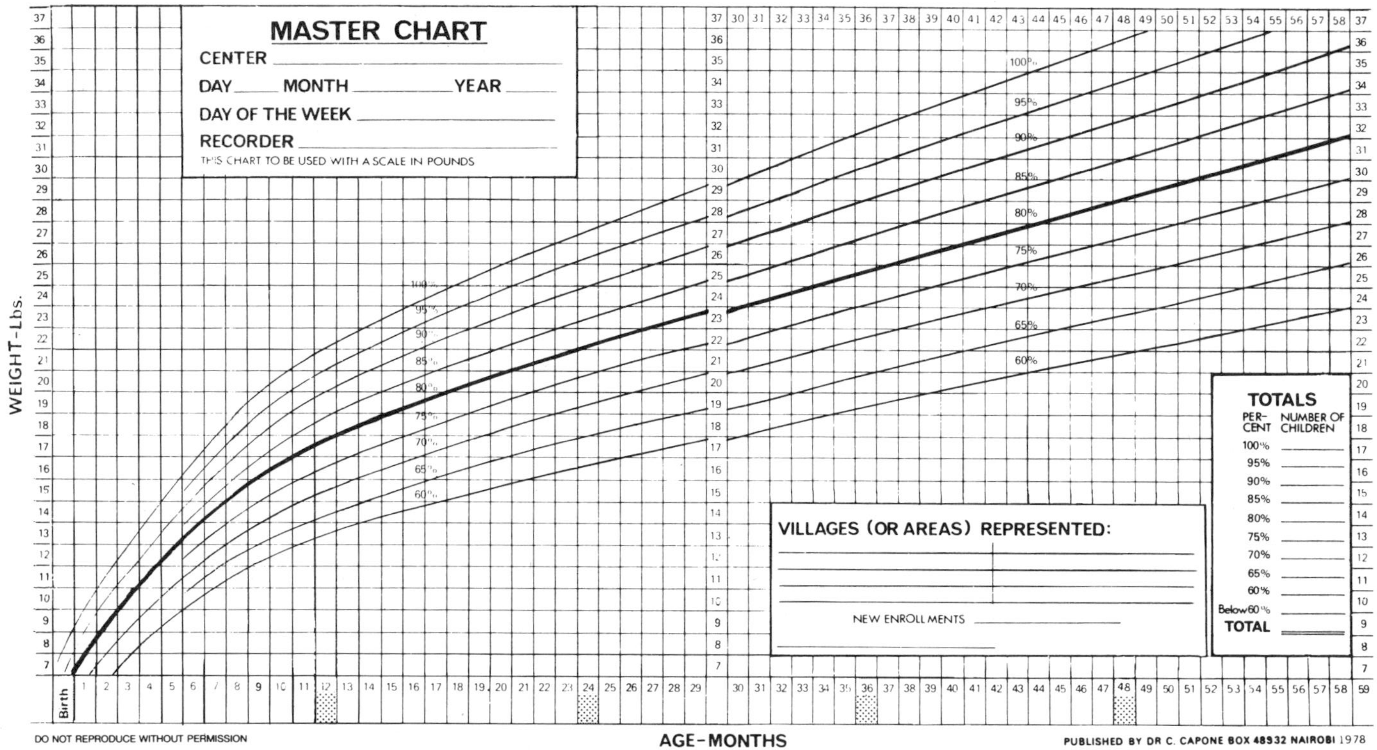

Fig. 5.28 Master chart, showing weight levels at 10 per cent intervals for use in collecting information from mothers attending clinic(s) or in an area. This could be simplified using reference (100 per cent), −2 SD (approximately 80 per cent), −3 SD (approximately 70 per cent), and −4 SD (approximately 60 per cent). (Courtesy of Dr C. Capone, Catholic Relief, Nairobi, Kenya.)

prepared with care. Both of these requirements can best be met if a simple, standardized system of training is adopted.

3. There are important savings in production costs if the records are simple and standardized. For example, duplication of time and effort is avoided.

4. In the future, the pooling of experience would be much more useful if identical systems of growth charting are used. Different workers' experience will be directly comparable.

Multi-line charts Many other types of growth charts have been used in various parts of the world. These can have four lines representing the Gómez classification of underweight (100 per cent, 90 per cent, 75 per cent, 60 per cent) of reference level (median), and are especially used in Latin America (Gómez *et al.* 1955). Some have three lines showing 100 per cent (50th centile), 80 per cent (3rd centile) and 60 per cent (Jelliffe 1966) (Fig. 5.29(a), (a)–(c)). Sometimes, such charts may have various colours indicating 'danger'. Red is often used for the 60 per cent-and-under level, but needs to be culturally appropriate, as in some societies other colours symbolize sickness and ill health — for example, yellow in Indonesia.

In areas where being overweight in infancy and early childhood can be a problem, an additional upper line can be added indicating +20 per cent (97th centile) for detection of children on the road to obesity. Such charts also vary with the amount of other information contained on them. Some contain what can be an overwhelming amount of verbal and visual nutrition educational information. Others include weight graphs showing both grams and pounds and ounces (which are too complicated), space for information on the timing and type of supplementary foods, immunization status, use of antimalarials, method(s) of family planning, local risk factors, 'developmental milestones', etc.

The advantages of charts showing percentage weight levels are that children can be immediately categorized based on weight-for-age (p. 122), while the percentage below 'standard' (reference level) appears to be understandable by primary health care workers (Segall 1979). The disadvantage is that the main importance of growth following the curve may not be emphasized enough, nor be so obvious. In most circumstances, a basic sexes-combined growth chart may be employed and retained by the mother.

Uncommonly, separate, more complex 'service charts' are also used, and can be made for both height and weight, separately for boys and girls. Usually, such charts have been used for research purposes. They use two measurements — weight and height — and require suitably trained staff to record and interpret the different levels achieved.

Single-line weight chart

In at least two countries, Zimbabwe and the Dominican Republic, a

(a)

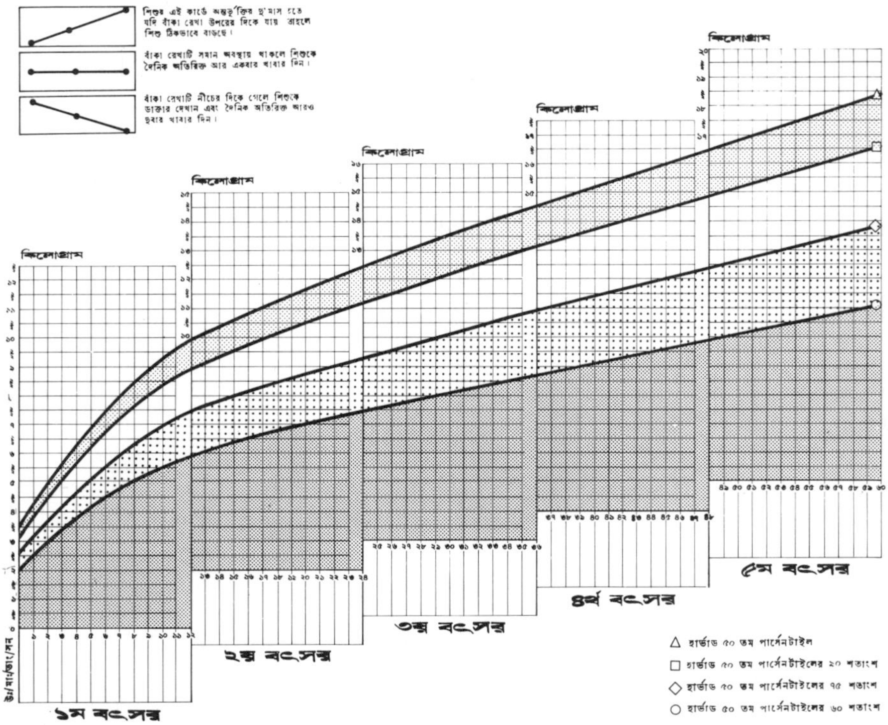

Fig. 5.29(a) Multi-line growth charts showing weight levels *below* reference level (80 and 60 per cent) from Burma. Designed for mothers to keep.

(b)

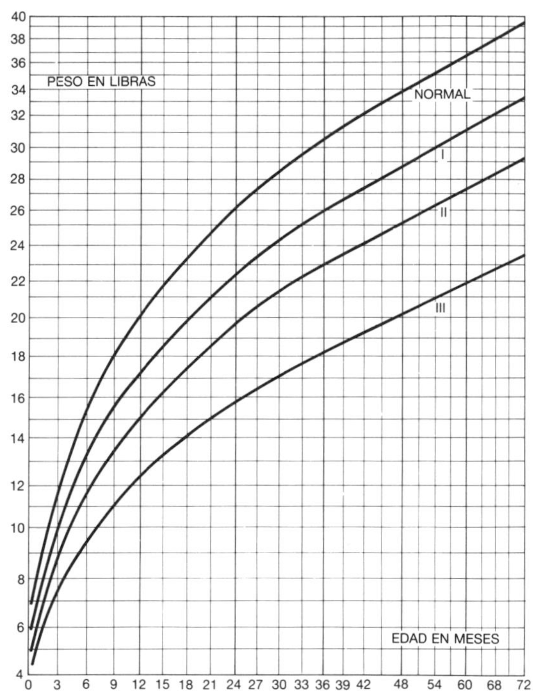

Fig. 5.29(b) Multi-line weight chart using the Gómez classification, indicating first, second, and third degrees (see text for explanation) (Hospital Infantíl, Mexico City).

(c)

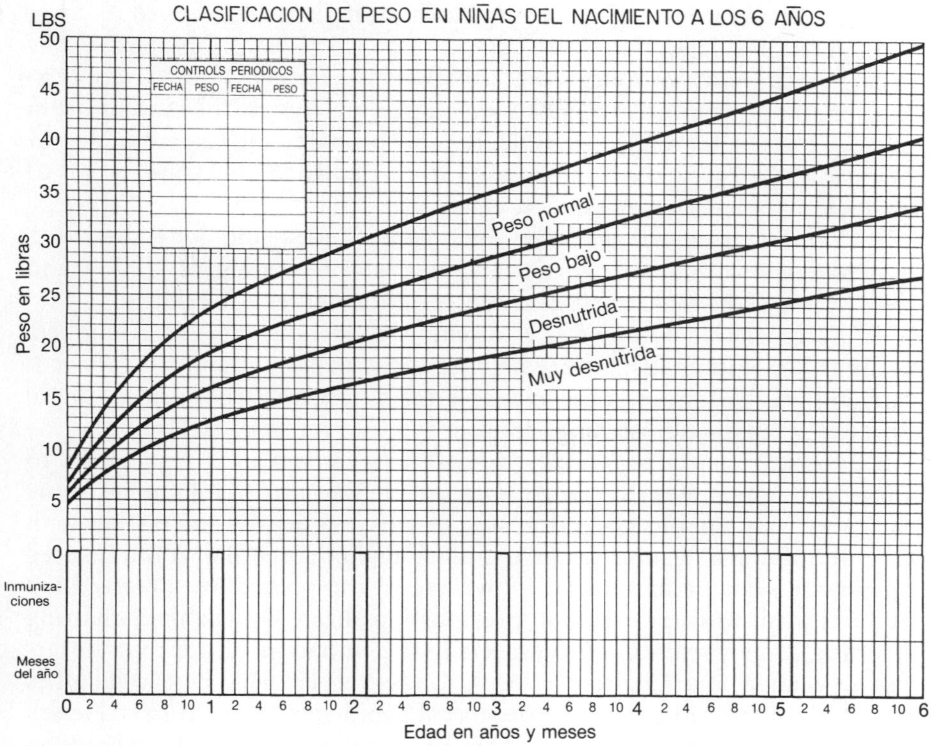

Fig. 5.29(c) Multi-line chart using the Gómez classification with added descriptive labels (*peso bajo* = low weight, etc.) (Colombia).

single-line weight chart has been employed. The line used is the 3rd centile NCHS level.

Recent controversy

In recent years, the practical usefulness, feasibility, and detailed design of growth charts has been questioned (Gopalan and Chatterjee 1985; Ghassemi 1985), at least as currently employed in primary health care services by community health workers (CHW), for the following reasons:

1. *More expensive than realized*: (a) Very limited national funds competed for by other ministries (e.g. trade, military, etc.); (b) public health service funds also competed for within health budget, and money for growth monitoring with other more clearly measurable public activities, such as immunization and oral rehydration; (c) cost of scales (including

repairs and replacements) and cards much more than appreciated to cover thousands of villages.[75]

2. *Educational limitations of community available health workers*: Marginally or semi-literate; not used to decimal system or reading from circular dial (Salter scale); 'graphic literacy' probably nil; uncertain degree of pictorial literacy concerning symbolism of 'Road to Health' type of concept or other information on chart.

3. *Variable support available*: Inadequate funds and long distances, limited inappropriately trained staff, etc., make training of CHWs and their supervision difficult. It also limits opportunities for referral.

4. *Large numbers of children*: Attempts to include very large numbers at appropriate intervals[76] overwhelm services, making monitoring inaccurate and greatly limiting time available for other activities, such as advice on diet, sympathetic listening, and appropriate referral, etc.

5. *Growth charts technically difficulty to understand.* This seems to vary from one part of the world to another. Recent careful studies show that relatively small-scale pilot studies are frequently successful, with careful training and supervision and much higher costs than could be used on a large scale or nationally. However, all the procedures involved are more difficult to carry out than previously realized — weighing, charting (plotting), interpretation, and especially the initiation of appropriate action (Gopalan and Chatterjee 1985; Ghassemi 1985). These difficulties have been increased greatly by the recent rapid spread of Primary Health Care (PHC) in many countries. This has entailed attempted coverage in greatly increased numbers by less trained, often less supervised staff.

6. *Difficulties with interpretation of details of growth chart.* This is not only for the educational and cultural reasons already mentioned, but also for technical and biological reasons — some of these are easily appreciated, but some are not. The latter include the following facts:

(a) Growth in normal children is not a smooth uninterrupted curve with *regular* gains in weight each month (Harrison 1984);
(b) 'Crossing of centiles', upwards or downwards is a normal occurrence in a significant percentage of normal well-nourished children (Davies and Williams 1983);
(c) Low-birth-weight babies who are small for gestational age (SGA) (especially chronic SGA) appear to have an inability to catch-up after birth, even if well-fed (Hofvander 1984);
(d) Deceleration of growth in the second 3 months of life is a normal

[75] With Salter scales at the 1988 UNICEF price (approx. US$30–35), the expenditure of over US$2 million would be needed to supply one to each of the 68 000 villages in Bangladesh.

[76] WHO (1986*e*) currently recommends monthly for the first year, 2 monthly for the second year, and 3 monthly for the third year.

variation, following the 'first trimester growth spurt' (Hitchcock and Gracey 1981; Whitehead *et al.* 1986; Stuff *et al.* 1987);

(e) Possible genetic differences in growth *patterns* (as has been noted in Hong Kong (Davies and Leung 1985).

7. *Detection of 'inadequate growth' difficult to define*, as opposed to 'no gain' or 'weight loss'.

8. *Action following detected growth failure is difficult to select and often not undertaken.* With multiple causes usually involved, selection of feasible, appropriate action can be difficult, especially for community health workers. This is made more so by having to try to deal with large numbers, and by an understandable (but overwhelming) tendency to include many other activities in the CHW duties, as indicated on the HBCR (Home-Based Child's Record). Training to assist in interpretation and action is much under consideration at the present time (Jelliffe and Jelliffe 1988*b*).

Needs

It is apparent that growth monitoring using weight charts as currently practised is undergoing a period of review at different levels, including international agencies. Fundamental questions to be answered include:

- What constitutes inadequate growth?
- How much over what period of time?
- How does this show itself on a growth chart?
- How are the main causes of any inadequate growth identified?
- What action needs to be taken? Where? How? By whom?
- What advice needs to be given to the mother?
- How can the success or otherwise of advice given be assessed?

Also, on a practical basis, the years to be covered on the chart, the frequency of weighing, the amount of educational material on the card, and the possibility of selective weighing (after initial screening by using the arm circumference) need consideration.

Improved practical training of community health workers is likely to be a major issue (Woodland and Kelly 1979; WHO 1985*a*; Jelliffe and Jelliffe 1988*b*), with emphasis not only on tasks, but also on the knowledge, attitudes, and skills needed for subtasks.

Cheaper, more appropriate scales (Burns 1986) (including the trial by WHO and UNICEF of the PATH solar-powered electronic digital read-out scale: estimated cost, US$15) *and* attempts to facilitate plotting as with the new TALC scale (cost US$5) (Morley, personal communication) also need testing (Fig. 5.30(a), (b)). Attempts are also being made to facilitate plotting on a weight graph. Examples include the 'Bubble chart'

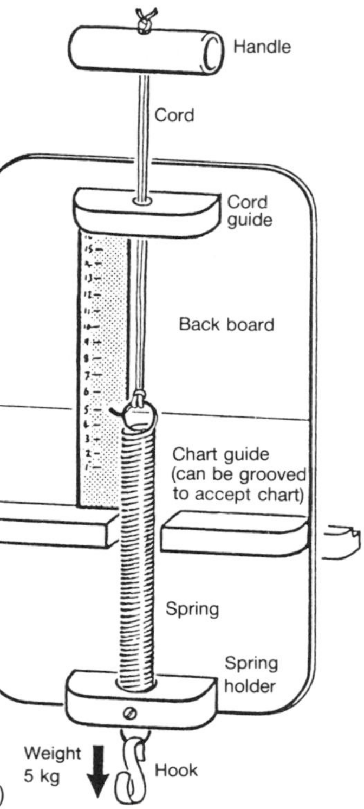

(a)

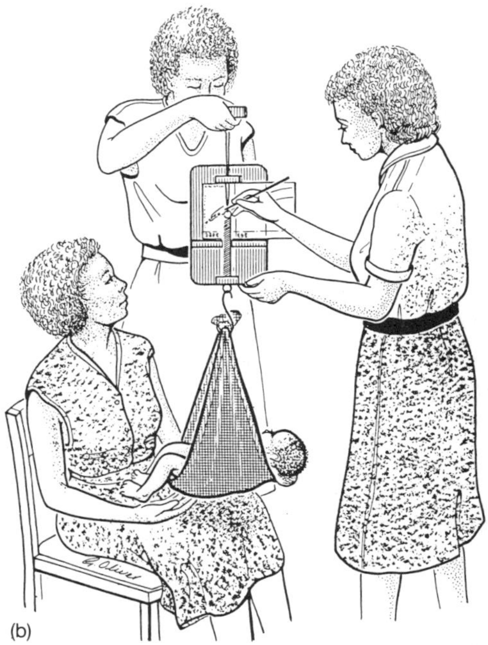

(b)

(c)

Name ______________ PHILIPPINE NUTRITION PROGRAM PROVINCE: ______________
Date of birth ______________ NUTRITION HEALTH CHART FOR BABIES MUNICIPALITY: ______________
BARANGAY: ______________

	MONTH	Birth month	1	2	3	4	5	6	7	8	9	10	11	12	13	14	15	16	17	18
	WEIGHT (kg)																			
	NUTRITION LEVEL	(PLOT MONTHLY WEIGHT IN CORRECT BLOCK TO DETERMINE NUTRITION LEVEL)																		
	1 healthy	3.1	3.8	4.5	5.1	5.7	6.2	6.7	7.1	7.6	8.0	8.3	8.6	8.9	9.1	9.3	9.5	9.7	9.9	10.1
MILDLY MALNOURISHED	2	2.9	3.8	4.2	4.8	5.4	5.9	6.3	6.7	7.1	7.6	7.8	8.2	8.4	8.6	8.8	9.0	9.2	9.4	9.5
	3	2.7	3.4	4.0	4.6	5.0	5.5	5.9	6.3	6.7	7.1	7.4	7.7	7.9	8.1	8.2	8.5	8.6	8.8	9.0
	4	2.6	3.2	3.8	4.3	4.7	5.2	5.6	5.9	6.3	6.7	6.9	7.2	7.4	7.6	7.7	8.0	8.1	8.2	8.4
MODERATELY MALNOURISHED	5	2.4	2.9	3.5	4.0	4.4	4.8	5.2	5.5	5.9	6.2	6.4	6.7	6.9	7.1	7.2	7.4	7.6	7.7	7.8
	6	2.2	2.7	3.2	3.7	4.1	4.5	4.8	5.1	5.5	5.8	6.0	6.2	6.4	6.6	6.7	6.9	7.0	7.2	7.3
	7	2.0	2.5	3.0	3.4	3.8	4.1	4.4	4.7	5.0	5.3	5.5	5.8	5.9	6.1	6.2	6.4	6.5	6.6	6.7
SEVERELY MALNOURISHED	8	1.9	2.3	2.8	3.1	3.5	3.8	4.1	4.3	4.6	4.9	5.1	5.3	5.4	5.6	5.7	5.8	5.9	6.1	6.2
	9	1.7	2.1	2.2	2.8	3.2	3.4	3.7	4.0	4.2	4.6	4.6	4.8	5.0	5.1	5.2	5.3	5.4	5.5	5.6
	10																			

Fig. 5.30 (a) TALC scale, showing individnal parts. (b) TALC scale in use, showing *direct plotting* on weight chart. (Details available from TALC, P.O. Box 49, St Albans, UK.) Further trials are needed in different ecologies and cultures. (c) Weight record using tabular form rather than chart. (Courtesy of Philippine Nutrition Program.)

(Griffiths 1986) and the 'Right-way Weight Plotter' (Jelliffe and Jelliffe 1989*b*).

From another point of view, the question of avoiding underappreciated cultural difficulties with graphic growth charts has been raised. For example, in the Philippines a non-graphic numerical chart or sequence of numbers has been introduced, which may be more easily filled in by community health workers (Fig. 5.30(c)). A similar method has been suggested as a 'growth action record' by Essex and Gosling (1987). However, this does not easily allow the 'curve' or slope of the child's growth to be visualized.

In some circumstances, growth monitoring by serial weighing may be impossible for one or more of the reasons given. If this is the case, various options are available, including 'targetting' those families or children 'at risk' or devising an arm band for illiterate community health workers with eight zones to enable approximates monitoring to be undertaken (Jelliffe and Jelliffe 1989*b*) to be made more precisely.

Height (length)

Measurements of composite skeletal, linear growth (stature) has become increasingly recognized as the most valuable cumulative *long-term indicator* of growth or its failure. Abnormal 'diminished' stature can be a reflection of chronically inadequate nutrition. However, unlike weight, the height is not a labile measurement and cannot *decrease* with malnutrition.

Supine length is usually measured with a length board up to the age of about 2–3 years, because of inability to stand with infants and understandable uncooperativeness in young children. After this or when the child can stand, the height is taken. The difference between height and length in an individual child can be 2 cm, so that the method used in obtaining reference data needs to be known.

Problems with measurements of stature include the surprising dearth of cheap, accurate, rugged apparatuses available commercially. Locally-made wooden length boards are usually required and, if carefully constructed, give accurate results (p. 82). Also, because the normal range of distribution of measurements of height is relatively small, accuracy is particularly important, but can be especially difficult to achieve in a frightened young child. Last, the interpretation of stature depends on knowing the precise age, which is a problem in many parts of the world.

Arm circumference

The midarm circumference was introduced as a public health index of protein–calorie malnutrition (now generally more commonly referred to as protein–energy malnutrition) in young children in a 1958 national survey in the Republic of Haiti, as was the basic formula: $c_2 = c_1 - \pi s$, for calculating the underlying muscle circumference (Jelliffe and Jelliffe 1960). The main reason for the trial of this measurement was that malnourished children have thin-to-wasted limbs, due to different degrees of depletion of both fat (calories) and muscle (protein). The arm was used because it is roughly circular, easily held (in a fractious child) and less likely to be affected by oedema than the lower limbs. Also, tape measures and arm bands are cheap, available, easily portable, and can be readily used by mobile community health workers. The non-dominant left arm is measured.

Since 1960, this measurement has been widely used in developing countries. A 23-author symposium outlining experience around the world was published in 1969 (Jelliffe and Jelliffe 1969). Numerous 'appropriate technology' devices (p. 361) have been suggested for approximate categorization of children in developing countries, including the Shakir strip (Shakir and Morley 1974), the '10-anna' bangle (Laugesen 1975), the *quipu* (Jelliffe and Jelliffe 1975), the MUAC-meter (Korte and Lambert 1975, personal communication), the insertion tape (Zerfas 1975, 1979), the four-colour arm band (Zeitlin *et al.* 1982), and the hand in the 'trained feel' (p. 95) (Morley 1979). Several of these have been tried in different parts of the world (p. 98), particularly the Shakir strip, which has been employed by village-workers and even by older siblings (in the CHILD-to-child programme) (Aarons *et al.* 1979).

The arm circumference — also termed the mid–upper arm circumference (MUAC or MAC) or arm girth — gives a rough composite gauge of stores of protein (muscle) and calories (subcutaneous fat). It correlates, approximately with changes in body weight in malnourished children (Buzina and Uemura 1974). Also, a low arm circumference has been shown to be a sensitive and specific indicator of risk of death in children in Bangladesh and Zaire (Briend *et al.* 1987). However, the usefulness of the arm circumference measurement depends on the purpose of the enquiry.

While reference data can be used for the appropriate year, the arm circumference has the advantage that there is little change from 1 to 4 years (12–59 months) (Fig. 5.31(a)) (Burgess and Burgess 1969), so that it can be used as a 'precise age-independent measurement' (p. 325) in communities where exact ages of children are unobtainable (p. 63). Alternatively, the arm circumference — a measurement of the labile tissues: muscle, and fat — can be correlated with skeletal measurements unaffected by recent malnutrition, such as the head circumference (Kanawati and McLaren 1970) or the height, using the QUAC (Quaker arm circumference) stick (Arnhold 1969; Lowenstein and Phillips 1973). As with many apparently new ideas, earlier, not easily accessible, literature

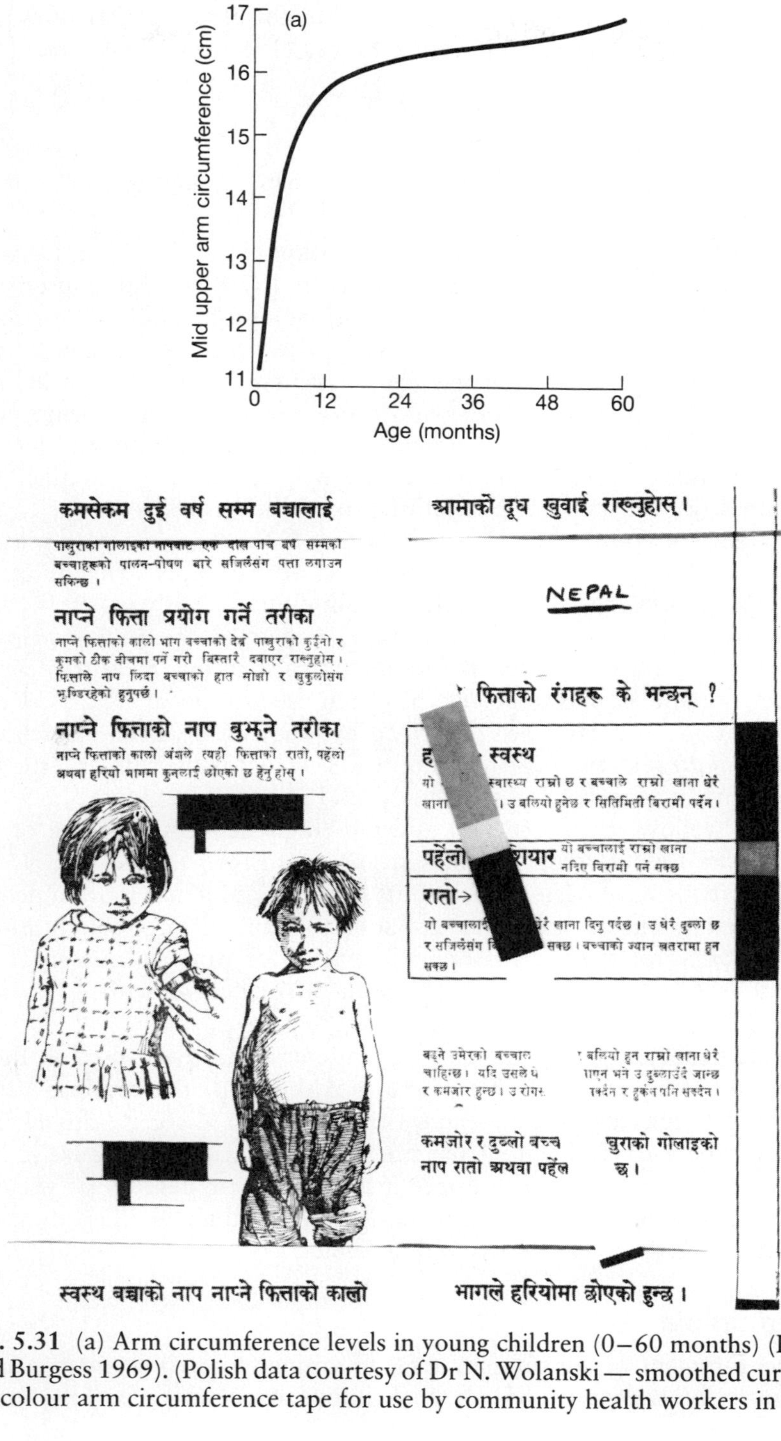

Fig. 5.31 (a) Arm circumference levels in young children (0–60 months) (Burgess and Burgess 1969). (Polish data courtesy of Dr N. Wolanski — smoothed curve.) (b) Tricolour arm circumference tape for use by community health workers in Nepal.

has indicated that others had previously thought along similar lines. For example, in the Indonesian literature, Klerks (1956) described the

$$\frac{\text{arm circumference}}{\text{height}}$$

(AC/H) index — termed by him as the 'ABC index' because of its simplicity.

Investigations in Iraq (Shakir 1979), in Colombia, Costa Rica, Dominican Republic, India, and Pakistan (Anderson 1979), in Fiji (Jansen and t'Mannetje 1982), in El Salvador (Trowbridge and Staehling 1980), and in Guatemala (Velbezoer *et al.* 1983*a*,*b*) used the arm circumference alone, with an age-constant reference to estimate nutritional status. All agreed that this index is as valid and more convenient in screening and surveillance than the arm circumference for age or the arm circumference for height index. Arm circumference growth charts are available, but rarely used (Zeitlin *et al.* 1982, Jelliffe and Jelliffe, 1989*b*).

Experience in young children suggests that it can be taken with reasonable accuracy at the *approximate* midpoint of the upper arm, or at the maximum circumference. This allows community health workers, with arm bands, such as the three-colour tape, known as the Shakir strip (p. 000), to categorize levels of arm circumference with one measurement. A practical example of this approach has been used in Nepal (Fig. 5.31(b)).

An ingenious arm tape was described by Voorhoeve (1983) which can categorize *both low and high* measurements — that is the thin and the fat. This has five colour bands: red (low), 12.5 cm; yellow (low), 13.5 cm; green line; yellow (high), 18 cm; and red (high), 19 cm. The use of the same colours for different extremes seems confusing.

Recent trends have been to record the arm circumference in millimetres. Also, different cut-off points seem advisable in various communities, possibly partly for genetic reasons and partly for practical purposes. In Bangladesh 11.0 cm (110 mm) has been advocated (Briend *et al.* and Zinicki 1985).

As noted earlier (p. 92), the calf circumference has been used in India (Visweswara Rao *et al.* 1978), where it was found, to correlate better with clinical signs of protein–energy malnutrition. Also, Zeitlin (1979) advocated the measurement of the mid-thigh, principally because it is a larger circumference than the upper arm, and lesser degrees of wasting give changes which will be more easily measurable. Neither of these alternatives seems to have been widely used.

Triceps fatfold

The measurement of subcutaneous fat in young children is most usually made over the triceps (p. 85). It gives information which parallels total body fat — that is, the subcutaneous layer and internal accumulations (e.g. omentum, perirenal, associated with muscle tissue, etc.). It is both a rough indicator of the body's depleted calorie reserves and is also needed for the calculation of underlying muscle circumference, area, and volume (p. 101).

However, it is the least used of the four main measurements. Observer measurement variation is much greater than with the other three, especially between different observers.

Fatfold measures require large-sized, expensive calipers originally designed for adults. There is a real need for 'appropriate technology' for the design of inexpensive, simple instruments to measure subcutaneous fat sufficiently accurately (p. 88) and to clarify results in terms of children's nutritional status. The recently developed cheap plastic fatfold calipers (p. 88), used in some countries, including the USA, for home self-assessment in weight control in adults, are in need of further trial in all age-groups, including young children in less technically developed countries.

Other difficulties with fatfold measures relate to genetic differences, demonstrated in schoolchildren of different ethnic groups (Eksmyr and Engsmer 1971), and the possible variation with fat compressibility at different ages which is unrelated to nutritional status. Also, the triceps fatfold can vary with the size of the underlying muscle, which, if relatively large, can be considered to 'stretch' the overlying subcutaneous fat.

Combined measurements

Based on the four measurements suggested, various combinations or ratios can be calculated, which either can give additional information concerning the quality or form of malnutrition present, or can provide 'precise age-independent' information, or both.

Weight-for-height

The relationship of body weight and height has long been recognized. Also, weight needs to be envisaged as three-dimensional, while height is unidmensional. For this reason, investigators have suggested various ratios which increase the mathematical 'power' of height. The earliest was the Quetelet Index: W/H^2 (Quetelet 1836), which was more recently supported by Cole (1979). This index correlated best with signs of protein–energy malnutrition in pre-school children in India (Visweswara Rao and Singh 1970). Dugdale (1971) suggested that for the pre-school age a ratio of $W/H^{1.6}$ be used.

For practical purposes, the World Health Organization recommended using the weight-for-height (W/H) for children (Keller *et al.* 1976), as being a simple, understandable approximation, which has already been used successfully in numerous field surveys.

Levels of weight-for-height have two special values in community assessment of protein–energy malnutrition in young children. First, as has been appreciated for some time, it is a method which can be employed when ages are not known.

Also, it is increasingly clear that underweight children are not a homogeneous group. Children can be underweight and undersized, based on reference data, but relatively proportional, active, and apparently well. These were often taken for younger than their true age, and termed 'nutritional dwarfs' or 'bonsai babies' (Downs 1964; Jelliffe 1959, 1966).

The classification by Waterlow (1972, 1973) clarified the situation. In this, young children are assessed by *both* weight and height. They can then be differentiated by weight-for-height and height-for-age into four categories:

Normal: above 90 per cent height/age,
above 80 per cent weight/height

Wasted: above 90 per cent height/age,
below 80 per cent weight/height

Stunted: below 90 per cent height/age,
above 80 per cent weight/height

Wasted and
stunted: below 90 per cent height/age,
below 80 per cent weight/height

The Waterlow classification can be visualized in a 2 × 2 diagram (Fig. 5.32). the clinical appearance of body size and proportions in various categories can be illustrated by silhouettes (Fig. 5.33). The differentiation arising from this system was well demonstrated by Mata (1978*a*), who contrasted the Gómez weight-for-age classification, used for decades especially in Latin America (Gómez *et al.* 1956), with the Waterlow classification (Fig. 5.34). In the illustration, both abnormal children would be considered Gómez state II, but have very different meanings when further analysed.

The categorization into stunted, wasted, and stunted and wasted is of practical significance. The *stunted (dwarfed) child* is usually the end-result of chronic, less severe, relatively 'balanced, inadequate nutrition' (Fig. 5.26). These children show relatively normal body proportions ('*bonsai* babies'), and on general inspection look younger than their actual age, except for their dental eruption. Such children are not such *immediate* public health priorities as wasted children and are not strongly associated with increased mortality in the near future. However, in several studies, a higher percentage of stunted children appeared to be at risk of developing severe clinical malnutrition than do normal children in the same commun-

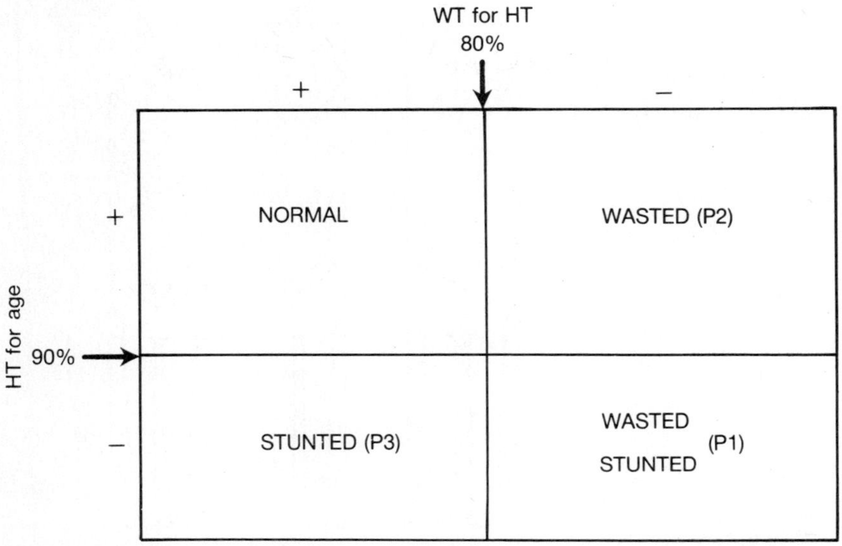

Fig. 5.32 Classification of protein–energy malnutrition based on weight, height, and age (2 × 2 diagram modified from Waterlow 1973). *Immediate* public health priorities: P1→P2→P3.

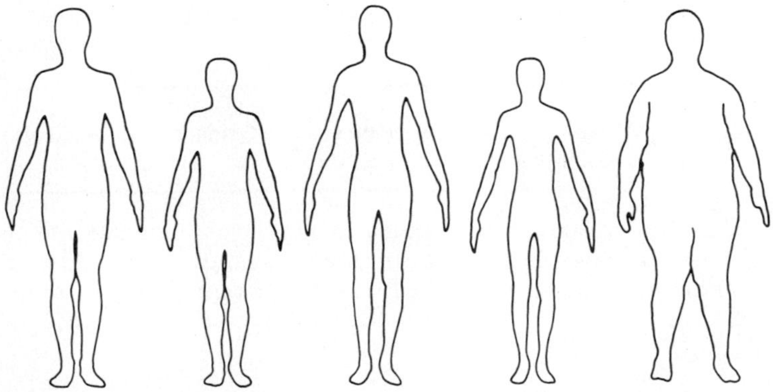

Descriptive Term	'Normal'	Stunted (Dwarfed)	Wasted	Stunted & Wasted	Obese
Wt/Age	100	<80	<80	<80	120
Ht/Age	100	<90	100	<90	100
Wt/Ht	100	100	<80	<80	120
Appearance	Proportional	Small, proportional, 'younger'	Thin limbs, large-seeming head.	Small, thin limbs, large-seeming head.	Fat limbs & abdomen

Fig. 5.33 Silhouettes and weight/height relationships in normal children of similar ages with the different forms of protein–energy malnutrition (stunted, wasted, stunted and wasted, obese). (Mata 1978*a*.)

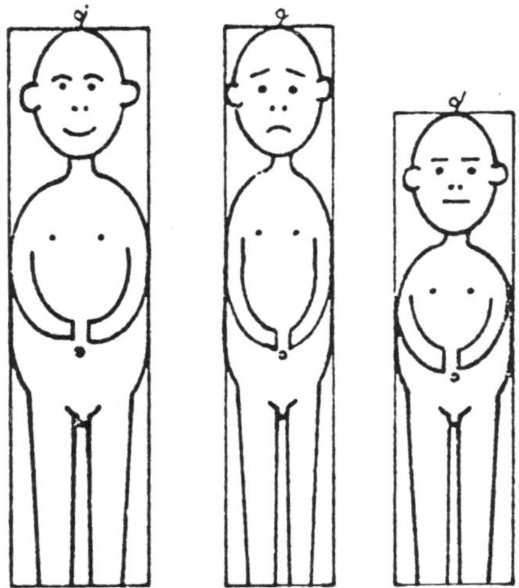

Wt/Age	100%	70%	70%
Ht/Age	100%	100%	<90%
Wt/Ht	100%	70%	100%
Waterlow Classification	Normal	Wasted	Stunted (Dwarfed)
Gómez Classification ([a])	Normal	Grade II	Grade II

Fig. 5.34 Interrelationships between weight, height, and age and comparisons of the Waterlow and Gómez classifications (adapted from Mata 1978). Gómez classification: weight/age: Grade I, 90–75 per cent; Grade II, < 75–60 per cent; Grade III, < 60 per cent.

ity (Scholl *et al.* 1979). Sufficient follow-ups of such stunted children have not yet been made to measure mental ability, as opposed to continuing stunted stature in subsequent adult life. Current views concerning the significance and prognosis of these children vary. One interpretation is that they may not reach their genetic growth potential, but will be otherwise little the worse for their small size ('adaptation'). Alternatively, Gopalan (1983) emphasizes that this view condones a continuing substandard damaged population as 'normal', who are 'maladapted' with permanent ill-effects and increased risks of mortality from infections (Gopalan 1987).

While this obviously does not have the *immediate* public health priority of more acutely malnourished children, emphasis on the differentiation of this form of protein–energy malnutrition is relatively new and further follow-up studies are needed. Certainly, the ultimate objective is for all children to achieve their genetic potential. Recent evidence suggests that the *small but healthy* classification of such children is not correct.*

The *wasted child* with more acute protein–energy malnutrition has a low weight-for-height, but relatively normal height (Fig. 5.25). On inspection, his body is thin, especially the limbs. If marked, the loss of subcutaneous fat and muscle also make the head appear to be large and the joints seem to be prominent. This type of child is in need of early attention. The body reserves of protein and calories are markedly depleted, so that there is a danger of the development of severe protein–energy malnutrition, either kwashiorkor or marasmus, especially if an infection occurs, which has an increased likehood.

The *wasted and stunted child* is suffering from acute malnutrition on a background of chronic malnutrition. Such children are not only small in stature, but also have thin limbs. They have the highest priority for urgent attention.

Comment While the Waterlow classification is to be recommended, there are three problems. First, two measurements have to be made needing two apparatuses. Second, two results have to be recorded and interpreted, with increased chances of error, cost and complexity. One of these — the length or height — needs careful attention if it is to be made accurately. The two pieces of equipment needed increase the cost of assessment. Third, the child's age has to be known.

Interpretation Reports of the analysis of the adequacy of weight-for-height can be undertaken with tables of different levels of sophistication (p. 441), which can be simplified for village use (Brown and Brown 1979*a*), with coloured zones fixed on to the clinic wall (Nabarro and McNab 1980) (p. 80), with nomograms showing weight and height (Dugdale 1971; Seaman 1978), or with electronic assistance, via an appropriate computer program (such as is available from WHO and the Center for Disease Control, Atlanta, Georgia), or using an inexpensive programmable calculator (Seaman 1978).

Difficulties often occur in knowing children's exact ages. It may be that more mothers in different parts of the world are becoming aware of the value to families of having this information available. At the same time, it seems likely that the majority of mothers in non-Western, largely rural cultures do not know the precise age of their children. It has little cultural

* This was the conclusion of a special symposium on '*Small but healthy*?' at the 1987 Annual Conference of the American Anthropological Association.

or practical significance. This means that the assessment of height-for-age is not possible. Under these circumstances, 'precise age-independent measurements', such as the weight-for-height or the midarm circumference (p. 325) can be employed.

Chest–head ratio

Classical paediatric teaching has emphasized that in well-nourished children the circumference of the chest usually becomes larger than that of the head after the first 6 months of life — and that this is certainly so by the second year. In children with protein–energy malnutrition, the chest seems thin, possibly mainly because of wasting or poor growth of the pectoral muscles and low levels of subcutaneous fat. By contrast, the head *seems* large. For this reason, a chest–head ratio of below one has been suggested (Jelliffe 1966) as a possible 'precise age-independent' method of rough assessment of less severe protein–energy malnutrition, requiring only a tape measure or even a piece of string. Unfortunately, subsequent tests of this approach have not found it to be sufficiently reliable or constant to be of value (Martorell *et al.* 1975).

Arm muscle measurements

From the measurements of the arm circumference and of the triceps fatfold it is possible to calculate the 'inner circle' (see earlier, Fig. 2.31) (p. 101) which is composed principally of muscle, with a small central core of bone. It is recognized that the bone is *relatively* constant in size, being only slightly affected by malnutrition in young children, and, in any case, not measurable without radiography.

The arm circumference itself is only an approximate gauge of nutritional status. Neither the arm nor the muscle mass are exactly circular; the underlying tissues include bone, nerves, muscles, fascia, etc., and the triceps fatfold is visibly much larger than the biceps fatfold.[77]

Also, muscle is a *three*-dimensional tissue. For this reason, a nomogram for arm muscle *area* was introduced (Gurney and Jelliffe 1973) (Appendix 3), which at least gave a *two*-dimensional measurement. More recently, a method expressing midarm muscle volume has been suggested (Jelliffe and Jelliffe 1979*b*). This is based on the fact that the main muscle mass in the upper arm overlies about one-fifth (20 per cent) of the length of the humerus, as judged by examination of soft tissue X-rays and study of modern tests on surface anatomy. Thus, the cylinder of midarm muscle volume can easily be calculated by multiplying the midarm muscle area (derived from the nomogram based on arm circumference and triceps fatfold) (Appendix 3) by one-fifth of the length of the humerus (mea-

[77] In some calculations, the *average* of the biceps and the triceps fatfold has been used (Fidanza 1975). This seems mathematically sound, but the triceps fatfold is more often employed by itself.

sured from the acromial process to the olecranon in the standard way) (p. 90). The result would only be an approximation, but could give comparable results between individuals and would reflect major muscle mass. The arm muscle circumference and area have been shown to parallel the increase in body muscle mass in children during recovery from severe protein–energy malnutrition (Reeds *et al.* 1978), as judged by laboratory tests.

Whether the additional measurements to calculate arm muscle area or volume are worthwhile is uncertain, as the amount of subcutaneous fat present in protein–energy malnutrition in young children is usually small. Further practical studies are indicated, including the devising of simplified reference data. (Also see: Addendum 1988.)

Arm calorie–protein measures

Attempts to use limb measurements to make composite or comparative estimations of fat and muscle date back some decades. In the 1920s, Von Pirquet developed the ingenious, complex, short-lived, composite 'Sacratama Index'[78] (which sought to assess *sa*nguis, *cra*ssitudo, *t*urgor, and *m*usculus) (Bigwood 1939).

Comparative muscle-fat areas can be calculated, as noted earlier (p. 505). Investigations in Guatemalan pre-school children showed energy reserves (subcutaneous fat) to be much more affected than muscle (Martorell *et al.* 1982).

Cuban investigators have devised the *E/P* (energy/protein) ratio based on the log transformation of the triceps fatfold and the arm muscle circumference (Amador *et al.* 1981, 1983).

Age considerations

Age assessment: General comments

Many persons living in technically less developed regions, mostly the tropics, do not know their exact age. Alternatively, they may employ a system of age classification or a calendar which differs from Western methods. This is understandable since precise age has little practical or cultural significance unless it has a recognized social value — for example, in relation to legal responsibility, admission to school, pension rights, etc. In some cultures, functional or physiological age-groups are recognized. These can include, for instance, 'big enough to be able to herd goats', or 'capable of carrying a younger sibling', or 'marriageable'.

In all cultures, transitions from one group to another are often recognized by special ceremonies and by the wearing of different clothes,

[78] Blood, fat, turgor (skin), muscle.

decorations, or hair style thereafter. These include initiation rites in some communities — for example, the elaborate ceremony and short-haircut carried out before a girl can enter the marriageable group among the San Blas Indians of Panama (Jelliffe and Jelliffe 1961).

For adults, all that may be useful is to consider the two sexes in broad age-groups — young adults, adults, elderly. However, differentiaton may sometimes be difficult in groups where the scalp hair is shaved, where there is no 'middle-aged' obesity, and where facial wrinkles may appear less prominent against a darker complexion, or, conversely, where women age rapidly with continuous child-bearing and too much hard physical work.

Estimating age

Knowledge of exact age becomes of greater importance in the anthropometry of young children, because of their rapid growth and because this is when the growth retardation associated with protein–energy malnutrition has its main incidence. When dealing with infants and preschool age children, ages should, ideally, be known to the month. For schoolchildren, assessment of ages to the nearest 6 months should be attempted.

Documentary evidence In field circumstances, age assessment in young children may be attempted in various ways. Uncommonly, documentary evidence may be available, including birth or baptism certificates, or, in some cultures, neonatal horoscopes. Careful prior enquiries need to be made and, wherever possible, the parents must be encouraged to make these important papers available.

However, in some developing countries, birth registration is likely to be delayed, leading to official ages which systematically underestimate the true ages (El Lozy 1976). Sometimes, the mother may not know the child's age, but may be able to recite the month of birth, and occasionally the day as well. If this is so, the mother will often recall details of the youngest child only, not those of the older siblings. If dates are known, they should be recorded as given and the ages calculated later.

In some communities, the period of the year in which the child was born can be recognized by the name given, e.g. 'born during millet harvesting', or as belonging to a certain ritual age-set; or there may be a local lunar calendar, as among the San Blas Indians of Panama, (e.g. iguana egg-laying moon, corn-sprouting moon, etc.) (Jelliffe and Jelliffe 1961). It may be possible to obtain information in relation to Muslim lunar months or other systems.

Local events calendar Often the only practicable method may be to construct a locally relevant calendar (Tukei 1963) based on events in the preceding years, including agricultural, climatic, and political and social occurrences (including festivals), as well as natural or man-made disasters (Table 5.14). However, such a calendar takes a long time to prepare and pre-test in the field, while its use in field circumstances is laborious, time-consuming, and most unsatisfactory with less sophisticated communities. Experience in Nigeria suggested that this approach is more accurate with regard to *months*, but that inaccuracies are more likely with years (Cobey and Cunningham 1968).

Calendars have to be specific for different communities. They have been tested out satisfactorily in Nigeria, in India (Pralhad Rao *et al.* 1973; Cobey and Cunningham 1968), in Afghanistan (Scanland 1976), in Tanzaniz (Burgess and Burgess 1975), and in the Congo (Brown and Brown 1979a). The calendar devised for Mweka in rural Zaire is simplified for local needs (Table 5.15). The calendar in Afghanistan was of special interest being based on local events (droughts, floods, etc.), national historical happenings and the 12-year cycle Chinese animal calendar also used in this country (Scanland 1976).

Deciduous dental eruption The eruption time of the 'milk teeth' varies somewhat from child to child. However, in *community studies*, it is sometimes possible to *categorize* young children into different rough age-groups.

Results of an international enquiry (Jelliffe and Jelliffe 1973) suggested that less severe degrees of protein–energy malnutrition usually had little delaying effect on primary dental eruption (Delgado *et al.* 1975). It appeared that the Bailey (1963*a*) formula — age (months) = 6 + number of erupted teeth[79] — could be useful for *roughly* grouping children in community studies into 'second dental year' (6–12 teeth) and 'first dental year' (less than 6 teeth) in areas, such as St. Vincent in the West Indies (Jelliffe and Jelliffe 1973). This approach can be of use, then, for such 'precise age-independent' measurements as arm circumference (p. 106), in which the general age category is all that is needed. Of course, the formula is of very little use for age assessment of individual children anywhere.

However, evidence has accumulated to suggest that *severe* protein–energy malnutrition does lead to delay in deciduous eruption, although with much less impact than on weight. This has been suggested by studies of hospitalized children in various countries, and possibly by a greater degree of retardation of dental eruption in more undernourished communities (Jelliffe and Jelliffe 1973) — for example, in Hyderabad, India (Visweswara Rao *et al.* 1973).

[79] Erupted with the crown of the tooth visible through the gums.

Table 5.14 Calendar for the assessment of young Buganda children (*Tukei 1963*)

Main events of the year	Rainy seasons	Month	Recalled seasonal or special events	Age on 31.12.1962 years	months
1959 Year of trade boycott (okubaliga ya kamya)		January	Beginning of New Year Picking and selling of cotton crop	4	
Queen Mother visited Uganda		February	Children go back to school End of cotton picking; selling continues Queen Mother visited Uganda	3	11
	Togo	March	Muslim Fast, ending with Id celebration *(okusiiba bya absiramu)*	3	10
	Rains	April	Easter (*paska*) celebrated White ants fly	3	9
		May	Early cotton planting	3	8
		June	Main cotton planting Weeding early cotton	3	7
		July	Main cotton weeding	3	6
		August	Main groundnut harvest	3	5
	Dumbi	September	Coffee picking	3	4
		October		3	3
	Rains	November	Kabaka's birthday	3	2
		December	Christmas *(Noeli)* End of year	3	1

1960 Year following the trade boycott		January	Beginning of New Year Picking and selling of cotton crop	3	
		February	Children go back to school End of cotton picking; selling continues	2	11
	Togo	March	Muslim Fast, ending with Id celebration *(okusiiba bya abasiramu)*	2	10
	Rains	April	Easter (*paska*) celebrated White ants fly	2	9
		May	Early cotton planting	2	8
		June	Main cotton planting Weeding early cotton	2	7
		July	Main cotton weeding	2	6
		August	Main groundnut harvest	2	5
		September	Coffee picking	2	4
	Dumbi	October		2	3
	Rains	November	Kabaka's birthday	2	2
		December	Christmas *(Noeli)* End of year	2	1
1961 Year when Buganda declared independence		January	Beginning of New Year Picking and selling of cotton crop Buganda declares Independence *(Okuwofeguwa Baganda)*	2	
Year when feasting for Kabaka's return from London Conference		February	Children go back to school End of cotton picking; selling continues	1	11

Table 5.14 (Continued)

Main events of the year	Rainy seasons	Month	Recalled seasonal or special events	Age on 31.12.1962	
		March	Muslim Fast, ending with Id celebration *(okusiiba bya abasiramu)*	1	10
Year of initial Congo refugees	*Togo*				
			Democratic Party win general elections, boycotted by Buganda		
Year which ended with bad floods closing many roads	Rains	April	Easter *(paska)* celebrated White ants fly	1	9
		May	Early cotton planting	1	8
		June	Main cotton planting Weeding early cotton	1	7
		July	Main cotton weeding	1	6
		August	Main groundnut harvest	1	5
	Dumbi	September	Coffee picking Very heavy rains and flooding of roads	1	4
	Rains	October	Kabaka went to first London Conference	1	3
		November	Kabaka's birthday General feasting for Kabaka's return from Conference	1	2
		December	Tanganyika became independent Christmas *(Noeli)* End of year	1	1

1962		January	Beginning of New Year Picking and selling of cotton crop	1	
The year Uganda became independent		February	Children go back to school End of cotton picking; selling continues		11
	Togo				
	Rains	March	Muslim Fast, ending with Id celebration *(okusiiba bya abasiramu)* Kabaka-Yekka won the Lukiiko elections		10
		April	Uganda People's Congress-Kabaka-Yekka won National Assembly elections Easter *(paska)* celebrated White ants fly		9
		May	Mr Obote succeeded Mr Kiwanuka as Prime Minister Early cotton planting		8
		June	Main cotton planting Weeding early cotton		7
		July	Main cotton weeding		5–6
		August	Main groundnut harvest		5–6
	Dumbi	September	Coffee picking		4
	Rains	October	Uganda became independent		3
		November	Kabaka's birthday		2
		December	Christmas *(Noeli)* End of year		1–0

Table 5.15 Abbreviated monthly calendar for age assessment (Mweka, Zaire). *(Courtesy of Drs J. and R. Brown)*

Mweka Calendar			
Jan.	Harvest maize and groundnuts Short dry season	Jul.	Dry season Cut forest for new fields Mango trees bloom
Feb.	Harvest groundnuts 2nd planting of maize	Aug.	Cut and burn forest Rains begin
Mar.	Harvest beans	Sept.	Plant maize, beans, groundnuts
Apr.	Harvest beans Eat flying ants	Oct.	Continue planting Eat ripe mangoes Flight of butterflies
May	Harvest beans and rice Rains end	Nov.	Eat ripe mangoes Gather and eat caterpillars
Jun.	Dry season Eat green maize Independence Day (30 June)	Dec.	Eat green maize Christmas (25 Dec.)

Stage of development The stage of psychomotor development by itself is usually of only partial value, as it is variable in healthy children, and particularly difficult to test in anxious children in the field. The picture may also be obscured by the muscle wasting and weakness characteristic of protein–energy malnutrition.

Family evidence The presence of older or younger siblings, or a pregnant mother, may provide further useful information in guiding age-assessment of the individual child. However, in some groups it is difficult for the passing observer in a prevalence survey to discover which children belong to which women. For example, among the Baganda, the sending of young children to stay with relatives is widely practised and, by local convention, the woman with whom they are staying may not like to admit that a particular child is not her own. A knowledge of children's ages is one of the advantages of long-term longitudinal studies and, on a more practical level, it usually will be known by community workers in primary health care services.

Combined methods A combination of a local calendar with other factors, such as dental eruption and physiological development, is often most useful (Brown and Brown 1979*a*). One use of this type of approach is summarized by Burgess and Burgess (1975):

A local calendar has been used successfully in Eastern Africa. The important thing is to list events which have a direct impact on the sampled population. The best way to use this calendar is to determine the stage of development of the child or fetus at a particular well-remembered local event (such as a typhoon or the visit of the president) and work back or forward from there.

The questioner must be familiar with the local idiom and also capable of cross-checking information and tallying it with a child's development, birth spacing, birth dates of children of friends, etc. This may need two people. After a little practice birth dates can be found quite quickly.

Example: Child born a few weeks after new road opened, the grass was burning, the mangoes were green and land ready for maize (mother remembers planting maize soon after baby was born). She thinks initiation ceremony was just over. Most likely birth date was September, 1969. Confirmed against another separately-assessed child born October, 1969 — matched dental eruption, height, and motor development.

Precise-age-independent anthropometry

Precise-age-independent anthropometry measurements for the nutritional assessment of young children are needed in many countries, of the world, where birth dates have little social significance and cannot be verified by documentations.

Measurements of this type may be of: (1) a tissue showing slight gradual change in the period under consideration, as, for example, the arm circumference during each year from 1 to 5 years of age (p. 309); or (2) ratio of a measurement of nutritionally labile tissues (muscle, fat) with a measurement of a tissue little affected by acute protein–energy malnutrition (e.g. skeletal bone).

In practice, the nutritionally labile tissues in protein–energy malnutrition are the protein and calorie stores — that is, skeletal muscle and subcutaneous fat, often assessed anthropometrically by arm measurments, including circumference (p. 91), the calculated muscle circumference (p. 10), the cross-sectional areas of subcutaneous fat and muscle (p. 505), or suggested by low or decreasing body mass (weight).

The most usual tissues selected as being less immediately affected are skeletal — height, head circumference, etc. An additional advantage is that these bony measurements are not affected negatively. They do not shrink in malnutrition.

Thus, the arm circumference (muscle, fat) has been compared with the height (skeletal bone), as in the arm circumference-for-height (Klerks 1956), or in the QUAC-stick method (Arnhold 1968; Bailey 1975) (p. 94), or with the head circumference, as described by Kanawati and McLaren (1970). As noted earlier (p. 80), the weight-for-height has become increasingly used as a practical precise-age-independent method for assessing protein–energy malnutrition (or obesity) at any age including young children, as well as for distinguishing 'stunted' from 'wasted'. However, in areas where ages are not known, weight-for-height *alone* will not differentiate the normal from the stunted (dwarfed), as for this the height-for-age is required (p. 312). In general, however, the *weight-for-height* and the *arm circumference* using an approximate 1–5-year mid-point standard (p. 94) are the most widely used precise-age-independent anthropometric measurements.

Selection of anthropometric measurements

Selection of the most useful of the basic four measurements — weight, height, arm circumference, and triceps fatfold, or combinations depends upon; (1) *epidemiological criteria*; (2) *biological significance*; (3) *practical considerations*; (4) *availability of verifiable age*; (5) *the target group*; and (6) *the purpose of the investigation.*

Epidemiological criteria

Selection has to be guided by epidemiological definitions of sensitivity, specificity, replicability, and other criteria given later (p. 508). This can add greater scientific precision and potential comparability between studies in different parts of the world (Appendix 4).

Biological significance

Different measurements reflect different changes in growth or body composition. For example, height is a non-labile indicator of cumulative skeletal growth during the child's life. The weight is a composite indicator of all body tissues, including bone, but with muscle and fat the most labile constituents in under- or overnutrition.

The arm circumference is an approximate, labile, composite indicator of body stores of calories (fat) and protein (muscle). It correlates well with body weight (or weight-for-height) because changes in weight are most usually due to increases or decreases in fat and muscle. However, the arm circumference does not give exactly the same information as body weight, because each measures different body components. This is one reason why a low arm circumference rate in a community is not the same as a low body weight rate.

The weight-for-height is mainly an indicator of labile body stores of fat and protein, in proportion to stature. Last, the triceps fatfold and calculated arm muscle circumference (or area or volume) are indicators of body stores of fat and protein respectively.

Practical considerations

The measurement used need to take into account their practicability in relation to cost, sturdiness, need for transportability of equipment, and simplicity for use, especially by trained auxiliaries or village workers in primary health care. Such measurements should be rapid, without causing anxiety, pain, or discomfort.

Availability of verifiable age

As noted earlier (p. 317), the measurements selected and their use will depend on the availability of verifiable age.

Target group

For use in early childhood, from birth to four years, anthropometric tests of nutritional status in early childhood have to be selected in relation to the age incidence of malnutrition, and its severity, chronicity, and aetiology (Habicht *et al.* 1979). For example, the arm circumference cannot be used as an age-independent indicator in areas where protein–energy malnutrition is found mainly in infancy, as the arm circumference normally increases rapidly in circumference in the early months of life.

Purpose of investigation

Anthropometric assessment can be undertaken for a wide range of different purposes. Scientifically, anthropometry may include multiple precise measurements of very carefully defined and selected samples of population to investigate patterns of growth in a particular ethnic group or to try to obtain locally appropriate 'reference data' (p. 110). Clinically, anthropometry usually focuses on the nutritional diagnosis of an individual and the response to treatment (p. 348). From a public health point of view, anthropometric nutritional assessment can be carried out for a variety of different purposes with differing objectives, including prevalence surveys, screening, surveillance, and evaluation of intervention programmes. In all such considerations, a key question is whether anthropometric measurements are made on a single occasion or serially (repeated at intervals).

The concept of *sequential anthropometry* is useful. In this, additional anthropometric measurements can be made as a sequence which gives increasing insight into the type and degree of protein–energy malnutrition or of obesity present, but with increasing cost in time and money for equipment. Thus, sequential anthropometry using all four of the common measurements is given in Table 5.16

In the public health use of anthropometry, Habicht (1979) rightly pointed out that various anthropometric indicators can have a wide variety of different functions imposed on them with a view to describing present, past, and future situations, and that there is:

> an unreasonable burden of expectations placed on these (nutritional) indicators. The same indicator, for instance arm circumference, is somehow thought to be of equal usefulness in calorie and in protein–calorie malnutrition (Bangladesh versus

Table 5.16 Diagnostic value of sequential anthropometry in protein–energy malnutrition in young children, when ages are known

	Indicators	Diagnostic value	Equipment considerations
Weight	Weight-for-age	Underweight children (mixed group)	One, simple measurement; weighing machine
Height	Weight and height for age	Differentiation of underweight (wasted and stunted)	Two measurements and more expensive equipment (length board)
Arm circumference*	Arm fat and muscle (combined)	Estimation of calorie and protein stores	Four measurements; two extra pieces of equipment (one cheap: tape; one expensive: fatfold calipers)
Triceps* fatfold	Calorie stores (fat)		

* Combination: estimation of calories and protein stores (fat and muscle areas) (see p. 505).

El Salvador), in acute and in chronic malnutrition [Nigerian civil war (QUAC stick) and El Salvador], and finally as a *reflection* of past or present nutrition as well as a *predictor* of undesirable nutritional outcomes in death or morbidity.

Reference data and presentation of results

NCHS reference data are given in this book in tabular form (Appendix 9) for weight, height, weight-for-height, arm circumference, and triceps fatfold. For young children, data for both sexes are combined.

As noted elsewhere, the weight and height data for young children probably will be appropriate for many ethnic groups, but not necessarily all. The procedure recommended if there is any doubt has been outlined earlier (p. 110). Greater uncertainty exists with regard to the widespread use of the NCHS reference data for arm circumference and triceps fatfold measurements. This is both for genetic reasons and because the NCHS population may have been over-fat, perhaps especially the adolescents and adults.

Results of investigations should be reported in tabular form in numbers and percentages of different measurements which are below or above the selected cut-off points, usually $\leq$ 2 SD (or $\geq$ 2 SD) or appropriate percentage levels of reference data, together with appropriate lower levels for more severe cases (see Appendix 9). Usually for young children, the data for boys and girls are combined. Reference data with both SD and corresponding percentage level cut-off points are given in Appendix 9. If separate results are needed for boys and girls, data for each sex for weight, height, and weight-for height, are available (WHO 1983a).

In addition, numbers and percentages of young children who are either stunted or wasted should be calculated in accordance with the Waterlow classification (p. 312).

Results are often presented in two age-groups — infants (0–11 months) and pre-school age children (12–59 months). If accurate age-assessment is possible, it is preferable to give findings by year. This indicates the time of maximal impact of malnutrition or risk period, and assists in suggesting practical preventive activities.

Anthropometric results also need combining with relevant clinical signs of protein–energy malnutrition, especially oedema. Other strongly suggestive clinical signs of the forms of nutritional deficiency (p. 493), ecological data, especially concerning food consumption (p. 198), and any biochemical findings (p. 496) should be given in relation to agreed-upon and clearly stated cut-off points.

It may also be possible to include information obtained from health services, including hospital admissions (numbers, 'case control' studies), out-patient attendances, and analysis of weight charts (indicating the number and percentage of children with inadequate growth, according to local definition).

Last, interpretation of the probable meaning of fingings should be attempted, together with suggestions concerning possible action (p. 449). However, despite current widespread use of anthropometry, Gopalan (1987) cautions against overreliance on body measurements alone:

> Data on the degree of growth retardation must be supplemented by other relevant data related to undernutrition, in order to enable us to arrive at judgements on the severity of undernutrition in an individual child or community.

In other words, as with all nutritional assessment, a 'navigational' approach or 'triangulation' is needed, with useful, but necessarily approximate, information from several sources being combined for corroboration.

School-age children and adolescents

> *'Thinness is the state of a person whose muscular flesh, not being filled out with fat, reveals the shapes and angles of his bony structure.*
>
> Brillat-Savarin (1755–1826)

Children of school-going age (usually 5–15 years) in any part of the world, including less technically developed regions, do not usually show significant signs or serious illness, still less mortality, from malnutrition. However, this can occur in disasters such as famines or with refugees (Fig. 5.35).

Individuals in this age-group have passed through the nutritionally dangerous years of early childhood. They are growing more slowly, and are able to compete for, and digest, the full range of the adult diet. In addition, in traditional rural areas, they may be able to supplement their diets with wild fruits, berries, insects, and small animals; in sophisticated urban areas, the influence of snacks and 'out-of-home' foods need consideration. Ordinarily, they will have achieved a substantial immunity against at least some of the more prevalent infections and parasites, including malaria. However, some infections of nutritional significance may persist — for example, hookworm or giardiasis (Loewenson *et al.* 1986).

On the other hand, schoolchildren in severely disadvantaged communities can show some signs of malnutrition, with occasional positive ('strongly suggestive') clinical signs (such as Bitôt's spots or mucosal pallor) (p. 23). They often have somewhat subnormal anthropometric measurements, such as stunting or a low weight-for-height and thin subcutaneous fat. Usually ill-effects are not severe enough to make them seek attention in the health services.

Nutritional inadequacy is particularly likely to occur when children walk long distances to school having had little, if any, breakfast, when no school meal is provided, and when assistance with physically demanding manual household chores, such as chopping wood or herding domestic animals, is expected of them when they return home in the evening. A general tiredness can, in fact, interfere with making the most of opportunities for learning at school.

In industrialized countries and the more wealthy, often Westernized minority in less technically developed countries, the emphasis may be partly on nutritional problems due to an overconsumption of calories in relation to energy output (obesity) and to a sticky sugary diet (dental caries). Conversely, problems related to self-imposed dietary restrictions in 'slimming regimens' (including anorexia nervosa and bulimia) or fad diets, to overreliance on processed foods of limited nutritional value or to teenage pregnancies need increasing consideration in some sophisticated groups.

School-age children should be included in any complete population sample examined in the course of a cross-sectional survey, or other family-based community nutritional investigation. In some circumstances, it can be useful to carry out a survey of schoolchildren alone. This can lead to the planning of a school health service, sometimes including a meal programme adapted to the local problems — nutritional, financial, and practical, if found necessary and feasible.

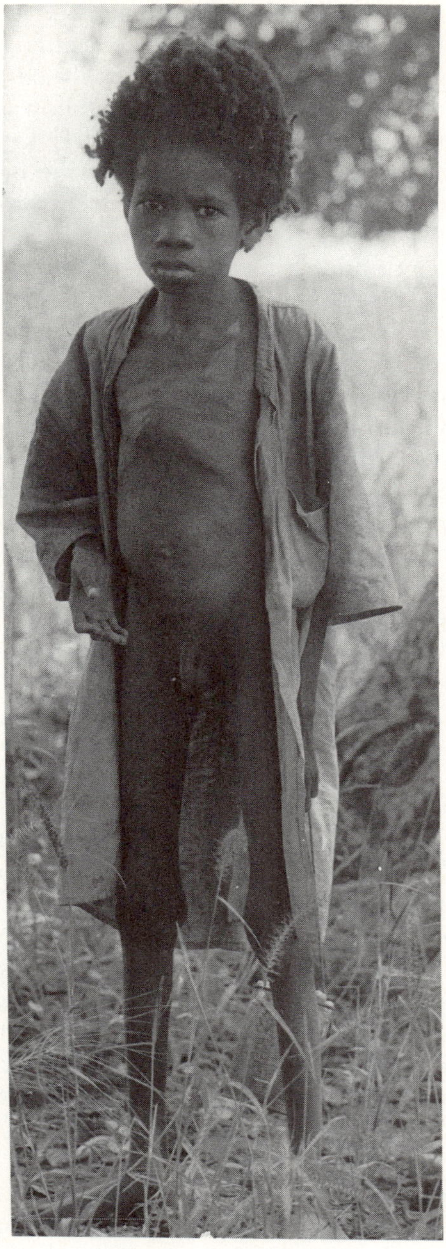

Fig. 5.35 Marasmus in school-age child, showing low weight-for-height and wasted subcutaneous fat and muscle during drought and famine in the Sahel in 1974. (Courtesy of WHO.)

A survey of schoolchildren offers the obvious advantage that the subjects are easily accessible at an existing collecting place, in buildings equipped with tables and chairs that can readily be adapted for examination purposes. Schoolchildren can also be followed longitudinally to assess growth. In fact, serial measurements of weight and height, undertaken by health worker or teacher, can usefully be included in a pupil's health record, when feasible. If such measurements are already available and are reasonably reliable, their analysis may yield valuable data. Obvious difficulties include adding to the teachers' already over-loaded schedule and the purchase of simple anthropometric equipment.

The disadvantages of this type of nutritional investigation survey are that it is directed at an age-group not markedly vulnerable nutritionally and which may not be representative of the school-age population as such. In many countries, often only a limited proportion of children will be attending school, with the remainder taking part in more traditional activities in the village, especially at times of high agricultural activity, such as harvesting, with somewhat different nutritional consequences. Results of such studies also need to be considered in relation to possible seasonal variation in food availability and to the nutritional consequences of absence from school for long holiday breaks.

Nutritional assessment

Direct assessment

Clinical signs (p. 13)

While varying in different parts of the world, some signs can occur in this age-group. All or, more usually, some of the following nutrition-related signs need to be looked for: Bitôt's spots; anaemia; angular cheilosis; dental mottling; caries; goitre; tropical ulcers; hepatomegaly; and splenomegaly. These signs are, of course, not all suggestive of nutritional deficiency as such, but include changes related to the diet itself (e.g. caries) and results of contributory or resultant infections (e.g. hepatosplenomegaly from past malaria; and tropical ulcers). Therapeutic scarification patterns may indicate treatment for previous illnesses in some cultures.

Anthropometry

That the physique of schoolchildren is related to environmental factors, including nutrition, is suggested, for example, by the improvement in the heights and weights of well-to-do Indian children in East Africa and Britain as compared with poorer children of the same genetic stock in India. Likewise, Bakwin and McLaughlin (1964) showed that the weights and heights of 'privileged' American schoolchildren in 1936 were matched by the measurements of children in the lower socio-economic groups in the same country in the early-1960s.

As with other age-groups, the basic measurements are weight and height. The arm circumference may be useful, especially as a screening procedure in emergency situations and, together with the triceps fatfold, to assess relative stores of protein and energy. Anderson (1975) employed the arm circumference related to height (employing locally-derived reference data) to classify children into 'normal' and 'below normal' in a school feeding programme involving over a million children in Sri Lanka.

Age assessment often presents problems in developing countries. Assistance may be available from records available from teachers and parents. Supportive evidence may be obtained from a local-events calendar (p. 318) and from the eruption of the permanent dentition. Ages should be determined as accurately as possible, at least to the nearest year.

Weight-for-height[80] has the advantage of being independent of knowledge of age, but canot detect children who are proportionally stunted ('nutritional dwarfs') (p. 312). However, interpretation of other measurements, including weight, height, arm circumference, and triceps fatfold, require the age to be known at least to the nearest year.

General reference data on the weight-for-height for each sex is given in (Appendix 9) (p. 524). The 'cut-off point' for an abnormally low weight-for-height ('wasted') is 80 per cent of reference level (approximately the 3rd centile or -2 SD below the median). Overweight is usually defined as 120 per cent of reference level (approximately the 97th centile or $+2$ SD above the median). When, as is usually the case, overweightt for height is due to obesity, subcutaneous fatfolds (p. 91) and the calculated percentage of body weight composed of fat will be increased.

As genetic variations in body size and shape become more marked after infancy and the 'pre-school age' period, local reference levels become more relevant and should also be used, if available. This has been suggested for schoolchildren in Thailand (Chavalittamrong *et al.* 1980), and needs consideration still more if several genetically very distinct ethnic groups are present in a country, as in Fiji, where the population is partly Melanesian and partly East Indian.

The height of school-age children is particularly useful, reflecting both inherent genetic factors and prior environmental influences, especially previous cumulative nutritional experiences. It has been termed an 'anamnestic indicator'.

As a community indicator, Bengoa *et al.* (1959), revived the earlier suggestion of Hundley and co-workers (1955) that height at a given age

[80] In India, a low W/H^2 has been suggested as the best age-independent indicator of undernutrition in children between 6 and 15 years (Babu and Chittani 1979), but this seems to represent an unnecessary refinement for general use.

in schoolchildren might serve as a suitable indicator of previous nutritional conditions in a population for the preceding years of life. This has been re-demonstrated recently in Panama (Parillon *et al.* 1987.) In particular, height at school entry can often be reasonably easy and convenient to collect. The height obtained would be expected to reflect a number of variables that influence early growth and development, and, as shown by secular trends, height appears to be a sensitive indicator. Bengoa also observed that height at 7 years of age correlates relatively well with indices of general socio-economic development. Prokopec (1977) compared the height of 7-year-old children in different parts of the world (Table 5.17).

The influence of the adolescent growth (height) spurt makes interpretation of growth changes very difficult at this phase of life, especially when comparing communities with different nutritional levels. The onset of puberty, especially as signalled by the clear-cut event of commencement of menstruation (menarche), is delayed by malnutrition. Conversely, the onset of menses is triggered in part by body weight, or possibly by body fat. In Papua–New Guinea, the latest recorded onset of menstruation anywhere in the world — 18–19 years — was noted by Malcolm (1970). For young females, the median age of menarche can itself be considered as an indicator of environmental influences, including the diet, level of physical work, and burden of infections. Secular trends in the USA and certain Western European countries have also shown a dramatically earlier onset of menarche in the past 100–150 years (Tanner 1962) to between 12–13 years in the early-1960s compared with the earliest record in Norway in 1840 of about 17 years. In practice, however, in developing countries the collection of information on the age of menarche is often difficult. Differing ages for the pre-pubertal growth spurt makes anthropometric data difficult to compare. For example, reference levels from early maturing American or European adolescents cannot necessarily be used for, say, less well nourished communities elsewhere in the world where the age of the pre-pubertal growth spurt and menarche occurs several years later.

In all parts of the world, adolescence can pose nutritional problems (Heald 1985). In more technically developed countries, 'fad' health-food diets and slimming diets (sometimes carried to dangerous limits as in anorexia nervosa or bulimia) can be compounded by increasing rates of early teenage pregnancy. Plainly, this is a nutritional hazard for girls, although, fortunately, the main pre-pubertal growth spurt occurs before the commencement of menstruation. Nutritional status can also be assessed in a school-age population by repeated measurements to test the rate of growth. This can be done with individual children or with groups. As growth is relatively slow, a fairly prolonged interval is needed between weighings to allow for a significant and measurable increase. The opti-

Table 5.17 Stature of 7-year-old boys in certain countries *(Prokopec 1977)*

Year of investigation or publication	Group	(cm)
1950	Norway	125.7
1951	USA	123.8
1947	Sweden	123.0
1960	Sofia	122.9
1947–1952	Murmańsk	122.7
1956	Poland	122.5
1960	Bulgaria (urban)	121.9
1956	Belgian Congo	121.9
1960	Holland	121.9
1958	Switzerland	121.5
1961	Czech distr.	121.5
1961	Estonia	121.1
1964	Bonn	121.0
1961	Bulgaria (rural)	120.8
1955	Toscana	120.7
1957	Bologna	120.4
1959	London	120.1
1956	Berlin E.G.	119.9
1965	Yugoslavia	119.8
1961	Slovakia	119.8
1950	France	118.6
1965	Rwanda Tutsi	116.9
1950	Rumania (urban)	116.0
1965	Rwanda Hutu	115.9
1950	Rumania (rural)	113.3
1960	India	112.5

mum time interval is 12 months, since this will also eliminate any possible effects of seasonal variations in growth due to diet, infections, climate, etc. (Robson 1964*a*).

Prior to the onset of the rapid growth of puberty, serial measurements can be employed to detect the adequate development of individual schoolchildren. To make the interpretation of measurements easier, Gurney

HEIGHT AND WEIGHT CHART ★

Name ______________________________ Date of Birth __________
(Last Name) (First Name) (M.I.) (Full Nan

Grade & Section											
Date when Ht. & Wt. Were Taken											
AGE** Years	6				7				8		
Months	1 2	3 4 5	6 7 8	9 10 11	1 2	3 4 5	6 7 8	9 10 11	1 2	3 4 5	6 7 8

NUTRITIONAL LEVELS												
HEIGHT	NORMAL	101.5	102.5	104.0	105.0	106.5	108.0	109.0	110.5	111.5	113.0	114.0
HEIGHT	UNDER-HEIGHT	101.0	102.0	103.5	104.5	106.0	107.5	108.5	110.0	111.0	112.5	113.5
WEIGHT	OVER-WEIGHT	20.8	21.1	21.4	22.1	22.7	23.3	23.9	24.5	25.2	25.7	26.4
WEIGHT	NORMAL	20.7	21.0	21.3	22.0	22.6	23.2	23.8	24.4	25.1	25.6	26.3
		17.0	17.3	17.6	18.1	18.6	19.1	19.6	20.1	20.6	21.1	21.6
WEIGHT — UNDERWEIGHT	MILD	16.9	17.2	17.5	18.0	18.5	19.0	19.5	20.0	20.5	21.0	21.5
		14.2	14.4	14.7	15.1	15.5	15.9	16.3	16.7	17.2	17.6	18.0
WEIGHT — UNDERWEIGHT	MOD-ERATE	14.1	14.3	14.6	15.0	15.4	15.8	16.2	16.6	17.1	17.5	17.9
		11.4	11.6	11.7	12.1	12.4	12.8	13.1	13.4	13.8	14.1	14.4
WEIGHT — UNDERWEIGHT	SE-VERE	11.3	11.5	11.6	12.0	12.3	12.7	13.0	13.3	13.7	14.0	14.3

*Based on FNRI studies **Age as of last birthdate

Fig. 5.36 Height and weight chart for school boys (Food and Nutrition Research Institute, Philippines). Separate charts available for girls: age range 6–14 years.

(1969) designed growth charts showing 'satisfactory', 'acceptable', and 'dangerous' height and weight line.

In the Philippines, the Food and Nutrition Research Institute has devised a tabular system for recording height and weight changes (Fig. 5.36).

As occurs in other age-groups, body fat stores are roughly gauged by the single measurement of the triceps fatfold (Appendix 9). Lower fatfold measurements have been found in apparently healthy schoolchildren in developing regions (Ferro-Luzzi 1962; Robson 1964*b*). This may be

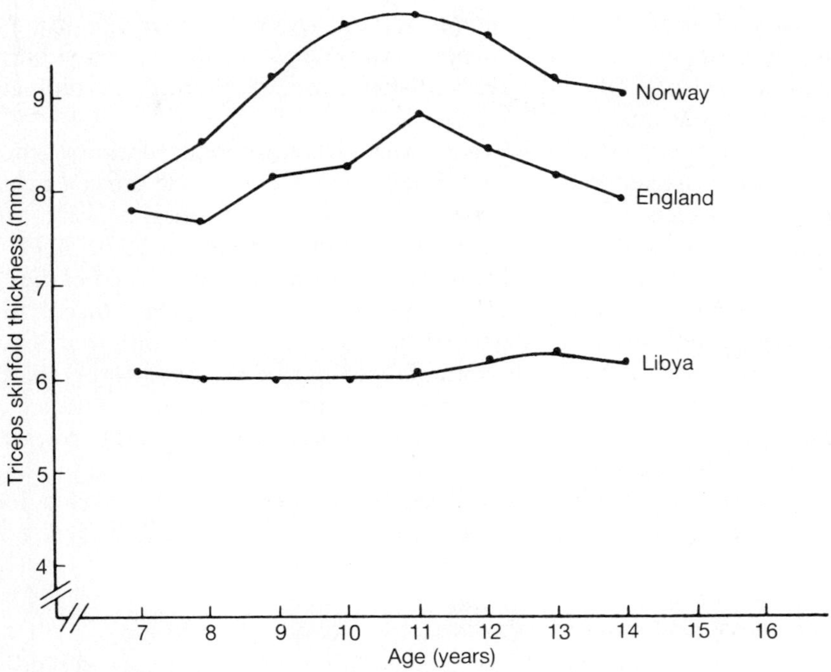

Fig. 5.37 Comparison of triceps fatfolds in children aged 7–14 years in Norway, England, and Libya (Andersen *et al.* 1978).

related to four interacting factors — a lower calorie intake, greater physical exercise, genetic variation, and perhaps an adaptation to a warmer climate, with a decreased need for insulating fat.

Genetic differences in subcutaneous fat distribution have been noted in Ethiopian compared with British school boys, in whom more subscapular fat was present than in the triceps area (Eksmyr and Engsner 1971). However, it seems probable that energy (calorie) intake and physical work are also responsible, as can be seen in comparative figures from triceps fatfolds from children 7–16 years old in Norway, England, and Libya (Andersen *et al.* 1978). The Libyan results remain the same throughout the period, with no fattening (Fig. 5.37).

In adolescents in Britain, Durnin and Rahaman (1967) have devised a formula based on the summing of four fatfolds — biceps, triceps, subscapular, and supra-iliac, which can give a crude estimate of fat as a percentage of body-weight, as an indicator of obesity. In the USA, Frerichs *et al.* (1979) have developed an equation derived from measurements of weight, height, and triceps fatfold which also estimates the percentage of the body weight composed of fat in children aged 10–14 years.

Selection of anthropometric reference data As with other age-groups, a range of different possible anthropometric reference data are available. As noted earlier (p. 110), all have statistical, methodological, or biological flaws or limitations.

To conform with the WHO recommendation, reference data for school-age children are as given for both sexes from the NCHS survey results, together with cut-off points. These include weight, height, weight-for-height, arm circumference, and triceps fatfold (Appendix 9, p. 524).

These data have various advantages and disadvantages noted earlier (p. 110). The NCHS study population included some obese children. Also, differing ages of onset of menstruation and actual genetic differences need to be taken into account. The data should not be assumed to be valid in non-Caucasian communities without testing their local relevance by measurement of a least 200 school-age children from a suitable referance group, usually the socio-economic elite.

For school-age children, it will usually be preferable to develop local reference data, if the NCHS levels are plainly not relevant, as will often be the case.

Biochemical and biophysical tests

Examination of the blood for haemoglobin concentrations should be included and, in less technically developed countries, stool examinations for ova and a thick blood film for malaria, may be undertaken if considered relevant for the particular community. In addition, various biochemical tests may be carried out on a sample of children to investigate known or probable local problems (p. 405). Although usually not relevant, dark-adaptation tests for vitamin A deficiency (p. 52) or dynamometry to assess muscle strength (p. 51) have been included in community studies for research purposes.

Adults

> *Tall is beautiful? Tallness is generally considered healthy, handsome, and desirable and it is indeed statistically correlated with intelligence, success, and social class (in 'Western' societies). In the United States, bishops are 4.5 cm taller than rural ministers, and presidents of major universities 2.5 cm taller than those of small colleges, in Scotland there is a 5.3 cm difference between upper and lowest social classes.*
>
> Barnes (1983)

This quotation probably indicates that those with a more privileged childhood and better nutrition grow nearer to their genetic potential. Also, in some parts of the world, there may be a subconscious bias towards selecting taller individuals for some types of responsible positions.

Special considerations

Growth cessation

In adulthood, most growth usually ceases at various ages usually at about 19 to 21 years. After this, the only physiological changes in body dimensions are those that result from ageing (if these can be termed physiological) or from muscular hypertrophy due to constant physical exercise. Nevertheless, selected anthropometric measurements in adults are useful in assessing past or present protein–energy malnutrition, or overnutrition from an excessive intake of calories (obesity). They can also be repeated in a community in successive generations, to reveal a positive or negative secular trend — that is, a change occuring over a number of years.

Biological variation

As emphasized in the monumental review by Eveleth and Tanner (1976), it is in adults that genetic biological differences in body proportions are most marked. This has been long recognized by physical anthropologists who have used some measurments for tracing past migrations of different groups (El Nofely 1978). For this reason, very great care needs to be taken before using reference levels from one part of the world for a genetically quite distinct community. For adults, there is a particular need for locally derived reference data, as evidenced, for example, in the demonstrated inapplicability of US reference levels for individuals in Northern Nigeria (Harries *et al.* 1985). This key issue has been elaborated elsewhere in this book.

Differing nutrient needs

Adult male and female nutrient needs differ, mainly in relation to body size, but also with higher calcium needs and iron requirements for menstruating women and for other nutrients in pregnancy and lactation (p. 226). The nutrient requirements of the elderly include a lower energy intake and probably somewhat higher levels of some nutrients, such as folic acid. Females after the menopause need less iron than previously.

Methods of assessment

Investigations to assess the nutritional status of adults often use a combination of methods previously described, including clinical signs (p.

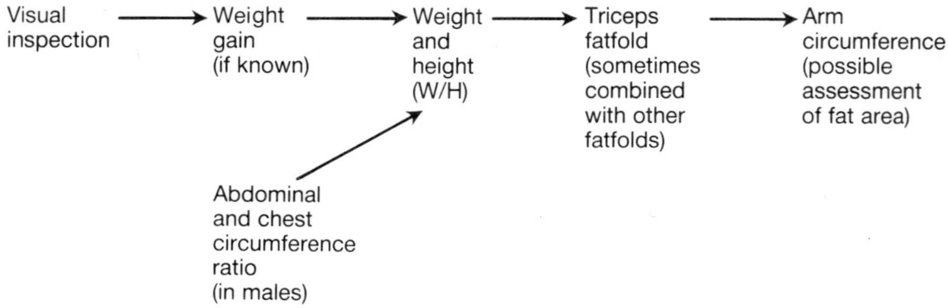

Fig. 5.38 Sequential anthropometry in obesity.

14), assessment of ecological factors (especially economic influences (p. 142) and estimates of dietary intake (p. 187)), haemoglobin (together with carefully selected laboratory tests (p. 14) for a subsample, if and when indicated, especially for nutrients likely to be deficient such as folic acid and vitamins C and B_{12}). As with other age-groups, anthropometric measurements are the most practical and economical. Routinely, these measurements include the weight and height, preferably associated with a measurement of the triceps fatfold and sometimes the arm circumference. Jointly, these give a useful guide to the general state of protein–calorie nutrition of adults. In both under- (p. 109) and over-nutrition (Fig. 5.38), *sequential anthropometry* is a useful concept and a logical, practical approach. Such a sequence is outlined in Fig. 5.38 for the investigation of obesity, which is the leading nutritional problem in adults in more technically developed countries (Powers 1980).

Reference data: general

Suggested reference data for haematological tests (p. 48) and laboratory examinations (p. 469) are given elsewhere. General difficulties with the selection of all anthropometric reference levels have also been considered earlier (p. 110), notably the need for genetically appropriate data, whenever possible. This is especially so for adults. The most usual method is to measure the weight and height, to check this with reference levels considered within the 'desirable' range of weight-for-height-for-sex and to express the result as a 'relative body weight'.

Weight-for-height levels are usually given for each sex for '25 years and over', because it is currently considered that the increase in weight in middle age commonly seen in well-fed communities is probably undesirable from the viewpoint of health and ageing. However, increases in weight-for-height level do not take into account the *components* making up the body weight (e.g. muscle, bone, oedema, fat, etc.), or the type of body build or frame (skeletal width). Nevertheless, in practice, increased weight-for-height in adulthood is usually mainly due to excess, partly visible, body fat. Overweight due to other causes, such as oedema or increased muscle bulk (as in weight-lifters or body-builders), is usually obvious on history, inspection, or clinical examination. More deceptively, a 'normal' weight-for-height in middle-age commonly can occur in 'creeping obesity', where muscle weight is replaced by fat weight. In the present publication, reference data are given from two sources — NCHS (1984) and Society of Actuaries (1959).

An attempt to classify body build into 'large', 'medium', and 'small' frame-sizes was made by the Society of Actuaries (1959), but has been used very little in practice because of difficulties in defining frame-size. Currently unavailable measures of laterality or breadth would be needed. As a practical approach, the elbow breadth has been suggested (Lindner and Lindner 1973; Frisancho and Flagel 1982), but needs further testing.

Selection of anthropometric reference data

Previously used weight-for-height reference levels (Jelliffe 1966) were derived from 'desirable' levels calculated by the US Society of Actuaries on the basis of a large-scale survey of body build, blood pressure, and other factors affecting longevity (Society of Actuaries 1959). The figures have been adjusted for people of average frame measured. Various problems with these figures have been discussed earlier (p. 110).

Currently, several sets of reference data are available for weight-for-height-for-sex from various countries. In the USA, there are at least four, including the Society of Actuaries (1980). All of these refer to recent American data and are mainly concerned with the detection of obesity and its later associated conditions, such as diabetes, hypertension, coronary heart disease, and life-expectancy. All are imperfect.

Considerable controversy has developed as to the significance of the heavier US males and lighter-weight females in 1980 compared with 1959, and levels below and above that are abnormal. Differences in life-styles and ideal cultural body-image need consideration. The decline in tuberculosis and the rise in incidence of cigarette smoking are also considered to affect the number of underweight individuals in different ways.

In view of the lack of consensus, the reference data given (Appendix 9) for adult males and females for weight-for-height, arm circumference, and triceps fatfold are those given by Frisancho (1981, 1984) for individuals considered to be of medium frame size. The main reasons for this selection are: (1) the data are from the same (or similar) population as the NCHS figures used for children; and (2) all measurements (weight, height, arm circumference, triceps fatfolds) are from the same population.

Again, *caution is needed*, especially with the arm circumference and fatfold data, as it is likely that this population includes many individuals who are unduly fat. To remove the concept of 'ideal', 'optimal', or 'desirable', median levels given in Appendix 9 are only labelled as 'reference', with cut-off points below and above.

For non-Caucasian groups, locally relevant reference data will be needed for the genetic group concerned, whether this be a country or larger region.

Expressing anthropometric measurements

Because height is a linear measurement and weight reflects a three-dimensional measurement of body volume, numerous ratios of weight to height^2, height^3, etc., have been suggested over the past 100 years. Two of the earliest seem to have been the *index ponderalis* (Livi 1897), quoted, by Bigwood 1939),[81] W/H (Bigwood 1939),[81] and Quetelet index W/H^2 (Quételet 1836). More recently, (as a revival of Quetelet's index) the body mass index W/H^2 (Bray 1978) has been suggested. Last, Abraham *et al.* (1975*b*) calculated the 'optimal power function of height in relation to weight' and suggested W/H^2 for men and $W/H^{1.3}$ in women. In practice, either the weight-for-height or the body mass index (W/H^2) are most commonly used for adults.

Measurement of total amount of body fat, including subcutaneous abdominal, peri-renal, etc., can be undertaken by a variety of sophisticated laboratory techniques (p. 56). Usually, the triceps fatfold is used alone (p. 89), or combined with the subscapular measurement (p. 89) Sometimes, fatfolds from other sites, particularly the biceps and supra-iliac, are summed with the triceps and subscapular measurements (Durnin and Rahaman 1967).

The midarm circumference (p. 91) has been used mainly in the detection of protein–energy malnutrition in young children. Previously quoted reference data for adults (Jelliffe 1966) were obtained from the only information that appeared to be available at that time. Frisancho (1974) published the results of arm circumference and triceps fatfolds from adult males and females in the United States (Appendix 9). Combining the triceps fatfolds and the arm circumference, Bray (1978) suggested the 'adipomuscular ratio'

$$(\text{AMR}) = \frac{\text{fatfold thickness}}{\text{arm circumference}}.$$

[81] In the League of Nations publication, Bigwood (1939) lists 12 somatometric indices suggested by various European workers in the 1920s and 30s. They do not seem to have been tested scientifically.

However, as stressed earlier, anthropometic data in adults should, if possible, be compared mainly with local genetically appropriate reference data, only using general reference data for comparative purposes, when required. Reference levels for weight-for-height, subcutaneous fatfolds, and arm circumference given in Appendix 9 are based on fairly recent measurements made on large samples of apparently healthy, well-fed (and possibly over-fed) American adults. They may neither be optimal nor genetically appropriate for some other groups. Discussion of the difficulties of selecting the most useful reference levels for any age-group has been given elsewhere (p. 110).

Malnutrition in the general population

With the exception of pregnant and lactating women (whose situation is considered elsewhere) (p. 226), adults are usually the least vulnerable segment of a population in so far as severe undernutrition is concerned. Only in such extreme situations as famines are the severe syndromes of protein–energy malnutrition (p. 272) — marasmus and kwashiorkor — seen. By contrast, in relatively well-fed communities, adults, especially women, often show high rates of obesity (p. 345).

In general medical practice, nutritional assessment needs greater attention, particularly a brief dietary history and the weight and height measurements (Margen 1979). Weight needs to be measured in minimal clothing on a frequently checked scale by someone who is aware of the test's importance. Last, the weight (and height) need interpreting in comparison with reference data (Appendix 9) (p. 524) and general inspection, taking into account genetic variation.

Protein–energy malnutrition

The clinical picture and anthropometric changes in adult protein–energy malnutrition vary with its duration (whether brief, prolonged, chronic, or lifelong), the degree of deprivation, associated deficiences (e.g. vitamin B complex), and the presence of complicating infections. Malnutrition may also be seasonal, as in the endemic, recurring decreased body weight and even occurrence of oedema seen in some regions during particularly severe 'hungry seasons'.

Investigations have been undertaken of extreme cases of protein–energy malnutrition seen in starvation during famines, in World War II volunteer experiments (Keys *et al.* 1950), in prolonged siege conditions (e.g. the Jewish ghetto in Warsaw in 1940) (Winick 1979), and among victims of concentration camps. All have shown severe weight loss with no alteration in height, save for that produced by stooping, presumably partly related to muscle wasting. Very low body weights, more than 50 per cent below the original level, have been observed in occasional extreme instances, and must, in fact, have been still lower, as water retention is a well-recognized feature, even in the absence of oedema. The skin in such circumstances is loose and inelastic. Muscle and fat wasting are strikingly obvious, and demonstrable quantitatively by the decrease in limb measurements, including the arm circumference. The head and the bony prominences appear to be enlarged because of the disappearance of muscle and fat 'padding'. The general appearance is that of a person 20 or 30 years older than the real chronological age.

In extreme food shortage, a clinical picture similar to that of kwashiorkor may occur occasionally in adults, including oedema, light-coloured hair, and skin. In famines, for example, kwashiorkor has been noted particularly in pregnant women and the elderly.

In severe protein–energy malnutrition in adults, the commonest clinical picture, with the exception of the 'famine oedema' of advanced cases, is identical with that of marasmus (inanition) in young children, including even the 'little old man' face. In view of the lack of a clinical label for this type of severe protein–energy malnutrition in adults — the use of the same generic term, adult 'marasmus' appears appropriate.

Examples of severe adult marasmus are not common, except in famines and similar disasters. However, in some developing countries less advanced protein–calorie malnutrition occurs among adults, particularly during the 'hungry season'. This is especially so among women and results from continuous nutritional maternal depletion from the drain of too frequent reproductive cycles of pregnancy and 'prolonged' lactation, commencing in their own girlhood and often made worse by restrictive and cultural attitudes and heavy physical labour.

A low body weight-for-height may be related to a number of factors, such as a light bone structure or a 'small body frame'. For practical purposes, however, it is principally a reflection of body thinness due to subnormal amounts of subcutaneous fat and muscle, the result either of poor development, or tissue wasting, or a combination of the two. Correction may be necessary to account for oedema, ascites, or even for grossly enlarged viscera (e.g. hepatomegaly), if present. A body weight-for-height of $<$ 80 per cent of reference level (median) can be labelled 'moderately severely malnourished'. Conversely, 120 per cent and above can be labelled 'overweight'. The rationale for the selection of these 'cut-off' points is given elsewhere (p. 122).

Calorie reserves are indicated by thickness of subcutaneous fat, usually measured, for convenience, at the triceps skinfold (or fatfold) site, for reasons discussed elsewhere (p. 89). Protein inadequacy is indicated clinically by thin musculature, due either to poor development or to wasting or both.

The arm circumference is a simple measurement and can be used to indicate both protein and calorie reserves (p. 91). In the USA, Ohlson *et al.* (1956) found a close correlation between arm circumference and underweight in Michigan adults. Apart from pregnant women (p. 236), this measurement has not been much used in nutritional assessment work among adults in developing regions, although it has been employed in New Guinea (Bailey 1963*b*).

However, nutritional 'categorization', using the arm circumference has also received attention recently in India, where Tibrewala and Shah (1978) used a coloured tape for women, similar to that devised for young children (p. 94). The levels they selected were > 22.7 cm, 22.7–20 cm, and < 20 cm. Again, genetically appropriate levels need to be determined and used.

Arm muscle circumference may be calculated from the arm circumference and the triceps fatfold measurements (p. 89), as can the muscle and/or fat areas and/or volumes in the upper arm (p. 101). The arm circumference and the calculated arm muscle circumference have begun to be used in the nutritional assessment of sick, in sophisticated hospital circumstances.

Recently, considerable effort has been given to trying to assess the immediate functional effects of malnutrition, especially protein–energy malnutrition and anaemia, on work capacity or productivity (Latham *et al.* 1982). This is discussed briefly elsewhere (p. 50), but obviously such investigations are very difficult to undertake and interpret, especially related to the degree of positive (or negative) motivation.

Obesity

Over-fatness (obesity), mainly associated with an excessive calorie intake in relation to energy output is widespread in adults (and children) in more privileged populations anywhere in the world. However, it affects a very small proportion of well-to-do persons in poorer technically less developed countries, but is on the increase among the privileged. The main cause is over-eating. This results mainly from easy accessibility to foods, especially high-calorie fats, sugar, and alcohol, together with insufficient physical work and exercise. 'Reactive overeating' may also be precipitated by general anxiety and stress. In some communities, such as in some West Indian countries, an obesity of 'relative poverty' is common in poorer women, who may be compensating for their unsatisfactory circumstances by eating excessively.

In some countries, obesity is culturally desired. In women, this can be a mark of beauty, for example, among the Zulus (Abramson *et al.* 1961). In either sex, it can be a symbol of wealth and prestige, as in the rulers of ancient Hawaii (Jelliffe and Jelliffe 1964) or modern Tonga.

In most societies, increasing fatness occurs with age. The optimal level at different age ranges is difficult to state with certainty. Indeed, this could vary, not only with cultural concept of beauty and ideal body-image, but also with life-styles. An abundant fat layer undoubtedly constitutes a vital store in societies with an annual 'hungry season'.

Overweight, as distinct from obesity, is defined in relation to reference data, such as those given in Appendix 9, or to tables of so-called 'desirable weight' which are usually prepared from insurance company information (Bray 1978). It is fair to say that obese people are usually overweight, but that not all overweight people are obese.

Obesity (over-fatness) needs differentiating from overweight. As noted earlier, increased weight-for-height-for-sex can be due to a large frame-size, to muscle bulk, etc. In fact, it is most usually due to obesity and is easily recognizable on inspection. This is especially so with increasing weight, although *very* rapid weight gain suggest water retention (subclinical or clinical oedema). The body mass index (W/H^2) has tended to be used as a more refined measure of overweight, and therefore, in most cases can be taken as a more sophisticated gauge of obesity.

Degrees of 'overweight' are most usually expressed in two ways:

1. *Relative weight*, which is the ratio of actual to desirable weight, expressed as percentages. These data can be derived from appropriate Tables (Appendix 9). Overweight can be defined as a weight-for-height measurement of $\geq$ 120 per cent of reference.

2. *Body mass index*. A second approach uses various ratios of height and weight, of which body mass index (Quetelet index) is the most widely used. This index is the weight (kg) divided by height (metres) squared (W/H^2) and can be obtained from Bray's nomogram (1978). Overweight is defined as a body mass index above 30. The correlation coefficient of body mass with other techniques for measuring body fat ranges between 0.7 and 0.8 (Bray 1978). The difficulty with weight-for-height measurements, as noted elsewhere (p. 79), is that they do not usually take into account the type of body frame nor abnormal muscularity.

Frank obesity is usually obvious on inspection, except in early creeping or 'replacement' fatness of sedentary middle-age. The chest/abdomen circumference ratio has been suggested for use in surveys for male subjects (Welham and Behnke 1942).

Bray (1978) gives the most succinct account of the assessment of obesity:

> By definition, obesity exists when fat makes up a greater than 'normal' fraction of total body weight. In males aged 18, approximately 15–18 per cent of body weight is fat, and for females 20–25 per cent. There is normally a gradual increase in the percentage of fat with age, but this may not be necessary or desirable. Obesity in women might be defined as body fat content greater than 30 per cent of total body weight; for males a comparable definition would be a body

fat greater than 25 per cent of total body weight (Bray 1978). Measurement of body fat requires sophisticated techniques which are not widely available. These techniques include measurements of body density, determination of fat or water by isotopic or chemical dilution, and the measurement of the naturally occurring isotope of potassium (K^{40}).

Assessment of body fat directly rather than by body weight can be made using fatfold calipers (p. 86). Subcutaneous fat thickness is relatively independent of height, so that a single level for each sex can be established above which obesity is suggested. Measurement of subcutaneous fatfolds is always difficult, with much potential for observer error, especially in the very obese. The most representative body site is in dispute (Bray 1978). However, the triceps fatfold is usually measured, largely because of its accessibility and convenience. As an approximation, obesity is probably present if this fatfold exceeds 15 mm in males and 25 mm in women. More detailed reference data are given in Appendix 9.

Various summations of different fatfolds have been suggested at various times (p. 91). None give identical results. None take into account variation in internal fat in the abdomen and in other sites.

Particularly in weight loss in obesity during dietary treatment, Bray (1978) prefers decreasing circumferences, in especially the abdomen and arm, rather than measurement of fatfolds.

As a combination of fatfold and circumference, Bray (1978) has suggested an 'adiposomuscular ratio'

$$\text{AMR} = \frac{\text{skinfold thickness}}{\text{arm circumference}} .$$

The biceps AMR in adult males is ≤ 0.21 and in women ≤ 0.48. Figures for the femoral AMR are ≤ 0.19 (males) and ≤ 0.63 (females).

In other circumstances, the body's 'lean body mass' (LBM) may be of more concern. Predictive equations have been given by Fuchs *et al.* (1978). In the latter, a minimum lean body mass (24 per cent) was needed in young adults males for acceptance into the US Air Force.

Recently, body composition, actually fat and lean body mass plus bone, have been assessed by electrical impedance (p. 85).

Vascular atheroma and diabetes

The interpretation of serum cholesterol is difficult, even though methods for comparing data from observers employing different techniques have been established. Concentrations can be raised or lowered in a short period by diets high in animal fat without reflecting the presence or absence of any associated atheromatous deposits in the coronary arteries. Also, the endogenous production of cholesterol by the body increases difficulties in interpretation. However, on these premises and subject to the reservation that the incidence of atheroma in a population has to be related to various aspects of the whole way of life, the probability of adults having a high rate of atheroma is greater if serum cholesterol concentrations levels are 'high' (250 ± 30 mg/dl) rather than low (120 ± 30 mg/dl) (US Department of Health and Human Services 1985). Other biochemical tests are indicated in special studies.

As regards coronary heart disease and other forms of atheroma, studies will usually include estimations of serum cholesterol and electrocardiographic tracings, sometimes taken in surveys from a sample of the population with a portable machine from persons between 40 and 60 years of age. Other nutritional or diet-related 'degenerative diseases' may need to be sought for in the assessment of communities or individuals. To screen for diabetes, urine examinations for sugar with easily transportable, chemically impregnated paper test-strips can be included.

Results have to be correlated with height, weight, and blood pressure determinations, taken by standardized methods, community surveys, the incidence figures of coronary thrombosis and diabetes cases in the area, as well as hospital autopsy findings from adult hearts.

Dental caries

This is also a condition with multiple causes, including a low fluoride content in the drinking water, genetic susceptibility, nutritional status, oral hygiene, and especially the oral effect of the diet itself. In particular, studies based on methods of geographical pathology have disclosed, among different peoples, a considerable incidence in groups whose diet is high in refined sticky sugars and flours, as distinct from communities subsisting on unprocessed animal and vegetable foods containing little free sugar and considerable cellulose fibre and roughage.

Caries is currently still a major problem in technically developed parts of the world, although it appears to be diminishing. By contrast, it is increasingly prevalent in children and adults in Third World countries, mainly because of dietary changes so often associated with urbanization and the cultural modifications it entails.

Caries should receive attention in general nutrition surveys, at least to the extent of determining its prevalence. The procedures recommended by the WHO Expert Committee on Dental Health (1962) and Wilson *et al.* (1964) are guides to more intensive, specialized community surveys.

Nutrition in sick adults

The question of inadequate diet and nutrition in hospitals in industrialized countries has been recognized intermittently for 40 years (Platt *et al.* 1963). However, only in the last 10 years or so have usually 'subclinical', poorly nourished chronically ill patients been recognized as occurring commonly on admission to hospital and/or during the course of their stay. Because of this increase, emphasis has begun to be given to the nutritional assessment and support of patients in hospitals.

This important re-emphasis needs to include consideration of *all* patients. Nevertheless, it will be focused on major conditions associated with nutritional deterioration from anorexia, depression, metabolic loss, diarrhoea, vomiting, complications of therapy, etc. These include, for example, patients with extensive burns, receiving radiotherapy, ulcerative colitis, malignant disease, etc., for whom nutrition is a major therapeutic weapon. In such cases, hyperalimentation (intragastric feeding with mixtures of nutrients, such as amino acids, etc.) or parenteral nutrition (intravenous feeding with mixtures of amino acids, fat emulsion, etc.) can be literally life-saving in appropriate cases.

Increasingly, nutrition support services are being developed at many larger hospitals in the USA, Britain, and elsewhere. Such services are excellent in that they draw attention to practical nutrition in general — still almost completely neglected in medical and nursing curricula, and to nutrition as a major and scientifically respectable aspect of prevention and therapy. These services also have the advantage of drawing together different disciplines in hospitals in a nutrition support committeee, including for example, surgeons, radiotherapists, dieticians, biochemists, nurses, gastroenterologists, etc. A disadvantage of this otherwise valuable 'movement' is that 'technological feeding', hyperalimentation, and total parenteral nutrition will be used excessively and when not actually needed, in part persuaded by the pharmaceutical companies concerned with the manufacture of these formulations. While life-saving in appropriate patients, the cost of this form of feeding is considerable and the dangers of using prolonged perfusion in major vessels, such as the external jugular vein, are significant. These dangers include sepsis and metabolic ill-consequences, some of which are still in the process of being identified, such as various mineral imbalances.

Various schedules for 'nutritional and metabolic assessment' can be undertaken for initial and sequential use in hospitalized cases. Such assessments can include varying combinations: *anthropometry* — weight, height, arm circumference, triceps fatfold, calculated arm muscle circumference; *haematological* — haemoglobin, lymphocyte count; *biochemical* — *blood* — total iron-binding capacity, transferrin albumin; *urine* — urea, creatinine; and *cellular immunity* — skin tests. In addition, estimations of pre-albumin, retinol-binding protein, mineral concentrations (e.g. zinc, magnesium, etc.) and tests for vitamin A, C, and folate may be included (Blackburn *et al.* 1977; Shenkin and Steele 1978). Enquiries concerning previous and present *dietary intake* should always be included as well as use of medications, which may result in drug–nutrient interactions.

Various similar regimens have been described (Kaminski and Jeejeebhoy 1979; Kaminski and Ruggiero 1979; Beck 1979). This approach to hospitalized sick individuals has been based on what has been termed their 'Anergic Metabolic Profile'. This is considered to include assessment of *'somatic protein component'* (weight-for-height, triceps fatfold, arm muscle circumference, creatinine-height index (p. 498), *'visceral protein component'* (serum albumin, transferrin, etc.), and *'cell-mediated immunity'* (total lymphocyte count, skin tests for 'common recall antigens', such as streptokinase–streptodornase (SK/SD), mumps, candida, and purified protein derivative) (Kaminski and Ruggiero 1979) (Fig. 5.39).

A logical sequence would seem to be: dietary history and recent medical history (especially weight loss) → inexpensive anthropometry → further expensive biochemical and immological tests, *if indicated.*

Nutritional monitoring of this type then needs to be used selectively with serial measurements, although the relative usefulness of each of these procedures in assessing nutritional status varies with the length of time over which measurements are envisaged (Shenkin and Steele 1978).

The Journal of Human Nutrition (1979) summarized current views as follows:

> Ideally, the patient's notes should contain a nutritional assessment data sheet that would bring together in one place all the relevant information. It would be the place for recording parameters such as height, weight, skinfold thickness, mid-upper arm circumference, and creatinine-height index, and it would include observations relevant to the assessment of energy requirements — bedridden/ambulatory, obese/cachectic — and a careful assessment of dietary intake before and/or during hospitalization as appropriate. It would also include information on diagnosis, treatment, and drug therapy that might influence nutritional status or nutritional requirements, as a summary of results of biochemical tests.
>
> The nutritional support programme would be planned and instituted on the basis of this collected information, and its success monitored by repeated measurements of relevant parameters at regular intervals. Continuous monitoring would highlight the need for flexibility in nutritional support, both in nutrient content and in the form in which it is provided. Monitoring the actual quantity of food eaten by the patient — as opposed to the quantity prescribed or served — would, for example, emphasize the important of food viscosity or consistency in the feeding of the very ill.

The advantage of nutritional assessment in hospital circumstances in a major centre in an industrialized country is that laboratory facilities are easily available and timed samples can be obtained (e.g. 24–48-hour urine specimens for creatinine excretion). Also, the functional significance of tests or measurements can be appraised, in relation, for example, to mortality and prognosis (Harvey *et al.* 1979; Donaldson and Lenon 1979), or to scientifically specialized techniques such as ultrasonics, or X-ray tomography of the arm to judge the area of muscle tissue directly

ANERGIC METABOLIC PROFILE

PATIENT ____________ ROOM ________ DATE ________

	PARAMETERS	VALUE	DEFICIT: SEVERE	MOD	MILD	ADEQUATE
	SOMATIC PROTEINS					
MARASMUS	WEIGHT/HEIGHT					
MARASMUS	TRICEP SKINFOLD (mm)					
MARASMUS	ARM MUSCLE CIRCUMFERENCE (cm)					
MARASMUS	CREATININE/ HEIGHT INDEX					
	VISCERAL PROTEINS					
KWASHIORKOR	ALBUMIN					
KWASHIORKOR	TRANSFERRIN					
KWASHIORKOR	TOTAL LYMPHOCYTE COUNT					
	CELL-MEDIATED IMMUNITY					

NITROGEN IN (g/day) ________

NITROGEN OUT (g/day) − ________

NITROGEN BALANCE (g/day) ________

NUTRITIONAL STATUS	**DEGREE**
□ ADEQUATE	□ NONE
□ MARASMUS	□ MILD
□ KWASHIORKOR	□ MODERATE
□ MARASMUS KWASHIORKOR MIX	□ SEVERE

STANDARDS	SEVERE	MODERATE	MILD
SOMATIC PROTEINS—% DEFICIT	>30%	>15–30%	>5–15%
ALBUMIN (g/dl)	<2.5	<3.0–2.5	<3.5–3.0
TRANSFERRIN (mg/dl)	<160	<180–160	<200–180
LYMPHOCYTE COUNT (No./mm^3)	<900	<1500–900	<1800–1500
CELL-MEDIATED IMMUNITY (mm)	<5–0	<10–5	<15–10

Fig. 5.39 'Anergic metabolic profile' suggested for selected hospitalized patients (Kaminski and Ruggiero 1979).

(Heymsfield *et al.* 1982). The scope of such procedures can include not only levels of nutrition, but also a rough appraisal of host resistance to infection as well.

Some of the methods used for assesment of hospitalized patients in Western countries have been adopted from techniques tried out in developing countries for years, or even decades — without an understanding or awareness of the debates, old and recent, concerning their usage, values, and limitations in developing countries. Also, terminology which is well-defined in nutrition in Third World countries is sometimes used with somewhat different meaning. Examples include categorizing 'marasmus' as protein–calorie malnutrition and 'kwashiorkor' as protein malnutrition (Blackburn *et al.* 1977). In addition, new terms are being used which are unfamiliar to those working in developing countries (e.g. 'acute visceral attrition', etc.) (Blackburn *et al.* 1977).

Last, as with Western medical practice as a whole, too little attention is given to relative costs, especially when it is proposed to undertake a wide range of tests repeatedly. Insufficient attention tends to be given to nutritional support via an improved diet, during sickness, convalescence, and prior to elective treatment (such as surgery, radiotherapy, etc.) by making every effort to supply individualized appetising and nutritious meals to suit the particular person's needs and tastes.

There is plainly a need for much greater interchange of information between those working in nutritional assessment in developing countries and in hospital nutrition support services in industrialized areas. There is much to learn from both sides. In particular, some detailed, serial technolgical investigations possible in well-equipped major centres can validate the necessarily uncomplicated methods feasible in Third World circumstances (Heymsfield *et al.* 1982).

The elderly[82]

Nutritional care for the elderly is clearly a bigger issue in technically more developed countries where longevity has increased greatly in recent decades. However, throughout the world, the elderly are increasing in numbers. They are susceptible to lesser degrees of protein–calorie malnutrition, as well as to vitamin (and mineral) deficiencies for a variety of reasons. These can include lack of teeth, diminished earning power, solitude, inability to cultivate the land (in agrarian societies) and collect or cook foods, diminished appetite, depression and apathy, and inadequate instruction and diet. The assessment of protein–energy malnutrition in

[82] Detailed consideration is given in *Geriatric nutrition* (1983) by D.A. Roe, and in *Handbook for nutrition in the aged* (1985) edited by R. Watson.

the elderly is complicated by uncertainty as to reference data for the 'physiological' range of changes in body compostion in weight, muscle atrophy, skin changes, the degree of malabsorption and recommended dietary allowances (RDAs), and the decline in height associated with ageing (Trotter and Glaser 1951). Also, it is difficult to disentangle the interacting affects of ageing, accompanying chronic disease, inadequate nutrition and decreased activity.

Concern with the nutritional status of the elderly is still mainly a problem of so-called developed countries, but is emerging with varying degrees of speed in urbanized populations in developing countries, with movement to a cash economy and with a breakdown of the support usually implicit in traditional extended families.

In the elderly in urbanized industrial societies, increased fatness is common, but may be masked by lighter bones, sometimes with osteoporosis and a decrease in muscle tissue (lean body mass). In a study in the USA, 42 per cent of elderly subjects were found to be obese (Yearick 1978); women are more often affected (Dibble *et al.* 1967). In less technically developed countries, increasing leanness is likely to occur with greater risk of intercurrent infection. In all parts of the world, height always becomes less, owing to the thinning of vertebrae and their discs, and some degree of kyphosis, together with osteoporosis in some post-menopaused women.

When obesity in the aged is an issue, difficulties can occur in weighing or measuring the height of bed-ridden individuals. For this reason, the abdominal girth has been suggested as a useful approximate indicator (Vir and Love 1980). This should be taken at the level of the umbilicus at the end of expiration, with the subject lying flat and relaxed. Over 90 cm has been suggested as being excessive, but this will vary with body size.

Deficiencies vary in different circumstances — iron, folate, vitamin C, and riboflavin deficiencies need consideration. Particular difficulties may occur in interpretation of clinical signs and biochemical tests. For example, purpura may be the result of mild trauma, deficiency of ascorbic acid, or vitamin K shortage from liver disease or side-effects of various medicines. Similarly, the results of biochemical tests have to take into account such factors as incontinence and renal impairment. Calcium and vitamin D deficiencies appear to be much more frequent than previously believed. This is especially the case in post-menopausal women. Presvious and continuing calcium and vitamin D inadequacy combine with declining oestrogen production to lead to osteoporosis, with brittle bones which are easily fractured. Recent reports indicate significant seasonal changes in vitamin D status in the elderly in Belgium (Bouillon *et al.* 1987)

An extensive bibliography on nutrition in the elderly has been compilled by Metress and Kart (1979), Roe (1983), and Watson (1985). However, appropriate reference data of all sorts need much further investigation and clarification, including for example, recommended dietary allowances (RDA).

Conclusions

In adults, as in children, the concept of optimal nutrition needs to be clarified by various types of 'functional classifications'. From a short-term point-of-view, this is already the goal of the different forms of training, including diet, employed in the rapidly developing field of sports medicine (Pariskova 1978). In this, assessment by anthropometry plays an important role, with a continuing scientific search for optimal body structure for the different functional stresses characteristic of such varying sports as long-distance swimming and basket-ball.

On a life-time basis, the relation of nutrition in childhood and early adulthood to health and survival in later life is difficult to resolve, as so many other factors influence an individual's 'life-light'. Functional classifications are needed for adults, especially concerning overweight and obesity, as indicated earlier (p. 345), in relation to immediate health with gross 'malignant obesity' and to the long-term associated effects of marked obesity ($\leqslant$ 140 per cent reference level), such as high blood pressure, coronary heart disease, and diabetes. An essential and controversial question remains the reference data selected (p. 110) and the need to develop appropriate data for different genetic communities as exemplified by the contrasting physiques of short, thick-set Eskimos and tall, slender Nilotic Africans.

7

Methods of data collection

General

Life cannot wait until the sciences have explained the universe scientifically. . .we cannot put off until we are ready

Ortega (1981)

The information needed for community nutritional assessment can be obtained by many methods through numerous channels, either singly or preferably in combination. These can be considered in the following overlapping categories — *existing services, surveys*, and *surveillance*. As noted many times, information from each is imperfect, but can best be used together to give a more complete picture and to complement deficiencies in all data.

The range of information to be collected, the resources available, and, in particular, the purpose of investigations can vary greatly. Extremes would include the rapid collection of approximate information in a refugee situation (Arnhold 1969) or a famine (Seaman and Holt 1975), through to the gathering of data from a carefully selected sample of the population (concerning dietary intake, economics, food availability, conditioning infections, etc.), as well as direct assessment by anthropometry, (clinical signs, haematology, etc.) (Pan American Health Organization 1972). Indeed, all such studies have individual 'personalities', because of differences in inherent difficulties, resources, and purposes, because of political and administrative considerations, and, less often perceived, because of the views, inevitable biases, and the degree and type of technical expertise of the investigators themselves.

In general, several trends have developed in the collection of this type of data in the last two decades. These include: the need for selectivity, simplicity, minimal cost, and speed in what has been termed 'rapid rural appraisal' (Conlin and Wiggins 1979); the importance of nutritional assessment being linked with action; the greater value of continuing surveillance rather than isolated, cross-sectional surveys; and the desirability of community participation (p. 424) at all stages and as much as feasible. The last mentioned can include, for example, village workers who screen, using appropriate technology (p. 361), such as tricolour arm tapes (p. 94), or community assistance in planning and organizing activities and assisting in their practical implementation. (Also see: Addendum 1988.)

From a different and in some ways contrary viewpoint, the need for as much mathematical exactitude as possible has been emphasized increasingly. Examples include statistically rigorous sampling (p. 405), quality control of anthropometry and other investigational methods (p. 101), and the epidemiological recognition of the sensitivity and specificity of nutritional indicators (Appendix 4).

Major aspects of these trends — simplicity and community participation — and epidemiological precision are all important. The practical problem is to combine them harmoniously and understandably in a workably useful blend with sufficient scientific rigour, within the limitations imposed by reality, and with the recognition that investigations of nutritional status of communities are always incomplete and imperfect, because of the complex and varying forces involved.

Existing services

The best is the enemy of the good.

Voltaire (1764)

Imperfect and incomplete information helpful in the nutritional assessment of a given community can frequently be obtained from existing published information and from data compiled by governmental agencies, particularly health services. This information can be overlooked, ignored, or under-used.

Before launching into the nutritional assessment of a community, a thorough search for existing information and methods needs to be made from a variety of sources.

Literature

Background information concerning a country, region, or community will often already be available, usually scattered through the medical, nutritional, public health, agricultural, economic, and social science literature — both in journals and books. Not infrequently this may be out-of-date or of limited accuracy or with a different focus or emphasis from that required. Sometimes information may have been collected together for particular countries concerning health and nutrition.[83]

Computer-aided bibliographic searches such as MEDLINE and

[83] Nutritionally relevant statistics are available in WHO and other UN agency publications and specialized publications such as *Agricultural development indicators* (International Agricultural Development Service, Washington, DC, 1980) or the *World's children* (World Bank, Washington, DC, 1979).

ORION are available in large libraries which comb the world's published literature in a week's time for a fee. More expensive specific literature searches can be undertaken by various private organizations. Monthly or quarterly listings of published articles on various aspects of nutrition are available through different journals, frequently helpfully indexed and annotated.[84]

There are various international non-governmental organizations, foundations (Ford, Carnegie, WHO, FAO, UNICEF, USAID) who have regional offices relevant to and accessible to the country of interest. Government ministries other than health may furnish relevant materials and many produce excellent reports. These are ministries of agriculture, fisheries, livestock, development, finance and economic planning, water, meteorology, and education. Often, there will be a bureau of statistics responsible for censuses, and, in some countries, for various multipurpose national surveys.

Discussion with individuals experienced in the area, both national and expatriate, should be sought out. However, as with the literature, subconscious bias or lack of knowledge of the rural or urban slum situation needs to be borne in mind.

Existing services

Much approximate, but useful, information can (or could) be obtainable through existing health services and through other governmental services and statistics. Some relevant data may be available without nutrition workers realizing that it exists. This can include, for example, information on changing food prices which may be available from the Ministries concerned with trade, economic planning, and/or agriculture.

Health services

Health services at all levels can supply some information and with slight modifications could furnish much more relevant data on an ongoing basis. In any case, annual reports of hospitals and health centres in the areas to be studied need to be examined.

Such data may be obtained at little additional cost. Sometimes information may, in fact, have been collected, but not analysed or used. As always, the possible accuracy of the methods used needs to be considered (e.g. weight measurements).

[84] Valuable examples include *Nutrition Abstracts* (Commonwealth Nutrition Bureau, Bucksburn, Scotland), *Courrier* (International Children's Centre, Bois de Boulogne, Paris), and *State of the World's Children* (annual publication by UNICEF).

Available data Hospital statistics can be of some value. Although they usually do not represent actual community conditions as regards the commonness, types, or severity of malnutrition, they do suggest that less severe subclinical cases are certain to be present in the community. This 'tip-of-the-iceberg' effect is the basis for the 'sentinel hospital' approach (p. 138). Less severe cases will be greatly underrepresented. Difficulties with interpretation — of numbers admitted or seen as out-patients — can arise from the inadequacy of local transport and communications, available bed space, the hospital admission policy, and the cultural attitudes of the local population to technological medicine, to the hospital itself, and to the causes of malnutrition and its treatment. At least, a rapid reconnaisance should be made to examine hospital records and to visit the wards and out-patient clinics.

Hospital data often fail to furnish as much information as they might, because protein–energy malnutrition in young children is rarely identifiable in the disease classification used, except for such very severe forms as kwashiorkor and marasmus. In addition, confusion often occurs with regard to the diagnostic labelling of malnourished children who are also suffering from multiple infections. What is usually recorded is the presenting or terminal illness. This is usually a serious infection, such as pneumonia or sepsis, which obscures and takes clinical and diagnostic priority over underlying inadequate nutrition. With some modifications and assistance by the hospital administration, recording of major nutritional diagnoses can be included and could furnish some very useful information. In particular, it would be helpful if *all* cases of kwashiorkor and marasmus were to be recorded at hospitals, and that secondary, probably causative, factors also be noted, especially contributory or associated infections. Again, this requires appropriate administrative action and education and motivation of staff, especially if they are to include information collection without adding too much to their usually heavy work load.

Annual figures for key nutritional disorders can best be reported as percentages of the total number of children under 3 or 5 years of age admitted to the wards. Similar records can be kept for out-patients. Care must be taken to try to avoid duplication of reporting if children with malnutrition are first seen in the out-patients' department and subsequently admitted. Ideally, such data should be broken down in relation to infants and 1–4-year-old children, and, if age assessment has been sufficiently accurate, figures for the latter can be analysed in yearly age-intervals. However, this is usually not possible.

Hospital admissions with kwashiorkor and marasmus can also be used to supply some insight into varying seasonal incidence and the geographical distribution in the surrounding area. If the population 'drainage or catchment area' of the hospital is known, it may be considered as a 'sentinel hospital'. The plotting of home sites of affected children on superimposed transparent nylon-acetate maps has been used to try to correlate with local ecological factors, including population distribution, urbanization, and staple food crop. However, this is obviously a time-consuming activity, only feasible as a special research activity.

Ideally, the weight and height of each young child admitted should be measured and subsequently analysed (p. 64). The inclusion of weights and heights as part of a hospital physical examination is by no means universal, not even in wealthy nations. Some hospitals have scales and weigh children that are being followed in the clinic or admitted to the hospital. However, many hospitals do not do so. Indeed, in Third World countries the problems of very limited staff usually make this very difficult. Nevertheless, whenever possible, the weighing of young children should be undertaken routinely and the data collected should be used in management of sick children and should be incorporated into national statistics.

Analyses of case histories and results of investigations of children admitted to hospital with severe forms of protein–energy malnutrition or keratomalacia can yield valuable information on important local nutritional and non-nutritional factors causing these conditions. For this, clinical histories concerning preceding infections and feeding practices are needed, including the method of 'weaning' (separation from the breast). Current infections also need investigation clinically, as well as by locally relevant, available tests, such as a chest X-ray, a stool examination for helminth ova, a thick blood film for malarial parasites, and a tuberculin skin test.

A more scientific approach of this type is the 'case control study'. This is based on the frequency of relevant causal factors in case histories of affected malnourished children compared with unaffected, apparently healthy individuals of the same age and background. These can include children admitted because of a traumatic accident, such as fracture cases. A similar approach is that used in comparing 'positive deviants' (e.g. unaffected) with affected children from comparable environments and backgrounds (Zeitlin *et al.* 1987*a*).

Mortality figures for various hospitalized cases of severe malnutrition, such as kwashiorkor, may be available. Of course, these give no indication of mortality from these conditions in the community. They are biased by the various factors common to all hospital data, and, in the case of kwashiorkor, by the contributory and associated infections common in the particular region and by the effectiveness of the treatment employed. Finally, where autopsies are obtainable, post-mortem evidence of protein–energy malnutrition and contributory and associated infections may be available, although this is not usually the case. When carried out, the final infection may be all that is recorded as the cause of death.

Useful, though biased, information concerning geographical distribution and seasonal incidence has been obtained occasionally by training staff, including auxiliaries, to recognize kwashiorkor and marasmus at health centres and to record cases attending with these conditions (Burgess and Dean 1962). Diagnostic signs should be simple, clearly understood, and taught to personnel by means of practical demonstrations and photographs or pictures. Kwashiorkor may be recorded for every young child with oedema, poor growth (low weight), and wasted muscles, and marasmus may be diagnosed by the clinical appearance of extreme wasting with marked loss of muscle and subcutaneous fat, with no oedema, and with a body weight <60 per cent of the reference level (median). In some areas, other signs may be recorded (e.g. Bitôt's spots) (p. 23). Recognition should be included in training and posters can be displayed in centres or clinics as reminders. Results can be expressed as percentages of children under 1, 3, or 5 years of age attending the centre, according to local need.

Additional information from health services Additional information on the prevalence (and incidence) of malnutrition and some of its causes can be gathered from other parts of existing standard health services (including nutritional rehabilitation units and home visits).

Examples of such reports from health services include data from a health centre in Colombia (DeGwynn and Sanjur 1974) and young child clinics in South Africa (Waldmann 1976) and in Indonesia (Harijono 1976).

In addition, information should be available increasingly from the community workers and village auxiliaries that form the basis of a primary health care service. Notably, it may be possible to collect information on *key aspects of infant feeding*, such as (length of exclusive or predominant) breastfeeding and age of introduction to items from the family diet (p. 203); *occurrence of well-defined, strongly suggestive clinical signs* (p. 23) (pallor of mucosae, Bitôt's spots); a *history of night blindness* (Sommer 1980); and *appropriate simple anthropometry* (arm circumference, weight charts for young childen (p. 296) and for pregnant women (Table 6.1) (p. 237)). However, simplified methods of assessment, recording and reporting will be required, and care taken to avoid trying to add unrealistic burdens to already overloaded community health workers.

Another opportunity for the collection of nutritional data under existing health services is to record and analyse birth weights in all hospital and health centre deliveries by nurses and trained midwives. Traditional birth attendants using colour-coded scales can be trained to obtain birth weights or to categorize into different levels, especially 'low birth weight'

Table 6.1 Examples of appropriate technology for possible use in nutritional assessment. Details are given in the text.

Direct assessment

Clinical
Signs: 'strongly suggestive' (e.g. Bitôt's spots, mucosal pallor) (p. 23)
Symptoms: Night-blindness (reported by mother) (p. 52)
Anthropometry
Single:
Weight-for-age (p. 68)
Weight-for-height (thinness chart) (p. 80)
Arm circumference
measurement (p. 91)
categorization (colour code) (p. 94)
Serial: weight charts (p. 296)

Assessment of causation

Parasitic infection: anal tube technique (p. 159)
Food intake
24-hour recall (? semi-quantitative) (p. 197)
Task analysis: food preparation cycle (p. 188)

(p. 252). Simplified pregnancy weight gain charts and other anthropometric charts are becoming available (p. 237).

Weight charts and growth surveillance The use of weight charts was discussed earlier (p. 296). Their interpretation can be used to give information on the nutritional status of children in a community and to compare the situation from one year to another. Definition has to be given to how best to carry out this type of analysis and is outlined elsewhere (p. 300).

Other relevant services

Data concerning what have been termed 'ecological variables' considered in the 'community nutrition level equation' (p. 143), may be available in appropriate governmental bureaux, ministries, units, research institutes, etc. These may include reports containing information concerning *economics* (p. 148) (basic wages, employment (rate, categories), per capita income, income distribution: cash, subsistence, and barter); *food considerations* (p. 175) (production and distribution of key foods and cash crops, cost of basic diet (especially staple(s), legumes, and cooking oil), food balance sheets (p. 178); *education* (p. 148) (literacy rates, percentage of children attending school; *demographic* (p. 162) (population increase, levels and forms of population movement, including migration, nomads, refugees); and *meteorological* (p. 172) (especially rainfall).

The limitations of such statistics are clear and were discussed earlier (p. 222). Their usefulness depends on the methods of collection, which are often inadequate in coverage, in sampling, in definition, and in general accuracy. Even when available, such centrally available data are usually at best concerned with large groups, even whole nations. Difficulties are usually encountered in 'disaggregation' — that is, breaking down such overall statistics into information from different geographical areas, income groups, subcultures, and/or age-groups.

Further consideration of the selection and longitudinal collection of such data, especially through existing services, is discussed in relation to the organization of nutritional surveillance (pp. 374, 551).

Surveys

> *Nutritional surveys and nutritional studies differ very markedly in scope, as in resources, in funding, in extent of personnel, and in facilities for data analysis and the preparation of reports. Many are truly minimal, making use of available personnel and with scanty laboratory support. Some few are extensive, involving multiple coordinated field teams, mobile laboratories, and backed by computer-analysts, biostatisticians, and professional report-writers. There is a tendency to confuse size with success and maximum funding with optimal results. Often, this is not the case.*
>
> Garn (1979)

A worthwhile, useful, and successful nutrition survey may not be large in terms of complexity of design or numbers covered (Table 6.1). However, it must have a well-defined purpose directed to the selected population or subgroup with specific nutritional objectives. Surveys require sufficiently large numbers of subjects in each age-group to provide useful and meaningful results. Selection of the indicators or measurements, be they anthropometric, haematologic, biochemical, or dietary, need to be limited to specific objectives and the available resources and not from a hypothetical idealized list.

The realities of the areas most in need of nutritional surveys, less technically developed countries, dictate the type of survey to be undertaken. There will no doubt be very limited funds available — the total per

Table 6.2 Oxfam 'mini' survey kit (OFK 4). Available from Oxfam House, 274 Banbury Square, Oxford, OX2 7D2.

1	25 kg hanging scale and pants
10	Fibre glass tape measures
2	Exercise books
1	Clipboard
10	Weight-for-height graph sheets + weight/height tables
1	Pack of graph paper
2	Pens
2	Pencils
2	Rulers
1	Pencil sharpener
1	Rubber
1	Box drawing pins
2	*Oxfam's practical guide to selective feeding programmes*
1	*Management of nutritional emergencies in large populations* (de Goyet *et al.* 1978)
2	*Oxfam's practical guide to refugee health care* by Dr Paul Shears
1	Weight/height wall chart
1	Pocket calculator and batteries
1	Rucksack

capita per year health budget in such areas is anywhere from US$0.50 to US$2.00 per person. There will be few highly trained staff available, and probably little in the way of suitable, least-cost, and reliable equipment.[85] Conversely, there may be considerable numbers of auxiliary staff or underemployed, perferably literate individuals available who can be trained for some aspect of survey work. Logistical problems include poor roads, lack of vehicles, and often great distances to be covered. Also, cross-cultural misunderstandings between the health and nutrition workers and the population concerned need to be avoided (p. 169). External resources and expatriate staff may be necessary (especially for training), if local funding and personnel are insufficient. The simplest and most effective methods are needed for the particular survey.

Basically, two kinds of surveys are used in nutritional assessment, with considerable variations and combinations to suit different purposes. These are *cross-sectional* and *longitudinal*, each with their own advantages and limitations.

[85] An economical kit is available from Oxford (Table 6.2).

Cross-sectional surveys

> *Even armed with such technological aids to objectivity as questionnaires, interview schedules, checklists, or even tape recorders and photographic equipment, the fact remains that by the very nature of RRA the person and personality characteristics of the individual or group carrying out RRA will have a crucial influence on the texture and quality of the RRA process and findings. The individuals concerned can truly be regarded themselves as 'tools' of the RRA process.*
>
> Feuerstein (1979)
> *Rapid Rural Appraisal*

The assessment of nutritional status of a community will most often be evaluated of necessity by short-term cross-sectional studies, plus information from health services, and perhaps some longitudinal data of a very limited nature. The degree of complexity of a cross-sectional survey[86] varies greatly. Examples are: national country surveys as carried out in four African countries by the UCLA Nutrition Assessment team (Zerfas *et al.* 1982) and of Nepal, Egypt, and other countries by the CDC (Center for Disease Control, Atlanta, Georgia); repeat cross-sectional studies in Kenya (CBS, Kenya 1976, 1979); rapid surveys of a few weeks duration, as in Haiti (Jelliffe and Jelliffe 1960), in times of emergency as in Bangladesh (Sommer and Lowenstein 1975); as a feasibility or pre-survey before a longitudinal study is planned and implemented. Cross-sectional surveys can be used as a baseline or as a periodic evaluation of a programme. They can be focused on a particular age-group or geographical urban or rural area where malnutrition is believed to be common, or they can be more general. They should be undertaken with as careful sampling procedures (p. 406) as possible, but may have to compromise with a convenient or supposedly representative sample. They can sometimes be combined with cross-sectional surveys into crop production, economics, etc. as in Kenya (Agenda, 1982) or with family planning practices (Anderson *et al.* 1987).

Classical examples of high-technology, very expensive, multidisciplinary surveys with heavy laboratory support were those carried out in the 1950s and 1960s by the US Interdepartmental Committee for National Nutrition Defense (ICNND 1963).

[86] Excellent summaries of practical issues in low-cost cross-sectional surveys have been given by Burgess and Burgess (1974), Bailey (1975), and Brown and Brown (1979*a*). An account of practical problems has been given by Scott *et al.* (1980) and Lutz (1981) has given a useful account of planning and organization.

Cross-sectional surveys can be repeated in the same or similar groups at prescribed intervals, particularly at different seasons of the year.

Advantages and disadvantages

Short-term prevalence surveys offer the obvious advantages of being relatively inexpensive, requiring few staff, and taking little time to carry out.

The limitations and disadvantages of these surveys are also clear. They are brief in duration and, unless supplemented by necessarily biased information from health services, reflect conditions during only one season of one particular year. They are short episodes and thus afford extremely limited opportunities for gaining a real insight into the way people live and the causes of their nutritional problems. Such studies detect stunting, only the more chronic conditions, such as fluorosis, or rickets and they tend to miss important acute, often lethal conditions of shorter duration, such as untreated infantile beriberi or kwashiorkor (compared with marasmus).

Lastly, it is a frequent and at times valid complaint that surveys easily become sterile academic exercises that fail to better the conditions in the community studied. Plainly, surveys should not be carried out solely to satisfy scientific curiosity. They should measure the size of problems and suggest logical means of improving the situation to politicians, administrators, and to the community itself.

Results of cross-sectional surveys should be combined with evidence from other sources, including local health statistics, long-term incidence studies (when available), and information collected by primary health care workers.

Prevalence surveys are not the complete answer for the nutritional assessment of the community. Their value can be increased if repeated, as they can indicate changes over periods of time, as in the Gilbert Islands (Roberts *et al.* 1981). Also, in Costa Rica, Mohrs (1978) found 7 per cent of young children to be below 90 per cent of expected height-for-age in 1975 compared with the much greater figure of 17 per cent in 1966.

Alternatively, repeated surveys can identify possible seasonal differences in nutrition and obtain a rough estimate of disease trends at selected periods of the year. This can give representative data related to climatic, agricultural, and financial cycles throughout the year and of other variations in community life, such as seasonal population movements for various reasons.

Types of prevalence survey

Nutrition prevalence surveys can vary greatly in complexity, scope, and purpose. They may include a wide spectrum of activities and resources. On one hand, small, unelaborate teams with limited objectives may rely mainly on rapid screening by clinical assessment, anthropometry, and field observation. An example of such a survey was undertaken in Haiti in 1958 (Jelliffe and Jelliffe 1960).

On the other hand, large multidisciplinary groups, including physicians, nutritionists, biochemists, dieticians, and dental experts may have sufficient funds and laboratory facilities for more comprehensive studies. An example of the latter is the national survey of Barbados in 1971 (Pan American Health Organization 1972).

Despite their many disadvantages, such cross-sectional surveys of different levels of complexity continue to be the mainstay of community nutritional assessment. For this reason, detailed consideration of sequences and ranges of action are given in full later (p. 384).

Rapid nutritional assessment

Ideally, the findings should be geared to immediate action. The goal is to identify and sort populations according to need and then intervene as required. This type of rapid assessment is particularly well-suited in times of disaster — natural or man-made (e.g. refugees, blockades, floods, droughts, earthquakes, locust plagues, etc.).

A simplified rapid nutritional assessment does not mean a simple-minded one. This type of cross-sectional survey needs to be well thought-out with adequate sampling and appropriate indicators with acceptable sensitivity, specificity, and validity (Appendix 4). There needs to be careful training to collect a few selected indicators which have to be of optimal reliability, and reproducibility, giving accurate results, but being inexpensive to gather. The hallmarks of these are that they are simple, readily analysed, and understood and portray the extent of the problem. An example was the evaluation of Nigerian children during the civil war with the QUAC-stick which uses arm circumference for height. This was used to estimate the presence of protein–energy malnutrition and especially to identify the children needing the most immediate intervention (Arnhold 1969) (p. 94).

The philosophy of the rapid survey, as also used in agriculture, is that it needs to be timely, low-cost, flexible, and have the ability to measure the problem. Instead of using a whole list of indicators, simpler proxies are used which need to be tested in the particular area. For example, rather than carrying out a detailed study of the economic condition of many communities, the presence or absence of a metal roof may be a short cut (or surrogate or proxy measure) for earnings, as only the wealthier people have such roofs. In quite different circumstances in an Arabian Gulf country, the number of servants was used as an indirect indicator of wealth.

An important, large-scale example of rapid assessments was in Kampuchea in South-East Asia. Here simple, rapid, inexpensive objective measures were carried out under difficult field conditions. The rapid surveys were needed to assess the need for immediate food relief intervention. Several methods were tried. Community workers were trained to detect the presence of kwashiorkor, as judged by oedema, hair changes, and other clinical signs, and to measure the arm circumference, height, and weight. Once again, the methods had to be reproducible, accurate, and simple to perform by unskilled, but trained workers. The method had to separate the severe from the moderately severe malnourished and had to be rapid and objective. In a few weeks, this programme screened one million individuals and identified those needing immediate intervention for severe protein–energy malnutrition.

Longitudinal surveys

> *Cross-sectional survey techniques may be the most efficient approach to an initial analysis of health and (nutritional) parameters in a population. However, longitudinal studies will generally be necessary to define cause and effect relationships and demonstrate the effectiveness of specific interventions.*
>
> De Sweemer *et al.* (1979)

Longitudinal studies have the advantage of demonstrating the *incidence* of malnutrition. Usually, selected members or families in a community are kept under observation for a relatively prolonged period. Such surveys enable more subtle and changing influences on the community to be recognized. This type of approach owes much to the initial work of Spence and his colleagues in Newcastle upon Tyne (Miller *et al.* 1960).

Longitudinal surveys are complex and expensive undertakings and there must be a very clear rationale for their being undertaken. Longitudinal surveys assess the incidence (over time) of certain events and the intervening factors and determinants associated with them. Families, households, and individuals are selected and kept under continuing, regular, systematic observation for a prolonged period.

Longitudinal studies are frequently undertaken on children to identify environmental influences on them. These can include the diet, infections, socio-economic levels, cultural practices, and education that may affect growth, health, and development, including mental development. They can also reflect the influence of seasonal changes, as they often continue for a minimum of a year and preferably longer. They attempt to study multiple, related, interacting factors over time and also try to indicate the interaction of such variables as diet, contributory (conditioning) infections, customs, and economics. In addition, they assist in selecting priority activities for preventive programmes. Longitudinal surveys entail close, prolonged contact with the people studied, resulting in an intimate knowledge and understanding of the community and its way of life.

Past examples in less technically developed countries have included: *Eastern Mediterranean* — Beirut, Lebanon (Harfouche 1965), Jordan (Pharaon *et al.* 1965); *Asia* — rural Hyderabad, India (Jyothi *et al.* 1963; Swaminathan *et al.* 1964); *Africa* — Keneba village, Gambia (McGregor *et al.* 1961), Imesi (Morley 1963), Aku'o village, Nigeria (Gilles 1964); *the Americas* — Mexico City (Ramos-Galvan 1966); *West Indies* — rural Jamaica (Standard and Miall 1965).

Few such planned longitudinal surveys have been undertaken in recent years, largely because of cost. Exceptions include surveys in Hong Kong (Field and Baber 1973), and predominantly anthropometric studies in Cuba and Venezuela.

Longitudinal surveys have often taken the form of research studies, particularly in less technically developed countries, as in the Danfa Rural Health and Family Planning Studies in Ghana (Ofosuh-Amaah and Neumann 1979), and the study by Mata (1978*b*) in Santa Maria Cauqué, Guatemala. Currently, a collaborative study called the Nutritional Collaborative Research Support Program, consisting of longitudinal studies is going on simultaneously in Egypt, Mexico, and Kenya to examine the effects of reduced energy intake on a variety of functions — growth, cognitive development, reproductive outcome, etc. (Also see: Addendum 1988.)

Some longitudinal data may be available from the 'defined areas' which may be present around some health centres. However, these are often demonstration, training centres and thus results may be atypical. Also, some longitudinal information may be collected over periods of time in the course of special activities, such as with an anthropologist resident in a community for months or years.

Of much more general practical significance, the spread of primary health care services can lead to the collection of some basic data by community health workers (including mothers) (Rohde *et al.* 1975). On a continuing basis this can give regular information on changes in services as well as in populations.

Advantages

Longitudinal investigations are usually carried on for at least one year and thus not only permit an annual incidence of malnutrition and disease to be determined, but show the seasonal variations caused by the climate, the availability of food, community activities, and other circumstances.

Most illnesses in early childhood are short-term episodes. In longitudinal studies, the incidence of such severe acute diseases as diarrhoea and respiratory infections, measles, or minor-seeming, but cumulatively important, skin infections, will be noted and can be correlated both with one another and with environmental changes. This contrasts with the short-term cross-sectional prevalence surveys, which miss most of the acute conditions and tend to over-emphasize chronic diseases.

Another advantage is that the ages of children born during the study will be known with accuracy, together with the dates and causes of death. Growth can be compared with reference data for age. Vital statistics such as the mortality rates and causes of death in the perinatal period, in infants, and in the 1–4 year age-group, have the potential for more complete assessment.

Above all, longitudinal studies permit an understanding of the dynamic interplay of factors at work, and in particular enable the identification of *locally* important causes of malnutrition, and logical preventive programmes.

Finally, the prestige attached to the research aspect of this type of investigation may help to attract young health workers, including physicians, to rural districts. Also, the detailed knowledge gained in the particular area should ultimately lead to its use for the field training of medical and auxiliary personnel, and, above all, help to plan long-term health services adapted to the local scene and involving the community.

Disadvantages

Long-term studies are not easy to organize. They are inevitably very expensive, and are by their nature time-consuming to undertake, analyse, and present to appropriate authorities for action. Often, by the time the results of a longitudinal study are complete and analysed, they may be out-of-date because the community itself or other circumstances may have changed.

Constant definitions and methods of examination and interview have to be maintained over the whole period and not be altered with experience. The ethical question of the degree of clinical responsibility to be assumed will have to be decided in advance, clearly defined, and adhered to throughout. This should be judged according to the circumstances of the particular study. In some surveys, it may be justifiable to limit the therapy and advice given to the minor, readily treatable, conditions and emergency medical care; in others more than this will be necessary. Moreover, 'any survey inevitably alters both the observer and the observed'.

Preparation of the population to be surveyed calls for careful thought and repeated explanation, obviously much influenced by the type of clinical care or other assistance that the surveyors may be able to offer.

Many practical difficulties may arise — logistical, technical (quality control) (p. 410), and social. For example, there may be seasonal or other movement of people between the town and rural villages, or a high proportion of defaulters due to indifference, boredom, or suspicion.

Last, suitably trained, well-motivated staff may be difficult to recruit, and still more so to retain for long periods of time during which monotonous, repeated measurements and observations are required. A large measure of patience, dedication, and team-spirit is needed on the part of the survey group. Also, they must fully appreciate that frequent periodic visits to households for questioning and observation can become an intrusion and a tiresome burden to families unless handled courteously and diplomatically, as exemplified in the Newcastle-upon-Tyne study.

Comment

According to Mata (1978), experience gained with the very successful Santa Maria Cauqué study distinguished at least seven fundamentals for this kind of field work. The first three related primarily to human relations, and in order of importance they were: (1) recruitment of a hard-working, capable, and loyal field staff; (2) establishment of good relations with the population concerned, together with continuing efforts to maintain or improve that rapport; and (3) provision of compensating services to the community in a systematic and reassuring fashion. The remaining four conditions were technical; (4) adequate physical and administrative support facilities (including finance); (5) full coverage of the designated population, whether a sample or the whole, in order to guarantee an adequate interpretation of results; (6) systematic supervision of field operations to ensure good quality information; and (7) organization of a system to manage the data collected.

Techniques

In the longitudinal surveys being undertaken in different parts of the world, numerous variations in technique and procedure are applied. These are often dictated by local circumstances and the special aims of the particular study, which must be clearly defined at the outset. Nevertheless, certain general principles seem to be common to many such investigations.

Sampling Special statistical guidance will be required with sampling in longitudinal studies regarding the selection of families, the number to be covered, the frequency of examinations, and the length of the study. Allowance must be made for a probable decrease in the total sample size during the observation period due to defaulting, to movement, and to deaths.

Some aspects of sampling are detailed later (p. 405). However, longitudinal studies have complexities which require guidance from a statistician experienced in field activities.

In view of the continuing concern with the nutritional problems of early childhood, longitudinal surveys often aim at observing a selected group of pregnant women, or of full-term babies, born by normal delivery, through the first 2 to 5 years of life.

Selection of area The selection of the community or households to be studied becomes complex and the community needs to be thoroughly prepared in order to ensure ongoing co-operation. The area selected should be as typical of the particular area as can be judged on the available general and statistical evidence. Frequently, a simultaneous survey may be made of contrasting socio-economic groups or ethnic communities. If one of the contrasting groups consists of children of the local elite, it may be possible to use the results obtained as a basis for local reference data for the growth and development (p. 110). In all cases, the advice of a statistician and an anthropologist should be sought.

Selection of places of examination Usually three types of examination sites need to be planned: a regular clinic for the survey children; systematic home-visiting; and some form of emergency clinic service for the acutely ill. Home visits are essential for the assessment of environmental and socio-economic circumstances, for explanation concerning defaulters, and for the investigation of any deaths that may have occurred. It is also important to arrange for transport for those attending the regular clinic, for home-visiting staff, and for emergency cases.

Useful, though incomplete and biased, longitudinal information exists already in many parts of the world in the records of health centres with an adjacent defined area and sufficient staff to permit home visiting and adequate record-keeping (Kark and Steuart 1962). The disadvantage of this information is that it is necessarily influenced by the health centre's activities, and hence not typical of areas lacking similar facilities.

Selection and training of staff[87] It is imperative to have local people involved in the survey, particularly when there are problems of custom and language. There will always be sensitive areas into which enquiries need to be made.

In large surveys, a full-time staff is needed for continuous employment throughout the whole period, preferably headed by a doctor or senior nutritionist with experience in public health and in paediatric nutrition for technical concerns, as well as a field administrator.

An adequate preliminary period must be devoted to the selection and training and to pre-testing methods, in particular the techniques of interviewing and home-visiting, often culminating in a pilot study.

Supervision is essential and it takes very experienced staff to train local

[87] Further details are given elsewhere (p. 194).

people how to be supervisors, as they may not like to criticize their colleagues and acquaintances. Supervision also involves immediate constructive feedback concerning performance and results both to the collectors of the information and those from whom data has been collected.

Other requirements Maintaining the co-operation of the population or groups being studied is a major challenge. A difficult dilemma is to decide how much to intervene in problems without changing the population under study, what incentives to offer, and ethical considerations of intervention for life-threatening situations.

There are problems with missing data, defaulters, and the migration of families seasonally and for longer periods. There may be difficulties with finding people at home during periods of intensive labour outside the household as at times of harvesting, planting, and on market days.

Unless there is adequate logistical support in terms of administration, personnel, and transport, and adequate living arrangements for staff, then the study is doomed. Data management, including editing, data entry, storage, and analyses, must be planned well in advance (p. 438).

The techniques of pre-planning, planning, sampling, and training are discussed elsewhere in greater detail (p. 405). In selection of the study area, it is essential that it should be an area of low migration. It must be typical and representative, and there must be a range of values for the key variables of interest.

Logistics will differ with the target area, which may vary from compact villages where people can be reached easily in a short time, contrasted to distant homesteads or farms necessitating long periods of walking between households or contacting mobile nomads. Adaptation of methodology and logistics must take place. Two-way radio may be needed for communications and bicycles or mules for feasible transport.

Type and frequency of investigations The methods used must have validity, sensitivity, and specificity (Appendix 4). They have to be thoroughly pre-tested in the local situation to see that they are workable.

Although the detailed arrangements vary, a longitudinal survey commencing at birth may often start with regular examinations held monthly for 3 months, and thereafter at 3-monthly intervals. Care should be taken to ensure that children are seen within a defined number of days of their scheduled appointment — for example, 3-monthly intervals ± 7 days.

Data collected during longitudinal surveys Indirect indicators include socio-economic information, climate, agriculture, market prices, and data on illnesses and deaths. Direct assessment includes anthropometry, clinical examination, and biochemical and food intake studies. These are the basic components of longitudinal studies. However, it is important to use modern epidemiological techniques to try to judge the significance of variables found, including those considered 'associated' or 'causative'.

Careful consideration has to be given to the desirability and feasibility of doing laboratory investigations. For example, if an area has a number of clinical cases that are suspicious of a particular nutritional deficiency, then it would be very worthwhile to check serum or urine levels of the particular nutrient in question, at least on a subsample. However, anything that involves blood drawing, processing, preserving (or freezing), and then transport to a distant site, increases the cost, complexity, and manpower of a survey very greatly. For example, in field work the simplest, most commonly used laboratory tests are for the detection of anaemia, with a finger-prick method yielding sufficient blood for haemoglobin or microhaematocrit determination.

Longitudinal surveys of children usually include the *serial collection* of some of the following data:

1. Anthropometric measurements — weight, height (length), circumference of the head and arms, skinfold thickness;
2. Clinical characteristics — general, nutritional stigmata, physical (psychomotor) development (milestones, sometimes radiological bone-age);
3. Biochemical data — haemoglobin, haematocrit, serum albumin;
4. Parasitological data — results of examining stools for helminth ova, etc., thick film for malaria;
5. Tuberculin test results;
6. Health history — type and duration of illnesses since last visit (e.g. diarrhoea, respiratory-tract infection), immunization;
7. Dietary history (p. 187) — types and approximate quantities of food given in previous period (often the preceding 24 hours).

Data on socio-economic circumstances of the family and cultural attitudes also have to be collected by methods suggested earlier (p. 144). Some may be obtained by questionnaire, but more personal details will only be learned later either by questioning when rapport has been established or by observation during home-visiting.

If practicable, a brief study of other family members should be undertaken, including the obstetrical history of the mother and a clinical and anthropometric examination of the parents and siblings.

Items of information collected in this type of survey require to be carefully pre-defined and graded numerically, so that they may lend themselves to analysis on punch cards or preferably, if available, by computer. Precise criteria for the retrospective diagnosis of past illness must be laid down. For example, diarrhoea may be defined as four or more loose watery stools in 24 hours. Likewise, the grading of socio-economic data must be defined. For example, this can be related to various types of housing, water supply, methods of transportation, or occupation.

Statistical techniques may be employed to obtain more detailed information on a subgroup of those being studied. It is particularly valuable if family food-consumption studies, made by actual measurement of foods cooked and eaten (p. 193), can be carried out on a randomly selected subsample. Similarly, more detailed biochemical tests, such as serum concentrations of vitamin A or the amino-acid imbalance test may be carried out on a subgroup.

Conclusion

Ideally, more longitudinal surveys are needed in representative rural and urban areas of the world, and the nutrition of the community must form a major aspect of all such studies. Unfortunately, in most places such long-term incidence studies will not be feasible, principally because of cost and shortage of staff. The assessment of the nutritional status of a community will often have to be evaluated by short-term cross-sectional prevalence studies, with information available from health (and other) services and some longitudinal data collected by primary health care workers.

The time needed to produce and analyse results may be too prolonged for their value and relevance as current data. There is a high cost for staff, logistics, and data analyses. A high percentage of the budget goes towards vehicles, particularly maintenance, tyres, and fuel. In addition staff must understand that maximum flexibility is necessary to respond to the daily schedule of the people under study. Also, over a long period of contact with the study population, the observer as well as the observed will change because of the survey. The staff concerned need continuing ongoing training, quality control, and constant supervision in order to remain technically competent and high in morale.

Surveillance

> *Surveillance, from the French 'surveiller', means to watch over with great attention, authority, and often with suspicion.*
>
> World Health Organization (1976)

Nutritional surveillance involves watching, on a continuous basis, those factors responsible for the nutritional status of populations and the early existence of inadequate nutrition. Surveillance permits timely action to be taken to improve nutritional status in a given population or to prevent its deterioration (Morley 1976; Foege 1976; Aranda-Pastor *et al.* 1983; Mason *et al.* 1984). Because of its broad scope, nutritional surveillance

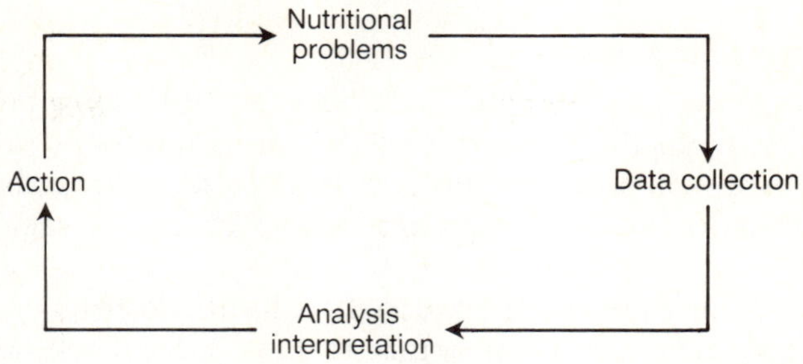

Fig. 6.1 The cycle of nutritional surveillance.

overlaps with health and epidemiological surveillance (*International Journal of Epidemiology* 1976) and cannot be readily separated from related disciplines such as economic, social, and agricultural studies.

Surveillance requires regular data collection from populations either specifically for surveillance or from available sources, or both. Such data must be presented in an understandable manner for informed decision-making (Lwanga 1983).

This section provides some guidelines for conducting nutritional surveillance, realizing there is no one standard method. Indeed, flexible approaches are needed to determine how this assessment method can most appropriately be applied to nutritional improvement of defined populations, without being too complex or too costly.

The cycle of nutritional status assessment for action involves identifying relevant problems based on appropriate (though often imperfect) data, and their analysis and interpretation (Fig. 6.1). Ideally, this leads to informed decisions and focused action. Nutritional surveillance repeats this cycle regularly; action results from changes shown by such information. Changes over time may be predictable (e.g. due to seasonal effects) or unpredictable. The type and extent of action will depend on available resources.

Applications of nutritional surveillance

Use in programmes

Nutritional surveillance may be used to assist the planning, implementation, management, and evaluation of programmes. Questions which must be addressed include whether the necessary services are provided as planned, particularly to target groups, as well as whether and why nutritional status is improving or not (Stinson 1983). Surveillance may occur before, during, or after programme goals and objectives have been identified; hence its content and scope must be directed to actions which satisfy these programme goals and objectives.

Use in policy and planning

Surveillance may also be used for policy and planning purposes with regards to resource allocations for specific programmes or projects or for other purposes such as legislation (e.g. food price controls, bottle feeding by prescription only). This often occurs at a central or regional government level.

Where decisions are made (national to local) determines the kind of surveillance structure. It is important to have a feedback mechanism to include programme recipients. Critical questions include who makes such decisions, how such decisions are translated into action, and what types (technical, administrative, political) and extent of information influence these.

Use in early warning systems

An early warning system is a special application of nutritional surveillance to assist in the prevention of acute food shortages due, for example, to crop failure or economic decline. Predisposing factors include severe poverty in populations susceptible to acute emergencies such as drought or war. Surveillance should provide staged signals to suggest timely sequential interventions and prevent or modify undesirable increases in malnutrition. Such an early warning system is a stop-gap procedure, not a substitute for solving long-term problems.

Foege (1976) provides broad guidelines for famine relief surveillance. Key elements include the evaluation of the efficacy of the surveillance system and the effectiveness of the response system. For planning, lessons from past experiences to prevent avoidable mistakes are essential (De Goyet *et al.* 1978).

Further details are given in Appendix 10.

Sequence of activities

Surveillance requires an initial assessment to identify need, advocate commitment, and assess available resources. This usually requires a cross-sectional survey. When seasonal effects influence nutritional status, the 'initial' assessment should include a one-year cycle, using appropriate service information, such as health service records, (Valverde *et al.* 1982). Setting up a surveillance system involves a sequence of pre-planning, planning, training, data collection, analysis, interpretation and report writing, similar in approach to that presented in sequence of activities (p. 384). However there are important, often critical, aspects to consider.

The first question is whether surveillance is needed. Have nutrition problems (current or potential) been identified and are they serious enough to warrant action? Will the information presented (however pertinent and detailed) influence or promote the appropriate action by in-

Table 6.3 Types of information needed for nutritional surveillance in largely rural, less technically developed countries

Climate	Timing, duration, and adequacy (or excess) of rainfall
Crops	The pattern of the crop calendar, the amount of crop produced, the presence of crop pests
Livestock	Pasture conditions, herd size, production, and condition
Water	Availability and adequacy for animals and humans
Market	Prices and flows of major food commodities and livestock; migration patterns
Nutrition	Food stocks held by families, dietary intake, and the state of nutrition
Health and vital statistics	Crude death rates, infant and child mortality rates, birthrates, disease prevalence

formation,? Are there sufficient resources (available or potential) to support programmes or interventions?

If surveillance is indeed required, can it be done effectively at affordable costs? This involves setting up and continuing a regular system for reporting timely, selective, and relevant information for a variety of users (i.e. decision-makers at every level) who influence (start, continue, modify, or stop) a variety of actions. It is important to determine at what level the major responsibility for each step in surveillance occurs and from where support will occur to indicate types of information needed (Table 6.3). Resources for surveillance must be balanced over the whole period of its use, rather than expending too much effort in a single phase, such as planning.

On a national basis involving several sectors (health, planning, agriculture, etc.) surveillance may require several full-time staff and may not become fully operational for years. At the community level, surveillance should be instituted and maintained quickly enough to satisfy programme requirements. In one sense, appropriate surveillance may be considered a prerequisite for satisfactory programme management.

Selection of indicators

Since resources for surveillance in developing countries are nearly always limited, both comprehensive and basic lists of possible health, agricultural, and socio-economic indicators have been presented WHO 1976; Mason *et al.* 1984). Mason (1978) groups agricultural indicators as follows: production data, census information, price reporting, single and multipurpose surveys.

Indicators must be kept to the minimum, emphasizing ease of collection, relevance, and interpretability, whether by technicians, policy-makers, providers, or the population of concern. Indicators also should be sensitive and specific to detect change (Habicht 1980).

In general, types of information may relate to cause or effect. Causal information will suggest why changes are occurring, whether they be due to social disruption, drought, unemployment, economic factors, etc. Effect or outcome indicators reflect the changes that occur; these include health and nutritional status, as well as food availability, cost, and consumption patterns. Information will also be required about health and other services provided and utilized, as well as the perceptions of such services by the populations concerned.

Sources of data

Available sources

Data may be acquired from available sources (e.g. administrative, health, or clinic records; vital statistics). Existing records from health and other services may provide regular information about programme recipients, but this is usually only a part of the target population of concern. The quality of the data may be suspect due to constraints of staff training and supervision. Moreover, although there is often plenty of data already collected, its lack of relevance and organization may defy useful analysis. The reasons for collecting such data may not be consistent with those for surveillance. Focusing on a limited number of indicators relevant to the programme and improving data quality may provide appropriate information for surveillance purposes. In addition, a random sample of the data will reduce the work load for analysis and not reduce the validity of the results. The use of specially selected 'sentinel' clinics, hospitals, or communities to give information for programme purposes is worth considering, provided that they reflect the other areas being serviced.

A special example of surveillance is the use of growth monitoring records, usually available from weight graphs on children's cards examined by mothers (Griffiths 1985; Yee 1985). Yee illustrates how growth monitoring data can be applied to levels of primary health care development (Table 6.4). It is a particular value that direct (anthropometric) information for nutritional status can be assessed for individual children and for growth changes over time, such as the presence or absence of weight gain. Summary results for communities or populations will then also reflect the progress of subjects (e.g. the proportion of young children with weight gain over a defined period of time) rather than just the overall change in undernutrition prevalence rates, perhaps reflecting different subjects. The approach bears some similarily to that for longitudinal surveys (p. 367). When growth monitoring is done at the community level, the information will tend to describe more the target sub-

Table 6.4 Illustration of how growth monitoring data can provide the basis for nutritional surveillance and the types of decisions that can be supported by the information at each level. *(Yee 1985)*

National summary	Policy decisions; resource allocations
District, provincial, or regional summary	Policy recommendations; resource allocations
Health centre summary	Programme management, monitoring, and evaluation
Village or community summary	Programme development and management
Individual growth charts	Health interventions; family decisions and actions

jects than just be limited to the service population normally attending clinics, etc.

Information on a growth card (e.g. reasons for being at risk, birth weight; and health inputs such as immunizations) if recorded and analysed systematically may provide useful information on health status and receipt of services.

Sources specifically for surveillance

Data may be acquired from repeated surveys (Martorell 1982). If ongoing surveys in sectors related to nutrition (e.g. health, agricultural, household income/expenditure) are already being conducted or planned, co-ordination of data collection and analysis (linkage) should be encouraged. Frequently, such linkage is applied to surveys of different households at different times, but using samples which describe the same or similar populations (Cornell Nutritional Surveillance Program 1984).

If linkage of surveys is done, an understanding of their design, definitions, content, and purpose is required. For example, household income/expenditure surveys may be more concerned with relatively urban areas, agricultural surveys with areas of food production, and family planning surveys with women of child-bearing ages. At whatever level, linkage must consider consistency in a common unit of analysis, usually the household. For this reason, nutrition surveys should use the household or family as the key unit of analysis (at least for sampling purposes) and not be entirely limited to individuals, such as young children and pregnant/lactating women.

In practice, linkage requires bureaucratic co-operation as well as technical co-ordination. In the USA, for example, during the last decade there has been no functional linkage between national surveys on food consumption and health/nutritional status, each done by different government agencies in the country. Only recently has a plan evolved to incorporate these two studies, perhaps using a single agency (*Nutrition Week* 1983).

Another major problem is that specialized surveys are often centrally co-ordinated and large-scale. Hence, their summary information cannot be readily applied for local purposes of surveillance. Ideally, any survey related to surveillance should summarize the information at each level of decision-making and action. Often, this may start at the community, particularly where participation in action is important.

Surveys are relatively costly and can only be done infrequently. However, they are an efficient way to corroborate and supplement information from other sources of data. One example is to compare the results from clinic records with those of the general population (Trowbridge and Stetler 1980). Quality control (p. 101) in surveys is usually better than for data from clinic and other routinely collected records, because of the more intense training and supervision.

It should be noted that formal surveys are not the only method to acquire information specifically for surveillance. Other methods include systematic informal observations, life histories based on small samples, group interviews, and unstructured interviews based on a general list of discussion topics ('focus group discussions') (Manoff 1985). Included in this group are rapid ecological visits, discussed more fully elsewhere in this book (p. 437).

Repeated cross-sectional surveys

Repetition of cross-sectional surveys involves a learning process for both doers (survey implementers) and users of the information. The lessons learned from the experiences and results of the initial survey will modify the approaches to later surveys.

Adequate documentation of the first survey is important. This includes field procedures and methods: lists, records, manuals, schedules, maps, reports (particularly those evaluating performance, logistics, and resources), as well as a detailed breakdown of actual costs and their justicfications. Methods of field editing, quality control, data entry and coding, analysis, and interpretations should also be reviewed and documented to provide a basis for later use.

Key personnel at all levels should be retained where feasible for future studies. Between surveys, some staff may be used for related assessments within the programme services (e.g. record entry, checking, and summarizing).

The results of the initial survey will guide later surveys. These include identifying areas and groups with greatest need (as shown by higher prevalence rates of malnutrition indicators) for more intensive focus, and by using these results for planning later sampling procedures. Modifications may involve sample design (selection of strata, type of sample) and sample size (based on the variability between and within clusters). In addition the choice of 'sentinel' communities might be considered. In this case, the sample should be sufficiently large to describe changes in each of these communities. Their representativeness will be based on their characteristics (especially those associated with malnutrition) as compared with those from the remaining population described in the first survey or from other means.

Repeated surveys for nutritional surveillance may differ from the initial one in content, focus, and scope. Changes will be dictated by the purposes of surveillance. With each successive survey, the use of other information (e.g. health clinic records, vital statistics) will be better clarified as well as the specific role of further surveys. For example, such surveys may assess change in populations in which programmes presently are directed as well as those in which programme expansion is anticipated. Usually, surveys will be required every 3 to 5 years, although smaller, more focused surveys may be considered in the interim.

Nutritional surveillance for programme management

Nutritional surveillance for programme management is directly related to community assessment. Ideally, surveillance should begin at the programme-planning phase to keep pace with goals and objectives. Often, however, surveillance develops with the programme to be modified as required.

The sequence of activities will be modified by the following:

1. Need to set up an infrastructure, including personnel and resources (physical, administrative, and technical);
2. Time frame for cycle flow, frequency, and duration;
3. Mechanism for review of surveillance activities.

Basic issues include: Are the purposes of surveillance activities being satisfied? Are the resources used for surveillance adequate and affordable? Can the programme itself afford the actions to which surveillance is directed?

Ideally, the costs for surveillance should be separated from other programme costs, although at times this distinction may be difficult (e.g. use of existing records collected for other purposes). The benefits of surveillance include improving programme efficiency, for example by better targetting of beneficiaries within and between population groups.

Key questions which should be asked in the planning phase have been considered elsewhere in this book. These include the types of nutritional problems, where they occur, their extent and severity, and who they involve (e.g. by age, socio-economic status), defined so that relevant solutions can be directed to populations at risk.

Programmes take time to start and develop fully. They may expand in content or in populations targetted. If surveillance includes those areas partially reached or as yet unreached by the programme, results may be used for future planning. In addition, those areas not yet served by the programme may be used as 'controls' for evaluation purposes. How the results are interpreted will depend on the reasons why certain areas are selected before others (i.e. the 'controls') and comparisons of their characteristics.

Programme management should consider a number of population groups within its area of responsibility (Habicht and Mason 1983; Miller and Sahn 1984):

1. The total population;
2. The targetted group[89] to which the programme is directed (based, for example, on geographic location, age, and biological status, occupation or other socio-economic indicators);
3. The needy[89] (identified by more specific criteria related to nutritional status, such as low weight for age or failure to gain weight);
4. The actual recipients of programme services.

Programme recipients will include a proportion of those targetted (i.e. coverage) and/or needy and those not. Data from programme records are limited to recipients. Data for the totals in other groups must be derived by other means, usually surveys. In programmes with relatively small populations, an initial census may be done, to identify targetted households and individuals within those households. This census may be updated as required (for births, deaths, and migrations) to monitor, evaluate, and study the overall effects of the programme.

Conclusions

Nutritional surveillance began as a formal entity in 1974 as a result of the World Food Conference. It is now being applied in several countries in different ways for different purposes. Some examples are given in Appendix 10. It should form an important basis for appropriate programme management. Nutritional surveillance involves ongoing assessment to provide limited, essential information to decision-makers.

It is important to first determine whether there is a need for surveillance and, if so, what types of information are required. Major limitations in this process include a lack of clarity about nutritional goals and objectives, where decisions are made, and what influences such decisions.

[88] Depending on the criteria used, the target groups may be identical to the needy.

If surveillance is indeed required, can it be done effectively at an affordable cost? Major obstacles include limited physical and human resources (e.g. due to a high turnover of key personnel); poor supervision; lack of decentralization of activities; uncoordinated data collection and use; and inappropriate indicators in terms of relevance and simplicity.

8
Planning and implementation I

All nutritional surveys are undertaken on the basis of a 'theory' about the structure of nutritional problems and their causes and how they may be altered by various means. This theory is seldom explicitly stated, and often it is denied by the person or institution undertaking a survey that they have any pre-set perception of the situation they are studying, thus claiming that they are 'objectively' assessing the nutritional situation.

The theory will always influence the design and execution of a survey and this fact should be recognized. This does not mean that the survey only will provide confirmation of a pre-set hypothesis, but it will govern what kind of background factors and relationships that may be exposed by the survey.

Mgaza and Ljunquist (pers. commun., 1978)

There remains a basic ideological dispute between the advocates of screening (for action)[90] *('evangelists') and the advocates of the (never ending)*[90] *scientific method ('snails').*

Sackett and Holland (1975)

General

The sequence and range of activities undertaken in nutritional assessment will obviously vary with objectives (Table 7.1) and the type of investigation proposed (Table 7.2), financial and other resources, and other constraints (geographical, time, weather). Most of the following section is concerned with relatively large-scale surveys in technically less developed countries.[91] However, a systematic approach is needed in nutritional assessment in all situations relating to both populations and individuals. **The contents and suggestions in the present chapter are mainly concerned with large-scale surveys. They need to be used selectively in other forms of nutritional assessment** (Fig. 7.1).

Special selection will be needed for more usual small-scale investigations in a single village or in a series of schools or in a refugee camp. Many such limited studies can yield invaluable information.

[89] Added by present authors for clarification.
[90] Recent references include Rose and Barker (1978), Casley and Lury (1978), Ross and Vaughan (1986), Kelsey *et al.* (1986), and Marks (1987).

Table 7.1 General aims of nutritional assessment: epidemiological considerations *(Zerfas* et al. *1985)*

— Record the extent and severity of malnutrition, relative frequencies between groups under investigation, and trends over time with or without intervention
— Predict the occurrence of malnutrition and its distribution within populations, by identifying 'at risk' groups
— Explain the causes of malnutrition, attempt to measure their relative significance and to differentiate them from 'associated' factors
— Measure reductions in malnutrition rates in populations using preventive and curative interventions, both those within the health care system, and elsewhere, such as in agriculture and economics

Table 7.2 Categories of nutritional assessment: epidemiological categorization *(Zerfas* et al. *1985)*

Type of design	Major purpose	Example
Ecological (group)	Explore possible causes comparing groups	Low birth weight and social development
Cross-sectional	Determine extent (prevalence) of problems and resources	National nutrition surveys
Repeated cross-sectional	Assess change in communities over time	Intervention evaluation Nutrition surveillance
Longitudinal (cohort, prospective)	Assess change in individuals (e.g. derive incidence of new cases)	Factors (e.g. diet) influencing heart disease-Framingham study
Retrospective (case control, case history)	Convenient, approximate test for suspected causes	Determinants of severe protein–energy malnutrition in hospital patients and controls
Experimental	Most specific and difficult test for suspected causes	Food supplementation in pregnancy and influence on birth weight

In large-scale community nutritional assessment, it is helpful to consider including the following in this rational development process — *the reasons for initiating activities, preliminary considerations*, including a *tentative* plan, *reconnaissance visits* for feasibility purposes, followed by a *detailed plan* based on major objectives and how they can be most efficiently satisfied.

Technical planning will include selection of methods for *data collection*

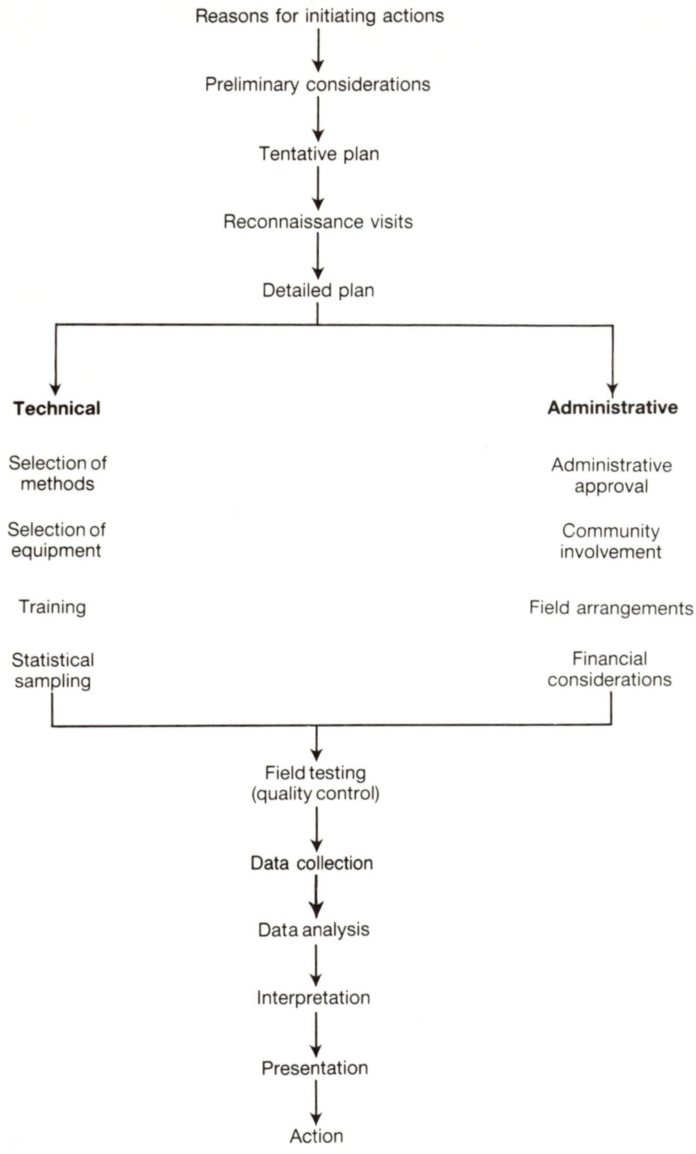

Fig. 7.1 Flow-chart of considerations often included in a large-scale nutritional assessment. It needs to be used selectively.

and analysis; statistical sampling, selection of equipment, recruitment and training of personnel, and *logistical requirements* (transport, time). Administrative planning will need to consider *government community, and public approval and involvement, field arrangements*, and *financial considerations*.

Following adequate field testing, the *nutritional assessment activity* should proceed (often as a community survey), with particular attention to *quality control*. As far as possible, data analysis should follow as soon as possible after the collection of field results, to prevent any backlog and unnecessary and frustrating technical, administrative, and political delays.

Interpretation and presentation of results

These need to be made in relation to agreed objectives, but always mainly concerned with their practical usefulness in effective action. With this in mind, data collected should usually be kept to the minimum required to give the information needed for action.

The extensive sequence of activities as presented here is given only as a guide — to be used selectively and modified flexibly as circumstances warrant. (**Fig 7.1**). Small projects will need to include only some of the items listed.

In general, the *goals* of such investigations should be directed to ultimate action. Goals should focus on how this complex process of information collection can be used to improve the nutritional status of the population. The *objectives* are more directly related to the information on nutritional status being obtained during the assessment process. For example, the goals of a cross-sectional survey may be to modify nutrition planning, policy, and programmes through appropriate, defined administrative or political actions. The objectives will include an estimation of prevalence rates of various types of malnutrition by area and among various at-risk groups, and at least suggestive information on some possible causes and at-risk groups. The objectives of such a community investigation should, when possible, include consideration of the available and potential services, and other resources in the area.

In addition, other available relevant information on the community (economic, food production, etc.) needs to be considered to provide an overall, if incomplete, picture of the state of nutrition in the particular area.

Results of such studies should provide technical facts to support any suggested actions, although administrative, financial, and political forces usually play a major role in ultimate decision-making.

There is always a continual struggle to balance objectives and limited resources. Resources are usually limited and fixed, but may be flexible. When fixed, objectives may have to be modified or restricted and activities planned accordingly.

Funds required will be determined by the scope, complexity, and duration of the activity and the requirements for personnel, equipment, and transport. Conversely, selection will have to be made from the wide range of options available depending on the usually limited funds. However, even when resources are limited, the *quality* of the data collected can still be kept at a satisfactory level, provided there is careful training and supervision is maintained.

Objectives will influence the design of the investigation. Examples of major epidemiological designs, their main purposes, and examples have been presented by Zerfas *et al.* (1985). The present account will be primarily concerned with large cross-sectional surveys, in which various personnel may be involved in the actual survey work. These may include senior investigators, supervisors, and surveyors, working together as a team.

The sequence of activities for other, often smaller community studies are similar in outline, but must be modified according to requirements, practical uses, and resources, including staff.

One potential future objective of every activity may be further investigations in the same situation for comparison purposes, including surveillance (p. 374), or in other areas, or with a different scope and content. Alternatively, other types of studies may be undertaken subsequently in the same community. These may include longitudinal surveys (p. 367) or more detailed tests (e.g. biochemical) (p. 31) of a statistically selected subsample, in order to obtain a better understanding of the possible causes of malnutrition and to identify at-risk groups, families, or individuals (p. 453).

However, such studies must avoid the 'further-research is eternally needed' syndrome — in which nothing positive is done, and the need for further investigation blocks any useful action.

An investigation of nutritional status of a community may be 'isolated' or incorporated into other studies, with similar or overlapping objectives. This includes 'piggy-backing' with other planned, funded health, socio-economic, or demographic surveys. Such co-operative ventures can lead to financial economies with regard, for example, to transport, statistical sampling, timing and duration of procedures, and choice of additional indicators. However, this type of combination can also cause difficulties, as the objectives and sequence of activities in the primary investigation will almost always be dominant. The challenge is to blend the two sets of objectives to supply mutually helpful information. This is often possible with diplomatic recognition of both groups' different, but often overlapping, needs, especially as regards sampling and transport.

Reasons for initiating activities

Information may be required for various reasons, including planning, policy-making, and evaluation of programmes by governmental and non-governmental agencies (Reutlinger and Selowsky 1976; Winikoff 1978; Joy 1973; Austin 1979; Berg 1981; Beaton 1982; Scrimshaw and Wallenstein 1982; Ghassemi and Teply 1983; Hruby 1983; McNaughton and Sabry 1983).

As part of the background in nutritional assessment, it is essential to understand the *general function and policies* of both governmental and non-governmental agencies, as well as those concerned with nutrition. This will enable a clearer picture of those who will be responsible for using the results of the investigation, as well as how and when decisions are made and who makes them. In turn, this may modify some details of the data collected and how results are presented.

Early enquiry is needed to appreciate the major reason (or, more usually, reasons) for suggesting action. Examples can include:

1. A government needs to know the extent and distribution of malnutrition throughout the country or region to decide on the most efficient allocation of limited resources (planning);
2. A primary health care programme requires information concerning its impact on the nutritional status of young children in the area served (evaluation);
3. A rural hospital is concerned about the reason why so many young children in their area are malnourished (investigation of causes);
4. A community (possibly influenced by a local health worker or a more educated and/or motivated citizen) wants to do something about malnutrition in the area (community programme development);
5. The Nutrition Division needs more funds and resources from government to undertake or expand specific programmes which have to be justified on a basis of factual and understandable evidence (administrative advocacy and policy development);
6. A politician wants to show that something is being done about malnutrition during his administration (political);[92]
7. A researcher requires information for scientific information and publication (increase scientific knowledge, personal academic advancement).[93]

Initially, it is necessary to review available information on the current nutritional situation, as well as existing and possible future policies, plans, or programmes relevant to the main nutritional problems. As much detail as possible should be obtained on such problems, including types of

[91] This can have the disadvantage that negative results may not be publicized, as witness the lack of publicity given to the deteriorating conditions in Ethiopia both in the 1970s and 1980s in quite different political circumstances.

[92] This remains an understandable motivation, whether stated or not. In less technically developed countries especially, field research by expatriates must *always*, but always, be (a) undertaken at the request of and with explicit approval by the administrative authorities concerned; (b) carried out, and published in partnership with national colleagues; (c) linked to public health priorities; and (d) never published without governmental approval.

malnutrition and populations at risk (e.g. age-groups, geographic areas, etc.).

Questions concerning additional information required in the course of nutritional assessment will have to consider: *where* it will be gathered and on *whom, what* should (and can) be the content, *how much* information is required and by *when*?

The need for rapid action occurring as a direct consequence of assessment varies with each situation. For example, in an acute emergency (drought, war), speed is essential. The methods used should be limited accordingly, even though care in attention to data collection and adequate planning are still required. For nutrition planning purposes, the link between assessment and ultimate action often may be prolonged, frequently depending on non-nutritional considerations, especially politics (p. 461). Nutritional investigations incorporated into programmes (e.g. evaluation) usually have a more direct impact in guiding or modifying activities, but may be difficult to undertake as 'evaluation' is often viewed exclusively as criticism.

Once issues concerning the reasons for assessment have been resolved, at least in principle, a thorough review is required to consider alternative practical and feasible methods to obtain needed information — some of which already may be available. Such methods can range from simple and inexpensive to costly and sophisticated. If a new study is needed, it is necessary to consider *who* will do it (including community participation) and *how* it will be undertaken, *when* it should begin, *how long* will it take, and, most important, the *total cost.*

When decisions have been made about any form of nutritional assessment, including community surveys, it is always necessary to consider the key question — *what will be done with the results*? Realistic consideration is needed as to the likelihood of appropriate actions; otherwise results will be filed and forgotten. This is too often the case. Positive governmental support, *rapid* analysis, and presentation of results in an understandable way often seem necessary ingredients (p. 449).

Preliminary activities

Initial discussions

Once a decision has been made on the method of nutritional assessment required, initial discussions should follow to consider the steps needed to develop and outline a tentative plan to clarify and define objectives. These objectives will then be submitted to the ultimate 'users' — all of whom will have been involved in prior discussions. These include administrators, representatives of health and other appropriate technical agencies, and members of the community itself. This outline or tentative plan should

Table 7.3 Some written sources of information

1. Published articles, books, reports
2. Non-published documents
3. Unreported data from prior studies
(a) Analysed
(b) Not analysed
(i) Edited
(ii) Not edited
4. Current studies

always refer to the key question: is this information necessary for appropriate decision-making?

Background information

A systematic search for existing information must be carried out (Table 7.3), as noted earlier (p. 146). Relevant data already may have been analysed and published for various purposes, which may be related (directly or indirectly) to the nutritional considerations in a community. Sources include publications (books, journals), either general or in the areas of nutrition, public health, medicine, sociology, anthropology, agriculture, economics, or demography. Unpublished reports of agencies, institutes, or meetings may be less readily available, but often present details of methods and procedures, as well as and other nutritional data. If further details are required, it may be useful to try to contact the sources of such reports. For example, summary tables may contain important data in a form that is not readily evident or sometimes not appreciated by the original compilers. Recourse to the original data and discussion with its authors sometimes can be useful for further understanding and analysis.

Relevant data may have been collected (perhaps coded and entered into files), but never analysed. This can often occur within busy agencies or institutes. It is important to know if such data is 'clean' (edited for obvious gross errors). Even data collected several years ago can be useful, especially as a basis of comparison, showing trends. Finally, ongoing studies in overlapping fields (such as family planning surveys) may have collected preliminary data of nutritional relevance — for example, on the pattern of breastfeeding. These may be made available, if the usefulness of the data is explained to the original investigators and if acknowledgement is assured.

Data obtained may be quantitative or qualitative. The former is most useful and technologically appealing, with numbers, rates, and proportions, provided its reliability can be judged. However, the qualitative information can also be useful, particularly where the observer indicates if the situation is usual or unusual. A detailed descriptive account can provide different and deeper insight into problems to complement numerical data.

The search for background information will include discussions with nationals, both within the country and abroad, such as university students, and with expatriates. Discussions should not be limited to the report writers or the senior people involved. Useful first-hand information can be obtained from available key individuals, such as trainers, supervisors, mappers, administrators, economists, epidemiologists, and statisticians. In this way, survey methods and procedures (manuals, interim reports, data sheets) can be reviewed.

Guidance from available information may have biases. For example, the educated urban elite of a country or a foreign physician working exclusively in a hospital may know little about the situation in rural villages or urban slums. There is also a need for awareness of the subconscious biases and/or technically limited vision of the investigators themselves. This can favour the selection of some sources of information, and minimize or disregard others. In all situations, a critical approach is needed.

Formation of a tentative plan

A tentative plan should provide an outline for the survey in preparation for a reconnaissance visit which can then test its feasibility in practice. Areas visited should be representative of the general population to be studied. Such a visit will involve consultation with local governmental authorities (including health service and agricultural extension officials) and with community or other leaders. The general methods and objectives of the investigation will need explanation in appropriate non-technical terms. The benefits that the community will receive need highlighting, but without exaggeration. Explanations are also needed concerning the assistance expected from the community, including accommodation for examinations and people to help with directing 'lines of flow' of individuals from one examination 'station' to another.

Reconnaissance visits

Initial field visits should follow administrative and political protocol, receiving advice, approval, permission, and advice from senior authorities. Initially the field visits require formal letters of introduction, with a brief official mention of why the study is being done and which agencies are represented. If possible, a senior local government representative should be present. This can improve the recognition and authority of the study, as well as exposing the senior agency representative to the field situation, which sometimes can be a novelty. On no account should the visit be misconstrued as threatening, e.g. related in people's minds to tax collection or conscription.

Explanations

The first meeting should deal with basic issues, especially the purpose of the survey. It should involve such local leaders and decision-makers, administrative and technical people (education, health, agriculture) as are available, preferably together, or separately. Before details of the survey are discussed, obviously some understanding of the type of community and its characteristics will need to be known. This should include the population structure, distribution of houses (e.g. villages or scattered), the major occupations, principal crops produced, socio-economic levels, etc. It is also useful to enquire if any other studies have been done, including information on their outcome and community reaction. If available, data from a recent census needs to be acquired.

The proposed content, timing, and duration of the survey should be briefly outlined. At the household level, clear explanations are required: who will be questioned about what and the importance of them being available on the appropriate day, who is to be examined and what records should be made available, if present (e.g. health cards, birth certificates).

In some larger surveys, further discussions may include the likely need for lists of household heads and their locations (if available) or the numbering of households for sampling purposes. If judged appropriate, the basic concept of sampling should be explained. It is obviously extremely difficult for lay people to understand why only certain households (often scattered and for no apparent reason) should be selected in the investigation.

The purpose and methods used in any potentially 'invasive' study or any 'frightening' methods must be explained. For example, finger-prick blood collection can be likened to malaria testing, if this is locally known. Even anthropometry (such as length and fatfold measurements) may be frightening to young children. For these reasons, demonstrating the equipment and its use in practice may be helpful, with older co-operative children as subjects.

Benefits to the community itself, both immediate (treatment or referral of sick individuals, feedback to the population of information concerning the results obtained), and the realistic possibility of long-term, future programmes, should be indicated when this is the case.

Feasibility

A critical question is whether the investigation can be carried out in a practical way, with 'minimal' encroachment on, and in co-operation with, the community itself.

Questions of feasibility should bear in mind the accessibility of households and individuals — both geographical (in distance and time) and cultural. A rough map showing roads, and locations of dwellings (villages or scattered) can be most useful in this context. It can also identify possible locations for examination points, if required, such as schools, churches, or mosques.

Knowledge of the climate to be expected is essential, particularly the time of the rainy season, its intensity, and the accessibility of roads, tracks, paths, and waterways during its course.

Understanding of community activities and events on a usual daily basis (times for farming, meals and snacks, schooling, etc.), during longer periods (market and religious days), and on a seasonal basis (farming and occupational cycles, local and distant migrations) is essential for organizing any surveys, especially those based on collection points, and in judging the most convenient time and duration for household visits.

Support

Support at the community level is important and should be encouraged. The more the community is involved and responsible for the survey, the greater their interest, co-operation, advice, and the greater the likelihood that community action will assist in subsequent programmes. Local people required may include at least one political representative (to assist protocol), organizers (to help direct people at collecting points), and educated individuals known to the community (teachers, public health inspectors) to assist in the preparation of such items as a local calendar of events, mapping, interpretation of questions used in the study, and the meaning of local vernacular terms.

Clerical assistance may be needed (e.g. in the preparation of an updated list of household heads for sampling purposes) in some surveys. A messenger for communicating between survey personnel or alerting households of forthcoming visits should be considered. Individuals to be included in the survey also should have been asked to be available on the particular day, and, when necessary, to have asked permission to do so from employers or school teachers.

Consideration also needs to be given to the personal requirements of members of survey teams. These will include local accommodation, food, and water (for washing and drinking). Local transport and availability of fuel may be discussed, especially if the community is large, sparsely populated, or separated by obstacles, such as rivers. Certain buildings or rooms may be required for temporary office quarters, examination sites, or overnight storage for equipment and supplies. If vehicles are employed in the study, they may require secure placement (locked compound or garage) or guards when not in use.

The question of some form of recompense must be considered. In general, services that involve costs (food, transport) or physical labour (porterage) usually have priority. Payment or otherwise for other services will depend on budget allocation, the agency represented, and the level of community participation.

Incentives for the people examined in the survey may have to be discussed, if funds are available. They may not be required nor permitted by governments, as they set a precedent for future studies. Before any commitment is made (as with those assisting in the study), it is necessary to find out discreetly whether community expectations are realistic. Any material incentives should not bias the population examined. A disadvantage, therefore, of including medical treatment is that it can attract those not in the sample, especially in areas where health services are sparse and inadequate. Under these circumstances, it is important to have someone present who can identify 'non-sample sick', who will then receive treatment or be referred without being included in the data that is subsequently analysed.

Detailed planning

Detailed planning involves an extension of the tentative plan, modified by feasibility (reconnaissance visit) and reviewed by peers (e.g. central planning committee.) Each revision should ultimately lead to a blueprint for formal field testing followed by further reviews (and perhaps retesting, if required) and training.

A formal commitment to goals, objectives (major, minor), the type of study, and the methods must be agreed upon. This commitment should be recorded for ready reference and review throughout all phases of the survey.

Definitions

Definitions are critical, both in technical and lay terms. For example, the uncertainties of interpretation in anthropometric indices, cut-off points, and sources of reference data must be resolved and agreement achieved.

Regarding a cross-sectional survey, such a documented statement may be: 'We consider protein–energy malnutrition (PEM) as defined by under a level of ______ of a reference value for __________ (source of data). PEM can be divided into wasting (low weight-for-height) and stunting (low height-for-age). Wasting indicates more recent onset (or acute) PEM and stunting is a reflection of prior episodes of PEM (or chronic)'.

Such definitions can be illustrated by photographs of individuals with protein–energy malnutrition and those without, including relevant histories, backgrounds, and likely outcomes based on prior studies, both local and non-local. Ideally, seeing affected children in a hospital setting is much more realistic and informative, especially as some administrators are unaware or forgetful that such conditions occur in their country.

Some questions may concern the numbers affected, with special reference to the prevalence in different areas of country.

Other problems with regard to definitions must be resolved by the technical investigators. These include differentiating causes from associations, identifying risk factors, and defining validity, reliability, etc. (Appendix 4). In discussion with non-technical individuals, such detail is rarely needed and should not be included. *It must be emphasized that the main report is primarily written for the users, not the doers of the study,* although publications of a more technical nature are also required. Details in the report should be directed to results and interpretations, complemented by their justification through accounts of the methods used, and quality control procedures used to insure accuracy. However, the report *should* anticipate key questions, such as was the sample adequate in size and quality? Were measurements done correctly?

Agreed definitions should be maintained throughout training, preparation of the report, and interpretation of the results.

Field methods

Planning for field work should take into account the choice of measures, methods, and organization of data collection, the selection of appropriate equipment and materials, sampling procedures, training and choice of personnel, logistical considerations, community co-operation, and cost requirements.

Choice of measures

Each objective must be accompanied by corresponding item(s) of information from which indicators (p. 395) and measures will be selected. For example, if the prevalence of under-nutrition is of concern, one item may be wasting. Its usual indicator will be the weight-for-height, related to the measures of weight and height for the appropriate sex and age.

Technical procedures

Techniques for procedures include those for organizational responsibilities ('protocol'), sampling, interview methods, and measurements. For protocol, an organizational chart can clarify responsibilities for field conduct, data collection, editing, supervision, and review.

Methods of measurement, units to be used and their precision, range, quality control procedures, and practicality will determine the equipment required, including especially the best use of appropriate technology (p. 96). Laboratory tests will depend not only on the availability of technicians and equipment, but also on the feasibility of collecting an adequate number of specimens, packaging, preservation, and timely transport to the laboratory (p. 32). For this reason, a field laboratory may be helpful, provided suitable energy (battery, electricity) and water sources are available and reliable (p. 35).

Organization of data collection

Site

Data may be collected from a central location (where subjects are assembled), during home visits, or in a combination. For example, the former may be more suitable for physical examinations and special tests, by senior technicians or professionals, as well as to help in supervision. The latter method is better for on-the-spot inspection of home conditions and for ensuring that all selected individuals are present.

In certain situations, such as camps (e.g. for refugees), institutions (workplace, hospitals, prisons), and schools, central points are plainly indicated, because of the convenience of working in such circumscribed, 'captive' populations. However, they are obviously not representative of communities at large. Even children examined in schools do not take into account those of appropriate age not attending because of distance, work at home, and/or poverty.

Household visits are obviously the most convenient for individuals or families, especially if distances, terrain, and lack of local transport are major obstacles. In addition, there may be prolonged waiting periods at the collecting point.

Mobile units parked as close as possible to the selected households (e.g. within a mile or further if transport is provided or available) may be a suitable compromise. However, this is expensive and depends on adequate roads for the units, more likely to be affordable in more technically developed countries. This is the method, for example, used by the National Center for Health Statistics in the Health and Nutrition Examination Surveys in the USA.

If an adequate listing of potential survey subjects and their residences is available, it may be possible to examine most of them at the collecting point and the rest at home. The closer the location (fixed or mobile) is to the households the better. Thus, if a cluster of adjacent households are selected, a central point for these may be considered. In some instances, it may be useful to have neighbours present for complementary information (e.g. verifying ages by comparing the age of their child with that of the subject's). In other circumstances, privacy of interview and examination will be necessary.

Collecting data during home visits has added advantages in ensuring response. Even if respondents are initially absent, local questioning may indicate their movements, so return visits can be appropriately planned. For repeated non-attenders, at least some basic information can sometimes be obtained (e.g. through neighbours). At times, visits to farms may be required. In these cases, practical limits for the greatest distance travelled and time spent by surveyors should be clarified. If adequate pre-survey information is available, localities outside this range may have to be excluded from the population to be sampled.

Telephone and mail interviews may be attempted in more technically developed countries. However, in such conditions, self-reporting of facts (e.g. body weight) may be unreliable and descriptions of food intake suspect. The further the separation from personal contact with subjects, their homes, and customary background, the more difficult it is to verify their responses directly or by inference from the home environment.

Procedures

If surveys are undertaken at central collecting points, 'lines of flow' need to be organized for a sequence such as registration, questions, measurements, clinical signs, laboratory, and other special tests. Space and time considerations for each activity will determine the most effective sequence. For young children, painful procedures should be avoided, or, if needed, are best undertaken last. Once decided, a time-and-motion trial using a few subjects should be done. The forms are best kept with the person being examined throughout the procedures or with a child's mother (or accompanying relative).

Even at the household level, a similar systematic sequence must be followed, modified by local circumstances. These include the availability of shelter from the sun, wind, and rain, of lighting at night, of activities during the interview and of structures for equipment (e.g. a sufficiently strong horizontal house beam or tree for hanging a scale). In the last situation, it may be more convenient to measure several children consecutively. When included, adults should be measured before children, with the two sexes dealt with in separate rooms or different times.

Appropriate times for visiting households during the survey need to be determined. In addition, market days, occasions for feast or fast, and other culturally-related events should be noted. Such a record overlaps with the monthly calendar of events, sometimes prepared to assist in the determination of the ages of young children.

Degree of detail Data collection may include rapid ecological visits, during which observation at the local level of various situations related to food availability and sources of infection can be undertaken. These include home gardens, food storage, village stores, methods of food preparation (p. 187), sanitation, water supply (p. 156), etc. Such observations are required to complement information from discussions with local leaders. Selection of the most useful sites to include in these rapid ecological visits can be decided in the planning phase.

More detailed methods of data collection include photographs, extensive descriptions, and even tape recordings or filming. These are difficult to systematize, but can be used to enhance the 'flavour' of the report. Photographs are useful tools to illustrate the usual or unusual, and to indicate visually the type of community being investigated. Also, they may strengthen or clarify important issues or messages in the report presentations, and make suggested programmes more realistic and understandable.

The anthropological methods of participant and non-participant observation may be feasible in certain situations (Pelto and Pelto 1978; Scrimshaw and Hurtado 1987). Child-following, for example, is an extremely detailed and prolonged procedure (Wilson 1979), but can provide insight into several aspects of nutrition, including sources of food and activity patterns (p. 210). This method is obviously limited by constraints of time and personnel and usually can only be done with a small sample.

In all such detailed descriptive accounts, the representativeness of the sample and difficulties with the analysis of often qualitative information must be borne in mind.

Recording procedures

Recording procedures involve the systematic documentation of observations, replies to questions, and findings at examination. Information concerning the locality (i.e. in a specifically defined area, such as a village) may require a special form. Items to consider may include the name of village (or community), the distance from services, such as market, schools, health centre, towns (both in kilometres and time of travel by usual transport), and type of local road. Such questions need then not be separately asked at the household level.

For households, a special form may be required for registration of members, their name, age, sex, occupation, whether present, etc. Such information is also needed for correct sampling, as well as a record of possible non-attenders.

The usual record for more detailed household and individual information is the questionnaire. Such questionnaires can be considered in terms of size, content, and design. Although usually not practicable, copies of the final product are desirable, (e.g. using 'copy sensitive' NCR) or carbon sheets, providing the copy is aligned properly). Both the content and the design of the questionnaire should be easily read and understood by the surveyor.

Computers have greatly facilitated from design. Conversely, all forms should be prepared with a view to computer analysis.

Draft questionnaires may be stencilled or photocopied; the final version should be printed, particularly if several hundred or more are required. Unless carefully done by an excellent machine, mimeographs are not recommended as they may be difficult to read and do not encourage quality work. For a small added cost, quality paper should be considered, usually white. For durability, thin cardboard has been used. However, copies cannot be made and similar firmness can be obtained with paper forms and a proper backing (e.g. a clipboard).

In preparing a questionnaire, the questions to be asked and measures to be recorded need listing in the appropriate order. It is then necessary to consider the logical procedure and sequence with which the subjects will be questioned and examined. For example, identifying information first, then essential demography, such as household size, followed by age determination, general nutrition, related topics (e.g. weaning habits), then specific ones, followed by measurements, signs, and special tests. Last, more detailed information may be required for a special investigation or group, (e.g. diets of young children), and conveniently placed on a separate page. Questions will usually need to be translated into the local language. They should then be tested by 'back-translating' by an indigenous English-speaking interpreter in order to test their understanding abilities.

Questions must be directed to the subject's own experiences. Brown *et al.* (1979a) list bad and good examples of questions. Words such as 'usually', 'often', 'sometime', etc. are vague and difficult to define. A specific, short, time period must be indicated (e.g. since this time yesterday; the past week, indicating the day of starting). Major weaknesses of cross-sectional studies are the completeness and reliability of such recall information.

In general, there should be no leading questions (i.e. that hint at an expected result). For example, 'do you (or you do) look after this child most of the day?' This might encourage a 'yes' answer from the mother, because she feels it is expected of her. This is reinforced by the tone of the question as well.

Close-ended questions anticipate a reply that can be directly coded. The simplest range of answers is 'yes', 'no', and 'don't know'. Other answers may be based on a prepared check list which anticipates most of the likely replies, those not being on the list being included as 'other' or the reply recorded as such.

Reading out a list of possible answers to the subject (e.g. local foods in a diet study) has the advantage of adequate coverage. However, it may also encourage false positive replies (i.e. 'yes' answers when truly 'no').

'Probes' are added questions which try to clarify the original query or answer. They are particularly important in dietary studies, where food items may be overlooked. For example, 'what foods has this child eaten since this time yesterday?' If the answer includes a stew, the probe would be 'what foods were in that stew?'

From what age the child can be questioned depends on whether an accurate response can be expected, based on the actual question and the local culture, education, etc. Generally, the mother or caretaker is the respondent, especially for pre-school age children. However, for certain information (e.g. food eaten outside the household and not known by the caretaker), direct questioning of older children may be required. Similarly, an older sibling may be a more appropriate respondent for such items about young children.

Coding and directions

Sufficient space must be allocated for coding and for presenting code numbers in a different way (e.g. italicized) to other numbers on the form to avoid confusion. Code sequences should end at 80 for punch card entry, but for direct computer entry may extend much further, to be clarified with the appropriate consultants. Numbering sections and questions have value for reference and training purposes, although code numbers may suffice.

Directions on the form should be confined to essential issues, and written in different print to the questions. It is necessary, for example, to decide what procedures are important enough to warrant frequent reminders, realizing that such directions will use up potential space for other items.

Design

The design of forms should be clear and unambiguous. Issues such as whether items and results read down or across the page will also depend on ease of understanding, space and coding requirements. When the same questions are asked of different subjects, a matrix design[94] may be most economical of space. Small print should be easily readable. It is essential to draft a few layouts, then pre-test them using mock interviews, before deciding on the most appropriate and readily understood design.

If data is collected by village workers, in certain communities, the design and format may have to be modified considerably (e.g. for illiterate recorders). The use of appropriate diagrams or illustrations has been

[93] Matrix design: questions and subjects are arranged in columns and rows.

tested in countries, such as Indonesia and Egypt, for village workers to send in simple information on morbidity and mortality.

Space should be left on such forms in case comments need to be made by investigator or supervisor. The forms should be 'computer-ready' (i.e. prenumbered for data editing, etc.).

Equipment

All requirements of field equipment must be listed in detail. The needs for training and for field supervisors must also be considered. For each item, information is needed on the numbers required; size, shape, and weight (for porterage and storage); cost; availability; repair and maintenance. Packaging needs should account for economy of space and protection from nature (rain, dust) and humans (being dropped or stolen). Boxes, bags, or thick plastic sheets may be required for wrapping.

The cost and maintenance of the instruments are not the only financial factors to be borne in mind. Others include salary of the measurer, special training required, and the 'correction cost'. This cost is related to the increased time and effort required to edit or repeat suspect measures caused by problems, such as inappropriate equipment or carelessness of workers.

Technical Description of technical equipment has been given elsewhere[95] (p. 64), including consideration of appropriate technology. In general, the hence surveyors or teams, the less total equipment is required, with lesser costs and constraints (e.g. of porterage). More sophisticated equipment and personnel may require central collecting points. For longitudinal studies where continuous data is needed, equipment may be left on site, providing it is properly secured and the population sample is conveniently located.

All equipment should be labelled with the name of the responsible person or team member. All items allocated should be signed for by the recipient. Rules must be clearly defined. For example, loss or damage to key items due to negligence may result in the deduction of pay or benefits for those concerned.

Anthropometric equipment ranges from bulky (height/length board) to small (tape). The local construction of boards must consider total length and weight for appropriate field use, apart from specific measurement concerns. For example, if surveyors need to carry the board by bicycle, hinges should be considered to reduce its total length. In other situations, the board itself can be used as a frame for packing of other items and carried on the head of a bearer.

[94] The OXFAM field pack is described elsewhere (p. 363).

The Salter hanging scale has a convenient shoulder bag for ease of carrying. At the opposite extreme, precise sophisticated scales may be damaged over rough terrain, even when carefully packed in vehicles.

More detailed dietary recall information requires local measures (spoons, cups, etc.) and, if available, and affordable, food models. Special weighing scales will be required if household food consumption is undertaken (p. 193). Blood collections not only need the basic equipment (e.g. stylettes, tubes, glass slides, etc.), but also cotton wool, alcohol for swabs, adhesive tape, labels, markers, and containers, both for unused equipment and the collected materials. The convenience of field analysis of laboratory specimens (overcoming transport problems back to base) must be balanced by the local need for a power source, running water, stains, microscope, and refrigerator, as well as field technicians (p. 32).

Records These include maps, manuals, and directives which must be available at all times. Protection from water, dirt, and dust is essential. Unused questionnaires should be arranged in suitable folders, perhaps with a clipboard, and, when completed, put in a large envelope, appropriately labelled. Notebooks, pencils, sharpeners, and erasers, as well as a felt pen (e.g. for marking the midpoint of the upper arms) are required.

Special forms may be needed, such as for messages or referrals. In large-scale surveys, a transport log needs to be prominently displayed in the vehicle and removed only when instructed by seniors (e.g. for review). Receipt books with carbon are necessary for records of cash disbursements.

A diary or log of daily activities is recommended. It can be compiled briefly at the end of the day following discussion with team members.

Medical Medical requirements include those for subjects to be examined, survey personnel, and the general population, (e.g. in an emergency). Common illnesses in the area and conditions felt to be important by the local populace should be reviewed. Drugs (e.g. aspirin, antimalarials) may be prepackaged in small envelopes or wrapped in paper, with appropriate labelling for ease of dispensing.

Tongue depressors for ointment applications, swabs for solutions (e.g. gentian violet) and appropriate containers (bottles, boxes) need to be available, as required.

The complexity of equipment and range of drugs depend on prior arrangements made for health care during the survey and the backgrounds of the surveyors. Treatment may be supplied directly by survey personnel or through referrals to the local clinics, preferably ensuring that these have been supplied with added drugs, etc.

Inducements, if any, may be provided on a locality (for chief or elders) or household basis. For the former, a culturally acceptable gift may be suitable. At times photographs of key leaders (with family) are popular. for subjects, soap, matches, pencils, or small notebooks may be appropriate, have local value, and are not directly health-related. The provision of sweets to children is a useful placator and minimizer of 'epidemic' crying.

In all circumstances, inducements should be consistent with local policy in not creating undesirable precedents for future studies.

For surveyors themselves, minor injuries and illnesses should be promptly attended to, before they reach a more serious stage. Paints, gauze, and adhesive plasters are required for skin cracks, fissures, and abrasions; crepe bandages for sprains. Locally effective malarial prophylaxis and a suitable supply of antibiotics and analgesics should be borne in mind, as well as provision for safe drinking water.

General The range of equipment needed for a survey obviously varies with local circumstances. It can often usefully include folding chairs, tables, provision for lighting (kerosene or hurricane lamps, torches, and batteries), and perhaps a power source (car battery or even a generator, as required). Adequate fuel must be assured for survey vehicles. If the study is conducted in the open, shelter from rain or sun may be necessary (tents, canopies). Central points for examination may require added equipment, such as partitions, and containers for filing or storage of forms, equipment, and specimens.

If surveyors and supervisors are responsible for their own personal requirements in the field, it is still wise to check whether their selection is appropriate. This includes the need for shelter (tent); food (local, prepurchased, cooking utensils, etc.); water; sleep (camp cots, mats, bedding); clothes and washing; basic recreation materials; and cash.

9

Planning and implementation II

The survey statistician is essentially an engineer, working to design and implement a product meeting as closely as possible the specifications of his client, the survey user. Like any other engineer, he finds his client specifying requirements which are not equally attainable: some can be met, some cannot be met, and some can be met only if others are dropped. This situation obliges him to return to his client for a more detailed specification, including an indication of priorities where requirements conflict. Thus, in the early stages at least, the role of the survey statistician is to engage in a dialogue with the survey user/sponsor; together they have to develop a plan for a product which can *be built and which satisfies as closely as possible the needs of the latter.*

Scott *et al.* (1980)

A figure is a delicate and sensitive thing which, put on the rack, will confess according to the desires of the torturer.

Alfred Savvy (1984) FAO, Rome, pers. commun.

Sampling[96]

There are two major considerations in sampling: *sample design* and *sample size*. Sample design involves the method of sampling and carrying it out. The need for a random sample with acceptable coverage and response rate is essential for cross-sectional surveys. Errors related to this are often difficult to estimate and may cause serious doubts concerning the acceptance of the sample data as reflecting the population of concern. Sample size, on the other hand, is concerned with the 'precision' of results, (i.e. how the results vary from that which would be obtained if the entire population were surveyed.) Hence, results from samples include as estimate and a range of statistical confidence ('confidence interval') (Appendix 4) around the estimate.

[95] Relevant systems of sampling are described in Castle (1979, pp. 25–40), Continua Productions (1975, pp. 45–70), Babbie (1979, pp. 73–112), Lwanga and Choo Yook-Tye (1986), Lutz (1982), and Bender *et al.* (1982.)

Sampling guidance

Invariably, some form of early and sustained statistical guidance will be required for sampling. The interrelationships between surveyors and statisticians is indicated in the first quotation given at the beginning of this chapter. Such a statistician must be experienced *both* in theory *and* in field work of a nature similar to the current investigation, to have a balanced view of what is mathematically 'correct' and what is practical.

Consultation should be available throughout the survey as plans may have to be modified and adequately defended. Complex formulae and statistical jargon must be translated into everyday language to ensure adequate understanding.

The statistician responsible for advice on sampling will require briefing on survey objectives; areas to be described (geographical, urban/rural, etc.); units of analysis (e.g. localities, households, individuals); type of study design (e.g. cross-sectional, longitudinal); indicators being used, with expected results (e.g. prevalence figures) and methods of presentation intended; resources (maps, listings); and constraints (time, funds, logistics, and personnel).

General and specific strategies both in sample design and size (with suitable alternatives) should be reviewed. This relates to delineation of the population to be sampled (study population or 'universe') (Appendix 4), excluding certain areas (e.g. for reasons of inaccessibility) and groups based on likely non-cooperation (e.g. for political or cultural reasons), or irrelevance to objectives (single-member households or those without young children, if these are the only subjects of interest). From this should be derived a sample frame (list of units to be sampled) which usually include sample sites (locations). Within these sites are sources of information for analysis (subjects or items of interest), such as households, individuals, and records (e.g. health centre growth charts).

Type of sample

Unless there are acceptable reasons to the contrary, the method of sampling must be random — that is, with an equal or known probability of selection for each unit, using a random numbers table or its equivalent. Only with a random sample can prevalence rates, resulting from the survey, be applied to the population of concern, from which the sample was selected. A random sample is usually, but not always, representative of the population. However, it is statistically correct and utterly defensible.

Types of random sampling include simple, systematic, multistage, cluster, and stratified.

Non-probability or non-random sampling may be of several varieties:

two include 'convenience' and 'judgemental'. The convenience method selects the most readily available subjects. For example, in emergency situations, due to time constraints and accessibility to populations, those nearest major roads ('tarmac surveys') or at food distribution centres may be selected. This also includes the impressions some dignitaries observe in people nearest their vehicle or in a few key areas visited. Often healthier, more mobile, or wealthier subjects are better represented unless there is a special reason for the ill to be present (e.g. expectations of treatment or free gifts, such as food).

A judgemental sample considers 'representative' groups or individuals, perhaps based on broad geographical or socio-economic considerations. However, such characteristics require more relevant detailed information about these groups, and how they differ from those not selected. Such judgements are often based in part on subjective criteria.

As a general rule, if random sampling is not done, the general features of the area or group should be described as thoroughly as possible, including similarities and differences from populations other than those sampled.

Information on population or 'universe'

Census data may be the only complete listing of a population available. It also should provide basic demographic information (e.g. names of subjects, age and sex distribution, occupations, and household size). For application to the population to which the survey is directed recourse may be needed to census subgroup descriptions not included in the major report, but sometimes available with systematic search of records. For young children, age may not be reliable, depending on the method of determination.

Data from a census loses value if not up-to-date. In some communities (e.g. transient, semi-urban), migrations, as well as births and deaths, may greatly modify a population listing after only a few years.

Other lists are likely to be incomplete and biased towards their specific purpose, such as a tax list for registered household heads; agricultural lists limited to landholders; and lists of telephone numbers limited to those with better socio-economic status.

Last, in some parts of the world, no census data will be available or in a suitably documented form.

Maps

Maps are essential for sampling procedures to determine population distribution and accessibility. They are also needed to delineate enumeration areas (EAs) or census tracts. These areas are defined geographically to encompass a population size, often from 500 to 2000.

The availability of maps include commercial (e.g. for tourists) and government (e.g. land and natural resources, military, census) sources, or maps from special studies (university, agencies) limited to the area of interest. Maps should be updated and relevant details included, such as roads requiring four-wheel drive vehicles, public transport routes, and the situation during the wet season.

Detailed maps of small areas will usually be unavailable. They require extensive preparation (aerial photographs or ground surveys) and specialized cartographic assistance for identifying individual households and detailed features of the area. Small-area maps need not be prepared unless sampling is done within that area. Even then, the type of sample (as described below) will determine the map size and degree of detail needed. Maps are invaluable for revisits for non-attenders, during both cross-sectional or longitudinal studies.

Methods of sampling

Simple random sampling is the most statistically correct method, but often is not used. It is too cumbersome to select individual units from a large total, and may tend to favour one part of an area due to chance.

Systematic sampling is more convenient than simple random sampling. It selects every nth unit after *randomly* choosing the first. Thus, if $n=10$, then the first selected would be between 1 and 10 (n), say 5, and the following 15 (5 + 10), the next 25 (5 + 10 + 10), 35, 45, etc.

Both simple random and systematic sampling requires enumeration of *all* units of analysis (e.g. households or subjects) prior to selection. This is clearly an impractical task for large samples.

Multi-stage sampling bypasses this problem, as the procedure is staged. Enumeration areas or specific population groups (e.g. villages) are first selected randomly ('primary sample unit') then subjects within these ('secondary sample units'). For each area only an estimate of the *total* population is required; only those areas selected need further enumeration. Within these smaller population groups, simple random or systematic sampling can be done more conveniently.

An even more practical method is *cluster sampling*, where groups are selected instead of units. For example, if the unit is a household and 20 are required in the sample, an area of 100 households can be separated into 10 groups, each of 10 households. Two of these 10 can be randomly sampled and *all* households within these chosen groups be included in the study. Another approach randomly selects the *first* household, then continues in a *pre-determined direction* (e.g. based on consecutive household numbers) until the total of 20 is obtained. This is better than selecting the nearest other households, which is based on convenience and favours more densely adjacent households.

The major disadvantage in cluster sampling is that units within the selected group tend to be similar in the characteristics studied. For example, malnourished children are more likely to belong to the same neighbourhood. This reduces the effective sample size required to estimate such characteristics.

Stratified sampling primarily pertains to the population which is to be sampled. This population is separated into parts (stratified), each part being sampled independently of the other (e.g. urban, rural). This has two major purposes: to reduce sample size needs and to enable complete descriptions of each part. Within each stratum selected, characteristics relating to the item of concern (e.g. protein–energy malnutrition) should be as uniform as conveniently possible. These include, for example, urban: high socio-economic status and relatively low prevalence of malnutrition; peri-urban (slum): poor health facilities, overcrowding; rural: subsistence economy, low level of health services.

Sample size

Results from a sample will always be an approximation to that of the population sampled. The greater the sample size the closer (i.e. more 'reliable') will be such results, given that measurement and other errors are similar. This reliability (or 'precision') is measured by a statistical term called 'confidence interval'. The greater the sample size, the smaller this interval and the more reliable the result.

For example, if the prevalence of stunting in a sample survey was 20 per cent, the expected ('true') result for that population might be 20 ± 5 per cent, for a sample size of approximately 250. Convention usually requires a 'level of probability' of 0.05. This means that if a random sample of similar size was repeated 100 times from the same population, the expected result would be outside 15 per cent and 25 per cent (20 ± 5 per cent) five times out of 100 (level of probability = 5/100). Thus in a single sample, the probability of this occurring is low — one can be 'confident' of this approximation.

If more reliable results are required (e.g. 20 ± 2.5 per cent), then the sample size would have to be greater (actually equal 1000) with increased work load and costs.

This reliability factor (or confidence interval) (Table 8.1) will also vary with the estimated prevalence. For example, a rare condition (i.e. with a prevalence of 1 per cent) would require a relatively small interval (e.g. 0.5 per cent) with closer approximation to the population result. This would require a relatively large sample size (about 1600).

Working out an acceptable sample size for a cross-sectional survey is

Table 8.1 Expected 95 per cent confidence limits* by sample size and disease prevalence simplified approach *(Burgess and Burgess 1974)*

Expected prevalence (per cent)	Confidence limits (per cent) for sample numbers of:			
	300	400	500	1000
2	0.9–4.2	1.0–3.8	1.1–3.6	1.3–3.0
5	2.8–8.1	3.1–7.6	3.3–7.3	3.7–6.5
10	6.9–14.0	7.2–13.4	7.5–13.0	8.2–12.0
15	11.2–19.5	11.7–18.9	12.0–18.4	12.9–17.4
20	15.6–25.0	16.2–24.3	16.6–23.8	17.6–22.6

* See Appendix 9.

usually an 'educated guess', because the prevalence of the conditions of interest (e.g. wasting, stunting, etc.) are not known and must be roughly estimated (Table 8.1). Because more than one estimate is usually required (e.g. prevalence of low height-for-age, weight-for-height, anaemia, etc.), each should be considered and a compromise made for a single sample size, taking into account their possible results and the 'acceptable' levels of precision required. It must be noted that if separate descriptions are required for parts of the sample (e.g. subsample, age groups of children by year) their precisions will be much wider, due to the reduced sample size in each part or subgroup.

For investigators with little statistical training, a knowledge of the terms used and general understanding of the methods employed are essential to permit satisfactory, meaningful dialogue with statisticians. At the same time, expert statistical guidance and advice are always needed to minimize errors. Also, information can be found in the books listed previously (p. 405).

Actually, in real-life circumstances in most large-scale surveys of nutritional assessment, sample size ultimately has to be a mathematically guided educated guess, compromised by such local constraints as geography and accessibility. Such facts need clearly noting in any report.

Training

Training extends far beyond the proper application of techniques for the collection of field data. The scope also includes correct conduct and attitudes towards officials and the individuals being assessed, recognition of logistical requirements and communication, and care of equipment and materials. It also includes methods of dealing with special problems. Some of these need to be anticipated, such as the comfort and health of the investigators, and non-attendance or non-cooperation of subjects. Almost inevitably, other problems will not and cannot be anticipated. These may necessitate referral for advice or action, or, in remote situations, the need for on-the-spot decision-making. In general, unplanned alteration of field procedures must be kept to the minimum.

In training, as in field work, the team approach must be emphasized. Details will vary with the type of study being undertaken and the size of the team. In large-scale, often national surveys, interaction between senior personnel, trainers, supervisors, and sureyors should be maintained. Formal and informal meetings with pertinent agenda and records of topics and discussions should be held occasionally to recognize and deal with technical, administrative, and personal matters.

Prior to training, questionnaires and methods to be used in the investigation must be finalized. This involves thorough field testing, preferably using as close to a full-scale rehearsal as possible. Such testing should include observation of the strengths and limitations of the surveyors. Many surveys entail prolonged field work under difficult and uncomfortable conditions.

Training should be practical and clearly understood and modified appropriately to the educational level of the surveyors, as well as the methods employed (equipment, time taken, recording, etc.). Systematic analysis of the tasks and subtasks to be performed is invaluable, including the knowledge, attitude, and skills for ('mental, manual, communication') (Abbatt 1980).

From the start of training, there should be no assumptions made of prior knowledge of the trainees. All too often, they may have acquired imprecise methods, such as with weighing, which require correcting. For example, some health professionals may belittle the care needed for an acceptable anthropometric measure, considering it to be routine, 'low-technology', and boring to do.

Training must be oriented at all times to the field situation, and the sooner field practice, supervision, and review occur, the better. Only in this situation can a true test for performance take place. Prior to this, field simulations with 'role playing' are practical alternatives.

Evaluation of performance must involve the whole training team. Trainees must learn to 'edit' (correct obvious gross errors) and review their own work. In large surveys, supervisors' key functions include assistance and checking of those working under their direction. However, no level of worker should be immune from evaluation. Hence, formal procedures for evaluation should be incorporated into training manuals and results tactfully made known to those concerned.

Sequence of training

Initial instruction will not only include techniques, but should emphasize the proper approach to the subjects and to the survey itself. This will

Table 8.2 General basic principles for survey trainees: a practical guide

(1) Follow the training instructions exactly
(2) Get all the information required
(3) Be very careful all the time
(4) Think about the answer when you write it down
(5) Practice as often as you can
(6) Show problems to your supervisor for discussion and advice

involve an explanation of objectives of the investigation, who needs the information, and what will be done with the results. It is important to stress the need for quality of data to be obtained and the surveyors' responsibility for this. This is of particular importance as it is an aspect of a survey that can be given greater certainty. Key survey items (equipment, methods, recording) must be outlined. A practical guide to general principles is useful (Table 8.2).

Practice will involve selected levels of field simulation. Ideally, this should move from classroom, school, clinic, and institution to representative field sites. At first, this should involve a few subjects, but later should include a larger number, especially sampling and logistical exercises. Supervision should include on-the-spot checks and corrections where necessary. This should be followed later by review of procedures, involving frank, supportive discussion between training personnel with a judicious balance of praise and criticism. Evaluation of training involves repeated formal and informal tests, with appropriate records for results.

The whole procedure for instruction, practice, supervision, review, and evaluation is repetitive and reinforcing. Even during the survey itself, review and retraining is often required. It is useful to allow for a short break for this review after the first few days of the survey proper. This is helpful in ironing out problems — technical, logistical, and personal.

Tables 8.2 and 8.3 need consideration when devising training for surveys and for ongoing activities.

In large-scale surveys, the supervisors should first be trained, the duration determined by the amount of time available. Obviously, their competence should be better than the trainees and they will require added skills for more complex procedures, such as sampling and a higher level of seniority to help with initial contacts with community leaders.

A detailed schedule for training should be prepared together with a training manual. The schedule should be realistic.

Selection of training personnel

Personnel may be available from several sources. This includes health services: physicians, nurses, public health inspectors, technicians (labora-

Table 8.3 Training: special considerations regarding community workers

Proposed function		
Recognition main issues	Illness Environment	Malnutrition Infections
Ability	Advise (includes higher education) Basic treatment Report Refer	
Level of Western-style education		
Literacy Pictorial literacy Mathematical literacy	Pre-test Method of reporting	
Practical		
Actual apparatus Field circumstances (role-playing)		
Adequate accuracy		
Quality control Supervision/check Refresher discussions		

tory and others), auxiliary workers, primary health care (community health care) workers, or students; agricultural services: extension workers; educational system: home economists, teachers, high school leavers. Nutritionists and dieticians, if available, are particularly required for obtaining dietary information, provided that they have had experience in community nutrition activities.

Often, there may be little or no choice in the availability of trainees. For that reason, in large-scale surveys it is wise to accept as many as possible for initial screening. At their interview, key questions include attitudes and motivation (e.g. 'Will you be prepared to stay overnight in a village?' 'Walk up to 10 miles in a day, if required and eat at unusual times?' 'Abide by all the rules for survey procedures?'). Age and sex are important in relation to cultural acceptance by the population being surveyed. For example, personal questioning of mothers and obtaining dietary information are usually best done by females. An older individual may gain more respect as a surveyor than someone younger. In studies involving diverse peoples and languages, multilingual surveyors will be essential. The degree of literacy required depends on the complexity of the questionnaires used.

Regular employees seconded to the study are preferred, as they are usually better motivated, often have a relevant background for the study, and are more likely to ensure continuity for future studies, such as a repeat survey or surveillance. However, their present job will need to be filled with a substitute, so that they may be readily available for the full duration of field work in an extensive survey.

Even after initial screening, the numbers of trainees accepted should be consistently greater than required. After a few days training, an interim evaluation should be conducted to exclude those obviously unsuitable for the tasks, if this is politically acceptable. Such tests should be practical and be on the tasks they will be expected to perform (Abbatt 1980).

Supervisors should be experienced in field studies and have an understanding of community nutrition. Responsible workers previously engaged in other studies, such as the census or general household surveys, are often suitable. If there is a lack of suitable supervisors, these may be selected from the trainees towards the end of the training period.

Training content

An example of a training manual outline used for a *large-scale cross-sectional survey* illustrates the content to be included (Table 8.4). Not only is a manual helpful for training purposes, it also provides a record of definitions, methods, and procedures for field work, which can be consulted when required. However, the tasks listed need to be broken down into practical subtasks and skills required (Abbatt 1980).

Purpose

The central and first focus of attention must be directed to the purpose (objectives) of the study — that is, who needs the information and how it will be used. The importance in collecting accurate data cannot be overstressed; otherwise results will be invalid and the work suspect. Even at this point, it is useful to indicate that there are methods of checking fieldwork (e.g. in data analysis) which will show errors of data collection traceable to the particular surveyor or trainee.

The trainee should be aware of the personal benefits of the study, both in experience and, perhaps, later advancement, providing the work is satisfactory.

Maps of area

A map of the area to be studied and a more detailed map of a survey site (with appropriate scales and headings) should make the trainees aware of

Table 8.4 Training manual: comprehensive table of contents, particularly suitable for large-scale, often national surveys. Selection of appropriate items is needed for smaller-scale assessment activities

1. Purpose of survey
2. Maps of area
3. Job descriptions
4. Training sites and facilities
5. Schedules for training and the field study
6. Definitions, abbreviations
7. Requirements for inclusion of subjects in the study
8. Human subject procedures
9. Study content-outline
    - Introduction to questionnaires
    - General instructions for completing forms
    - Survey items
    - Formcheck; editing
10. Field procedures
    - Transportation
    - Communication
    - Survey responsibilities
11. Mapping
12. Sampling
    - Registration of households
    - Approach to absent subjects
13. List and diagrams of equipment and supplies (anthropometric, dietary, laboratory, general)
14. Referrals for ill persons
15. Coping with problems
    - Personal
    - Administrative
    - Technical
16. Evaluation of training
    - Criteria for selection of surveyors and supervisors
    - Critical performance tests
    - Standardization tests
17. Appendices
    - Local calendar of events

the scope of the exercise and the logistics involved — both between the areas to be visited and within them. In addition, such maps will be in constant use during the study.

Job descriptions

Job descriptions should be clearly outlined, leaving no doubt as to what is expected of all those in the study and clarifying training objectives.

Training sites and facilities

A brief description of the training sites and facilities is useful to introduce trainees to methods of presentation and materials used, both in the classroom and in the filed. It also provides no excuses for people being lost during training! A more detailed outline for evaluation of training may be presented later in the manual.

Schedules

Preliminary schedules for training and for the survey proper should be presented. These will help to clarify the availability of both trainees and instructors. Sufficient time should be allowed for rest periods and for trainees to attend to their personal needs. Unlike training, schedules for field work must be oriented to survey needs, and may involve, for example, starting the working day very early.

Definitions and abbreviations

Definitions should be brief and restricted to the content and objectives of the survey. A list of abbreviations appearing in the manual or on the questionnaire may also be required (e.g. NA — not applicable, ID — identification number, cm — centimetre, HH — household).

Requirements for inclusion of subjects in the survey

There should be clear indications which villages, households, and individuals are to be included in the study. For example, these may include one or more of the following: selection in the sample, permanent resident (definition required), consent given, within the correct age range, and not seriously ill.

Human subject procedures

Human subject protection procedures need to be considered for the particular area. Those being used must be explained. The actual method used will vary with the community, especially with the level of literacy. Special care is required for 'invasive' procedures, such as blood-taking.

Survey data

The data to be collected in the survey should be first outlined. This will stress that the information may be obtained by questioning individuals (name, occupation), by observation (physical state of the house, kitchen facilities, and method of cooking), by direct examination (clinical signs, anthropometry), and by examination of records (birth certificates, health clinic data). A general review of questionnaires used will indicate who is being examined or questioned and the type of information required. It should be stressed that the layout of the form and its directions have specific purposes (e.g. question order, probes, etc.). General methods for filling the particular forms used should be explained (where to write words and numerals, make checks, put added information for open-ended questions, etc). At the same time, the form should not be unnecessarily complex and confuse trainees.

Survey items that are to be included in the study must then be considered in more detail, either individually (e.g. age determination, anthropometry) or in groups (e.g. questions about recent health and treatments sought). Major sections in the study can be considered as modules. Thus, anthropometry would include not only the techniques for measurements, but also methods for field checks and quality control, as well as the care, maintenance, and replacement of equipment.

Measurement procedures and techniques are presented in detail elsewhere in this book, together with potential errors in making measurements (p. 56). The manual should list these in a manner readily understandable to the trainee. Each measurement ('task') should be given in steps ('subtasks') with perhaps a maximum of 10 such steps (Abbatt 1980). Too many steps makes comprehension difficult and reduces the proper continuity of the procedure. Trainers should emphasize the correct method, pointing out errors of measurement as they occur and explaining the reasons for such errors.

Illustrations and diagrams for methods are helpful for introductory and reference purposes, but cannot replace practical 'hands on' experience. However, it is useful to include diagrams of the equipment, indicating moving parts, screws, hinges which may need repair or replacement, as well as the reading area (e.g. of anthropometric equipment) to indicate the graduations and units. The latter is of great importance to prevent reading errors, a serious problem producing unexpected or unlikely results.

Common problems in form-filling include failure to enter an answer or measure, either through obtaining information (often negative) and forgetting to fill it in or not even attempting the question; and unclear writing, particularly of numerals. During supervision of interviews, other problems may be apparent. These include not keeping to the correct wording or order of questions; not following directions precisely; giving leading questions when not indicated; filling in the form where no answer or result was elicited; and ignoring checking and editing procedures.

Field procedures

This section should briefly describe the administrative and logistical procedures for visits to survey sites. If there are multiple sites with large distances between them, staging areas may be required. Facilities (accommodation, food) need to be described at each area and methods of transport indicated from central to staging area to field sites. Often, surveyors may need to stay in communities for some days. For this reason, attention to personal needs should be emphasized. Bedding, basic cooking utensils, clothing, soap, and other essentials may have to be taken, depending on local arrangements and facilities.

Surveyors must be made aware of rules for drivers, especially as regards speeding, alcohol, and unauthorized trips. If public transportation is used, regular routes and schedules need to be indicated.

Communication between supervisors and more senior personnel may be required on a regular basis. Depending on local circumstances, this can include the telephone, cable, radio, mail, or hand-delivered messages using survey, public, or other transport. A procedure for sending urgent messages should be agreed upon.

A system for local purchases needed for survey purposes has to be developed. This will include the management of receipts, cash security, and reporting. Methods of payment of salary and *per diems* must be clear — how much, where, when, and by whom.

Surveyors must know precisely what they are expected to take with them and do from their departure to the survey site, at the site and on their return. This includes who they must meet with (e.g. arrangements with community leaders, teachers, etc.) and for what purpose. Details will depend on the type and scope of the study.

It is useful to provide a list of equipment and materials required for each field visit. Each item can be checked to ensure nothing will be forgotten. Where practical, certain equipment and materials should be taken in excess to allow for loss, or damage by humans or nature, such as rain (e.g. 20 per cent extra study forms).

In many studies, particularly where supervision is difficult, surveyors should keep a brief daily log, indicating their activities, how long they worked, and the problems that arose. This will greatly assist review and indicate, for example, where added support is required and if survey fatigue is imminent.

Mapping

At times, maps may be available for large areas. However, those at the local level will usually have to be drawn. This can best be done by competent staff prior to training. Even then, surveyors should be able to read a map correctly and be able to interpret scales and signs. This can be difficult for those not long familiar with this type and procedure. Understanding can best be reinforced during the field training exercise, where sampling procedures will also be demonstrated and practised. Maps prepared by surveyors should be as basic as possible with special attention to practical concerns with the feasibility of movement in the field. Thus, they should show areas accessible by road, track, or path; obstacles, such as rivers; key landmarks; and directions; as well as an approximate scale, and buildings (dwellings and others). Details required on maps will depend on the methods of sampling and type of survey. For example, cluster sampling (p. 408) usually requires individual dwellings, but only within the boundaries of the selected cluster.

Sampling

Only the essentials of sampling should be presented as they relate to the surveyors' responsibilities. Minimally, they should realize that *only* the households selected must be visited — and re-visited if the occupants are unavailable or absent. If this is not done, *all* the survey results will be questionable and may not even be accepted. Procedures for contacting absent subjects (e.g. await return from market or farm, see next morning early, visit work place, etc.) must be delineated. If all efforts are in vain, there should be clear instructions for visiting pre-selected alternative households. Even then information should be sought (e.g. from other occupants or neighbours) about who was absent and why, with available demographic information such as age, sex, and occupation.

Usually, senior survey personnel, with the appropriate statistical guidance, will select the sample. On-the-spot sample corroboration may be most conveniently done by a supervisor, if available. Clear, simple, dogmatic directives are required. In actual practice, it may be necessary to compromise the best 'theoretical' sampling procedure to ensure completion of the study within the allotted time. A modified method for random selection (e.g. spinning a bottle to determine direction) may be required; otherwise a basic understanding of a random numbers table is essential. All sampling procedures and alternatives should be listed, in order to minimize unplanned field decisions. A sampling field exercise is usually required for final evaluation and must include maps to trace movement from one household to the next.

List and diagrams of equipment and supplies

It is helpful to have a complete list of all equipment and supplies.

Surveyors will be accountable for checking each item on receipt, both for its presence and correct functioning, prior to taking these to the field. If done systematically, such items are less likely to be forgotten and responsibility is clearly identified.

Referrals for ill individuals

The procedures for ill individuals must be clarified. This includes general criteria for on-the-spot treatment (first aid, aspirin, antimalarials), or referral. The latter should be accompanied by a pre-prepared form or handwritten note. The extent of care available — from the survey team and through referral — will already have been decided upon with local administrators, community leaders, and health facilities. Surveyors must understand that the community should not look to the study as an extension of the health service (e.g. conduct local clinics) — otherwise survey attendance may be biased towards the sick. At the same time, ill individuals need attention for humanitarian reasons and for general acceptance by the population. A fine balance has to be achieved, which is often difficult to do, especially in areas with poor health services.

Coping with problems

There should be a clear recognition of expected field problems — personal, administrative, and technical. The inevitable delays may be due to injury or illness, vehicle breakdowns, heavy rains, equipment failure, uncooperative individuals, or a combination of factors. Wherever possible, such problems should be prevented — or sufficient resources and time allocated for contingency purposes, including inevitable unexpected problems.

The surveyor should understand which problems can be addressed and which require referral. For example, a minor equipment malfunction may be temporarily repaired until return to base; others may require ceasing measurements until a replacement is available. Minor illnesses may be controlled with readily available medication, such as aspirin; others may force a surveyor to stop work and be replaced by another.

The morale of workers is extremely important. Their expectations for performance should be fair and realistic, so that their level of support is continuous and enthusiastic.

Evaluation of training

Trainees must be informed about the criteria for their evaluation. These include general aspects, such as punctuality and attendance, reliability and courtesy, proper attitude to officials, household heads, and people included in the survey, and ability to follow instructions and work smoothly with the rest of the team. Technical aspects include a reading and writing level consistent with requirements, interview techniques, and correct form-filling, as well as adequate performance in anthropometric and other field procedures.

One method to determine competence in measuring is an anthropometric standardization exercise. Up to 10 subjects are independently measured by trainees and supervisors as well as a proven adequate measurer ('expert'). The results for each observer are compared for each individual examined. Thus, subtracting the result by the 'expert' from that of the trainee gives a difference which can be taken to estimate performance for that subject. Methods for analysing results have been documented (Habicht and Mason 1983), and a manual has been published on checking continuous measurements (Zerfas 1986). As an approximate guide for 10 measurements, there should be no more than one difference greater than the following: 0.1 kg for weight, 1 cm for height or length, 0.5 cm for head or arm circumference, and 2 mm for fatfold. These figures apply to subjects up to 5 years of age. The guides may be altered according to the age of the subject, equipment used, and type of study required.

Appendices
Brief descriptions for the methods used (e.g. local calendar of events, how to determine age in months) should be included in the appendices.

Supervisor training
In addition to training of surveyors, supervisors must learn and apply procedures consistent with their own job descriptions. In general, they should not take over trainee functions, but assist them and be the key contacts for review and advice during the survey. Field editing procedures must be emphasized — that is, the correction or deletion of gross errors. In addition, supervisors have a special role as contacts with officials and community leaders, in sampling and in field decisions in case of unpredicted events, which are bound to occur.

Logistical considerations

Logistics includes the movement of personnel, equipment, and supplies from central base to and within field areas and back. Provision must be made not only for the study itself, but its preparation (reconnaisance), planning (preliminary field trials), training (pre-testing), and evaluation (quality testing) and follow-up.

Transport

Methods of transport may include foot, bicycle, animal (horse, donkey, camel, etc.), motor vehicle (bus, four-wheel drive, van, car motorcycle), boat, or aeroplane. Some may be available through private or public sources. Others may have to be purchased or rented, or borrowed for a limited period when required (public or health centre transport). Local transportation may be used, if available (e.g. carts, porters for equipment).

It is wise to have an alternative, contingency method readily available if the proposed transport is disrupted (fuel shortage, motor breakdown, sudden unexpected unavailability). Bulky items (fuel, water, furniture) need to be transported and securely stored on location, with ready access to the field. A mobile field laboratory adds an extra dimension to demands and is almost never feasible.

All vehicles require a standardized, strict preventive maintenance programme, enforced by senior drivers, mechanics, and supervisors. Strict rules for vehicle upkeep and careful driving must also be followed, for safety and keeping to schedules.

An adequate supply of basic tools and spare parts should be kept in each vehicle, with sufficient reserves at base for ready replacement. If possible, at least one mechanic should accompany vehicles, or, more usefully, driver/mechanics employed, if available.

Provision for adequate insurance for vehicles and personnel must be obtained. Apart from extreme circumstances, study personnel (e.g. surveyors) should not drive, for reasons of safety, insurance, and fatigue. When not in use, the security of vehicles must be adequate. Thus, where convenient, drivers return their vehicles and keys to the senior field officer or appointee at the end of each period or day. There must be clear indications which people outside the study are allowed transportation in survey vehicles (e.g. local dignitaries, very ill survey subjects). Unauthorized trips should be forbidden or at least accounted for.

The same driver should keep to his own vehicle. Clear markings on each vehicle are recommended (e.g. Ministry of Health Nutrition Survey) to indicate its official nature. In addition, a large number on the front, back, and each side panel door is useful in identifying the vehicle and driver at a distance, thus allowing easy recognition.

Adequate records are needed for each vehicle with regards to places of travel, time and mileage, trip authorization, and perhaps personnel carried; for fuel and oil purchases or use; and for maintenance/repairs. These must be checked regularly. A waterproof map of the area studied must remain in the vehicle.

When a single vehicle is responsible for several surveyors working in different areas, the drop-off and pick-up locations need to be clearly indicated. A contingency plan for irregularities (e.g. surveyor fails to appear at pick-up site at the agreed time) should be developed.

Communications

Communications may involve the personal transfer of messages through the existing or other transport system or via radio, telephone, etc. It also includes publicity for the study through newspapers, radio, television, and brochures.

Regular lines of communication, often with government assistance (e.g. administrative posts, hospitals, police stations), are required for field arrangements (e.g. for meetings) with officials and community leaders, taking heed that this is a two-way process. In certain rural areas, a follow-up message, often through the local health staff, may be useful for confirmation and as a reminder. However, as mentioned earlier, personal contact by senior study members or representatives is most important in the initial preparations.

Regular communication is also needed to ensure smooth running of the study, especially if direct supervision is limited due to personnel, time, or transport constraints. Such needs include location of surveyors for on-the-spot checks (announced or without warning), as well as brief field reports on study progress.

All studies have field problems; thus ready communication is required for contingencies. These include: urgent supply replacement for items forgotten, lost, or damaged; illness of personnel; or technical problems, such as difficulty with sampling.

Time considerations

Appropriate timing and duration of the study is critical for success in field assessment. Even so, it is better to add a reasonable buffer to the projected duration of the study and achieve later praise for earlier completion. It is imperative to have sufficient time for planning. As far as the user is concerned, the date for receipt of information, once agreed, is relatively inflexible, particularly if required for a scheduled programme, conference, or plan.

Although duration encompasses all phases of the study, time-related costs are often greatest while carrying out field work. This depends on the scope of the study and its content, travel costs, personnel salary, and *per diem* allowance, as well as the inevitable delays. The duration (and cost) of data analysis and report writing is often underestimated. The work pace should never exceed a reasonable expectation of the capabilities of personnel, otherwise lack of motivation, boredom, fatigue, and carelessness will ensue.

By the time of detailed planning, an organizational chart should be refined to include estimated timing and duration of activities. Phasing the study so that data collection, analysis, and report writing overlap reduces the total duration and provides unique opportunities to modify or contract the rest of the study as required. If required, an interim, guarded, informal early communication of survey progress may be justified.

If approximately the same amount of time is spent at each locality or sample site, an estimate of total duration of the survey may be derived from the equation:

$$D = \frac{s \times d}{t}$$

where D is the total duration of the survey, s the number of localities to be visited, d the duration in each locality, and t the total number of teams on the survey. Often, however, the duration between and within localities will differ because of varied time spent travelling and local organization and co-operation.

In studies covering several locations where subjects are selected (sites), it is useful to plan procedures according to whether shorter, average, or longer duration is anticipated. This may be based on population density and remoteness from central or regional bases, as regards both distance and difficulties with transport (Zerfas 1979).

The proportion of time for travel rises and for the interview falls with increasing sparsity of population in an area. This might suggest that an increase in duration and depth of the interview in sparsely populated areas would be an efficient procedure, considering the time taken to reach the survey subjects. This would depend on a sufficient number being selected in these areas. Added training time would be required for the extra information. Alternatively, the extra time for the interview may be best allocated to validating and checking procedures. Also, in sparsely populated areas, the education of the person interviewed may be relatively poor, and the age of young children, difficult to determine.

Total time-related costs may be reduced by decreasing the total number of localities or the duration of time spent in each (particularly travel). Increasing the number of teams is limited by training problems, their field support, supervision, and, above all, funding. In addition, an increased number of teams introduces problems of observer variability between teams. This is particularly important if the results from different areas of the survey need comparing.

Community co-operation and participation

Realistic co-operation is required from individuals included in the survey as well as the remaining (unsampled) local population, both for initial registration and for reinforcing support and assistance in the area. The benefits from the survey may be immediate as a result of community or individual inducements (usually treatment or referral of the sick), or long-term, via action intended based on the results.

Relevant letters or reports, reinforced by public announcements should be sent to community leaders to express appreciation and to help with continued motivation.

The survey itself may be beneficial if it includes training of community workers in basic techniques, which can be used in future surveys or programmes, such as screening using simple anthropometry. This can also help develop greater community awareness, participation, and responsibility. The more the community senses it is their survey, done for and by them, the greater the co-operation, as well as concern about their health/nutritional status and, when possible, its causes. This is particularly true when the community itself is the user (at least in part) of the results, and when the community is involved in discussion and advice-giving during the planning phase of a field study.

Each community has its own political infrastructure, which must be respected, used, and not bypassed (e.g. by short-cut methods, such as appointing key community representatives for the study without full agreement by leaders). At times a special committee may be formed for the study with the responsibility for local publicity; arrangements for hire of community workers, visiting subjects, and keeping to planned schedules; and care of survey workers (e.g. shelter, food, porterage, and storage of equipment). These important details need to be worked out individually for the particular circumstances.

Publicity

Publicity includes meetings, messages, or even local dramas (e.g. in emphasizing survey benefits). These methods may be reinforced by central dissemination of information to communities by well known or respected sources, through radio, newspapers, or even specially prepared brochures.

Field arrangements

These are outlined later in the reconnaisance section (p. 428). It is wise to sense the general community attitudes to the survey and its workers as well as local resources, before requesting assistance (e.g. for shelter, water, food, etc.) and availability and willingness of the people to be examined (e.g. when they are least occupied in their fields or place of work).

If there is any local suspicion concerning the purpose of the survey, it is best to proceed cautiously, and to reassure community leaders. At the other extreme, if the community is well motivated and co-operative, it may be regarded as an insult to refuse key items of help.

Schedules

Before arranging schedules, the community's concept of time must be understood. Schedules, like other arrangements, should be as clear and precise as possible, yet allow for inevitable delays. For example, advance information to subjects about the household visit should be done in stages. At first, a general message may be given through community leaders to household heads regarding the day and time of the visit, perhaps done a few days before, followed by a repeat message the day before. In certain situations, as a reminder, a local messenger may visit the site or household to be surveyed about an hour before the arrival of the survey team.

This degree of preparation depends on the regularity of the subjects' activities, the geographical area covered, and likely co-operation. On no account should survey members make an arrangement and not keep it, or come late, even if community members themselves are unreliable or tardy. In practice, it is advisable to make contingency plans, particularly if certain uncontrollable situations occur, such as a breakdown of transport or heavy rains.

Costs

Costs may be direct or indirect, non-recurring or recurring. Direct costs are those clearly related to and for the survey, such as purchase of equipment. Indirect costs are those primarily incurred elsewhere, but part of their service is made available for the survey. This can include free loaning of equipment, use of agency training quarters, or health facility for referral of ill persons encountered. There may not be a clear dividing line between direct and indirect costs and the latter may not be included in the budget. However, it should be taken into account for recognition of assistance. In addition, if such services become unavailable, the cost of replacements should already be estimated.

Recurring costs are those which recur in every costing cycle, hence are usually related to duration (e.g. vehicle hire, fuel, staff salaries). Non-recurring costs are those which occur infrequently (often only once), such as for purchase of some equipment, etc.

When the survey is prolonged (e.g. longitudinal) or there is a long time between planning and implementation, inflation must be considered. This can include increased travel costs, future purchasing of equipment, rise in staff salaries, etc. For services or equipment requiring foreign exchange, rates between countries are often difficult to project. Graphing those for the past year by month may sometimes give some indication of the trends.

The budget should be clear, comprehensive, and in a sensible order. If certain funding agencies require a special (perhaps illogical) presentation, the original budget can be re-arranged to suit their special format. Other modifications may be required when more than one agency supports the study or when there is a subcontract for some part of the investigation.

The organization of budget line items is often based on: personnel; equipment/supplies; services; travel; contingency.

Within these headings, it is useful to have subheadings, according to the phase of the survey (i.e. preliminary activities, planning, training, field testing, implementation, data analysis, report writing, and review). Although overlap will occur, this method allows a continuous, logical appraisal of the budget throughout each phase.

Personnel should include the duration and percentage of time for work, and rate of pay, including benefits and vacation. *Per diems* are often best listed separately.

Equipment is sometimes defined as more 'permanent' and expensive than supplies. A practical point for including this separately is that the equipment may be used after the survey by the health or nutrition workers or even the communities. In general, supplies will be used only for the duration of the study.

Services can include such diverse items as office rent, copying, printing (questionnaire forms, report), data entry, computer expenses, freight, and communications (e.g. postage, telephone, cable).

Travel can include both international (where *per diems* also need to be listed) and within-country. For the latter the cost of vehicles (purchase, hire) and accessories (jerry cans, drums), spare parts, fuel, oil, repair, maintenance, and insurance costs should be included. Local enquiries may indicate an operating cost by kilometre, depending on type of vehicle and terrain.

Indirect costs may be added, especially by an institution (e.g. company, university) whose services (facilities, personnel) are not included elsewhere in the budget. This may range from 20 to 50 per cent of all costs incurred through the institution, except purchases of equipment.

The costs of data editing, analysis, and report writing are often underestimated. Even with the use of 'packaged' computer statistical programs an experienced person will be required to assist in most analyses.

Contingencies are based on the increase in costs over time (e.g. inflation) and an allowable 'buffer' for unexpected added costs. If funding agencies do not allow this item, plans must be made to incorporate such contingencies within other budget line items. Thus, inflationary and other extra costs, as applicable should be anticipated, and, where reasonable, extra equipment and supplies for loss, breakage, or disuse also included. Time-related costs are major budget components, hence a realistic appraisal of duration of work and travel is required.

Submitted budgets should be 'healthy', neither 'lean' nor 'fat'. However, there is always a temptation to 'overbudget' to a funding agency to acquire the maximum funds possible and allow extra for negotiations. This is inexcusable when there is a fixed sum for a total programme, of which the study is just one component. On the other hand, in competitive contracts from donor agencies, underbudgeting is the rule.

Budget rationale

This comprises a justification for the type, number, and cost of items, particularly unusual ones or those expected to be queried. The budget must be consistent with objectives, recommendations (e.g. from committees or peers), and documented evidence for costs. The reasons why certain items or services are required overseas and not locally should be explained.

Not only should absolute costs be considered, but also relative ones. This includes the percentage of total cost for each section (e.g. personnel, travel) and of the survey to the total programme.

Implementation: preparatory field work

Field work in survey areas incorporates planning (reconnaissance visits, pilot to full-scale field testing), and implementation (i.e. carrying out the actual survey). There may be overlap, particularly in phased or prolonged surveys where revision of planning may be required during implementation.

Initial field trials may be conducted in stages, each for specific purposes (e.g. testing major survey items, appropriateness of workers, schedules). The first trial (for convenience) may be carried out in an accessible and co-operative community. Later trials should reflect more the communities in the actual survey, where conditions may vary considerably by local culture, language, education, and population density.

During trials, supervision must be ample with adequate records and comments as well as time for discussion and review, involving all personnel. Each surveyor or team must be assessed for at least all key items and procedures. Replicate or check measures (e.g. anthropometry) may be done to reassure surveyors or indicate differences and why. Hence, the number of people examined may be limited to allow sufficient time for evaluation.

As in training, a decision should be made whether to correct performances on the spot or later, so as not to disturb the flow of procedures. Often, a judicious mixture of both is required.

Field testing for sampling procedures may be best done separately, as sampling procedures often involve a larger area with more subjects than do trials for survey items.

During evaluation, supervisors should systematically check each item tested. This can be conveniently done on the questionnaire form, such as a tick or cross for satisfactory, a query for poor, with reasons why. Such reasons may be related to competence of the examiner, co-operation of the subject, or appropriateness of the particular item. In the same way, there should be a check-list for specific procedures (e.g. registration, sampling, and results; approach to household head and subjects, care of equipment, and supplies).

In this connection, it is useful to consider some form of time–motion exercise, to indicate the duration of procedures in sequences and reasons for delays. From this a clearer insight into schedules can be derived.

Once procedures are satisfactory, a full-scale dress rehearsal should be undertaken. This incorporates all items and may involve a complete area. If the survey involves overnight stays in villages, this should also be considered during the rehearsal.

Study implementation

In large-scale cross-sectional surveys (p. 364), it is useful to start in a community which is relatively easy to supervise (e.g. densely populated) and close to the central base for logistical (transport, communication) convenience. The same principle applies towards the end of the survey, when field workers may be tired and require more support. For example, this period can sometimes be reserved for measurements of an 'elite' population or special group, usually more readily accessible near the capital city, and sometimes needed for comparison purposes with internationally available reference data (p. 000), especially for young children. The sequence of field activities should also consider local factors affecting timing, such as climate, crop cycles, holidays, and market days.

Procedures, such as those involved with logistics and supervision, will vary depending on whether a 'caravan approach' is used. In this method, several teams may work in the same locality or area, and move together to the next area. This has the advantage of better communication between survey teams and senior members. In addition, observer variability between teams, may be similar from one area to the next, hence less likely to affect results when different areas are compared.

However, the caravan method limits the total period within each area and may compromise the time required for local preparation (e.g. local calendar of events) and follow-up (e.g. revisits for absentees). In contrast to this method, one team can be assigned to a specific area for the duration of the field work. This may be required because of the in-depth nature of a questionnaire, which may contain many recall questions concerning attitudes and behaviour.

Implementation: household surveys

Ideally, most surveys should be carried out by means of home visiting, which offers the advantage of seeing the family together in their domestic setting, of not missing sick individuals, such as children with kwashiorkhor, who may be kept at home, and of causing the least disruption of normal life and behaviour. Moreover, a study by house-visiting may be necessary where it is not culturally permissible for the population, particularly for women, to attend a public meeting-place.

Proper timing is essential to ensure that household members are available. Not only is advance information for the visit required, but use of local messengers the day before or early in the morning of the day's study will assist co-operation.

In some cultures, it is imperative that the household head or elder be first approached on the team's arrival, even if most of the information is required from the mother. Thus, several visits to the same household may be necessary. For surveys with prolonged interviews, such as those including dietary intake and feeding habits, a decision must be made whether a single comprehensive visit or multiple briefer visits are more suitable.

Implementation: collecting point surveys

In a community nutrition survey, as distinct from a survey of 'ready-made' groups such as schoolchildren and armed forces, the major problem often is how to collect the sampled population of the particular age-range under investigation from the defined, selected geographical, or administrative unit.

In some parts of the world, no villages exist, and people live instead in scattered homesteads with adjacent cultivation areas. In such circumstances, the sampled population must assemble on a selected day at a suitable point, which should be so situated as to enable everyone, including mothers with children in their arms, to attend with a minimum of inconvenience. Clearly, this cannot be arranged without the full co-operation of the local authorities. Great difficulty in this respect arises with nomadic or pastoralist peoples, and still more with hunter–food gatherer groups, such as the Hadza of northern Tanzania (Jelliffe *et al.* 1962).

If villages or similar population groups exist — as on small islands — there may be little difficulty, provided that the community leaders understand and support the project. Suitable assembly points may be arranged at the health centre, the chief's compound, the community hall, or other socially familiar focal point, such as the church or mosque or the village square.

However, in countries where there is a shortage of doctors, the prior announcement of the survey team's arrival may mean that sick persons, including those suffering from malnutrition, will be brought into the villages from the surrounding countryside, thus giving a false impression of the health situation. In such a circumstance, the village mayor, headman, or other official who can recognize, and exclude from the main survey, persons from outside the area, can help greatly. Hopefully, appropriate arrangements and publicity will prevent such an occurrence, and enable adequate enumeration and identification of individuals included in the sample.

Frequent movements of village populations, such as those occurring during market days in Haiti (Jelliffe and Jelliffe 1960), also create problems. In every case all persons who may be absent, whether visiting relations or working in industry or agriculture at distant points, must be taken into consideration. It should also be borne in mind, in the assessment of malnutrition and disease prevalence, that sick persons may have been admitted to local hospitals or hidden at home. They should be looked for and included in order that the findings in the community be complete.

Slum areas are of increasing relevance in the urbanizing tropics, but present peculiar difficulties, unless low-cost housing estates exist and are treated as population units. Understandably, the inhabitants are often uncooperative or, at best, indifferent. Furthermore, because of overcrowding, uncertain community boundaries, and inadequate identification of subjects (e.g. from constant in- and out-migrations), examinations at collecting points may not be possible.

In every case, surveys carried out at collecting points must be complemented by visits to homes, kitchens, cultivation sites, shops, etc. — i.e. rapid ecological visits.

In surveys at collecting points, the sequence of activities needs organizing. It is indispensable, though difficult, to organize a smooth, continuous line of flow from one 'station' to the next. Without this, the team's field work will become progressively more confused as the day advances — to the point where the results may have to be abandoned.

To help in the preliminary organization and to supervise its continuation throughout the day, the co-operation of a school-teacher, the chief, the village mayor, or similar official, accompanied by his assistants, is essential.

Before the day of the survey, the local authorities must know how many 'stations' will be required, where they should be situated, and what each should comprise.

The 'stations' may be set up in rooms in a single building or adjacent buildings, or in the open, in the shade of a tree. The site chosen will depend on local circumstances, including the probable degree of wind, rain, or sunshine. If shade is available, some stations, including those for the clinical examination and anthropometric measurements of children, may best be located out of doors. They will be cooler and have better light than a dark crowded room. If necessary, the open-air stations can be surrounded by a rough 'fence' of string and sticks brought by the team for the purpose. It is usually better to set up the laboratory station, where blood samples are taken, in an enclosed room so as not to frighten children waiting their turn.

Problems of modesty arise in connection with the clinical examination and anthropometric measurement of adults or older children. As already noted, weighing is best carried out with subjects lightly clothed or nude, but since this is not usually possible, adults may have to be weighed in their clothes, subject to an appropriate adjustment for the known weight of clothes usually worn.

Clinical examinations of entire populations can be carried out either by setting up one 'station' for men and older boys and another separate one for girls, women, and their young children, or by making a combined visit to a family group. In either case, examinations will have to be carried out in rooms or, in some parts of the world, in *ad hoc* screened-off areas of thatch or palm-leaf. Of these two methods, the visit to the family group is often preferable, as the family composition can be observed and only one station is required, making for greater simplicity in the line of flow. Whichever is chosen, undressing rooms or screened-off areas are required. In the family-group examination, two to three 'rooms' are needed in order to ensure a continuous flow.

Even where privacy has been arranged, a further problem will arise if urine samples are collected. Either separate urine-passing rooms or screened-off areas will be needed for each sex.

The requisite number of stations and the line of flow will have been determined in the planning phase. The degree of simplicity of each station will depend upon its function and on the facilities available. Improvization will clearly be called for. A certain amount of basic furniture will be necessary for each station, such as four chairs (two for the team, one for the person to be examined, and one for the local assistant/interpreter) and one or more tables (e.g. a small table for the clinical examination and one or two large tables for laboratory specimens with a bowl and towel for the specimen taken).

'Stations' should be so placed that they are in the actual line of flow. They should not be near enough to one another to cause possible confusion and noise, or so far apart as to give rise to difficulties in directing people.

Examples of lines of flow: community child health surveys in East Africa

As an example, the line of flow normally applied in the community child health surveys in East Africa will be described. These surveys were carried out on young children, so that questions of modesty did not enter into the clinical examinations, which were often undertaken in the open air under shady trees.

Five stations were ordinarily employed, in the following sequence: (1) identification; (2) anthropometry; (3) clinical assessment; (4) laboratory specimens; (5) dietary inquiry.

Identification station

At the first station, a survey form was issued to each person on which was listed the survey date and number, the person's name (and, if this is not culturally specific, other data, such as 'child of'), sex, age, group, or tribe, religion, if relevant, and village, town, or area.

This form had to be kept by the individual, or the child's mother, until the last station had been reached; it was then collected. It was most important to ensure that the data obtained at each station were consistent — i.e. that they referred to the same subjects. At each station the form had to be checked before examination, in order to obviate any confusion with the numbering, which can occur very easily and, once it has developed, prove difficult or even impossible to sort out in a crowded rural survey.

The station was manned by one team member, assisted by one or two clerks who had been shown the routine, but who needed to be supervised closely if errors in numbering were to be prevented. A local policeman or other responsible person could usually be persuaded to control the flow of persons so that they present themselves one at a time. Another local volunteer could carefully direct the person to the next station after the form has been completed.

If it proved difficult to make an accurate age-assessment, this was attempted by means of an 'events calendar' at the first station, in which case an additional team member familiar with the local language was required.

If some of the team members did not speak the local language, those who did were deployed where they were most needed (e.g. age-assessment and dietary inquiry). In addition, where language problems existed, as many as possible of the local volunteer assistants were bilingual.

Anthropometry station

At the second station, anthropometric measurements were carried out. Again, two local volunteers were required — one to direct the line of persons waiting, and the other to guide people to the next station.

Platform weighing machines and length-measuring apparatus were set up on flat surfaces. A length-board for young children was sometimes placed on a large table, when care had to be taken to avoid falling. A suitable beam or tree branch was required for hanging scales.

For the measurement of adults, two persons were needed: a team member to do the measuring and a trained clerk or assistant to record it. For young children, two more volunteer assistants were needed, to hold the child while the measurements, etc. were being taken. The results were announced clearly, frequent checks being made to ensure that they had been correctly recorded.

Clinical assessment station

Two local volunteers were used, to control the queue and direct people to the next station.

Clinical assessment was carried out by a suitable health professional or trainee, who had at hand a list of the signs to be looked for. These had been typed, in the order in which they were to be sought, on a piece of paper affixed to a sheet of cardboard and protected with cellophane. the examiner could then check through the list (e.g. oedema — present; Bitôt's spots — absent; etc.). Each sign and its result were read aloud by the assessor and marked as positive or negative on the clinical assessment sheet by a trained clerk or assistant, whose work was continuously scrutinized.

The person being examined had to be in a good light and wearing as few clothes as possible. In the case of adults and school-age children, this usually consisted of shorts or drawers; young children were examined naked. An approximately head-to-toe sequence of inspection was best followed, with palpation (e.g. spleen, muscle wasting, pre-tibial oedema, etc.) done after this. Auscultation was not usually needed, and, in any case, it is difficult to hear sounds such as cardiac murmurs in the noise attending most surveys. However, the examiner wore a stethoscope in case it was needed for a particularly sick person — for example, a child with possible pneumonia.

Signs were reported as 'present' or 'absent'; the recording of grades of posivitity was not used. In addition, unexpected findings were briefly noted in the space reserved for this purpose.

In the case of young children, the state of eruption of the teeth was recorded, as an aid to confirming the estimated age.

A minimum of equipment was needed. Apart from a stethoscope, only the check-list of signs, pencils, one small table, and three or four chairs were usually required. A pocket torch and a box of wooden tongue depressors were at hand for the examination of the mouths of uncooperative young children.

Laboratory station

At the fourth station, samples were taken for subsequent biochemical or other tests. It is at this station that cross-cultural clashes are most likely, as the taking of a 'piece' of the body, especially blood, may be considered, in some rural groups, to be intended for an occult purpose, particularly if blood is taken by a woman wearing lipstick. However, misunderstanding may sometimes help, as in Haiti, where finger-prick blood collection for thick-film examination for malarial parasites was equated with a popular and highly successful penicillin anti-yaws campaign that had been carried out in preceding years (Jelliffe and Jelliffe 1960).

It may be found expedient in the first place to examine, and take samples from, the local dignitaries (in Africa, for example, the chief's family) and educated people, such as the schoolteacher, both as a matter of courtesy (especially as they will usually be helping the survey team) and as an example. Should any of the procedures prove unacceptable, especially the collection of blood samples, they may have to be deleted and the programme modified.

The taking of samples for laboratory tests was, wherever possible, carried out in the privacy of a room, partly to allay the fear of waiting children and parents. A sweet or a lump of sugar was given to each child at the end; otherwise the fear experienced was likely to be communicated to other children waiting in line and to intensify their anxiety and resistance.

Flies, which can rapidly ingest a blood sample from a slide, could complicate the taking of thick blood films for malarial parasites, as could wind-blown dust.

Whatever the number and type of samples taken, the collecting apparatus — needle or syringe and correct containers — was at hand in the proper place on the table used in the field as a laboratory bench. Similarly, equipment for sealing or closing tubes or containers, items for labelling (e.g. grease-proof pencil, ball-point pen), and boxes or thermos flasks for specimens were readily available.

The detailed routine for taking specimens was guided by field testing. Minor differences in practical technique can mean an increase in efficiency, as judged by the fatigue of those engaged in collecting the samples and by the numbers that can be dealt with in a given period.

Each member of the laboratory group had to know his detailed function and how to carry it out speedily, with economy of movement and a minimum of interference with his co-workers.

Ideally, two laboratory workers were used — one to take the sample and the other to have the container ready and seal it, to label it and place it in the appropriate box or thermos flask, and to record the tests taken from the person, both on the survey sheet and in a record-book.

Stool samples may be brought in by families in containers that have been distributed at least the day before. With illiterate groups, there was the difficulty that the containers could not be labelled in advance by the survey team or by educated local volunteer assistants, nor could they be labelled by the subjects themselves. There may thus be confusion in identifying the samples. There could also be a lack of co-operation, so that few stool samples were brought in. This could be due to misapprehension, suspicion of witchcraft, distate for the task, or a cultural prohibition of contact with excreta. On receipt, the stool samples had to be correctly labelled, and without delay — in any event on the same day. Stool preservative (10 per cent formol saline, etc.) was added to a small specimen of stool the size of a pea or other locally known objects of similar size.

For young children, a stool sample was best obtained by means of the anal-tube technique (p. 159). This is not advisable in the case of infants, especially in the first 6 months of life, as the stool is too liquid or semi-solid. In pre-school age children, a practised operator can obtain samples from about 75 per cent of the children. The disadvantage of the method is that the specimen is very small. After removal of the tube from the anus, the core of stool was poked out of the tube with a wooden applicator into a small flat-bottomed screw-capped vial, containing 1 ml of 10 per cent formol saline.

Urine sampling was always difficult. As noted earlier, random samples may be collected from adults in the privacy of the clinical assessment, special rooms may be set aside, or an available latrine used for the purpose. For young children, special collection techniques may be employed, particularly for males, but they are very difficult to apply at a crowded survey site. Alternatively, mothers may be asked to 'catch' a specimen in a plastic jar supplied to them at the survey site. With the practical difficulties, fasting samples of urine were impossible to obtain.

The laboratory samples taken from each subject were checked on the survey form by means of ticks at the side of the appropriate space. The laboratory results were filled in later when they are available.

Apart from the two laboratory workers and the two local volunteers for directing and controlling the flow, a further local assistant, preferably bilingual, was often required for explaining, reassuring, and, in the case of frightened young children, assisting the mother to restrain the struggles of her child.

One or two large tables were required, together with a minimum of four chairs. A plastic basin, soap, towels, and a light plastic jerry can of water were brought by the team to the station, together with a bowl and towel for handwashing by the specimen collector.

Dietary enquiry station

This station dealt with the questioning of sampled mothers about the diets of their children and the family diet, usually over the past 24 hours. This had to be done by a trained, culturally acceptable (often adult female) team member, fluent in the local language and, if possible, belonging to the same ethnic group.

A suitable form for this rapid dietary inquiry was based on adequate background knowledge of local foods, cooking practices, and feeding habits. A range of local measures and utensils was at hand — spoons, cups, bottles, and gourds — to help the mothers reply concerning quantities of food eaten.

Mothers were asked solely about their children's recent diet (24-hour recall), without reference to the diet in the past. Direct questions were avoided, as replies were considered likely to be approximate and inaccurate. One aspect of infant feeding that could be verified by observation at the survey site, at least in some traditional societies, was whether the child was still receiving breast milk or not.

In addition, at this station treatment was given when really indicated, according to expectations and availability, based on the written instructions of the clinical assessment station. The survey form was collected from each person and placed in a large envelope.

The staff for this station consisted of one team member and a junior medically-trained assistant to dispense drugs and give other treatment. Both had to speak the local language. One local volunteer assistant was required to direct the flow. Apart from dietary enquiry forms and medicines, one or two small tables were required, together with three chairs.

General remarks

It is evident that the stations and line of flow will vary in detail from one survey to another. In planning the line of flow, it should be borne in mind that the activities at certain stations (e.g. collection of laboratory samples; dietary enquiry) take much longer than at others (e.g. clinical assessment). The time required at each station should be tested in advance of the survey. A selective system may have to be introduced, whereby only a random sample of those attending go to the stations at which the examinations, etc. are relatively prolonged.

The question of operator fatigue is of importance, and where practicable, team members should have rest periods.

Rapid ecological visits

Concurrently with examination at collecting points, in East African studies, rapid ecological visits were carried out, photographs taken, and outline information obtained from local hospitals and health centres. Often, this was the only opportunity to collect such data concerning impressions on ecological variables.

Quality control

Quality control procedures are more difficult when subjects are studied at the household level. When supervisors or senior staff accompany surveyors, direct supervision is possible. However, if feasible, repeat measures may be more suitable after the surveyor's visit, providing subjects have been forewarned and are co-operative. This will ensure independence of the second measure and will not unduly delay surveyors.

Unannounced spot checks are especially useful, in evaluating surveyor's work because they are less conditioned to inspection. The content, scope, and timing of procedures will depend on the type of study, geographic spread of the sample, number of teams per supervisor, available time, and transport.

Repeat soft-tissue measures should not be unduly delayed. For example, nutritional status itself, as measured by weight, arm circumference, or fatfold, may vary within a week or so, particularly in young children exposed to acute infections and diarrhoea. This means that the difference between the initial (surveyor's) measure and the repeat one may not reflect an error in measurement after this length of time.

Checking interview items (such as age determination by calendar of events (p. 318) and 24-hour dietary recall) presents difficulties. Even then, repeat measures by a senior, more experienced individual can indicate data quality, but not necessarily observer competence.

At a collection point, check measures are usually done after the measures are completed by the observer. In some circumstances, such as for anthropometry and clinical signs, it may be more convenient to do 'check measures' in advance — for example, while subjects are waiting prior to or just after registration. Subjects may be more available and co-operative at that time, rather than towards the end of an often prolonged session.

Data analysis[97]

The purpose of data analysis is to organize information mathematically to answer questions based on the objectives of the survey or nutritional investigation. The scope and complexity of such analyses will be influenced by several factors, including the number of items of information collected (variables) and transformations (or new variables derived from the original ones), the number of subgroups described (e.g. differing geographical areas, age groups included, etc.), the sample size, and the complexity of statistical information acquired (including correlations and associations).

Other limitations include the resources available, including relevant computer hardware and software (e.g. package programs), trained personnel, time, and funds.

It is essential to plan for the analysis before data collection begins. If practicable, a simulation of methods should be carried out, taking into account the factors listed above, perhaps using 'dummy' data, or data acquired during field testing, or during the early phases of the study. Unless these preliminary trials are undertaken, analysis may become misdirected (involving much unnecessary work later), and/or incomplete (so that some of the essential results from the study are missing).

In some smaller studies, basic analysis may be undertaken manually,

[96] Mathematical and epidemiological details of survey data analysis are available in many publications, including a recent WHO (1986*f*) manual.

using a regular hand calculator or, more usefully, a programmable calculator. Nowadays, with the spread of microcomputers and more sophisticated models, this will certainly be increasingly unusual (Bertrand 1985; Frerichs 1988). (Also see: Addendum 1988.)

Data entry

Entry of data into the computer should be from clearly coded sheets or from the numerical codes on the questionnaire forms. Whenever possible, entry should be repeated for all measures to check their accuracy (validation). With very extensive data, this may only be feasible on a small sample.

'Editing' after entry

Grosser errors, such as a birthweight of 10 kg, will usually have been detected earlier by inspection. Once the data is entered into the computer, results which are plainly widely outside acceptable bounds can be identified, and probably eliminated. Consultation with the statistician will indicate if appropriate computer software is available to assist in such 'editing'.

Comparing results with reference data

Tabulations of internationally available (NCHS/WHO, etc.) data are available for some findings, especially anthropometric (Appendix 9). A basic hand calculator can then readily determine percentage of reference median. At this stage, it is more precise to enter the actual result (e.g. 75.6 per cent) rather than as a category (e.g. 70–79 per cent). This enables average percentages of median for groups to be estimated and can be later used for establishing modified cut-off points, if required.

Without a calculator, tables using percentage of median can be consulted and numbers and percentages in each category can be determined.

Equations for programmable calculators are available to estimate percentage of median and standard deviations (including Z-scores) without the need to consult tables. Depending on the user, they may be more convenient or more complex than methods already outlined. They require care in use, and should be cross-checked manually on a sample of the data.

Lastly, the Centers for Disease Control (CDC) have developed packaged programs (subroutines)[98] for weight-for-age, weight-for-height, and height-for-age indices, based on recent NCHS/WHO reference data

[97] Given a child's age (or date of birth and date of visit), sex, weight, and height (or recumbent length), the CDC Anthropometric Software Package (CASP) evaluates the weight-for-age, weight-for-height, and height-for-age expressed as centiles, Z-scores, and percentages of the median. Available: Centers for Disease Control (CDC), Nutrition Division. Atlanta, Georgia, USA.

(Appendix 9). They may be used with certain large (mainframe) computers and more recently with IBM compatible microcomputers. These programs also allow the inclusion of other variables, if cross-tabulation and associations are required.

Analytic approaches

Analysis needs to be directed to the objectives and major purposes of the particular large- or small-scale study. Thus, if a cross-sectional survey is intended to assess the prevalence of undernutrition in particular age groups in a defined area (national, regional, or community), this must have priority. Definitions of undernutrition should have been agreed upon at the planning phase (p. 395). The percentage frequencies of undernutrition, defined on a basis of both anthropometry and other variables (such as food intake), thus need to be calculated and presented in appropriate ways (written, tables, graphics).

The degree of exactness (confidence interval) (Appendix 4) for each measure of prevalence of undernutrition (percentage frequency) will be based on sample sizes for single communities or from the variation found between several areas or sites. This will provide estimates of the prevalence and total numbers undernourished in the population from which the sample was taken. Such information is often of major interest to policy- and decision-makers.

Further tables should examine the prevalence of nutritional status according to other ecological variables of interest, including geographical or administrative areas, socio-economic or ethnic groups, as previously agreed in the planning phase. Such analysis must consider the question: Is there a difference in nutritional status within each group? Or is one area (or group) in greater need than another? Hence, comparisons can be made, bearing in mind practical and statistically significant differences, which will have been discussed at the planning stages.

Analysis of differences between groups is intended to allow targetting of resources to those most in need (based on prevalence of undernutrition or greater total population affected). The objectives of the survey will determine how these groups are defined, including anthropometric, clinical, dietary, and other information. The programme must be able to readily identify such groups, for example, according to geographic/administrative areas, age, and occupation. This helps to indicate where differences occur and who is principally affected. Results may also provide clues regarding the possible reasons why the prevalence of malnutrition is different between such groups. Subdividing groups by age is particularly important because of the known variation of nutritional status with age. For example, children aged 6 to 24 months often have a much higher prevalence of wasting than those aged 2 to 5 years.

Expression of results

Data from nutritional studies are largely concerned with the results of anthropometric measurements, food intake, clinical signs, and biochemical tests. Results can be expressed in the following ways.

Anthropometry

Results from nutritional anthropometrical measurements should be reported in two ways: (1) mathematically; and (2) in relation to reference data (Appendix 9).

Mathematical reporting Whenever possible, measurements in figures should be given for each relevant age-group and sex as the mean plus or minus twice the standard deviation (± 2SD). These mathematical figures are required in order to ensure an understanding of the results by other workers and, if need be, to permit further interpretation and analysis or comparison of the findings to be made in the future.

Reporting in relation to reference data (Appendix 9) Anthropometric measurements should also be expressed in terms of reference data. As noted earlier (p. 120), it may be helpful for anthropometric measurements to be compared with two types of reference data—internationally available and local.

The methods of expressing the degree of inadequacy may have to be on several levels—first, easily understandable to junior staff and simple to calculate, and, second, scientifically expressed, with appropriate detail.

For these reasons, it is suggested that anthropometric measurements in community prevalence surveys should be reported in relation to previously agreed upon cut-off points below and (when indicated) above the reference data. These are noted in earlier sections on assessment in different age-groups (p. 122) and indicated in standard deviations or percentage levels in Appendix 9.

Clinical signs

The 'strongly suggestive' clinical signs (p. 23) found should be reported initially as 'percentage of positives' for each sign in the total population examined, and in each broad age-group, e.g., infants, pre-school age children, school-age children, and adults. A further breakdown of results into smaller age-groups and by sex will often be required, especially for adults, because the cumulative strain of continuous reproduction often results in severe malnutrition in women.

As noted earlier, no diagnostic conclusion can usually be drawn from the high prevalence of a single sign. However, in order to assist interpretation, positive signs may be considered together in two ways. First, the positive signs present should be listed together in accordance with the grouping of signs suggestive of various deficiencies (p. 18). Second, the percentages of the total population, or of specific age-groups, which show combinations of three or more suggestive signs listed in the different groups may be useful—for example, in community surveys for rickets.

Dietary assessment

Where detailed food-consumption studies have been carried out, Reh (1962) recommended that the results should be given as the difference for the group between observed consumption and the suggested allowances for all nutrients, expressed as percentages. She advised against the labelling of groups as 'undernourished' or 'malnourished' in respect of one or more nutrients on the basis of food-consumption studies alone. This advice remains correct.

If outline information has been obtained by means of a questionnaire and observation during rapid ecological visits, the results can be expressed as percentages of persons or families stating that they eat certain foods. In young children, analysis can often be made in 3-month groups for the first year (e.g., birth to 3 months; 4 to 6 months; etc.), and in 6-monthly periods thereafter. In all cases, it must be stressed that this information is at best only qualitative, giving an extremely approximate outline of the general dietary pattern.

Biochemical tests

The results of biochemical tests should be presented for the total population investigated, if appropriate, and also broken down into the main age-groups and for both sexes, especially for adults.

The results should be expressed mathematically as the mean plus or minus twice the standard deviation. In addition, they are often presented as percentages of the population falling into different ranges of values. These may be given tentative labels (e.g. 'low', 'deficient'). However, with the exception of a low haemoglobin, the labels given must be interpreted cautiously in view of the inadequate state of knowledge concerning possible variability in different ecological circumstances, especially in relation to prolonged adaptation to dietary patterns. Suggested guides to the interpretation of biochemical and haematological findings are given elsewhere (pp. 498 and 502).

Other ecological data

Similarly, other information concerning ecological variables, including conditioning infections, cultural influences, socio-economic factors, and food production, gathered by means of observation and questionnaire, can be expressed as percentages of families or people in different age-groups having certain characteristics. Again, the superficial and approximate nature of findings obtained in this way must be stressed.

Interpretation

Interpretation of data obtained in investigations of communities or individuals depends on the purposes of the nutritional enquiry. Some major purposes of nutritional assessment in communities and in individuals are given in Tables 8.5 and 8.6, respectively. As indicated, the objectives influence both the source of data and methods employed, as well as the interpretation of findings required to define the actions needed.

Nutritional surveys

Cross-sectional investigations of population groups are the commonest method of nutritional assessment employed in less technically developed countries, as emphasized throughout this book. Some questions concerning interpretation of findings need re-emphasis.

Such surveys—both prevalence and incidence studies—are epidemiological investigations of varying degrees of sophistication into the nutritional status of a population employing various direct and indirect methods, together with an evaluation of the determinant ecological factors in the environment. These have been detailed earlier. Some are summarized in Table 8.7, from which an appropriate selection has to be made for the particular study.

They are attempts to make a community diagnosis, and, as with the diagnosis of illness in an individual, information obtained by several methods is usually required. Thus, while in clinical medicine a diagnosis may very occasionally be made on the basis of one pathognomonic sign, such as the rash in herpes zoster, more usually information obtained by several means is required, including the history, clinical examination, radiology, and biochemical and haematological tests.

Similarly, the diagnosis of certain limited types of malnutrition in the community can occasionally be strongly suggested on the basis of one clinical sign only, as with iodine deficiency and goitre, or of one test, as with a low haemoglobin and iron deficiency. Yet, even with these examples, the possibility of factors other than nutritional deficiency, including goitrogenic substances in the diet and malaria (respectively), has to be considered. Moreover, at times, advanced syndromes of a particular deficiency may be readily identifiable, such as kwashiorkor and nutritional marasmus, but give no idea of the prevalence of more common, less advanced forms of protein–energy malnutrition of early childhood.

All the methods that can be used for the assessment of the nutritional

Table 8.5 Some common major purposes (objectives) of community nutritional assessment

(1) Identification of problems, causes and activities needed

- Existing sources
- Surveys
  - Rapid (screening)
    - Community
    - Emergency (cf. refugees)
  - Combined methods
  - Epidemiological (causes)
- Special studies (cf. therapeutic trials)

→ 'At risk' factors; Planned interdisciplinary food and nutrition policy and programmes

(2) Early recognition of need for urgent new activities

- Surveillance
  - Existing sources (national and international)
  - Limited surveys

→ Selected indicators (cf. famines) → Rapid targeted response

(3) Evaluation

- Direct nutrition activities
  - Breastfeeding programme
  - Supplementary feeding
  - Nutrition education
  - Xerophthalmia prevention
  - Agricultural policy
  - Food aid
  - Co-ordinated activities
- Development activities
  - Levels of living
  - National development plan

→ Selection of most effective, least expensive programme(s)

Table 8.6 Some common major purposes (objectives) of individual nutritional assessment

Technically more developed country

Hosptial ward
- Detection of clinically inapparent malnutrition (combined methods)
- Diagnosis of clinical malnutrition
  - → Need for special feeding programmes

Paediatric clinic
- Early detection of growth abnormalities (including obesity)
  - Weight (centile graphs)
  - Height

General (medical supervision or self-assessment)
- Weight–height–sex
- Fatfold(s)
  - → Mostly related to obesity

→ Dietary modification

Technically less developed country

Young child clinic (or) home visits
- Early detection of malnutrition
- Recognition of
  - Clinical signs
  - Serial anthropometry
    - Weight chart
    - Arm circumfernce

→ Appropriate management (nutrition education, supplementary feeding, oral rehydration, etc.)

Prenatal clinical
- Early detection of malnutrition
  - Clinical signs
  - Haemoglogin
  - Weight chart

Nutrition rehabilitation unit — Recognition of recovery

Paediatric unit
- Clinical diagnosis
- Detection of moderate protein–energy malnutrition
- Suggest prognosis
- Recognition of recovery
- Subsequent catch-up growth

→ Recognition of non-severe protein–energy malnutrition and other forms of malnutrition

Dietary modification

Table 8.7 Information useful for assessment of nutritional status in communities

Sources of information	Nature of information obtained	Nutritional implications
Agricultural data Food balance sheets	Gross estimates of agricultural production Agricultural methods Soil fertility Predominance of cash crops Overproduction of staples Food imports and exports	Approximate availability of food supplies to a population
Socio-economic data information on marketing, distribution and storage	Purchasing power Distribution and storage of foodstuffs	Unequal distribution of available foods between the socio-economic groups in the community and within the family
Food consumption patterns Cultural–anthropological data	Lack of knowledge, erroneous beliefs and prejudices, indifference	
Dietary surveys	Food consumption Distribution within the family	Low, excessive, or unbalanced nutrient intake

Special studies on foods	Biological value of diets Presence of interfering factors (e.g. goitrogens) Effects of food processing	Special problems related to nutrient utilization
Vital and health statistics	Morbidity and mortality data	Extent of risk to community Identification of high-risk groups
Anthropometric studies	Abnormal growth or body composition	Effect of nutrition on physical development
Clinical nutritional surveys	Physical signs	Deviation from health due to malnutrition
Biochemical studies	Levels of nutrients, metabolites and other components of body tissues and fluids	Nutrient supplies in the body Impairment of biochemical function
Additional medical information	Prevalent disease patterns, including infections and infestations	Interrelationships of state of nutrition and disease

* Adapted from WHO Expert Committee on Medical Assessment of Nurtitional Status (1963).

status of a community are individually imperfect, inaccurate, and subject to their own technical errors. It is, therefore, particularly important to avoid drawing sweeping conclusions based on limited evidence. The literature is full of examples of the unwarranted use of survey results.

Although valuable information can certainly be obtained with less than an extensive range of methods, which usually are not feasible in most prevalence surveys, the probability of obtaining a valid picture of the nutritional condition of the community in its widest sense increases if several approaches can be employed in conjunction. The different methods are aimed at assessing quite diverse aspects of human nutrition, ranging from dietary intake to abnormal growth (anthropometry) to food availability.

The evaluation of the combined information gathered from several methods of assessment should be aimed at delineating, as thoroughly as the complexity of the survey warrants, the following:

1. The principal deficiency diseases in the community in different age-groups, and their priority;
2. The probable causative factors.

In the more usual short-term, cross-sectional surveys with which this publication is principally concerned, prevalence figures will be obtained, together with approximate incidence data at hospitals and health centres.

Statistical and epidemiological guidance will be needed for the interpretation of the findings. At the same time, it is salutary to note the comment of Gordon (1963), the acknowledged father of nutritional epidemiology: 'Modern methods of machine tabulation, computer analysis and statistical manipulation have obvious value in dealing with projects with many data, but the interpretation of results remains rooted in the value judgements of workers in the field.'

10

Stimulating action

Tension arises between those who want to define the problem better, and carefully work out what to do—which takes time and money for absolutely no allevation of the problem; and those who want to do something now, based on best guesses and 'doability'. A divorce thus arises between 'data' and 'action'.

Mason *et al.* (1984)

Data is political. Analysis is a political act as much as it is prescription. But so too is prescription.

Schaffer (1984)

Introduction

It is sometimes assumed that the presentation of the carefully reasoned results of well-planned nutritional assessment activities will automatically result in action. This is not the case (Jelliffe and Jelliffe 1987).

To stimulate action at governmental and community levels, following large-scale nutritional surveys or smaller assessment activities, requires analysis, interpretation, and the presentation of results in ways which are understandable and which motivate the particular audience. The main groups requiring conviction and motivation are governmental decision-makers—that is, politicians and senior administrators in several ministries, and other agencies and non governmental organizations (NGOs or PVOs), whose activities need to be combined in what UNICEF has termed the 'Grand Alliance' to improve child health and nutrition (Grant, 1988). In addition, different considerations need to be borne in mind and highlighted for other groups. These range from scientific and technical leaders, to the population of the particular community.

Psychosocial and political considerations need to be taken into account as well as technical relevance (Table 9.1). In addition, their intended influence on nutritional activities needs to be incorporated into the process of selecting, gathering, analysis, and interpretation of data (Table 9.2), whether this be in the assessment of nations, communities, or individuals.

Practical categorization

The purpose of the investigation and the methods used need explaining (or re-outlining). The data obtained will have been analysed (p. 438) and,

Table 9.1 Technical and psychosocial considerations needed in all activities concerned with community nutrition assessment

Technical	
Practicability	Appropriate technology Affordable Logistically feasible Easily analysable Politically permissible
Understandability	Investigators Investigated Administrators
Relevance to main problems	Scientific Political Community
Scientifically-based	Equipment Techniques Statistical (sampling) Analysis Interpretation
Psychosocial	
Understanding Support Involvement Motivation Non-dependence	Family Community Health and other services Nation

as noted earlier, need to be presented *mathematically* (means, standard deviations, etc.) for scientific colleagues, for subsequent reference and possible further analysis, and for technical publications. For the politician–administrator, data needs practical categorization and presentation — that is, numbers of individuals (often young children) and the percentages below (or, less commonly, above) defined 'cut-off points', which will be technically understandable to the audience. For example, it is inappropriate to talk in epidemiological technical terms to politicians or administrators. They will want to know the numbers and approximate percentages in different age-groups who are severely or moderately malnourished (especially in their own districts), as judged by what criteria (including reference data and cut-off points) used and compared with results from elsewhere. They will also expect to be advised of the meaning

Table 9.2 Relating information to potential action at all stages — selection, gathering, analysis, interpretation, and presentation

	National	Community	Individual
Selecting information	Guidance from appropriate ministries	Guidance from community, including leaders	Trial of method in actual culture with relevant people (mothers, CHWs, individuals)
	Within framework of national/ party objectives Joint planning	Felt needs Health needs Field trial in actual ecology	
Gathering information	Tangible assistance from appropriate ministries: Information Transport Staff	Involvement Community PHCW Organization Data collection ? Inclusion of benefits ? Treatment ? Referral	Appropriate practical training Health staff PHCWs Mothers Individuals
Analysing information	Co-operative analysis		Interpretation Individuals Groups
Interpretation and presentation (findings, recommendations)	Co-operative presentation of results and interpretation: Speedy, brief, understandable Joint, national, and international staff Joint publication (when permitted) Repeated follow-up activities	Presentation to community Speedy, brief Understandable Relevant to health needs Relevant to PHC	Interpretation Understandable Feasible for practical action(s)

Table 9.3 Five principles usually involved in selecting priority problems (unwanted outcomes): a number of ways of combining these criteria are available to establish local priorities *(Backett* et al. *1984)*

— Considerable weight should be accorded to community priorities, preferences, and concerns
— The more common problems should have a higher priority than the more rare
— The more serious problems should be given higher priority than the less serious
— The more easily preventable health problems of mothers and children should have a higher priority than those that are more difficult
— Health problems whose frequencies show upward trends in time should in general be given higher priority than those that are static or declining

---

and importance of these findings, the main reasons why this seems to be so, and probably to hear suggestions concerning practical actions.

Lastly, but importantly, it is desirable for over-all results to be made known to field workers and the community that has been investigated together with suggestions concerning improvement. Ideally, this should be followed by later visits with information or programmes developed to improve the situation.

Interpretation for action

To interpret the data presented, it is important to know as much as possible about several measurements of nutritional status and a range of possible causes. The former is needed for corroboration — the latter to suggest possible methods of improving the situation.

From a practical point-of-view, it is necessary to try to sort out the causative versus associated factors. This requires a blend of common-sense observation and mathematical interpretation, such as multivariate analysis (Kune 1980). Priority problems need to be selected (Table 9.3) and 'risk factors' identified, preferably from a wide interdisciplinary point-of-view, including, for example, food availability, family economics, and the prevalence and significance of contributory infections (p. 156). In practice, the selection of what variables should be sought for as potential risk factors is more arbitrary and is usually headed by items considered likely to have some influence and believed be amenable to prevention.

Some 'risk factors' have been recognized for centuries. However, until the past 10 years or so, accounts of these have been mainly 'descriptive' — that is, based on observations alone rather than their statistical analysis.[99] They have been grouped as biological, environmental, and cultural (International Union of Nutritional Scientists 1977).

For example, a study in five UNWRA camps showed the following risk factors in families of malnourished young children matched with those of households of healthy children: illiterate mothers; history of malnutrition in siblings; marital problems; mother's marriage before age 17; occurrence of another pregnancy in mother before previous child was aged 1 year; female sex, low-birth-weight, or born pre-term; not breastfed at all; early bottle-feeding (before age 3 months); failure to gain weight; repeated ill-health; and repeated diarrhoea (Al Dabbagh and Ebrahim 1984). As a 'mirror-image' approach, investigation of 'positive deviants' — that is, individuals in similar situations *without* malnutrition — promises to be rewarding (Zeitlin *et al.* 1987*a*).

Various scoring systems have been suggested, intended to rank the relative importance of risk factors. Some of these have used rather arbitrary 'scores' in which risk factors were summed, without attempting to give any differential weighting to the significance of different factors.

At a descriptive level, risk factors are usually obtained by general observational information, including community assessment, health service data, etc. For example, some risk factors were suggested by Shah (International Union of Nutritional Scientists 1977) for rural India (Fig. 9.1) and for Costa Rica by Pradilla (International Union of Nutritional Scientists 1977) (Table 9.4).

As a more analytical approach and in order to obtain greater precision in judging the priority of risk factors often based on 'sometimes conflicting factors as prevalence, seriousness, preventability, trends in time and local concern' (Backett *et al.* 1984), *priority ratings* have been devised. In particular, the concepts of 'relative risk' (Fig. 9.2) and the population 'attributable risk' (Fig. 9.3) are epidemiological methods of estimating the relative significance and commonness of various 'risk factors' in the particular community (Backett *et al.* 1984) (Appendix 4). In this way, it is possible to suggest nutritional priorities in preventive programmes or interventions. In all cases, modification will need consideration as activities succeed, fail or meet unexpected difficulties, such as economic problems (Grant 1987*b*). All situations differ and unexpected changes may be expected.

Data needed to provide a comprehensive preventive programme obviously have to include 'non-medical' considerations, such as income distribution and accessibility of locally important foods. Some, but not all, of these aspects are given in Table 9.5, with regard to the main vitamin and mineral deficiency problems of young children in less technically developed countries.

[98] Details of this method are given in a practical form in Backett *et al.* (1984).

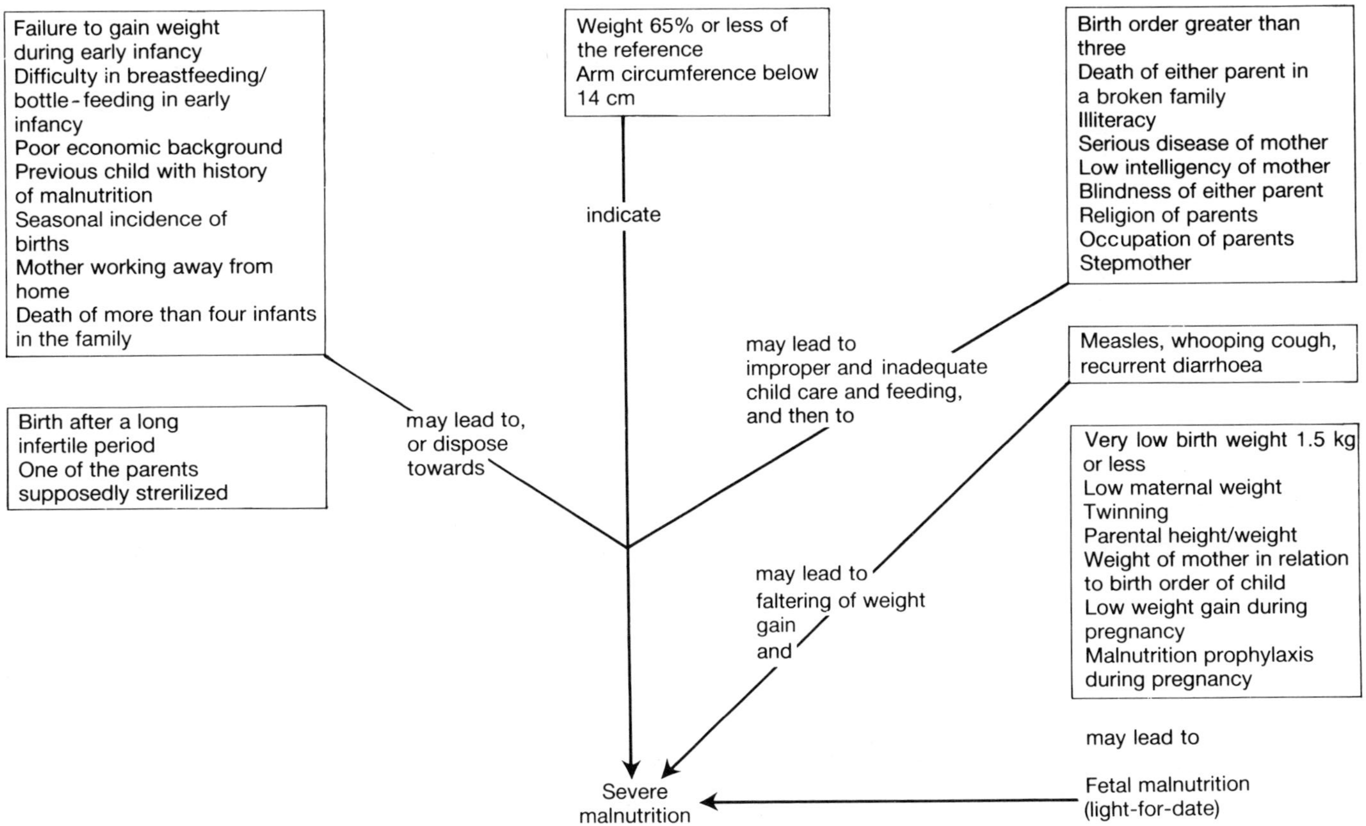

Fig. 9.1 Risk factors and malnutrition in early childhood in rural Bombay (P.M. Shah) (International Union of Nutritional Scientists 1977).

Table 9.4 Different types of risk factors for malnutrition in young children in different regions in Costa Rica *(Pradilla — in International Union of Nutritional Scientists 1977)*

Demographic
General mortality
Infant mortality
Percentage of deaths under 5 to general mortality
Number of dependents
Percentage of population in rural areas
Environment
House classified as good (per cent)
Excreta disposal (any kind per cent houses)
Public water (per cent houses)
Income
Percentage of the population with more than 5000 cólon
Coefficient of land distribution
Health coverage
Population covered by CCSS-MPH (National Health Service)
Education
Houses with radio
More than 2 years of school

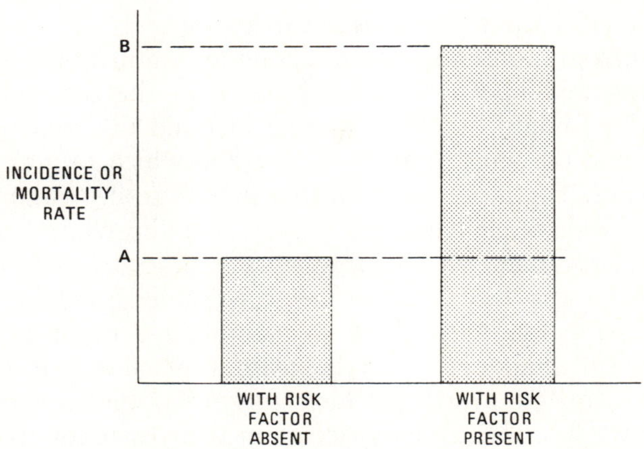

Note: The relative risk is sometimes called the "odds ratio". In the example it is $\frac{B}{A}$.

Fig. 9.2 Relative risk or odds ratio. In the example (B/A) shows the odds are three times greater of developing illness or dying from it in those with the risk factor than in those without (Backett *et al.* 1984).

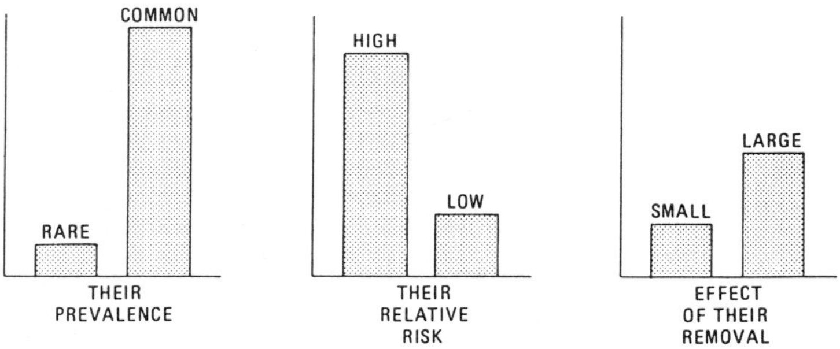

Fig. 9.3 Attributable risk (impact of a risk factor on the community related to prevalence (commonness) *and* relative risk) illustrating effects on the community of the removal of two different risk factors (Backett *et al.* 1984). Note: Attributable risk is based on the assumption of a causal relationship between risk factor and outcome.

With this type of approach, it is possible to consider in an approximate way the main risk factors and to assign different levels of priority to them as 'preventable antecedents' (Al-Dabbagh and Ebrahim 1984).

Presentation

Any presentation should follow an introduction covering the reasons for the investigation and how it was carried out.

Results from different forms of community nutritional assessment have to be presented in ways understandable to the particular group. The presentation should be made bearing in mind the sometimes brief time available and the most appropriate ways in which to make an impact on the audience. For more sophisticated presentations, summary hand-outs and visual aids (e.g. diagrams, graphs, and flip charts) will be helpful. In all circumstances, photographs and/or slides of malnourished individuals can be very helpful since they have understandable emotional impact. Occasionally, it may be both possible and useful to demonstrate a malnourished child. This can be helpful when senior administrators–politicians are not aware (or have forgotten) that severe malnutrition, such as kwashiorkor, actually occurs in their own country.

Such presentations should aim at arousing awareness that priority problems are present, but also how these can be improved *with attainable resources* (Table 9.6).

Guide to presentation (Jelliffe 1966; Burgess and Burgess 1975)

The presentation of data may often be organized at two levels. First, in order to speed up any action that may be considered necessary, a short,

Table 9.5 Assessment of nutritional status and main ecological factors: more common vitamin and mineral defiencies in young children

Direct examination				Indirect information			Food considerations				Assessment of ecological factors		
												Cultural influences	
Clinical	Biochem.	Anthrop.	Biophysic	Hospital data	Community knowledge	Late effects (older age group)	Nutrient availability	Nutrient affordability cost/income cost/nutrient	Nutrient consumption	Nutrient absorption	Major contributing infections	Pregnant and lactating mothers	Young children
Vitamins A Bitôt's* spots	Serum retinol < 10 μg per 100 ml	—	Night blindness: practical tests	Keratomalacia	Local names: Bitôt's spots (or) night blindness	Blindness in early childhood (beggars, institutions)	Each nutrient in relation to both mother and young child				Measles Roundworm Diarrhoea	Cultural restriction on vitamin A (retinol) and/ or carotene-containing foods	Avoidance of colostrum Non-breastfed Cultural restrictions: vitamin A and/or carotene containing foods
C Spongy*† swollen bleeding gums	Serum vit. C < 0.1 mg per 100 ml	—	—	Infantile scurvy	—	—				Boiling procedure (heat labile)	—	—	Non-breastfed cultural restrictions: vitamin C-containing foods
D Epiphyseal* enlargement	Serum alkaline phosphatase > 20 Bodansky units	—	X-ray wrists	Clinical rickets	—	Bow legs Knock knees				Phytates	—	Cultural restriction on vitamin D-containing foods Limitation of skin exposure to sunlight	Non-breastfed Cultural restrictions: vitamin D-containing foods, limitation of skin exposure to sunlight
Minerals Iron Pallor*‡ (conjunctiva, mouth)	Haemoglobin**	—	—	Severe anaemia (paediatric ward; laboratory records)	—	—				Vitamin C and animal protein	Hookworm (malaria)	Cultural restriction of iron-containing foods	Cultural restriction of iron-containing foods, non-breastfed practices with umbilical cord (haemorrhage, placental transfusion)
Iodine Cretinism Mental deficiency	Urinary iodine low	General growth retardation	—	Not helpful	—	Possible permanent mental impairment	Iodine deficient soil → Foods, Water				Not known	Not relevant	Not relevant

* 'Strongly suggestive' indicators only.
** If low, further tests needed.
† Only after dental eruption.
‡ Inspection or visual comparison (p. 000).

Table 9.6 Some information needing inclusion in the presentation of results to decision-makers

Existence of problem(s)	
Dimensions	Type Severity Extent Frequency
Distribution	Region Urban/rural Age-groups
Causes	
Level of priority*	
Existence of solutions	
Practical Low-cost Feasible Visible	Selection of alternatives

* Mortality, cost of treatment versus prevention, social consequences (including handicapping and burden to family and society in recovered cases).

(preferably, 1–2 page), lucid, typewritten summary report of the main findings (Table 9.7) should be sent as soon as possible to the appropriate authorities in the country. Sometimes, two brief reports are needed — one for administrators and one for technical colleagues. Often, an initial draft report is circulated on a limited basis to key personnel for review. This is particularly important when results may be considered as politically 'sensitive'.

Detailed analysis of data always takes time, and, if a preliminary report is not presented, further extensive delays will occur before the final draft, with tables, graphs, etc., is ready, and 1–2 years may pass before the report is finally published and reprints made available.

Second, a fully and more detailed report of the survey is needed, whether published or not. This main report should be clear and logically developed, with figures for the most part kept out of the text and incorporated in tables, graphs, or histograms. It should be as detailed as possible, although editorial policy often insists on limiting the text to the essentials.

Obviously, the method of presentation will vary with the purpose and

Table 9.7 Suggested basic layout for brief summary report

Detailed index: date of survey; map; agencies involved	1 page
Objectives	1 paragraph
Description of area	2 pages
Sampling methods	1 page
Survey methods	1 page
Summary of results	2-4 pages preferably on different coloured paper so it is easily found. The summary should be complete in itself so that it can be given out to the layman and the community.
Results	Basically this is a series of tables with a short comment on each which draws attention to main points and mentions any test of significance done.
Discussion (including interpretation and programme suggestions)	
Recommendations	
References	
Acknowledgements, including names of all staff involved and their duties	

scope of the survey, with the object and range of the report, and with individual preference regarding style and emphasis.

In general, however, the report should contain the sections described in the following paragraphs.

Background data

These will comprise a brief account of the area, often illustrated with a map, containing information about the particular community, including its culture patterns and ethnic groups; the geography, climate, and communications; the socio-economic status (including level of education and school; economics); food production (including processing and storage); health facilities; and demographic data (especially the population and its age and geographic distribution, and morbidity and mortality statistics).

Purpose of survey

A general definition of the purpose of the survey is required, perhaps with an explanation of the reasons for carrying out the particular study in the area selected.

Methods employed

This section will contain a description of sampling procedures, practical methods used in field work, and the details of the techniques employed in: (1) the clinical assessment (including definitions of signs looked for and control of observer error); (2) the biochemical estimations (with references to the published accounts of the techniques); (3) the anthropometric measurements, with special mention of the instruments used; (4) the dietary investigations (as well as the food-composition tables and recommended dietary allowances used); (5) the assessment of ecological factors; and (6) the gathering of information concerning local health statistics. Copies of questionnaires used should be attached.

Presentation of results to decision-makers

These are usually best presented in tabular form under the heading of the particular method of assessment (clinical, biochemical, etc.) broken down into appropriate age-groups and by sex, where necessary.

The tables showing the results of the *clinical examination* should show the numbers examined and the percentages positive with different signs, especially 'strongly suggestive signs' (p. 23), whose significance needs explaining.

Biochemical results, including haemoglobin levels, need to be shown numerically, as indicated earlier (p. 48). In addition, presentation should indicate numbers and percentages of individuals who fall below defined levels as *tentatively* labelled groups, e.g. low, deficient, etc.

Anthropometric measurements should also be expressed in a simple understandable way by means of percentages of the population examine that are at various levels below (or above) the reference. For young children — the most common target groups — various results may be presented. In addition to weight- and height-for-age, classification into 'wasted' and 'stunted' (p. 312) is often also used to separate malnutrition into acute and chronic, giving a more complete picture for decision-makers.

Data on *ecological factors* may be presented in tables. Often some of the information is qualitative. This needs to be presented descriptively, as well as in tabular form, and reinforced by slides or photographs, if possible.

Photographic illustrations in subsequent fuller reports are often of value in describing various ecological circumstances, showing examples of the types of malnutrition, and illustrating techniques and methods. Their reproduction is, however, costly, and they take up considerable space. Perhaps the main value of a limited number of photographs is in supplementing the descriptive account of the local people and their way of life, and ensuring that the reader receives and impression of the subjects and the site of the survey.

Discussion

Correlation of evidence Essentially, this will be concerned with a consideration of both positive and negative findings and the collective evidence they provide of the presence or absence of different types of malnutrition in the particular age-groups in the community investigated. Occasionally, it may prove impossible to attempt anything beyond a forecast requiring fuller investigation (e.g. therapeutic trials or additional biochemical tests).
Ecological diagnosis The deductions must be correlated with the ecological factors that appear to be aetiologically relevant or causetive in the particular region. From analysis of all the data available, suggestions can be made for future action.

Recommendations for future action The aim of public health investigations is to improve the health of the public. They should not become mere academic exercises undertaken in a spirit of scientific curiosity. Responsible officials and administrators need to be associated with the investigations at an early state, and a summary of findings, interpretations, and suggestions should be sent to them without delay.

Action

Follow-up surveys may be necessary to note the development of certain nutritional trends (e.g. changes in infant feeding or an apparent increase in incidence of some form of malnutrition) or to assess the effects of recommended preventive measures.

Apart from follow-up surveys, further investigation may occasionally be desirable in order to clarify some of the results obtained. Therapeutic trials or more detailed and specific biochemical tests on selected groups may be indicated. The aetiological factors may have to be identified with greater precision (especially to differentiate can see from associated factors), or the value of the preventive measures investigated more scientifically.

Specific recommendations for action as regards policy and programmes must be realistic in terms of needs; cultural, social, and economic considerations; existing and potential resources; and health and educational services. They should be clearly set forth in order of priority. Thus, the prevention of doubtful subclinical deficiencies should not receive undue emphasis if severe forms of malnutrition with a high incidence and mortality are common in some age-groups.

The range of recommendations may vary widely. They should be aimed at the most important potentially preventable causes responsible for the particular forms of malnutrition. Detailed consideration of possible recommendations for intervention programming is beyond the scope of this book. Some of the following are likely to merit consideration: improvement of health services, especially for mothers and children; agricultural improvements including increased local production of the main nutritious foods (and their storage, processing, preservation, distribution, and marketing); health education (MCH services, schools, etc.); legislation, including protection of mothers during pregnancy and lactation, fortification of foods, rationing, price subsidies, and minimum wage levels; selective supplementary food programmes for young children, pregnant and lactating mothers, and school meals; the prevention of infectious diseases, through immunization, improved water-supplies, anti-malaria measures, etc.

Motivation for action

Various levels and types of motivation for action need to be borne in mind at all stages of nutritional assessment. This applies in very different circumstances to nations, communities, and to individuals. Indeed, although the emphasis in this publication is on nutritional assessment in Third World communities, the situation regarding the nutritional assessment of individuals anywhere can have messages of wider significance. These can include, for example, non-nutritional motivation concerning culturally preferred 'body image' for the individual in Western countries.

For individuals, the main objective will be to try to persuade and motivate to behavioural change (Table 9.8). For example, in primary health clinics for young children, this may be directed towards persuading mothers to introduce semisolid foods earlier or making more use of available dark-green leafy vegetables. Motivation will usually be hard to devise because of different cultural concepts concerning the causation of malnutrition and classification of foods. Useful approach may be by practical, visible demonstration through improved weight gain on growth charts in clinics or in nutrition rehabilitation units, as a result of dietary change.

In more affluent areas, self-assessment may be undertaken at home by individuals. This is usually concerned with reducing or avoiding obesity, mainly measured by weight-for-height and/or fatfolds. Home-kits are available in some countries, including the USA. The motivation is partly cultural — that is, a striving for the currently preferred non-obese, muscular, or very lean 'body image' — as well as concern with nutritional status, health, and 'fitness'.

On a large scale, whether community or national, motivation is initiated and continued by *involvement* of decision-makers at all stages,

Table 9.8 Motivation for action following nutritional assessment needed at different levels for communities and individuals

	National	Community	Individual
Target populations	Politicians and decision-makers (interdisciplinary)	Community leaders	Mothers/parents Individuals Appropriate health staff
Motivations	Humanitarian Economic Food sufficiency Political National/party priorities National image Personal (or) political reputation Security (military)	Apparent community benefit in relation to Felt needs Newly-appreciated problems Incorporation of appreciated, non-nutritional motivation	Health benefit to individual Incorporation of appreciated non-nutritional motivation (e.g. culturally preferred body-image)
Main objectives	Governmental policy and programmes	Joint action by community	Behavioural change by individual (or mother)

including the planning phase and with *tangible* support (finance, equipment, staff) for the assessment activity (e.g. survey etc.). Such involvement should be interdisciplinary, whenever possible, including the ministries or governmental agencies involved with agriculture, trade, education, and finance, as well as health. Subsequent policy and programme developments will almost always have to involve several disciplines and sectors.

If nutrition assessment is carried out by a 'mixed' team, the national and foreign members can have complementary parts in presenting and interpreting results to government authorities and decision-makers. National investigators should have the major role, with short-term international team members playing a supportive part, including validating the whole endeavour in their capacity as visiting 'experts'. *Joint* presentation of data in subsequent publications (if permission is given) is essential.

Motivation by decision-makers depends on many factors as well as humanitarian concern for the prevention of illness and death from malnutrition. Policy decisions are inevitably influenced by economics, questions of self-sufficiency in food production, and political considerations. Health workers, including nutritionists, are usually not trained to consider these or to automatically understand their relevance. However, effective stimulation for action can only rarely be based on nutritional or health considerations alone. Politicians are not without human feelings, but economics and personal and/or party politics are usually also to the forefront in planning and stimulating action in generating and sustaining governmental policy and programmes.

Acknowledgements

The opinions expressed in this book are those of the authors alone. At the same time, the writers are deeply indebted to many colleagues working in all parts of the world. In particular, the following have generously given their time and advice in the preparation of this publication at various times in recent years.

A

Dr Sydney Abraham, Nutrition Statistics Bureau, National Center for Health Statistics, Maryland, USA; Dr Hutton Addy, Department of Community Health, University of Science and Technology, Accra, Ghana; Dr Kamaluddin Ahmad, Institute of Nutrition and Food Science, University of Dacca, Bangladesh; Dr Anna Alisjahbana, Department of Child Health, University of Padjadjaran, Indonesia; Professor Manuel Amador, Instituto Superior de Ciencias Medicas de la Habana; Dr G. Arroyave, formerly Institute of Nutrition of Central America and Panama (INCAP); Dr A. Arteage, Departamento de Nutrición, Facultad de Medicina, Universidad Católica, Santiago, Chile.

B

Dr K.V. Bailey, World Health Organization, Brazzaville, Republic of the Congo; Dr Robert C. Bailey, Department of Anthropology, Harvard University, Cambridge, Massachusetts, USA; Dr G. Beaton, Department of Nutrition and Food Science, Faculty of Medicine, University of Toronto, Canada; Dr I. Beghin, Institut de Médecine Tropicale, Antwerp, Belgium; Dr Moises Behar, formerly World Health Organization, Geneva, Switzerland; Dr José M. Bengoa, CONICIT, Caracas, Venezuela; Mr D. Bernard, Stanley-Mabo, Paris, France; Dr C.W. Binns, School of Community Health, Western Australian Institute of Technology, Australia; Professor W.H. Boon, University Department of Pediatrics, Singapore General Hospital, Singapore; Dr Robert B. Bradfield, International Nutrition Associates, Orinda, California, USA; Mr Art Braunstein, US International Development Cooperation Agency, Washington, DC, USA; Dr George A. Bray, Department of Medicine, UCLA, California, USA; Drs Richard and Judith Brown, Norfolk, Virginia, USA; Dr R. Buzina, Department of Nutrition, Institute of Public Health of Croatia, Zagreb, Yugoslavia.

C

Mr Sol Chafkin, formerly of The Ford Foundation, New York, USA; Mr Richard Charkin, Oxford University Press, Oxford, England; Dr Miriam Chavez, Instituto Nacional de Nutrición, División de Nutrición, Mexico

City, Mexico; Dr Lincoln C. Chen, formerly Cholera Research Laboratory, Washington, DC, USA; Dr Xue-Cun Chen, Institute of Health, Chinese Academy of Medical Sciences, Peking, People's Republic of China; Dr Y.H. Chong, Division of Nutrition, Institute for Medical Research, Kuala Lumpur, Malaysia; Dr May E. Cochrane, Health Sciences Center, Department of Pediatrics, University of Arizona, Tucson, Arizona, USA; Dr Tim Cole, MRC Dunn Nutrition Unit, University of Cambridge and Medical Research Council, Cambridge, England; Professor. Jeannine Coreil, University of Texas Medical Branch, Galveston, Texas, USA; Ms Catherine R. Crean, Metropolitan Life Insurance Company, New York, USA; Professor E.K. Cruickshank, University of Glasgow, Glasgow, Scotland.

D

Mr Peter David, Ideas Forum UNICEF, Geneva, Switzerland; Dr David P. Davies, Faculty of Medicine, Chinese University of Hong Kong, Hong Kong; Dr Warren Day, School of Public Health, Division of Environmental Health, UCLA, California, USA; Dr Carlos Daza, Pan American Health Organization, Washington, DC. USA; Dr Rajammal Devadas, Science College for Women, India; Mr Wallace C. Donoghue, Creative Health Products, Michigan, USA; Ms Gwennole Dorange, Coultronics France S.A., Margency, France; Dr Burris Duncan, Department of Pediatrics, Health Science Center, University of Arizona, Tucson, Arizona, USA; Professor H. Dupin, École Nationale de la Santé Publique, France; Dr Jose Ed. Dutra Dutra de Oliveira, Faculdade de Medicina, Riberao Preto, Sao Paulo, Brazil.

E

Dr Katherine Elliot, formerly AHRTAG, London, England.

F

Dr Frank Falkner, School of Public Health, University of California,. Berkeley, California, USA; Dr F. Fidanza, Universidad degli Studi di Perogia, Italia; Ms Laurie Finch, McGaw Laboratories, California, USA; Dr Preethi Fonseka, Cornell Nutrition Surveillance Program, Cornell University, Ithaca, New York, USA; Mr Robinson Fulwood, Division of Health Examination Statistics, Department of Health, Education, and Welfare, Maryland, USA;

G

Dr Rafael Galvan, Instituto Mexicano Del Seguro Social, Mexico; Ms Louise P. Galyon, Munsell Color, Maryland, USA Dr Manuel Garcia, Instituto Superior de Ciencias Medicas de la Habana, Cuba; Professor Stanley M. Garn, Center for Human Growth and Development, University of Michigan, Michigan, USA; Dr Shanti Ghosh, Department of Paediatrics, Safdoring Hospital, India; Dr James Goldsby, Center for Disease Control, Atlanta, Georgia, USA; Dr Harvey Goldstein, Department of Statistics and Computing Institute of Education, University of

London, London, England; Dr C. Gopalan, Nutrition Foundation of India, New Delhi; Dr Claude de Ville de Goyet, Emergency Preparedness and Disaster Relief Coordination Unit, Pan American Health Organization, Washington, DC, USA; Dr Michael Gracey, Princess Margaret Children's Medical Research Foundation, Perth, Australia; Dr Philip L. Graitcer, Nutrition Division, Department of Health, Education, and Welfare, Georgia, USA; Dr Peter Greaves, UNICEF, New York, USA; Ms Marcia Griffiths, Manoff International Inc, New York USA; Dr Michael Gurney, World Health Organization, Geneva, Switzerland.

H

Mr Charles Habis, US International Development Cooperation Agency, AID, Washington, DC. USA; Dr L. Hambraeus, Department of Nutrition, University of Uppsala, Sweden; Dr Ronald E. Hammond, Physiology Department, Carolina Biological Supply Company, Burlington, North Carolina, USA; Professor J. Hansen, Department of Paediatrics, University of Witwatersand, Johannesburg, South Africa; Dr Masazumi Harada, Institute of Constitutional Medicine, Japan; Dr Joseph Hautvast, Department of Human Nutrition, Agricultural University, Wageningen, Netherlands; Dr Roger Hay, Oxford, England; Dr Steven B. Heymsfield, Emory University School of Medicine, Atlanta, Georgia, USA; Dr James W. Hicks, Deputy Director, Division of Nutrition, Center for Health Promotion and Education, CDC, Atlanta, Georgia, USA; Dr Yngve Hofvander, Department of Pediatrics, Medical School, University of Uppsala, Sweden; Ms Mary Ruth Horner, Universidade de Brasilia, Brasilia, Brazil; Professor N. Hoyosa, Department of Nutrition, University of Tokyo, Japan; Dr H. Hussaini, Nutrition Research and Development Centre, Bogor, Indonesia.

I

Dr Maarten D. C. Immink, Division of Nutritional Sciences, Cornell University, New York, USA; Dr Bjorn Isaksson, Institute of Clinical Nutrition, Sahlgren's Hospital, Sweden; Dr Raymond B. Isely, Water and Sanitation for Health Project (WASH), Arlington, Virginia, USA.

J

Dr Seymour Jablon, National Research Council, Washington, DC, USA; Professor G.J. Janz, Departamento de Epidemiologia, Instituto de Higiene e Medicina Tropical, Lisboa, Portugal; Ms Christina Joe, National Food and Nutrition Committee, Fiji.

K

Professor Henry Kamin, Chairman, 1980–1985 Committee on Dietary Allowances, FNB; Professor Jamal K. Harfouche, formerly School of Public Health, American University of Beirut, Lebanon; Dr D. Karyadi, Departemen Keslehatan R.I. Bogor, Indonesia; Dr W. Keller, Nutrition Research, World Health Organization, Geneva, Switzerland; Professor E. Kerpel-Fronius, 2nd Department of Paediatrics, Semmelweiss Medical

School of Budapest, Hungary; Dr John Kevany, Department of Social Medicine, University of Dublin, Ireland; Dr S.H. Khamic, Statistics Division, Food and Agriculture Organization, Italy; Dr Kendall W. King, formerly Research Corporation, New York, USA; Dr Joe Kopple, School of Medicine, UCLA, California, USA; Dr R. Korte, formerly Division of Health, Population, Development, and Nutrition, German Agency for Technical Co-operation Ltd, Frankfurt/Main, West Germany.

L

Dr James M. Lansche, Neurosurgery Associates, Pennsylvannia, USA; Dr Michael Latham, Division of Nutritional Science, Cornell University, New York, USA; Dr. Aaraon Lechtig, Instituto de Nutrición de Centro America y Panama (INCAP); Professor Munro Lee, Department of International Medicine, Seoul National University, Seoul, Korea; Ms Susan Eastman Leone, Helen Keller International Incorporated, New York, USA; Mr Edward A. Lew Society of Actuaries, Florida, USA; Dr Helen Lewis, Senior Paediatric Registrar, Northwick Park Hospital, Harrow, England; Dr Peter G. Lindner, The Lindner Clinic, California, USA; Dr Christopher Lomax, AHRTAG Ltd, London, England; Dr Paul Lunven, Food and Agriculture Organization (FAO), Rome; Professor R. Luyken, Central Institute for Nutrition Food Research, Netherlands.

M

Dr T.N. Maletnlema, Tanzania Food and Nutrition Center, Dar Es Salaam, Tanzania; Professor Michel Manciaux, Centre International de l'Enfance, France; Dr J.P. Manshande, Sint-Pieters-Leeuw, Belgium; Professor J. Masek, Metabolism and Nutrition Research Centre, Czechoslovakia; Dr John B. Mason, Cornell Nutritional Surveillance Program, Division of Nutritional Sciences, Cornell University, Ithaca, New York USA; Professor Leonardo Mata, Department of Microbiology University of San Jose, Costa Rica; Dr John McKigney, Formerly Offices of Nutrition, US Agency for International Development, Washington, DC. USA; Professor Donald S. McLaren, University of Edinburgh, Scotland; Dr Stewart McNab, formerly UNICEF, Nepal; Dr Jack Metcoff, Department of Pediatrics, University of Oklahoma, USA; Mr Alan J. Morgan, Weighing Equipment Ltd, England; Professor D.D. Morley, Institute of Child Health, University of London, England; Mr James A. Muehlenbein, Health and Education Services, Novel Products Inc, Addison, Illinois, USA; Dr Gerald F. Murray, Center for Population Studies, Harvard University, Massachusetts USA.

N

Dr David Nabarro, Department of Nutrition and Public Health, London School of Hygiene and Tropical Medicine, London, England; Dr D. Neal, British Indicators Ltd, England; Mr Robert O. Nesheim, The Quaker Oats Company, Chicago, USA; Ms Nancy Newton, Program for Appropriate Technology in Health (PATH), California, USA; Professor

Olcay Neyzi, Istanbul Tip Fakultesi, Cocuk Sagligi ve Hastaliklari Jursusu Capa Istanbul, Istanbul, Turkey; Dr Milton Nichaman, Department of Health Education and Welfare, Center for Disease Control, Atlanta, Georgia, USA; Professor K.R. Norum, Institute for Nutrition Research, University of Oslo, Oslo, Norway.

O

Dr T. Oiso, International Medical Foundation of Japan, Tokyo, Japan; Dr Ulrich Oltersdorf, Institut für Ernahrungswissenschaft 1 der Justus-Liebig-Universität, West Germany; Dr A. Omolulu, Department of Human Nutrition, University of Ibadan, Ibadan, Nigeria; Dr R. Orraca-Tettah, Department of Nutrition and Food Science, University of Ghana, Legon, Ghana.

P

Dr Kanti Pakrasi, Anthropometry and Human Genetics Unit, Indian Statistical Institute, Calcutta; Dr Jana Parizkva, Charles University, Prague, Czechoslovakia; Dr Leonard Payne, Department of Nutritional Sciences, University of California, Berkeley, California, USA; Dr Michel Pechevis, Departement des Enseignements, Centre International de l'Enfance, France; Dr Maija Pekkarinen, Department of Nutritional Sciences, University of Connecticut, Storrs, Connecticut, USA; Dr Pensri, Ramathibodi Hospital, Bangkok, Thailand; Dr J. Perissé, Food and Nutrition Assessment Service, Food Policy and Nutrition Division, Food and Agriculture Organization, Italy; Dr Susan Pettis, Helen Keller International, New York, USA; Mr Edward G. Pfister, Pfister Import–Export Inc, New Jersey USA; Dr D. Picou, National Institute of Higher Education, Trinidad and Tobago; Professor Antonia Polychronopoulou-Trichopoulou, Athens School of Hygiene, Athens, Greece; Dr Alberto Pradilla, World Health Organization, Geneva, Switzerland; Dr Lem Pross, International Child Health Unit, Department of Paediatrics, Uppsala University, Uppsala, Sweden.

R

Dr J.M. Rideout, Division of Clinical Chemistry, Clinical Research Centre, Harrow England; Ms Gina M. Ries, State Department of Health, Des Moines, Iowa, USA; Rockefeller Study and Conference Centre, Villa Serbelloni, Bellagio, Como, Italy; Dr Jon Rohde, Rockefeller Foundation, Indonesia; Dr H.A. Ronaghy, former Department of Health Sciences, Shiraz University, Iran; Dr J.E. Rossouw, National Research Institute for Nutritional Diseases of the South African Medical Research Council, South Africa; Dr Robert Russell, Human Nutrition Research Center, Boston Massachusetts, USA.

S

Dr Z.I. Sabry, School of Public Health, University of California, Berkeley, California, USA; Dr John Seaman, International Disaster Institute, London, England; Dr Carl C. Seltzer, Harvard University, Cambridge,

Massachusetts, USA; Dr Beatrice J. Selwyn, School of Public Health, University of Texas, Houston, Texas, USA; Dr P.M. Shah, MCH, World Health Organization, Geneva, Switzerland; Dr Haif El Shazali, Department of Paediatrics, Medani Hospital, Medani, Sudan; Dr Maurice Shils, Memorial Sloan-Kettering Cancer Center, New York, USA; Mr Irwin Shorr, Division of Nutritional Sciences, Cornell University, Ithaca, New York, USA; Ms Mary-Jo Sier, American Thermometer Co, Inc, Dayton, Ohio, USA; Dr Richard Snyder, Biomedical Department, Institute of Science and Technology, Ann Arbor, Michigan, USA; Dr Florentino S. Solon, Nutrition Centre of the Philippines, Philippines; Dr Alfred Sommer, Nutritional Blindness Prevention Project, Indonesia; Professor P. Soysa, Department of Paediatrics, University of Sri Lanka, Sri Lanka; Dr S.G. Srikantia, formerly National Institute of Nutrition, Indian Council of Medical Research, India; Dr J. Paget Stanfield, formerly Department of Child Health, Royal Victoria Infirmary, Newcastle-upon-Tyne, England.

T

Professor James Tanner, Institute of Child Health, 30 Guilford Street, London, England; Professor Robert Tarjan, Institute of Nutrition, Gyali-Ut 3 9, Budapest IX, Hungary; Dr Carlos Tejada, formerly Director, Instituto de Nutrición de Centro America y Panama (INCAP), Carretera Roosevelt Zona 11, Guatemala; Dr Carlos Teller, Division of Applied Nutrition, Instituto de Nutrición de Centro America y Panama (INCAP), Carretera Roosevelt Zona 11, Guatemala; Dr. Frederick Trowbridge, Division of Nutrition Center for Disease Control, Atlanta, Georgia, USA; Professor A.S. Truswell, Nutrition Unit, University of Sydney, Sydney, Australia; Dr M. Turner, British Nutrition Foundation, 15 Belgrave Square, London, England.

V

Professor Aree Valyasevi, Institute of Nutrition, Ramathibodi Hospital, Bangkok, Thailand; Dr J. Vuylsteke, Department of Nutrition, Prince Leopold Institute of Tropical Medicine, Amsterdam, Netherlands.

W

Dr Napoleon Wolanski, Laboratory of Human Ecology, Polish Academy of Sciences, Warsaw B6, Poland.

Z

Dr Marian Zeitlin, School of Nutrition, Tufts University, Medford, Massachusetts, USA.

Appendix 1
Clinical signs: Descriptive list and suggestive grouping

The following descriptive list of physical signs is based on the 1963 report of the WHO Expert Committee on the Medical Assessment of Nutritional Status, but has been modified based on experience in the past 20 years. It was given as an aid towards achieving uniformity of terminology and the standardization of results obtained by different investigators.

Most of the signs given are believed to be of value in the clinical assessment of malnutrition (Group 1) that occurs commonly in poor, ill-fed communities. Those indicated with an asterisk (*) are considered to be relatively easy to identify and 'strongly suggestive' of a particular nutrient deficiency and have been referred to earlier (see Table 2.4 p. 23). A few are included which are of uncertain significance nutritionally (Group 2); others are probably not nutritionally significant, but require to be differentiated (Group 3).

In this list, no attempt is made to link particular signs with specific nutrient deficiencies; other non-nutritional causes are mentioned. Suggested groupings of signs according to nutrient deficiency are also presented (p. 492).

Hair

Group 1: Potentially nutritionally significant

Lack of lustre

The hair is dull and dry. As with all hair changes, comparison has to be made with local healthy people. The effect of scalp disease, such as extensive fungus infection or impetigo, of certain cultural practices, especially the use of oil on the hair, and of some environmental factors, such as exposure to salt water and a very hot dry atmosphere, must also be taken into account.

Thinness and sparseness

The hair may become thin — that is, fine and silky in texture — and sparse — that is, covering the scalp less abundantly and completely, and with wider gaps between hairs. Allowance must be made for local practices in the treatment of hair; as, for example, with the sparseness that can result in adult women in parts of Africa ('tension alopecia') from the tight braiding of hair into many short pigtails. A similar frontal baldness appears to occur in older Chinese women, possibly as a result of the traditional combed-back hair style.

Straightness

In some ethnic groups, with normally curly hair, malnutrition may produce pathological straightness. This is especially noticeable in children of African ancestry for whom normal healthy hair is thick and thightly curled. Colour changes and 'easy pluckability' are usually also present.

Dyspigmentation of the hair

The hair shows a distinct lightening of its normal colour, usually evident at the tips. The normal range of colours will vary with the particular ethnic group; sometimes the mother, if well-nourished and young; may be immediately available as a living colour standard for her children. The sign is a common feature of some forms of protein–energy malnutrition in young children, and is due to disturbance is melanogenesis. Normal hair colour returns following dietary treatment. The term 'dyspigmentation' is employed rather than 'hypochromotrichia' as there may be, in some instances, an abnormal pigmentation as well as a lightening of colour.

Various changes of colour may be found. In subjects with black hair, the changes, usually seen in decreasing order of frequency, are: dark brown; light brown; red-brown; blonde; and grey. Difficulties with precise estimations of shade of hair are related to observer error and to the occurrence of a gradation of colour changes.

It is not usually necessary to group the different types of colour change seen. Where this is required — as it may be for research purposes — attempts have been made to grade the hair colours seen with colour charts used by paint manufacturers, artists, wool firms, and even beauty salons. None has been found to be satisfactory, as the colours displayed do not approximate to those seen in malnutrition. It may be more satisfactory to prepare a local hair-colour guide made up of clear-cut specimens of the most usual shades of dyspigmented hair seen. These can be stuck to a piece of white carboard with transparent cellotape, and used on the survey.

Dyspigmentation of the hair is a *variable* sign and is not found even in all children with kwashiorkor. It is most marked in chronic, and hence often less severe, cases. it reflects changes occurring during the preceding weeks or, more usually, months, as hair grows about 0.2 mm per day.

Numerous problems arise in the assessment of dyspigmented hair. It may be customary for children of one or both sexes to have their hair cut

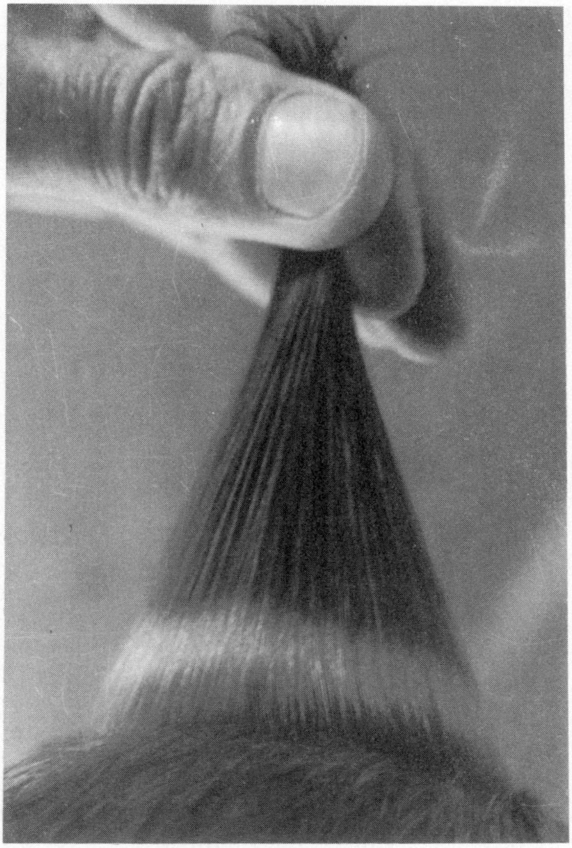

Fig. AP1.1 Flag sign (*signo de bandera*), a light-coloured band indicating a past episode of kwashiorkor.

short or shaved, so that the hair colour is not apparent. Local factors may be important, such as dyeing (e.g. with henna, cow's urine, etc.), the effects of sunshine, salt-spray, and dust, genetic factors (especially ethnically mixed communities, such as the West Indies), and the habitual use of oil.

Confusion has arisen between different workers because some have recorded this sign as positive when only the tips of the hair or the fringe of scalp hair ('fair frontal fringe' or 'halo effect') are affected.

Flag sign (Fig. AP1.1)

This hair change, found in young children and first reported from South America as *signo de bandera*, is usually uncommon, but has attracted undue attention because of its striking appearance. It is characterized by alternating bands of light and dark colour along the length of the hair, and reflects alternating episodes of protein–energy malnutrition and cure. It has been described in Arab children, and especially in South and Central America. It does not appear to have been reported frequently elsewhere.

Easy pluckability

In this sign, a small clump or tuft of hair can be easily pulled out with moderate force and without pain. In extreme examples, this looseness of the hair is a striking finding, easily demonstrated. In less advanced cases, it is often most marked in the temporal region, but is a difficult sign to judge objectively, as it plainly depends on the force applied to the clump of hair by the examiner's thumb and forefinger. Recently, an apparatus has been devised to measure the force needed (p. 54).

It is usually accompanied by other hair changes, such as dyspigmentation, thinness, and sparseness, and occurs in kwashiorkor and other forms of protein–energy malnutrition in early childhood. The easy pluckability and the sparseness are both related to a looseness of hairs in their follicles.

Face

Group 1: Potentially nutritionally significant

Diffuse depigmentation

A general lightening of colour of the pigment of the skin of the face can occur, and may sometimes be exaggerated by associated underlying anaemia. In protein–energy malnutrition, it is usually first and most easily noticeable on the face, centrally rather than laterally. As usual with estimations of colour change, lesser degrees are difficult to determine precisely. Genetic influences may sometimes be relevant. Its aetiology is probably similar to that of dyspigmented hair — that is, interference with melanogenesis. Both can occur in protein–energy malnutrition in young children, especially in kwashiorkor, in which condition the skin slowly darkens following dictary treatment.

Moon-face (Fig. AP1.2)

This is a peculiar rounded prominence of the cheeks, which protrude over the general level of the naso-labial folds. Pitting does not occur on pressure. The mouth presents a pursed-in appearance. This condition is encountered mostly in the pre-school age child with protein–energy malnutrition of the kwashiorkor type.

Conjunctival xerosis (WHO code:X1A)

This condition is almost always bilateral and is characterized by marked dryness. There is also a lack of lustre and transparency of the bulbar conjunctiva, especially on the most exposed part of the eyebal. A few seconds' exposure by drawing back the lids will aid in its identification. Some workers have used 1 per cent Rose Bengal or 1 per cent Lissamine Green eye drops to identify early conjuctival xerosis. This is not usually practicable nor very helpful (Sommer 1982).

Small, more or less vertical, dry folds of the conjunctiva can best be demonstrated by wrinkling up the loose temporal conjunctiva against the outer canthus with the eye in full external movement. The xerotic conjunctiva is not wetted by tears ('unwettability'). The process is due in part to keratinization affecting the cells of the conjunctival epithelium.

**Bitôt's spots (WHO code:X1B) (Fig. 2.3, p. 23)*

These are usually well-demarcated, superficial, dry greyish, silvery, or chalky-white foamy plaques, often triangular or irregularly circular in shape, more often confined to the regions lateral to the cornea. They are usually bilateral, and are composed of keratinized epithelial debris, which can be removed by wiping, revealing a xerotic conjunctival bed with a rough surface. They are also known in Russian literature as 'Iskerkii's patches'.

Bitôt's spots may accompany other ocular manifestations of vitamin-A deficiency, and the subject is most commonly a pre-school child. However, Bitôt's spots are also frequently observed, usually in school-age children and adults, as isolated and often minimal lesions in subjects with no other current evidence of vitamin A deficiency. In India, where *kajal* (carbon-oil cosmetic) is often used by mothers to outline their children's eyes, Bitôt's spots may present as black patches — the result of this material getting on to the conjunctiva and adhering to the dry areas.

Bitôt's spots are recognized in some cultures where they are common (e.g. in parts of Indonesia) and given special descriptive names, often referring to their appearance (e.g. fish scale) (p. 167).

Corneal xerosis (WHO code:X2) (see Frontispiece)

The cornea is hazy or opaque, frequently with a bluish milky appearance, usually most marked in the lower central area. It has a dry, roughened, often pebbly appearance (Sommer 1982). This appearance is due in part to cellular infiltration of the cornea. Corneal xerosis is usually accompanied by conjunctival xerosis. Both cornea usually show change, sometimes to a widely varying degree. Photophobia, pain, and inflammatory congestion are not usually present.

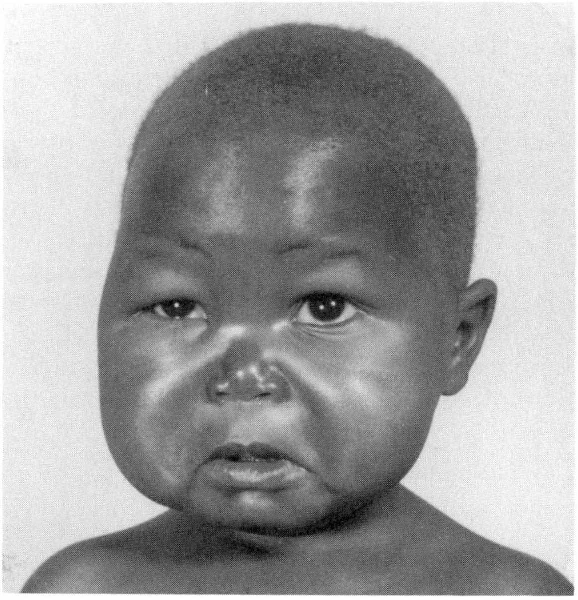

Fig. AP1.2 'Moon-face' in classical kwashiorkor (Uganda).

Group 2: Possibly nutritionally significant

Perinasal veins

Usually bilateral and possibly associated with exccessive alcohol intake.

Eyes

Eye signs have to be considered in relation to the possible effects of chronic ocular trauma from a combination of bright sunlight, dust, wind, smoke, and infection. Eye signs have their greatest value in the identification of anaemia and xerophthalmia (Sommer 1978, 1982). Current WHO views on their significance in vitamin A deficiency and abbreviated labelling (e.g. X1A, X1B, X2, etc.) are given elsewhere (p. 266).

Group 1: Potentially nutritionally significant

**Pale conjunctiva (Fig. 2.4, pp. 24 and 25)*

This sign is positive if there is pallor of the conjuctiva, which can be roughly gauged by clinical inspection or by direct colour comparison (p. 25). It is principally a clinical reflection of anaemia, whether nutritional in causation or due to non-nutritional causes, or both.

Keratomalacia (WHO code X3A and X3B) (see Frontispiece)

This consists of a characteristic softening of the entire thickness of part or more often the whole of the cornea, leading to perforation and prolapse of the iris.

Keratomalacia usually affects both eyes, but often with unequal involvement. Xerosis of the conjunctiva is usually, though not invariably, present. The condition is essentially quiet and insidious, with no pain or other complaints, and no secretion or discharge. It can occur 'behind closed eyelids' (McLaren 1963). Keratomalacia is especially sinister as it is 'white and quiet', compared with inflammatory lesions (Sommer 1982).

The process is a rapid one, the corneal structure melting into a cloudy gelatinous mass, which may be dead-white or dirty-yellow in colour. Extrusion of the lens and loss of vitreous may occur; in untreated cases, generalized infection usually occurs.

Angular palpebritis (angular blepharitis)

The sign is characterized by rawness and fissuring of the outer side of the eye and is sometimes associated with angular stomatitis (p. 26).

Group 2: Possibly nutritionally significant

Corneal vascularization

This is due to an invasion of the whole of the edge of the cornea by fine capillaries. Early changes can be defined only by biomicroscopic examination. It is caused by congestion of the normal limbal plexus, is non-specific, and can occur in any inflammatory or irritative process affecting the cornea.

Conjunctival infection and circumcorneal infection

The terms are self-explanatory.

Corneal arcus

This presents as a light-coloured ring around the outer edge of both irises. It is partly a phenomenon of ageing, but a relationship with high blood cholesterol has been suggested, especially if occurring in earlier adult life. Biochemical tests for blood cholesterol and low-density lipoproteins (LDP) are indicated.

Xanthomata

Yellowish-white, often rounded plaques in the skin, frequently beneath the eyes bilaterally, suggestive of high blood cholesterol.

Corneal scars (WHO code:X5) (see Frontispiece)

Their nature (fine or dense, deep or superficial) and position (which quadrant of the cornea) should be noted. Corneal opacities and scars of varying density may result from previous infection, including ophthalmia neonatorum, trachoma, and congenital syphilis, from trauma or from malnutrition, especially from past avitaminosis A (Sommer 1982).

Group 3: Not nutritionally significant

Pterygium (Fig. 2.1, p. 19)

This lesion, so-called because of its wing-shaped appearance, is produced by a fleshy double fold of conjunctiva, growing progressively, laterally across the cornea. Its cause is unknown, but appears to be related to prolonged irritation, as from sun-glare. It has no nutritional significance, and occurs in both poorly- and well-nourished adults who have been subjected to prolonged exposure to sun and wind (e.g. seamen).

Lips

Group 1: Potentically nutritionally significant

**Angular stomatitis (Fig. 2.7, p. 26)*

The term is used to describe sodden and excoriated fissures at the angles of the mouth. The fissures may be shallow or deep, confind to a small area of the angles of the mouth or extending into the buccal cavity and a few millimetres on to the skin outside. Milder lesions are discerned more easily with the mouth half open. The sign should be reported as positive only if both angles of the mouth are involved.

Angular scars

Healed angular stomatitis may result in pink or blanched scars at the angles of the mouth, depending on the interval since the acute episode. In older children, the possibility that the scars are healed rhagades of congenital syphilis must be considered.

Cheilosis

This lesion is characterized by vertical fissuring, later complicated by redness, swelling, and ulceration of the lips, other than the angles. The centre of the lower lip is most usually affected. Climatic factors, such as cold and wind, may sometimes be responsible.

Group 2: Possibly nutritionally significant

Chronic depigmentation of the lower lip

This is usually central and may, in some cases, represent the site of an old, healed cheilosis.

Tongue

Signs in the mouth affecting the tongue or gums must be considered in relation to local trauma, as from spicy foods and false teeth, as well as to nutritional deficiency.

Group 1: Potentially nutritionally significant

Oedema of tongue

This can be detected by the indentations made by pressure of teeth along the edges of the tongue.

Scarlet or raw tongue

The tongue is bright red in colour, usually of normal size or slightly atrophic, denuded, and very painful.

Magenta tongue

The tongue is purplish-red in colour; numerous morphological changes may coexist.

Attempts have been made to measure colour changes in the tongue by comparison with plates or swatches in the Reinhold Colour Atlas (Friedman and Hodges 1977). They note that the colour is also influenced by different haemoglobin concentrations, hypoxia, and thickness of epithelium on the tongue.

Atrophic papillae

The filiform papillae have disappeared, giving the tongue an extremely smooth appearance. The distribution may be central or marginal. Permanent records of the lesion can be made with 'tongue prints', although this is rarely practicable or necessary.

Group 2: Possible nutritional significance

Hyperaemic and hypertrophic papillae

The papillae are hypertrophic and red or pink, and give the tongue a granular or pebbly appearance (red strawberry).

Fissures

Cracks on the surface of the tongue with no papillae on their sides or floors. These must not be confused with the congenital ridging and convoluted appearance known as 'scrotal tongue' which has no nutritional significance.

Group 3: No nutritional significance

Geographic tongue

The tongue has irregularly distributed patchy areas of denudation and atrophy of epithelium. It is painless and symptomless. Its aetiology is obscure and no treatment appears to be effective.

Pigmented tongue

Punctate or patchy areas of blue–black mucosal pigmentation are present, sometimes associated with similar patches on the gums. These have no significance. They are the oral equivalent of the blue–black areas of increased pigmentation (misnamed 'Mongolian spots') seen in darker ethnic groups, usually on the skin of the lower back and especially visible in the newborn before full adult pigmentation has occurred.

Teeth

Group 1: Potentially nutritionally significant

**Mottled enamel (Fig. 2.12, p. 30)*

The teeth are mottled with white and brownish patches, with or without erosion or pitting of the enamel, usually best seen in the upper incisors. This sign is characteristic of fluorosis.

**Caries*

The presence of decayed, missing, or filled teeth (DMF) is often used to record the amount of caries present in a community, although teeth may be missing for other reasons, including chronic pyorrhoea and trauma.

In children in most developing countries with inadequate dental services, only the presence of decayed teeth with cavities can be recorded. The method of examination must also be noted. For observers with no dental training, this will usually be by inspection alone.

The prevalence of caries is suggested by the percentage of the adult population with one or more teeth decayed or missing or filled (DMF), or, in the case of young children, of those with one or more teeth decayed or filled (DF). The intensity of caries in a community is calculated by the average number of DMF teeth per person, preferably in 12-year-olds. The prevalence of caries has increased greatly in the past 20 years. It is now estimated that the DMF index is now greater in many urban areas in Third World countries than it is in Europe or North America. This has considerable significance as regards suffering, dental services, and the nutritional consequences of loss of teeth (Geissler and Bates 1984).

Malnutrition in the pregnant woman may play a part in the aetiology of caries in the first dentition. However, caries in both deciduous and permanent teeth is more related to the local effects of foods consumed, especially to the dietary content and frequency of ingestion of sugar (especially more sticky preparations), over-milled flour, and other highly-refined carbohydrate foods.

Attrition

The cutting borders of incisors and molars may be worn down and flattened. This seems to be related to the toughness of the diet, especially hard foods requiring prolonged mastication. It is, therefore, more common in rural communities who eat traditional diets.

Enamel hypoplasia

Defective formation is usually generalized over the tooth surface, especially the medial third. Linear hypoplasia of deciduous incisor teeth has been noted in under-privileged, older pre-school age children (Sweeney *et al.* 1971; Jelliffe and Jelliffe 1971*a*). The characteristic appearance is a 'carved-out' erosion affecting adjacent sides of the deciduous incisors, especially in the upper jaw. A relationship to maternal malnutrition in pregnancy has been suggested.

Enamel erosion

The term describes the sharply defined areas, usually around the gum margin, where the tooth enamel has become eroded.

Gums

Group 1: Potentially nutritionally significant

**Spongy, bleeding gums (Fig. 2.6, p. 26)*

Purplish or red spongy swelling of the inter-dental papillae and/or gum margins, which usually bleed easily on slight pressure.

This sign can occur with prolonged use of certain drugs, including the hydantoinates used in the management of some children with epilepsy. It is absent even in cases of severe lack of ascorbic acid in young children (infantile scurvy) until the teeth have erupted. Bleeding gums without hypertrophy are usually caused by periodontal infection (pyorrhoea).

Group 2: Possibly nutritionally significant

Recession of gums

Atrophy and recession of the gums occur sometimes, exposing the roots of the teeth. This is usually secondary to pyorrhoea.

Table AP1.1 WHO classification of goitre: revised version *(Delange et al. 1986)*

Stage 0	No goitre
Stage 1-A	Goitre detectable only by palpation and not visible even when the neck is fully extended
Stage 1-B	Goitre palpable but visible only when the neck is fully extended (This stage also includes nodular glands, even if not goitrous)
Stage 2	Goitre visible with the neck in normal position; palpation not needed for diagnosis
Stage 3	Very large goitre which can be recognized at a considerable distance

Group 3: Not nutritionally significant

**Pyorrhoea (periodontal infection)*

Infection of gum margins, which are red and bleed easily with no hypertrophy.

Glands

Group 1: Potentially nutritionally significant

**Thyroid enlargement (Fig. 2.8, p. 27)*

The gland is visibly and palpably enlarged. The enlargement may be diffuse or nodular. Inspection and palpation while the subject swallows may be helpful in diagnosis.

For more specialized endemic goitre surveys, the technique and classification revised by WHO should be used, as detailed by Sommer (1982) (Table AP1.1).

The lack of specificity of even such a clear-cut sign as goitre is indicated by the results of the Ten-State Survey in the USA. Just over 3 per cent of adults had goitres, but these had no association that suggested iodine deficiency. In a few areas of the world, endemic goitre occurs commonly with high intakes of iodide in the diet. This has been termed Hokkaido goitre or, in China, coastal goitre (Tai 1982). Also, in other areas with no evidence of iodine deficiency, such as parts of the USA, goitre is being reported. It is possibly caused by water pollution with resorcin.

In addition, in severely iodine-deficient areas, such as the New Guinea highlands, a high incidence of large goitres in pregnant women leads to fetal damage in the form of endemic cretinism, or fetal brain damage and mental deficiency (Fig. 2.9, p. 274). Thus, in future studies into IDD (iodine deficiency disorders), locally appropriate methods of detecting these conditions will need to be considered.

Parotid enlargement

This sign is positive if there is a chronic, visible, non-inflammatory swelling of both parotids. The glands are firm, non-tender, and painless. The overlying skin is unchanged. If the swelling is marked, the lobules of the ears are hidden when the subject is viewed from the front. It is most usually seen in schoolchildren and adults. Parotid enlargement is usually recorded as positive, without grading according to size.

Group 2: Possibly nutritional significant

Gynaecomastia

Bilateral, visible, and palpable enlargement of the nipple and glandular subareolar breast tissue in males.

Skin

Group 1: Potentially nutritionally significant

Xerosis

Generalized dryness with branny desquamation. Factors to be considered when interpreting this and other skin signs are environmental, such as dirt, lack of washing, a dry, hot, windy climate, and the habitual use of oil on the body, and, more rarely, genetic, as in the case of the uncommon condition, congenital ichthyosis.

Follicular hyperkeratosis

Type 1 In this type the lesion consists of hyperkeratosis surrounding the mouths of hair follicles and forming plaques that resemble spines. It is readily detected by the spiky feeling it gives when the palm is passed over an area of affected skin. Its distribution is frequently confined to the buttocks, thighs, and especially the extensor aspects of the legs and arms, particularly the elbows and knees. The surrounding skin is dry and lacks the usual amount of moisture and oiliness. In early literature on the subject, the condition was termed 'phrynoderma' (toad skin).

Type 2 In this type the lesions have a similar appearance, but the mouths of the hair follicles contain blood or pigment, and have a surrounding pink halo, the perifollicular haemorrhage (Hodges 1971). The intervening skin is not usually dry. The condition is seen mostly in adults. The distribution is usually over the abdomen and the extensor aspects of the thighs. The sign is less obvious in darker-skinned persons.

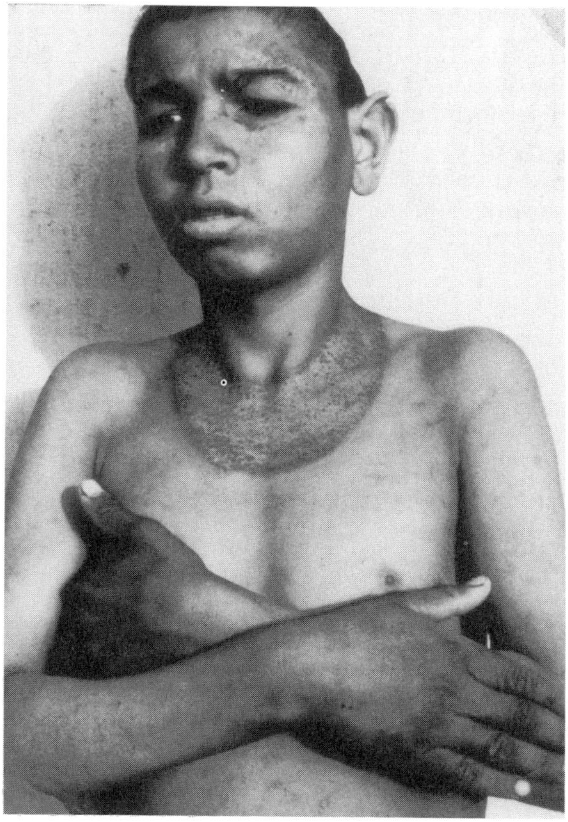

Fig. AP1.3 Typical pellagrous dermatosis with 'Casal's necklace' (Egypt).

Petechiae

Small haemorrhagic spots in the skin or mucous membranes, which are difficult to see in darker-skinned people. As a clinical test, the application of a blood pressure tourniquet may sometimes produce additional petechiae.

Pellagrous rash or dermatosis (Fig. AP1.3)

Typical pellagrous skin lesions are symmetrical, clearly demarcated, hyperpigmented areas with or without exfoliation. The lesions are common in parts of the body exposed to sunlight, including the cheeks and the forearms; when they appear around the neck the condition is called 'Casal's necklace'.

In acute cases, the skin is red, slightly swollen, and may show vesiculation, exudation, and cracking. The lesion itches and burns. In chronic cases, the dermatosis occurs as a roughening and thickening of the skin with dryness, scaling, and brown pigmentation.

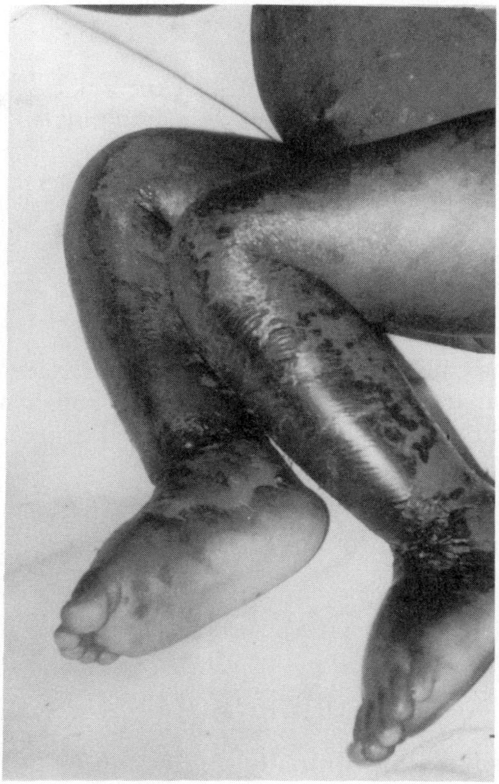

Fig. AP1.4 Flaky-paint dermatosis in classical kwashiorkor (Uganda).

Flaky-paint rash or dermatosis (Fig. AP1.4)

Extensive, often bilateral hyperpigmented patches of skin which desquamate to leave hyperpigmented skin or superficial ulceration, often resembling a second-degree burn. It can occur anywhere, but characteristically on the buttocks and the back of the thighs. The lesion was once termed 'crazy-pavement dermatosis'.

Scrotal and vulval dermatosis

A desquamating lesion of the skin of the scrotum or vulva, often highly itchy. Secondary infection may supervene.

Group 2: Possibly nutritionally significant

Mosaic dermatosis

Large thin mosaic plaques, firmly adherent in the centre, but showing a tendency to peel at the periphery, present bilaterally on both shins.

Thickening and pigmentation of pressure points

Diffuse thickening, with pigmentation of the pressure points, such as the knees, elbows, and front and back of the ankles. The knuckles may also be involved. The affected areas may be wrinkled, with or without fissuring.

Nails

Group 1: Potentially nutritionally significant

Koilonychia

Bilateral, spoon-shaped deformity of the nails in adults, suggestive of iron-deficiency anaemia. Slightly spoon-shaped nails can be found commonly, affecting the toenails only, in barefooted communities; the condition appears to have no significance.

Group 2: Possibly nutritionally significant

Transverse ridging or grooving of nails

This should be recorded if present in nails of more than one extremity.

Subcutaneous tissues

Group 1: Potentially nutritionally significant

Bilateral oedema (Fig. 2.10, p. 29)

Usually first apparent over the ankles and feet, it may extend to other areas of the extremities. It may involve genitals, face, and hands. In the early stages, it can be detected by firm pressure for 3 seconds with one digit on the lower portion of the tibia. The sign is taken as positive if there is a visible and palpable pit that persists after the pressure is removed. It is significant only if present bilaterally.

Subcutaneous fat

An approximate estimate of any excess or depletion can be seen or estimated by palpation of a skinfold. If indicated, detailed measurements with calipers can also be made (p. 85).

Muscular and skeletal systems

Group 1: Potentially nutritionally significant

Muscular wasting

This can be detected by observation and palpation of the upper arm, especially the biceps or the trapezius muscles. More detailed assessment of muscle tissue should be carried out wherever relevant by anthropometry (p. 101).

In children, particularly, muscle wasting, accompanied by poor muscle tone, can result in pot-belly, lordosis, and winged scapulae. In severely affected children with protein–energy malnutrition, including kwashiorkor, the degree of muscle wasting can be roughly tested by testing the child's ability to hold up his head when pulled gently from a lying to a sitting position.

Craniotabes

This sign consists of areas of softening of the skull, usually involving the occipital and parietal bones. Affected areas dent on pressure and spring back after the pressure is removed ('ping-pong ball' areas). The sign is positive only in infancy, especially in young babies.

Frontal and parietal bossing

Localized thickening and heaping up of the frontal and parietal bones of the skull occurs. Bossing may have a nutritional cause, but it can also occur in older children of African ancestry with sickle-cell anaemia and in other communities where thalassaemia is a common genetic problem. It appears to be recognized by some communities as a possible familial characteristic. It has also been noted rarely in older children suffering from very chronic iron deficiency.

Persistently open anterior fontanelle

This may be defined as an anterior fontanelle which is open on palpation after the age of 18 months. The sign is not specific for rickets and can be found in hydrocephalus and other conditions.

**Epiphyseal enlargement (Fig. 2.11, p. 29)*

Enlargement of the epiphyseal ends of long bones, particularly affecting the radius and ulna at the level of the wrist, and the tibia and fibula at the level of the ankle. Measurement of the width or circumference of the wrist can be undertaken (Snyder *et al.* 1977), and the use of an 'epiphysometer' (screw gauge) or some similar technique has been suggested to give a more objective field diagnosis of rickets (Jelliffe 1971) (p. 000). In the assessment of this sign, allowance must be made for the degree of subcutaneous fat present. In wasted persons, including young children with marasmus, the ends of the long bones appear unusually prominent because of the loss of fat padding.

Beading of the ribs (Fig. AP1.5)

A symmetrical nodular enlargement of the costochondral junctions, producing a 'rosary' effect. It is essentially a special, localized form of epiphyseal enlargement.

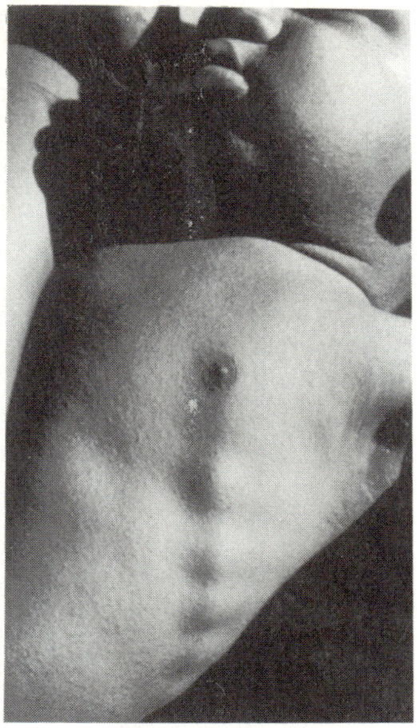

Fig. AP1.5 Beading of the ribs in rickets in a young child (West Indies).

Knock-knees

This condition (genu valgum) also occurs in India (Krishnamachari and Krishnaswami 1974; Srikantia 1984), and may be due to additional trace mineral deficiencies.

Bow-legs (Fig. AP1.6)

In some areas, these deformities occur not infrequently due to orthopaedic conditions quite unrelated to the late effects of rickets (Oyemade 1977)

Widespread or local pelvic skeletal deformities

Deformities of the thorax The two most important are Harrison's sulcus — an indentation running around both sides of the chest — and pigeon chest. However, many common thoracic deformities are unrelated to malnutrition (e.g. funnel chest).

Musculoskeletal haemorrhages Larger haemorrhages may occur as: (a) intramuscular haematoma, usually of the calf or thigh; (b) haemarthrosis; (c) subperiosteal haemorrhage. These may be suspected clinically, but can be confirmed only by detailed clinical examination and by special tests, such as aspiration for haemarthrosis, and radiology for subperiosteal haemorrhage.

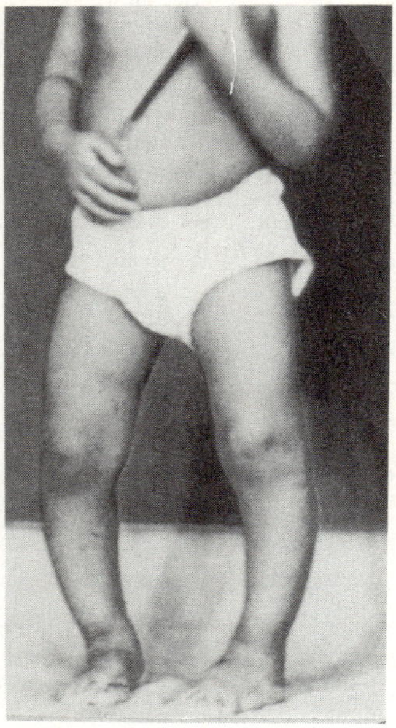

Fig. AP1.6 Bowing of legs — a late and residual sign of rickets (India).

Internal systems

Group 1: Potentially nutritionally significance

Gastrointestinal system: hepatomegaly

The abdomen should be palpated in a standard position, that is, with the subject lying down, with the hips and knees flexed, if it is intended to measure size of liver enlargement. This can be recorded in centimetres below the rib margin.

In the case of a young child, if the exact size is not to be recorded, examinations can be carried out with the child semi-reclining on the mother's lap, which reduces the likelihood of struggling.

Hepatomegaly in young children can occur solely as a result of a low-protein, largely carbohydrate diet. It was at one time particularly common in the West Indies. However, the enlarged palpable livers found in young children in many tropical regions usually appear to have mixed causes, including chronic malaria, malnutrition, and possibly the result of migration of helminth larvae through the liver.

Nervous system: mental change

Listlessness can occur at any age, but is most strikingly seen in severe protein–energy malnutrition of early childhood. This is especially so in kwashiorkor, when the child is apathetic, withdrawn, and lacking in liveliness and interest in his surroundings. It is difficult to measure exactly, but can be crudely tested by watching the reaction to a brightly coloured object or light, as well as the response to the examiner. In pellagra in older children, mental disorientation and psychosis can occur.

Clinical tests of the central nervous system

These may include sensory loss, motor weakness, loss of position sense, loss of vibration sense, loss of ankle or knee jerks, and calf tenderness.

These tests are extremely difficult to carry out with any accuracy under field conditions. Even in hospital the problem of obtaining accurate repeatable results with knee and ankle jerks is well-recognized. With apprehensive subjects examined in a rural survey, it is impossible, especially when testing for calf tenderness and vibration sense.

From the practical viewpoint, on the rare occasions when testing is included on a subsample, the tendon jerks should always be reinforced, tested in two positions, and verified by a second examiner. Only absolute and bilateral loss should be reported (ICNND 1963).

If required, vibration sense can be tested with a tuning fork of 128 vibrations per minute (ICNND 1963). Motor weakness in adults is classically judged by the 'squatting' test, that is, the ability to squat and rise four times successively.

Subjective symptoms suggestive of possible neurological involvement, such as paraesthesia, are even less reliable, and, on the whole, history-taking in developing countries has to be undertaken with great caution, owing to the many problems of language, cultural interpretations, and witness reliability.

However, recently Sommer (1982) has found that the mother's observation of her child's 'night blindness' correlates well with biochemical evidence of vitamin A deficiency, in communities where this condition is common. Also, history-taking may sometimes be helpful if a particular nutritional sign of disorder has a specific name in the local language.

Cardiovascular system: cardiac enlargement

The simplest test of value in survey work is an examination by palpation to assess the presence of cardiac enlargement. However, with the practical exceptions of anaemia and beriberi, causes of cardiomegaly are essentially non-nutritional.

Cardiovascular system: tachycardia

The resting pulse rate may be of value in a nutritional status survey, because tachycardia can occur in anaemia, beriberi, and certain (probably) nutritional cardiopathies. The rate must always be compared with 'normal' values for the appropriate age-group. It will, of course, be very difficult to obtain a resting pulse under survey conditions.

Group 2: Possibly nutritionally significant

Cardiovascular system: blood pressure

If the blood pressure is taken, the technique employed must be carefully standardized.

Guide to the interpretation grouping of clinical signs

Grouping of clinical signs suggestive of various nutrient deficiencies are given in Table AP1.2. The presence of more than one sign in a particular group increases the likelihood of a correct diagnosis. However, this is much more likely to occur in severe cases, which are usually seeking treatment in hospital.

TABLE AP1.2 Grouping of clinical signs *suggestive* of nutritional disease

Deficiency	Hair changes	Facial changes	Eye changes	Buccal changes	Glandular changes	Skin changes	Skeletal changes
Vitamin A			Bitôt's spots, conjunctival xerosis, keratomalacia			Xerosis, follicular hyperkeratosis (type 1)	—
Riboflavin		Nasolabial dyssebacea	Corneal vascularization, angular blepharitis	Angular stomatitis, cheilosis, magenta tongue, atrophic lingual papillae		Scrotal or vulval dermatosis	
Thamine						Oedema	Motor weakness, calf muscle tenderness *Other signs include:* sensory loss, cardiac enlargement, and tachycardia
Niacin				Raw scarlet tongue, atrophic lingual papillae, fissuring of tongue		Pellagrous dermatosis, pigmentation of supraorbital and malar regions	
Vitamin C				Spongy bleeding gums		Follicular hyperkeratosis (type 2), petechiae, ecchymoses	Epiphyseal enlargement, haematoma in muscles and beneath periosteum of bones

Vitamin D							1. *Active rickets*. Epiphyseal enlargement, beading of ribs, open fontanelle, Craniotabes, muscular hypotonia 2. *Healed rickets*. Bossing of skull, deformation of thorax, Harrison's sulcus, bow legs, knock knees.
Iron			Pale conjunctiva	Atrophic lingual papillae			Additional signs include: Deformities or ridging of nails (koilonychia)
Vitamin B_{12}			Pale conjunctiva				
Iodine					Goitre		
Protein–energy malnutrition (i) young children	Dyspig-mentation, easy, pluckability, sparseness, and straightness	Moon-face			Diffuse dyspigmentation of skin, flaky-paint dermatosis, oedema.		Muscle wasting *Additional signs*: Hepatomegaly, psychomotor change
(ii) Adults and schoolchildren					Parotid enlargement	Oedema of ankles	Muscle wasting, fat wasting

Appendix 2
Further laboratory tests

Collection of specimens

Blood samples

Plasma is required for examinations for albumin, vitamin A, carotene, ascorbic acid, and alkaline phosphatase, and will have to be prepared from oxalated whole blood by centrifugation. Fresh whole blood or blood preserved with appropriate anticoagulant, such as sequenstrene, is used for the determination of haemoglobin and haematocrit, and for the preparation of thin and thick blood films, if these are to be included. The technique for drawing blood must be thoroughly known and practised.

Blood samples are collected into stoppered or screw-capped glass vials, containing an appropriate anticoagulant, such as dried oxalate or heparin lithium, if required. Each container should have a previously affixed blank label.

Many of the biochemical tests used for nutritional appraisal can be carried out by micromethods. These methods are particularly important where young children are concerned. Blood obtained by finger-prick can be collected in heparinized capillary tubes, and sealed by heating in a flame or by using commercial clay, specially prepared for this purpose.

All blood samples must be kept chilled until tested. In the field, this is achieved in thermos flasks, in plastic cooling bags (with tins of freezing mixture), or, rarely, in mobile refrigerators. In the laboratory, the specimens are kept in an ordinary household refrigerator.

Urine samples

Difficulties in collection from adults are largely related to modesty. For young children, only boys can have this undertaken easily by fixing a test-tube (preferably of plastic) to the penis, although a relatively expensive plastic disposable collecting device, which sticks to the perineum, can be used for little girls. Sometimes, however, it may suffice for plastic jars to be given to mothers for them to 'catch' a specimen during the survey period.

For the commoner urinary analyses (e.g. urea, thiamine, riboflavin,

* Special thanks are due to Dr Howerde Sauberlich for reviewing this Appendix. His book (Sauberlich *et al.* (1974). *Laboratory tests for the assessment of nutritional status.* CRC Press, Cleveland, Ohio.) gives further details.

N-methyl-nicotinamide), fasting samples passed in a definite time-period are ideal, but not usually practicable under field conditions, especially with children. Single random specimens are usually the best that can be obtained.

Urine should be collected in sturdy screw-capped glass or, preferably, plastic bottles containing hydrochloric acid as a preservative and as an inhibitor of bacterial growth. The amount of hydrochloric acid should be such as not to dilute the sample greatly: one drop of concentrated hydrochloric acid should be enough for about 25 ml of urine. The specimen can then be kept at room temperature or stored in a refrigerator.

Protein–energy malnutrition

Other liver proteins

The concept of 'visceral depletion' emphasized by those concerned with the nutritional status of hospitalized patients in industrialized countries (Blackburn *et al.* 1977) has further drawn attention to the possibility of measuring serum concentration of proteins, other than albumin, which are synthesized by the liver. In particular, the usefulness of including tests of both serum proteins with a relatively long half-life (albumin — about 20 days) and with a shorter half-life (pre-albumin — 1 to 2 days) Shenkin and Steele 1978) has been suggested.

A number of different serum proteins which are synthesized by the liver have been analysed, including *transferrin, prealbumin, caeruloplasmin, retinol-binding protein, beta-lipoprotein, plasma thyroxine, binding pre-albumin*, and *2HS glycoprotein*, *somatomedin C*, *fibronectin*.

Some seem to have special advantages. For example, beta-lipoprotein is reduced in kwashiorkor and not in marasmus (Coward *et al.* 1971); pre-albumin and transferrin have a greater percentage reduction in kwashiorkor than does albumin (Ingenbleek *et al.* 1972). They are all affected by severe malnutrition contrasted with healthy normals. They can be used with varying effectiveness to gauge the degree of severity of kwashiorkor, but cannot diagnose less marked degrees of protein–energy malnutrition (p. 000). Factors other than protein deficiency may need consideration, in particular the relative influence of iron status on transferrin levels (p. 000). If deficiencies of both protein and iron occur at the same time, there may be difficulties in interpretation (Cook and Skifne 1982). Similarly, retinol-binding protein levels may be affected by deficiency of protein or vitamin A or liver damage (Rask *et al.* 1980).

Unfortunately, none have been evaluated sufficiently in lesser degrees of protein–energy malnutrition, and, apart from completely inhibiting practical considerations in community studies, such as complexity, cost, and availability of laboratory resources, their value remains unclear and at best, marginal. Their use in hospital nutritional assessment is also a matter of debate (Golden 1982; Carpentier *et al.* 1982). Currently, retinol-binding protein and pre-albumin seem to be considered most useful.

Urinary creatinine

Muscle depletion is a characteristic feature of severe protein–energy malnutrition, occurring both in kwashiorkor and marasmus, and 'lean body mass' can be measured by several sophisticated laboratory methods (p. 99). Creatinine is a breakdown product of creatine, nearly all of which is contained in muscle, and a decrease in total body muscle mass has been estimated from the 24-hour excretion of urinary creatinine in children with protein–energy malnutrition in metabolic wards (Arroyave and Wilson 1961). Also, Trowbridge *et al.* (1982) correlated creatinine secretion with mid-upper arm muscle area. Although the estimation of creatinine is simple and can be automated (Alleyne *et al.* 1977), a 24-hour timed sample is needed. Indeed, in the recent usage of this method in hospitalized patients, mainly adults, in industrialized countries, it has been recommended that all urine be collected for 3 consecutive days (Shenkin and Steele 1978) and that specimens be collected with precise timing, as differences of 15 minutes may lead to significant variation in results. In special studies, timed samples of 3 hours have been used as a compromise (Satyanaraya *et al.* 1981). Unfortunately, even such timed samples are not usually feasible, so that the method remains for one hospital usage, when it is expressed as a creatinine-height index (CHI). Various factors, including fever, stress, and renal failure can affect creatinine excretion, as can a recent meal of cooked meat, so that other methods need to be looked for to estimate body muscle mass (Heymsfield *et al.* 1982).

3-methylhistidine excretion

The excretion of this substance in the urine may partly reflect muscle mass and partly myofibrillar protein turnover (Bagepalli *et al.* 1973). It is reduced in seriously malnourished children, but has not been evaluated in less marked protein–energy malnutrition. It also has the disadvantage of needing a 24-hour sample of urine.

Amino acids in hair

The possibility of analysis of hair for amino acid composition, including cystine content, has been suggested by several workers in the past, but results, have shown too much variation to be useful.

Growth retardation

Urinary hydroxyproline

Growth retardation is a fundamental feature of protein–energy malnutrition, and the excretion of hydroxyproline — a product of collagen metabolism — in the urine has been shown to vary with rate of growth, to be low in malnourished children and to rise as growth restarts following treatment. As only random, non-timed samples of urine can usually be obtained in community studies, the hydroxyproline index relating the amount of this substance present in the urine to creatinine excretion is the best that can be obtained. The simplest form of the urinary hydroxyproline/creatinine (HOP/C) index (Alleyne *et al.* 1977) is

$$\frac{\text{mg hydroxyproline/ml.}}{\text{mg creatinine/ml}}$$

Standards for the HOP/C have been estimated biochemically for children of different ages. Unfortunately, as noted by Alleyne *et al.* (1977) the HOP/C has been shown to have many problems, including variation at different times of the day, normal levels in some actual cases of kwashiorkor, possibly affected by malaria and other infections (Wenlock 1977), relationship to riboflavin deficiency, etc. Also, its estimation is a 'somewhat tedious and time-consuming task, suitable only for relatively well-equipped and staffed hospitals' (Wenlock 1977). Other limitations are fully discussed by Sauberlich (1974).

Metabolic changes due to tissue malnutriton

Serum amino acids

Marked alterations in amino-acid metabolism in kwashiorkor have been recognized for years. The main finding is a decrease in the plasma concentration of some essential amino acids — valine, leucine, isoleucine, threonine, and methionine — while such non-essential amino acids, as glycine and serine, are unaltered or increased in concentration (Alleyne *et al.* 1977).

Based on this biochemical change, Whitehead and Dean (1964) introduced the amino-acid imbalance test. This is a semiquantitative method in which the 'distortion' of the amino acid pattern was measured by comparing the concentrations of two groups of amino acids measured by paper chromatography

$$\text{Ratio} = \frac{\text{glycine} + \text{serine} + \text{glutamine} + \text{taurine}}{\text{valine} + \text{leucine} + \text{isoleucine} + \text{methionine}}.$$

Malnutrition was characterized by a raised ratio; in normal children the mean value was 1.5, in subclinical malnutrition values ranged between 2.0 and 4.0, and in frank kwashiorkor they were above 3.5, with a mean of 5.0. The main attraction of this method in Uganda was its sensitivity to malnutrition at an earlier stage than serum total protein or albumin. But highly sensitive measurements have inherent problems as well as virtues; the amino-acid ratio, for example, returns to normal soon after the restoration of an adequate diet when, by clinical, anthropometric, and even other biochemical criteria, the child still is severely malnourished. Thus, the method is subject to false normals and these are a considerable disadvantage in a public health context (Whitehead and Dean 1964; Saunders *et al.* 1967).

Other problems have emerged, such as the test being unaffected in areas where marasmus is the main form of protein–energy malnutrition or where acute diarrhoea is a common precipitating infection. This is particularly unfortunate as the test can be undertaken on a blood sample taken by finger-prick and is independent of age. However, the difficulties mentioned, together with the need for a sophisticated laboratory, have meant that this method is not suitable for practical use in community surveys or other forms of assessment of the nutritional status or population groups in developing countries.

Serum ribonuclease

The concentration of serum free alkaline ribonuclease has been found to be diminished in severe protein–energy malnutrition (El Sawedy *et al.* 1978; Sigulem *et al.* 1973). The method needs testing in less advanced cases, and the need for a technically advanced laboratory makes its widespread practical use most unlikely.

Relative adequacy of dietary intake

Urinary urea/creatinine ratio

This test can be undertaken on a random sample of urine, and the ratio is of the amount of urea (mg/ml) divided by creatinine (mg/ml) or by creatinine nitrogen (mg/ml) (Alleyne *et al.* 1977). As with other methods, large numbers of problems have become apparent with this test. It is currently the consensus that its only value in practice is that of checking if individuals have actually consumed a dietary protein supplement or not (Lechtig *et al.* 1981) in community research projects involving supplementary feeding.

Thiamine

Estimations of urinary excretion of thiamine have been undertaken widely and reflect the intake of this nutrient. Despite an apparent marked decline in incidence of beriberi in less technically developed countries, thiamine deficiency can occur in chronic alcoholics and in individuals, especially active teenagers, on restricted fad diets. The 24-hour output, the 1-hour excretion on fasting, or the thiamine content of a random sample per gram of creatinine can be used. A specialized tissue test can be undertaken on red blood cells by estimating erythrocyte transketolase concentrations (Leevy 1980).

Riboflavin

In field surveys, riboflavin may be determined in a single random urine specimen, preferably collected from a fasting subject. The following reference concentrations for young adult males have been suggested (ICNND 1963):

1. Riboflavin per 6 hours: 'low' 10–29 μg, 'deficient' < 10 μg.
2. Riboflavin per gram creatinine: 'low' 27–9 μg, 'deficient' < 27 μg.

Normal values for young children are uncertain, although it is stated that excretion is 2–3 times as great as in adults when expressed per gram of creatinine. A specialized tissue test can be done on red blood cells by estimating erythrocyte glutathione reductase, which is now the preferred method.

Niacin

This water-soluble vitamin differs from others of the B complex because an amino acid, tryptophan, serves as its precursor in man, and because it is not secreted in the urine as such, but is metabolized to at least two derivatives, N′-methylnicotinamide and N′-methylpyridone.

In field surveys, excretion of these niacin metabolites in the urine over a timed interval — e.g. 6 hours, or, more usually, in a single random (preferably fasting) urine sample, expressed per gram of creatinine, provides information concerning the dietary intake of niacin and tryptophan.

As about equal quantities of the two metabolites are excreted, an assay of N′-methylnicotinamide is recommended, as this is technically less time-consuming than an assay of N′-methylpyridone. The suggested concentrations of urinary excretion for young adult males are:

1. N′-methylnicotinamide per 6 hours: 'low' 0.2–0.59 mg, 'deficient' < 0.2 mg)
2. N′-methylnicotinamide per gram creatinine: 'low' 0.5–1.59 mg, 'deficient' < 0.5 mg.

Pyridoxine

Vitamin B_6 (pyridoxine) is not usually considered in the assessment of nutritional status of the community in developing countries. Increased needs for this nutrient in women taking oral contraceptives and in individuals being treated for tuberculosis with INH (isonicotinic acid hydrazide) may occasionally indicate such studies. Urinary excretion rates and blood concentrations can be clarified by a number of specialized tests, such as tryptophan load and blood cell transaminase activity measurements (Sauberlich *et al.* 1974).

Table AP2.1 Suggested guide to interpretation of some biochemical determinants in adults in descriptive categories (*Kanawati 1976*)*

	High	Acceptable	Low	Deficient
Blood				
Total plasma protein (g/dl)	7.0	6.5–6.9	6.0–6.4	< 6.0
Serum albumin (g/dl)	4.25	3.52–4.24	2.80–3.51	< 2.80
Haemoglobin (g/dl)				
Men	15.0	14.0–14.9	12.0–13.9	< 12.0
Women	14.5	11.0–14.4	10.0–10.9	< 10.0
Haematocrit (PCV)%				
Men	45	42–44	36–41	< 36
Women	43	38–49	30–37	< 30
Plasma ascorbic acid (mg/dl)	> 0.60	0.50–0.59	0.20–0.29	< 0.20
Urine				
Thiamine (μg/g creatinine)	≥ 130	66–129	27–65	< 27
Riboflavin (μg/g creatinine)	≥ 270	80–269	27–79	< 27

* A more extensive review of adult 'normal or acceptable values' has been drawn together by Sauberlich (1983).

Lipids

Nutritional assessment in technically more developed countries should include tests of 'malnutrition plus', including obesity, using anthropometry (p. 345), screening for diabetes (glycosuria), and serum concentrations of various lipids. A similar approach is also needed with the more affluent in the cities of developing countries. The main lipids tested for are serum total cholesterol and serum high-density lipoproteins. High-risk concentrations of cholesterol in realtion to atheroma development are currently considered to be above 240 mg/dl, whereas concentrations of high-density lipoproteins above the normal range of 30–60 mg/dl for males and 40–70 mg/dl for females are considered to be protective against atherosclerosis and heart disease (Glueck 1982).

Reference data

Suggested reference data for some biochemical tests are given in Tables AP2.1 and AP2.2.

Further haematological tests

Community nutritional assessment will usually only include haemoglobin estimations. However, this only gives the prevalence of anaemia, without identifying nutritional and/or other causes, and also does not demonstrate lesser degrees of iron deficiency. In individual patients, and specialized surveys (or on a sample of the population in general community

Table AP2.2 'Normal' values of some biochemical tests of nutritional status in children (*Neumann* et al. *1982: compiled from various sources*)**

Nutrient	Approximate volume (ml)	Normal values	Comments
Albumin	0.1	≥ 3.0 g/dl	Simple radial immunodiffusion
Transferrin	0.1	> 200 mg/dl	
Pre-albumin	0.1	≥ 20 mg/dl	
Iron	1–2	≥ 40 μg/dl	
Transferrin saturation	1–2	≥ 16%	All serum
Ferritin	1–2	≥ 10 ng/ml	
Vitamin A	1	≥ 20 μg/dl	Serum or plasma
Carotene	1	≥ 100 μg/dl	Serum or plasma
Vitamin D (alkaline phosphatase)	1	< 40 King–Armstrong units < 15 Bodansky units	
Vitamin E	3	≥ 0.7 mg/dl	Serum
Vitamin K (prothrombin time)	5	11–18 s	Prothrombin time
Folic acid	0.5	≥ 3 ng/ml	
Red blood cells	0.5	≥ 140 ng/ml	Serum
Thiamine*	0.1	< 15%	Erythrocytes used
Riboflavin†	0.1	< 1.2%	Erythrocytes used
Pyridoxine‡	0.1	< 1.25	Erythrocytes used
Vitamin B_{12}	1	≥ 150 pg/ml	Serum
Vitamin C	0.4	> 0.3 mg/dl	Serum
Zinc	7	> 80 μg/dl	Serum

* Erythrocyte transketolase.
† Erythrocyte glutathione reductase.
‡ Erythrocyte transaminase.

** Smaller volumes in micromethods available

studies), further haematological tests may be included.

Analysis of finger nails for iron concentrations has been tried (Sobolowski *et al.* 1978), but does not seem to have been pursued.

Iron deficiency tests

A sequential range of tests can be undertaken to detect earlier stages of depletion of body iron stores. Details can be found in Sauberlich (1983) (Table AP2.3). Several recent studies have confirmed the value of low serum transferrin saturation (< 15 per cent) and of serum ferritin (< 10–12 ng/dl) in the detection of pre-anaemic iron deficiency (Derman *et al.*

Table AP2.3 Sequential changes in the development of iron deficiency *(Hillman and Finch 1974)*

	Normal	Iron depletion	Iron-deficient erythropoiesis	Iron deficiency anaemia
RE marrow iron	2.3+	0.1+	0	0
Transferrin IBC (μg/dl)	330 ± 30	360	390	410
Serum ferritin (ng/ml)	100 ± 60	20	10	< 10
Iron absorption (%)	5–10	10–15	10–20	10–20
Serum iron (μg/dl)	115 ± 15	115	< 60	< 40
Transferrin saturation (%)	35 ± 15	30	< 15	< 10
Sideroblasts (%)	40–60	40–60	< 10	< 10
RBC protoporphyrin (μg/dl RBC)	30	30	100	200
Erythrocytes	Normal	Normal	Normal	Microcytic/ hypochronic

1978). In sophisticated laboratory circumstances, an iron-screening algorithm with computerized control has been used to decide whether to undertake more detailed analyses on blood samples (Beck *et al.* 1979).

On a simpler basis, thin blood films, stained with Wright's stain, can be examined for cell morphology, especially for the presence of characteristic microcytes, hypochromia, anisocytosis, and poikilocytosis.

Other nutritional anaemias

Megaloblastic anaemias, due to folic-acid or vitamin B_{12} deficiency, are suggested by a low haemoglobin, associated with a thin film showing macrocytes, hypersegmented (5–7 lobed) neutrophil polymorphs, and reduced numbers of platelets, and with no lowering of haematocrit values. Leyland *et al.* (1979*a*, *b*) stressed the need to define local reference levels. Other specialized tests are summarized in Table AP 2.4. They may need to be followed by appropriate therapeutic trials, both on severely affected individuals and on a sample in the community itself.

Non-nutritional causes

Some community nutrition investigations may also need tests for non-nutritional causes of anaemia. In addition to haemoglobin (and haematocrit), studies may include a thick blood film (stained with Giemsa to show intensity of infection with malarial parasites and residual pigment), thin blood film (cell morphology), a stool sample (which can be taken from young children with a glass or plastic anal tube, stored in 10 per cent formol saline as a preservative, and later examined for occult blood, for the ova of hookworm, and for a rough estimate of approximate worm burden, although recent work has shown this to vary between stool samples in the same individual) (Hall 1981). In African populations, a test for sickling should be included. This may be done by the standard method

Table AP2.4 Tests for vitamin B_{12} and folic acid *(Hillman and Finch 1974)*

	Normal	Possible deficiency	Deficiency
Vitamin B_{12}			
Serum B_{12} (pg/ml)	> 200	100–200	< 100
Urinary methylmalonate (mg/24 hours)	< 4	4–10	> 10
Gastric acidity after histamine (pH)	< 3.5	—	> 3.5
Schilling test (8-hour plasma conc % close/ 1% body weight)	> 2	1.2	< 1
Folic acid			
Serum folate (ng/ml)	> 6	3.6	< 3

of a coverslip ringed with vaseline and examined 24 hours in the field, and by microelectrophoresis of the packed cells remaining in the capillary tube after micro-haematocrit estimations, if these have been made and if laboratory resources permit.

Iodine

A decreased availability of iodine to the thyroid may be the result of an inadequate intake, or, uncommonly, the effect of goitrogenic factors in the food.

Field surveys are usually based entirely on the detection of the principal physical sign of iodine lack — thyroid enlargement, especially in accessible age-groups likely to be affected, e.g. schoolchildren, pregnant women. Greater attention needs to be given to simple clinical methods of identifying individuals, especially children, with endemic cretinism and other manifestations of fetal iodine deficiency (p. 273).

Tests for urinary iodine related to creatinine can be undertaken, and 'low concentrations' have been given as below 50 μg/g creatinine (Trowbridge *et al.* 1975). Many other specialized tests have been included in detailed endocrinological studies, including serum thyroxine, protein-bound iodine, and plasma inorganic iodide.

Trace metals

Hair analysis can be undertaken to estimate the concentrations various trace metals, especially zinc (Klevay 1970) but also copper (Bradfield *et al.* 1980).

Hair has the advantage of giving a picture of mineral status, over preceding weeks or months, while serum concentrations indicate recent intakes and can be affected by a reduction in carrier proteins (cf. copper-transporting serum caeruloplasmin in protein–energy malnutrition). The use of scalp hair for such studies is relatively new, but has the advantages of ease of non-invasiveness, collection, preservation, and transport (including airmail postage to distant specialized laboratories). However, problems may arise in some cultures who are suspicious of witchcraft. Already it has become apparent that consideration needs to be given to the effect of different scalp medications and air pollutants in interpreting results of hair analysis for trace methods. These methods deserve further trial (Orfanos *et al.* 1981; Hambridge 1982).

Appendix 3
Nomograms: muscle and fat arm areas

Figures AP3.1 and AP3.2 are arm anthropometry nomograms for children and adults, respectively.

To obtain muscle circumference from these nomograms:

1. Lay ruler between values of arm circumference and fatfold;
2. Read off muscle circumference on middle line.

To obtain tissue areas from the nomograms:

1. The arm areas and muscle areas are alongside their respective circumferences;
2. Fat area = arm area − muscle area.

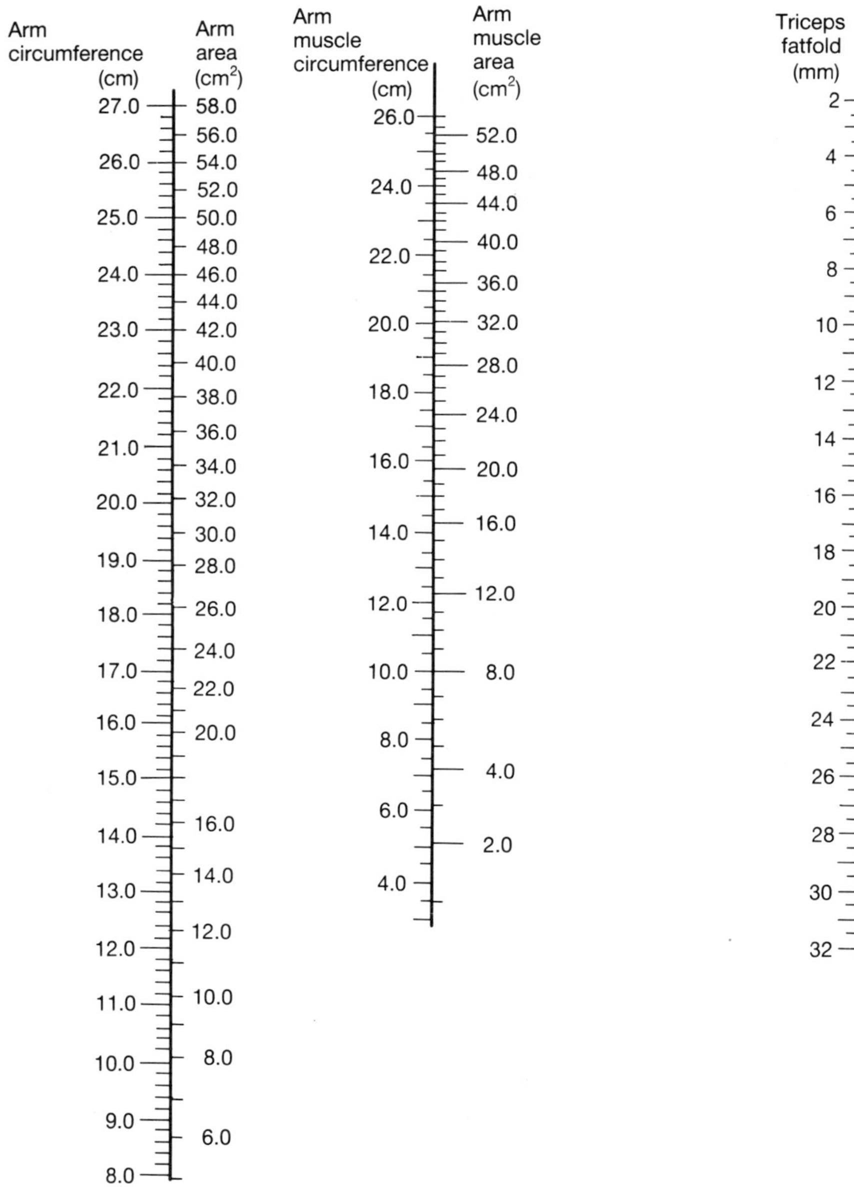

Fig. AP3.1 Arm anthropometry nomogram for children (Gurney and Jelliffe 1973).

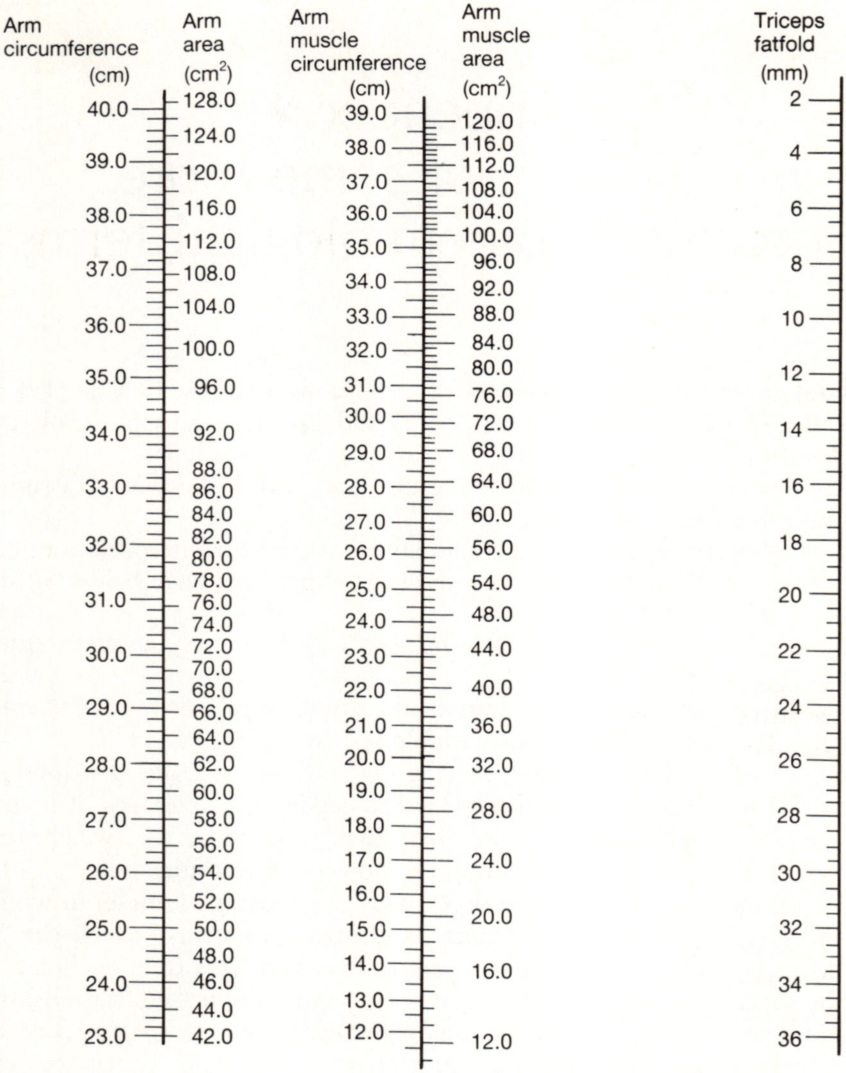

Fig. AP3.2 Arm anthropometry nomogram for adults (Gurney and Jelliffe 1973).

Appendix 4
Glossary of some more common epidemiological terms

Useful general reference books giving definitions are those by Last (1983), the British Medical Association (1979) and Lwanga and Cho-Yook Tye (1986).

Accuracy — Reflects the 'true' result (see also **Validity**) — assumes specific criteria for 'truth'.

Analysis — Arrangement and combination of data for interpretation; e.g. analysis of weight-for-age data showed 30 per cent were below 80 per cent of reference median.

Analysis, bivariate — Analysis using two variables, e.g. age distribution by sex.

Analysis, multivariate — Analysis of the effect of two or more variables on a separate or **Dependent** variable, e.g. using regression.

Analysis, univariate — Analysis using one variable, e.g. age distribution.

Analysis of variance — Analysis which compares the averages of a continuous variable across more than two subgroups, e.g. weight-for-height by low, medium, and high socio-economic status.

Area sample — A type of sample (usually a multistage sample) in which the sampling units are individual land areas (segments) which can be defined on a map. The segments cover the entire area to be included in the survey; the segments do not overlap; and, in most applications, the boundaries of each segment must be clearly defined so they can be recognized and identified by enumerators in the field. Often the segments are clusters of the units of analysis; for example, clusters of farms or housing units. Each unit of analysis must be associated with one and only one segment

Association — The relationship between two variables (also called **Correlation**).

Association: causal — The relationship is due to the direct effect of one variable on another within the correct time sequence.

Association: non-causal — The relationship is due to chance, errors, or is indirect (due to the influence of other factors).

Bias — The difference between the stated and the 'true' result — that is, a measure of inaccuracy.

Binomial distribution — A distribution in which there are only two possible results (e.g. present or absent).

Case control — A study which selects two groups : cases (those with a condition) and controls (those without), and collects past information to help compare relevant antecedents in each group (also called **Retrospective**). (For example, 'the case control study examined past morbidity with recent mortality.')

Census — Each individual in the population is studied, i.e. no sample.

Cluster sample — Groups (clusters) are selected rather than individual units. After this, some or all units may be further selected.

Cohort study — *Repeated observations of the same* subjects over time (also termed **Longitudinal, prospective, follow-up**); e.g. the cohort study observes children who enter the programme after 1 January 1986 for a period of one year.

Confidence — Compares the result, e.g. prevalence of undernutrition, from a sample to that of the 'parent' population from which the sample is taken. The sample result or estimate has a range (**Confidence interval**) bounded by limits (**Confidence limits**) — e.g. prevalence of undernutrition was 28 ± 3 per cent; i.e. 25 to 31 per cent.

Constant — Any quantity that does not vary, i.e. has the same value.

Cross-sectional — A study done at one point in time.

Data — Results expressed in a way that allows analysis.

Data: clean — Data fully edited.

Data: edit — Alter data to improve the efficiency of analysis, e.g. to modify or exclude errors, both proven and suspect.

Data: raw — Data which has not been analysed.

Data: round off — Contract a number to the nearest last digit of interest (e.g. 11.77 to 11.8). By convention 0.05 becomes 0.1.

Data: smooth — Modify data to a pattern which can be expressed mathematically, e.g. as an equation.

Data: sort — Arrange data in an order, often done from one extreme to another, i.e. highest to lowest.

Data: truncate — Contract a number by chopping-off (truncating) unwanted digit(s), e.g. 11.77 to 11.7.

Decision analysis — Analysis of alternative approaches which uses probabilities to forecast and compare outcomes (often expressed graphically as a decision tree).

Distribution — Presentation of data, e.g. by graphs, tabulations, which shows how results are distributed.

Distribution (frequency) — Results grouped according to the frequency in each category.

Effect modification — A situation where a variable modifies the effect of another variable on an outcome, e.g. the presence of wasting will influence the severity of measles, with an increased likelihood of mortality.

Enumeration areas (EAs) — A defined geographic area identified by a number for census purposes.

Experimental study — Applies a regimen to one group (treatment or exposed group) and not to another (control) to confirm a suspected causal relationship. This study is under the direct control of the investigator; e.g. the experiment examined the effect of Vitamin A on mortality.

Goal — What is hoped will eventually occur as a result of a study; e.g. reduce the prevalance of undernutrition by improving the efficiency of a programme.

Incidence — The number of new events (or cases) in a defined population and time interval.

Index — Usually a variable derived from combining two or more other variables, e.g. weight-for-height index.

Indicator — A variable or index which has a specific meaning for interpretation e.g. weight-for-height is an indicator for wasting.

Information — Interpretable and usable data, either for individuals or groups.

Interaction — The combined effects of two variables differ from the sum of their separate effects, e.g. poor diet and infections interact to increase the likelihood of undernutrition.

List — A population in which the sampling units have been numbered or otherwise identified; the list of units can be the basis for the selection of a sample. See also *Sampling frame.*

Logistic model — A mathematical model which uses logarithms (e.g. to predict an individual's risk of disease according to a risk factor.)

Multiple logistic model — A logistic model based on more than one risk factor.

Multistage sampling — Selection is done in stages up to the final sampling units, e.g., households or individuals. For example, the first stage may select villages, and the second stage, households within selected villages.

Non-participant observation — The observer merely observes and does not participate in activities.

Non-sampling bias — Errors in a study unrelated to random sampling methods, e.g. due to measurement or ambiguous questions.

Normal (or Gaussian) distribution — A continuous symmetrical frequency distribution whose shape is completely determined by its mean and standard deviation.

Null hypothesis — Assumes any difference (no association between variables) can be explained by chance alone — **Not guilty (no difference) until proved otherwise.**

Objective — What it is hoped a study (or project, programme, etc.) will provide, e.g. Prevalence of undernutrition according to a variety of situations, such as area, age, etc.

Optimum allocation of sample — The system of selecting a sample in such a way as to produce the minimum standard error for a constant sample size or for a constant cost. It is used in both stratified sampling and cluster sampling.

Parameter — A measure derived from a population (as compared with that from a sample).

Participant observation — The observer participates in the activities of the observed.

Population — Any clearly defined set of units (or elements) for which estimates are to be made. The elements can be persons, farms, households, blocks, countries, businesses, and so on. (Most of our discussion deals with sampling from a *finite* population, containing a finite number of elements.)

Positive deviant — A subject who is healthy in spite of an apparently detrimental environment.

Power — The ability of a statistical test to detect a difference when a true difference actually exists (see also **Type II error**).

Precision — Degree of exactitude, e.g. weight expressed to the nearest 0.1 kg is more precise than to the nearest 0.5 kg.

Prevalence — The total number of events (or cases) at any one time e.g. the prevalence of undernutrition in January, 1986 was 28 per cent.

Primary sampling unit (PSU) — The units making up the sampling frame for the first stage of a multistage sample.

Probability of selection — The chance each unit has of being included in the sample.

Probability proportionate to size (PPS) — The probability of selection of sample units is known and proportional to a measure of size. The size of a unit is believed, in advance, to be most appropriate for the statistics to be estimated.

Quasi-experimental — A study with the intentions of an experimental study, but not under control of the investigator (e.g. no random allocation of groups).

Random error — (see **Sampling error**).

Randomized controlled trial — An experimental study where groups are randomly allocated.

Regression analysis — An equation which allows a prediction of one variable ('*Y*' or dependent) from another ('*X*' or independent). **Multiple regression analysis** involves more than one '*X*' variable in the equation.

Reliability — Stability of a variable's result in a study, e.g. vitamin A intake using 24-hour recall is unreliable as it tends to vary greatly from day to day.

Reproducibility (replicability or repeatability) — Stability of a variable's result given similar conditions, e.g. weight measurement is more reproducible using different observers than fatfold measurement.

Risk factor — Something which increases the likelihood of an event or disease.

Risk (population atributable) — The number of people in a defined population likely to develop an event or disease which can be attributed to a risk factor, e.g. 100 cases of marasmus are likely to occur in the first year of life for bottle-fed infants.

Risk (relative) — The ratio between two risks. It is used to provide evidence of causality, e.g. the risk ratio for marasmus in the first year of life is 10:1 for bottle-fed as compared with non-bottle-fed infants.

Sample — A subset of a population. A *probability sample* selects each element in the population with known probability.

Sample: stratified — Divide (stratify) a total population into groups and separately sample each group.

Sample: universe — Population from which the sample is taken.

Sample weighting — Adjusting in analysis to account for known but different chances of selection.

Sampling bias — Resulting from incorrect method(s) in random sampling.

Sampling error — The difference in the result from a sample compared with the expected result in the population from which the sample is taken. This depends on the degree of confidence required (see **Confidence**). Also called **Random error.**

Sampling frame — The totality of sampling units from which a sample is to be selected. The frame may be a listing of persons or housing units; a file of records of punch cards; a subdivided map; etc.

Sampling unit — The units to be selected. These may or may not be the same as the units of analysis. For example, to obtain information on persons, one might use a complete listing in a Census, or a register, and select a sample of persons directly. However, one could select a sample of households and include in the survey all persons in the selected households. Similarly, one could select complete buildings, and include all persons in the sample buildings. The choice of the most efficient sampling unit is an important consideration in the design of a survey.

Sensitivity — Ability to detect the presence of a condition or disease.

Sentinel — A study group or area chosen for a special reason; e.g. representative of a larger group on the basis of judgement and available information.

Significance: statistical — An expected association between variables is unlikely to have occurred by chance alone. The 'P' value indicates the level of unlikelihood.

Simple random sample (also called unrestricted random sample) — The simplest type of sampling system. For a sample of size n, each of the possible combinations of n elementary units that may be formed from a population of N units has the same chance of selection as every other combination of n units. Moreover, every element will have the same chance of selection as every other element.

Specificity — Ability to indicate the absence of a condition or disease.

Standard error — A measure of the extent to which means from various samples differ from their expected value. With a reasonably large sample, the distribution of sample results for all possible samples is approximately the normal distribution, and probability statements can be made about how close the sample can be expected to come to the expected value — the probabilities being expressed in terms of the standard error.

Standardize — Modify the results of a variable or index to allow ready comparison with a reference, e.g. weight and age modified to weight-for-age.

Statistic — A measure derived from a sample.

Stratification — The process of dividing a population into groups for the purpose of selecting a separate sample from each group. Each group is usually made as internally homogeneous as possible. The groups are called *strata*, with each one referred to as a *stratum*.

Systematic sampling — A method of sample selection in which the population is listed in some order and every k^{th} element is selected for the sample.

Type I (alpha) error — Results from the sample show a difference (rejects the null hypothesis); for example, the treatment has an effect, but this difference could be explained by chance alone.

Type II (beta) error — Results from the sample show no difference (accepts the null hypothesis); for example the treatment has no effect, but fails to reflect the true result in the population (see also **Power**).

Unit of analysis — A unit for which we wish to obtain statistical data. The units may be persons, households, farms or business firms, or any records (e.g. from hospitals, clinics, etc.).

Universe — See **Population**.

Validity: external — Validity based on inferences from the study to its own (target) or other populations.

Validity: internal — Validity based on the actual study (see also **Accuracy**).

Validity: measurement — Ability of a measurement to reflect what it is meant to measure.

Validity: study — Correctness of a study based on design, methods (including sampling), analysis, and interpretation.

Variable — Any quantity that varies, i.e. can have different values.

Variable: confounding — A variable which distorts an assumed relationship between two other variables; e.g. the relationship between diet and nutritional status is influenced by the presence of infection.

Variable: continuous — Variables whose values have equal intervals, whose size is determined by the precision of measurement (e.g. weight). Also called **Interval or ratio** variables.

Variable: dependent — A variable that depends on other variables (i.e. it varies according to their values) — also called **Outcome variable.**

Variable: independent — A variable that influences a dependent one (also **Explanatory variable**).

Variable: nominal — A variable defined by name alone (i.e. no ordered numerical relationship) — e.g. sex as male/female.

Variable: ordinal — A variable whose components can be ordered, but with ill-defined intervals, e.g. high, medium, and low socio-economic status.

Variable: outcome — Identifies a result of interest, e.g. a change in nutritional status.

Variable: proxy — A variable that substitutes for another.

Variable: ratio — An interval variable whose lowest value is zero (in practice, equals an interval variable).

Weighted option — To modify the effect of some of the data on analysis, e.g. when stratified sampling is used.

Z score — The Standard Deviation value, e.g. — 2 Z equals — 2 SD from the median.

Appendix 5
Nutrient–cost nomogram for foods

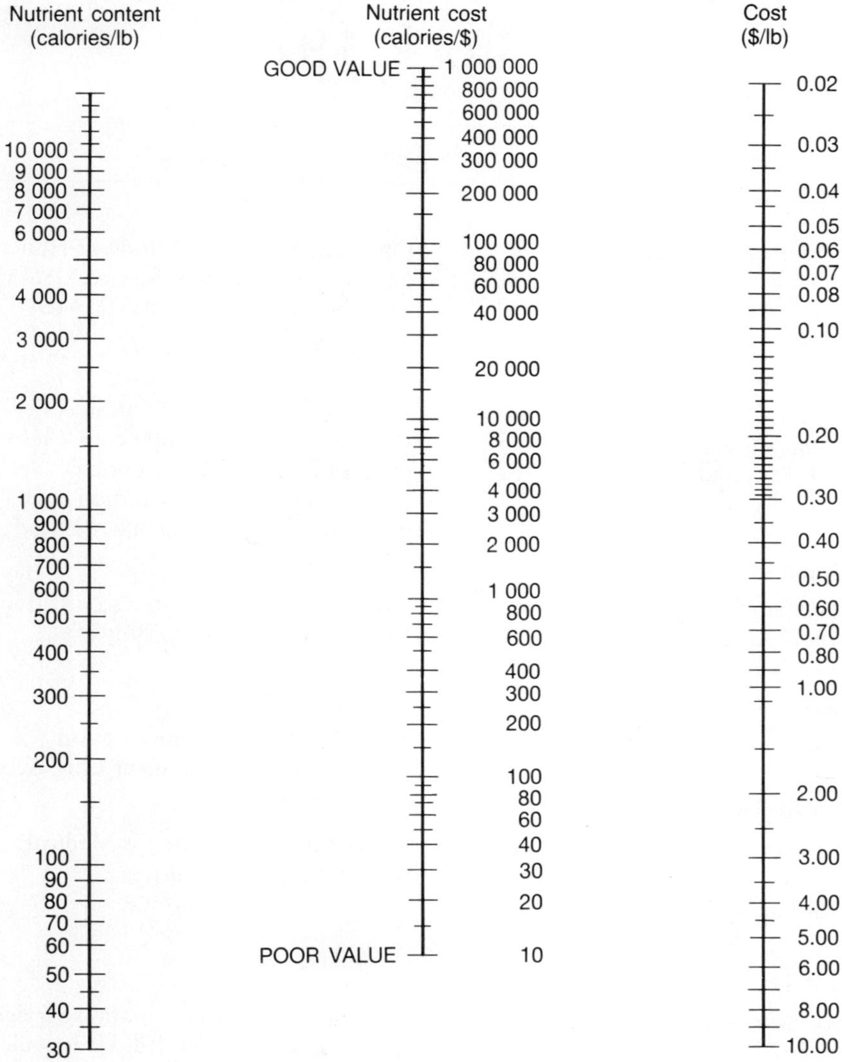

Fig. AP5.1 Nomogram to classify foods from 'good' to 'poor' value as judged by cost and nutrient value, showing nutrient content in calories as an example (Gurney and Jutsum 1980).

Appendix 6
Various food composition tables (From Davidson, Passmore, and Brock 1972)

Food tables	Source
AFRICA	
Food composition table for use in Africa Woo-Tsuen Wu Leung *et al.* (1968)	Obtainable from FAO, Italy or Human Nutrition Information Service, USDA, 6505 Belcrest Rd, Hyattsville, MD 20782, USA
West Africa	
Aliments de l'ouest Africain — tables de compostion Toury, J., Giorgi, R., Favier, J.C., and Savina, J.F. (1965)	Organisation de Coordination et de Coopération pour la lutte contre les grandes Endemies-Organisme de Recherches sur L'Alimentation et la Nutrition Africaines, Dakar, Senegal
Ethiopia	
Food composition table for use in Ethiopia Agren, G. and Gibson, R. (1968)	Obtainable from Children's Nutrition Unit, Addis Ababa, PO Box 1768
Ghana	
Food composition table (1969)	Food Research Institute — Food Research and Development Unit, Accra
South Africa	
Studies on the chemical composition of foods commonly used in Southern Africa Fox, F.W. (1966)	South African Institute for Medical Research, Johannesburg
ASIA	
East Asia	
Food composition table for use in East Asia (1972)	Human Nutrition Information Service, USDA, 6505 Belcrest, Rd, Hyattsville, MD 20782, USA *or* FAO, Food Policy and Nutrition Division, Rome, Italy.

Food tables	Source
India	
Nutritive value of Indian foods Gopalan, C., Rama Sastri, B.V., and Balasubramanian, S.C. (1974)	National Institute of Nutrition, Indian Council of Medical Research, Hyderabad 7
Japan	
Standard tables of food composition in Japan (1963)	Resources Bureau, Science and Technology Agency, Tokyo
The amino acid composition of foods in Japan Tamura, E. (1966)	Resources Bureau, Science and Technology Agency, Tokyo
Pakistan	
Nutrutive value of foodstuffs and planning of satisfactory diets in Pakistan. Part I, Composition of raw foodstuffs Chughtai, M.I.D. and Waheed Kahan, A. (1960)	Division of Biochemistry, Institute of Chemistry, Punjab University, Lahore
Philippines	
Food composition table recommended for use in the Philippines. Handbook I, 3rd revision (1964)	The Food and Nutrition Research Centre, National Science Development Board, Manila
AUSTRALIA	
Tables of composition of Australian foods, revised edition Thomas, S. and Corden, M. (1977)	Australian Commonwealth Department of Health, Nutrition Section, Canberra
EUROPE	
Denmark	
Fodevare-og ernaeringstabeller Rich Ege-Nyt. (1969)	Nordish Forlag. Arnold Busck., Copenhagen
Finland	
Ruoka-Aine-Taulukko Turpeinen, O. and Roine, P. (1967)	Department of Biochemistry, College of Veterinary Medicine, Hameentie 57, Helsinki
France	
Tables de composition des aliments Randoin, L., Legallic, P., Dupuis, Y., and Beradin, A. (1961)	Institut Scientifique d'Hygiene Alimentaire, Centre National de la Recherche Scientifique, Paris
Hungary	
Food composition tables, 7th edition Tarján, R. and Linder, K. (1972)	Medicinakonyvkiado, Budapest

Food tables	Source
Italy	
Composizione in alcuni principi nutritivi e valore calorico degli alimenti comunemente in Italia (1968)	National Institute of Nutrition, Rome (for internal use of the Institute, not published)
Netherlands	
Nederlandse Voedingsmiddeln Tabel, 30th edition (1977) (revised regularly)	Voorlichtingsbureau voor de Voeding, Lean Copes van Cattenburch 44, Den Haag-2011
Norway	
Nacrings Middel Tabell, 3rd edition (1966)	Pub. Landsforeningen for Kosthold of Helse, Oslo
Poland	
Tabele skladu I wartosci odzywczych produktow spozywczych Szczygla, A. (ed.) (1972)	Panstwowy Zaklad Wydawrietw Lekarskich, Warsaw
Sweden	
Fadodmnes-Tabeller Abramson, E. (1971)	Svenska Bokfōrlaget, Bonniers, Stockholm
West Germany	
Die Zusammensetzung der Lebensmittel: Nāhrwerttabellen Souci, S.W., Fachmann, W. and Kraut, H. (1973)	Wissenschaftliche Verlagsgesellschaft MBH, Stuttgart
United Kingdom	
McCance and Widdowson's The composition of foods, 4th revised edition Paul, A.A. and Southgate, D.A.T. (1978)	HMSO, London.
USSR	
Tabulky Kalorickych a biologickych Kudnor potravin, 2nd edition Muller, S. (1969)	SPN, Bratislava, Czechoslovakia
NEAR EAST	
Food composition tables for the Near East (1982)	FAO, Rome, Italy and the Human Nutrition, Information Service, USDA, 6505 Belcrest Rd, Hyattsville, MD 20782, USA
Iran	
Food composition tables Hedayat, H., Mermillod, M.J., and Hormazdyary, H. (1965)	Ministry of Health, Food and Nutrition Institute, Tehran

Food tables	Source
Israel	
Tablaoth Herkev Hamsonoth Guggenheim, K. (1964)	College of Nutrition and Home Economics, Ministry of Education and Culture, Jerusalem
Turkey	
Gida Komposizyon Cetvelleri Koksal, O. and Baysal, A. (1966)	School of Public Health, Ankara
AMERICA	
USA	
Amino acid content of foods US Department of Agriculture, Home Economics Report No. 4 Orr, M.L. and Watt, B.K. (1957, reviewed 1968)	Obtainable from Superintendent of Documents. US Government Printing Office, Washington, DC 20402
Composition of foods, raw, processed, prepared Agriculture Handbook No. 8. Watt, B.K. and Merrill, A.L. (1963) Revision 8-1: *Dairy and egg products* Posati, L.P. and Orr, M.L. (1976) Revision 8–2; *Species and herbs* Marsh, A.C., Moss, M.K., and Murphy, E.W. (1977).	Obtainable from Superintendent of Documents, US Government Printing Office, Washington, DC 20402
Canada	
Nutrient value of some common foods Health and Welfare, Canada (1971)	Nutrition Division, Department of National Health and Welfare, Ottawa
Latin America	
INCAP-ICNND Food consumption table for use in Latin America Woo-Tsuen Wu Leung and Flores, M. (*1961*)	Obtainable from INCAP, Apartado Postal No. 11–18, Guatemala City, Guatemala.
Caribbean	
Food composition tables for use in the English speaking Caribbean (1974)	Caribbean Food and Nutrition Institute, P.O. Box 140, Kingston 7, Jamaica
OTHERS	
South Pacific	
Some tropical South Pacific Island foods Muaj. M., Pen F., and Miller, C.D. (1958)	University of Hawaii Press, Honolulu, Hawaii, USA
Tropical countries	
Tables of representative values of foods commonly used in tropical countries (MRC Special Report Series No. 302) Platt. B.S. (1962)	HMSO, London

Appendix 7
Recommended dietary allowances (WHO/FAO 1974)

A discussion on the usefulness, variations, and limitations in recommended dietary allowances is given elsewhere (p. 220). More recent figures are available for some nutrients, but those listed are considered most generally useful, especially in Third World circumstances. Local modifications are often made, adapted to countries' presumed needs. RDAs from round the world vary. They have been compared and reviewed by Truswell (1983*b*). Modifications in energy and protein RDAs have been reviewed recently (WHO 1985*b*).

TABLE AP7.1 World Health Organization recommended intakes (Quoted from Davidson, S., Passmore, R., Brook, J.F., and Truswell, A.S. (1979). *Human nutrition and dietetics*, p. 153. Churchill Livingstone, Edinburgh and New York)

	Body weight (kg)	Energy[a] (kcal)	Energy[a] (MJ)	Protein[a,b] (g)	Vitamin A[c,d] (μg)	Vitamin D[e,f] (μg)	Thiamin[c] (mg)	Riboflavin[c] (mg)	Niacin[c] (mg)	Folic acid[e] (μg)	Vitamin B_{12}[e] (μg)	Ascorbic acid[e] (mg)	Calcium[g] (g)	Iron[e,h] (mg)
Children	7.3	820	3.4	14	300	10.0	0.3	0.5	5.4	60	0.3	20	0.5–0.6	5–10
	13.4	1360	5.7	16	250	10.0	0.5	0.8	9.0	100	0.9	20	0.4–0.5	5–10
	20.2	1830	7.6	20	300	10.0	0.7	1.1	12.1	100	1.5	20	0.4–0.5	5–10
	28.1	2190	9.2	25	400	2.5	0.9	1.3	14.5	100	1.5	20	0.4–0.5	5–10
Adolescents (Male)	36.9	2600	10.9	30	575	2.5	1.0	1.6	17.2	100	2.0	20	0.6–0.7	5–10
	51.3	2900	12.1	37	725	2.5	1.2	1.7	19.1	200	2.0	30	0.6–0.7	9–18
	62.9	3070	12.8	38	750	2.5	1.2	1.8	20.3	200	2.0	30	0.5–0.6	5–9

Adolescents	38.0	2350	9.8	29	575	2.5	0.9	1.4	15.5	100	2.0	20	0.6–0.7	5–10
(Female)	49.9	2490	10.4	31	725	2.5	1.0	1.5	16.4	200	2.0	30	0.6–0.7	12–24
	54.4	2310	9.7	30	750	2.5	0.9	1.4	15.2	200	2.0	30	0.5–0.6	14–28
Adult man (moderately active)	65.0	3000	12.6	37	750	2.5	1.2	1.8	19.8	200	2.0	30	0.4–0.5	5–9
Adult woman (moderately active)	55.0	2200	9.2	29	750	2.5	0.9	1.3	14.5	200	2.0	30	0.4–0.5	14–28
Pregnancy (later half)		+350	+1.5	38	750	10.0	+0.1	+0.2	+2.3	400	3.0	50	1.0–1.2	i
Lactation (first 6 months)		+550	+2.3	46	1200	10.0	+0.2	+0.4	+3.7	300	2.5	50	1.0–1.2	i

[a] *Energy and protein requirements:* Report of a Joint FAO/WHO Expert Group, FAO, Rome, 1972.
[b] As egg or milk protein.
[c] *Requirements of vitamin A, thiamin, riboflavin and niacin:* Report of a joint FAO/WHO Expert Group, FAO, Rome, 1965.
[d] As retinol.
[e] *Requirements of ascorbic acid, vitamin D, vitamin B_{12} folate and iron:* Report of a Joint FAO/WHO Expert Group, FAO, Rome, 1970.
[f] As cholecalciferol.
[g] *Calcium requirements:* Report of a FAO/WHO Expert Group, FAO, Rome, 1961.
[h] On each line the lower value applies when over 25 per cent of calories in the diet come from animal foods, and the higher value when animal foods represent less than 10 per cent of calories.
[i] For women whose iron intake throughout life has been at the level recommended in this table, the daily intake of iron during pregnancy and lactation should be the same as that recommended for non-pregnant, non-lactating women of child-bearing age. For women whose iron status is not satisfactory at the beginning of pregnancy, the requirement is increased; and in the extreme situation of women with no iron stores, the requirement can probably not be met without supplementation.

Appendix 8
International institutes concerned with specific crops and livestock (From AID Resources Report, US Bureau of Science and Technology, Washington, DC, USA)

Centre	Location	Date of initiation	Research	Coverage
IRRI (International Rice Research Institute)	Los Banos, Philippines	1960	Rice under irrigation, multiple cropping systems, and upland rice	Worldwide, special emphasis on Asia
CIMMYT (International Centre for the Improvement of Maize and Wheat)	El Batan, Mexico	1964	Wheat, triticale, barley, and maize	Worldwide
CIAT (International Centre for Tropical Agriculture)	Cali, Colombia	1968	Cassava, field beans, rice, and tropical pasture	Worldwide in lowland tropics, special emphasis on Latin America.

IITA (International Institute of Tropical Agriculture)	Ibadan, Nigeria	1965	Farming systems, cereals, cowpeas, soyabeans, lima beans, pigeon peas, cassava, sweet potatoes, and yams	Worldwide in lowland tropics, special emphasis on Africa
CIP (International Potato Centre)	Lima, Peru	1972	Potatoes (for both the tropics and temperate regions)	Worldwide, including linkages with developed countries
ICRISAT (International Crops Research Institute for the Semi-Arid Tropics)	Hyderabad, India	1972	Sorghum, pearl millet, pigeon peas, chick-peas, farming systems, and groundnuts	Worldwide, special emphasis on dry semi-arid tropics, non-irrigated farming
ILRAD (International Laboratory for Research on Animal Diseases)	Nairobi, Kenya	1974	Trypanosomiasis, theileriosis (mainly east coast fever)	Africa
ILCA (International Livestock Centre for Africa)	Addis Ababa, Ethiopia	1974	Livestock production systems	Major ecological regions in tropical zones of Africa
IBPGR (International Board for Plant Genetic Resources)	Rome, Italy	1973	Conservation of plant genetic resources	Worldwide
WARDA (West African Rice Development Association)	Monrovia, Liberia	1971	Regional co-operative effort in adaptive rice research among West African countries	West Africa
ICARDA (International Centre for Agricultural Research in Dry Areas)	Aleppo, Syria	1976	Barley, lentils, broad beans, and farming systems including animal husbandry	Emphasis on dryland farming and arid areas in Near East and North Africa
IFPRI (International Food Policy Research Institute)	Washington, USA	1975	International food policy and food distribution	Worldwide
ISNAR (International Service for National Agricultural Research)	The Hague, The Netherlands	1979	International service organization	Worldwide

Appendix 9
Anthropometric reference data

Guide to the use of anthropometric reference data

Reference data are given for young children (birth to 60 months), older children, and adults for weight, height (length), weight-for-height, and arm measurements (circumference, triceps fatfold).

Appropriateness for varying genetic (ethnic) groups needs considering (p. 110). Data for older children, adolescents, and adults are given for general guidance and information. More recent data are probably from a heavier and more obese population than previously.

Data are given *both* in percentage levels above and especially below the reference level and in standard deviations when practicable, with special reference to widely used cut-off points.

Comments on the sources and usefulness of the reference levels used were given earlier (p. 110); most reference levels are derived from the NCHS/WHO data (p. 112).

Weight and height tables

Young children (0–60 months; sexes combined)

Weight-for-age is given in Tables AP9.1 and AP9.2. *Length (height)-for-age* is given in Tables AP9.3 and AP9.4.

Children (5–9.5 years; sexes combined)

Weight-for-age is given in Table AP9.5. *Height-for-age* is given in Table AP9.6.

Children (10–18 years; sexes separate)

Weight-for-age is given in Tables AP9.7 and AP9.8. *Height-for-age* is given in Tables AP9.9 and AP9.10.

Weight-for-height tables

Children (49–120 cm; sexes combined)

Weight-for-height is given in Table AP9.11.

Table AP9.1 Weight-for-age for young children (birth to 60 months; sexes combined) in kg (20 per cent levels and in standard deviations above and below reference (NCHS/WHO data)

Age (months)	As percentage of reference					As standard deviations				
	140%	120%	Reference	80%	60%	+4SD	+2SD	Reference	−2SD	−4SD
0	4.5	3.8	3.2	2.6	1.9	5.0	4.1	3.2	2.3	1.4
1	5.7	4.9	4.1	3.3	2.5	6.7	5.4	4.1	2.9	1.7
2	6.9	5.9	4.9	3.9	2.9	7.9	6.4	4.9	3.4	1.9
3	8.0	6.8	5.7	4.6	3.4	8.9	7.3	5.7	4.0	2.3
4	9.0	7.7	6.4	5.1	3.8	9.8	8.1	6.4	4.6	2.8
5	9.8	8.4	7.0	5.6	4.2	10.6	8.8	7.0	5.2	3.4
6	10.5	9.0	7.5	6.0	4.5	11.3	9.4	7.5	5.7	3.9
7	11.2	9.6	8.0	6.4	4.8	12.0	10.0	8.0	6.2	4.4
8	11.9	10.2	8.5	6.8	5.1	12.5	10.5	8.5	6.6	4.7
9	12.5	10.7	8.9	7.1	5.3	12.9	10.9	8.9	6.9	5.0
10	12.9	11.0	9.2	7.4	5.5	13.4	11.3	9.2	7.3	5.3
11	13.4	11.5	9.6	7.7	5.8	13.8	11.7	9.6	7.5	5.6
12	13.7	11.8	9.8	7.8	5.9	14.2	12.0	9.8	7.8	5.8
13	14.1	12.1	10.1	8.1	6.1	14.5	12.3	10.1	8.0	5.9
14	14.4	12.4	10.3	8.2	6.2	14.9	12.6	10.3	8.2	6.1
15	14.8	12.7	10.6	8.5	6.4	15.1	12.8	10.6	8.4	6.2
16	15.1	13.0	10.8	8.6	6.5	15.4	13.1	10.8	8.5	6.3
17	15.4	13.2	11.0	8.8	6.6	15.6	13.3	11.0	8.7	6.4
18	15.7	13.4	11.2	9.0	6.7	15.8	13.5	11.2	8.8	6.5

Table AP9.1 (Continued)

Age (months)	As percentage of reference					As standard deviations				
	140%	120%	Reference	80%	60%	+4SD	+2SD	Reference	−2SD	−4SD
19	16.0	13.7	11.4	9.1	6.8	16.0	13.7	11.4	8.9	6.6
20	16.1	13.8	11.5	9.2	6.9	16.3	13.9	11.5	9.1	6.7
21	16.4	14.0	11.7	9.4	7.0	16.7	14.2	11.7	9.2	6.8
22	16.5	14.2	11.8	9.4	7.1	17.0	14.4	11.8	9.4	7.0
23	16.8	14.4	12.0	9.6	7.2	17.3	14.6	12.0	9.5	7.1
24	16.9	14.5	12.1	9.7	7.3	17.8	15.0	12.1	9.7	7.2
25	17.2	14.8	12.3	9.8	7.4	18.3	15.4	12.3	9.9	7.3
26	17.5	15.0	12.5	10.0	7.5	18.8	15.7	12.5	10.0	7.4
27	17.8	15.2	12.7	10.2	7.6	19.2	15.9	12.7	10.2	7.5
28	18.1	15.5	12.9	10.3	7.7	19.5	16.2	12.9	10.3	7.6
29	18.3	15.7	13.1	10.5	7.9	19.8	16.5	13.1	10.4	7.7
30	18.6	16.0	13.3	10.6	8.0	20.1	16.7	13.3	10.5	7.8
31	18.9	16.2	13.5	10.8	8.1	20.5	17.0	13.5	10.7	7.9
32	19.0	16.3	13.6	10.9	8.2	20.8	17.2	13.6	10.8	8.0
33	19.3	16.6	13.8	11.0	8.3	21.1	17.4	13.8	10.9	8.1
34	19.6	16.8	14.0	11.2	8.4	21.4	17.7	14.0	11.0	8.1
35	19.9	17.0	14.2	11.4	8.5	21.6	17.9	14.2	11.2	8.2
36	20.2	17.3	14.4	11.5	8.6	21.9	18.1	14.4	11.3	8.2

37	20.3	17.4	14.5	11.6	8.7	22.2	18.4	14.5	11.4	8.3
38	20.6	17.6	14.7	11.8	8.8	22.5	18.6	14.7	11.5	8.4
39	20.9	17.9	14.9	11.9	8.9	22.7	18.8	14.9	11.7	8.4
40	21.0	18.0	15.0	12.0	9.0	23.0	19.0	15.0	11.8	8.5
41	21.3	18.2	15.2	12.2	9.1	23.3	19.2	15.2	11.9	8.6
42	21.6	18.5	15.4	12.3	9.2	23.6	19.5	15.4	12.0	8.6
43	21.7	18.6	15.5	12.4	9.3	23.9	19.7	15.5	12.1	8.7
44	22.0	18.8	15.7	12.6	9.4	24.1	19.9	15.7	12.3	8.8
45	22.3	19.1	15.9	12.7	9.5	24.3	20.1	15.9	12.4	8.8
46	22.4	19.2	16.0	12.8	9.6	24.6	20.3	16.0	12.5	8.9
47	22.7	19.4	16.2	13.0	9.7	24.8	20.5	16.2	12.6	9.0
48	22.8	19.6	16.3	13.0	9.8	25.1	20.7	16.3	12.7	9.0
49	23.1	19.8	16.5	13.2	9.9	25.4	21.0	16.5	12.8	9.1
50	23.2	19.9	16.6	13.3	10.0	25.7	21.2	16.6	13.0	9.2
51	23.5	20.2	16.8	13.4	10.1	26.0	21.4	16.8	13.1	9.3
52	23.7	20.3	16.9	13.5	10.1	26.3	21.6	16.9	13.2	9.4
53	23.9	20.5	17.1	13.7	10.3	26.5	21.8	17.1	13.3	9.5
54	24.1	20.6	17.2	13.8	10.3	26.8	22.0	17.2	13.4	9.6
55	24.4	20.9	17.4	13.9	10.4	27.1	22.2	17.4	13.5	9.7
56	24.6	21.1	17.6	14.1	10.6	27.4	22.5	17.6	13.7	9.8
57	24.8	21.2	17.7	14.2	10.6	27.7	22.7	17.7	13.8	9.9
58	24.9	21.4	17.8	14.2	10.7	28.0	22.9	17.8	13.9	10.0
59	25.2	21.6	18.0	14.4	10.8	28.3	23.1	18.0	14.0	10.0
60	25.5	21.8	18.2	14.6	10.9	28.6	23.4	18.2	14.1	10.1

Table AP9.2 Weight-for-age (kg) (0 to 60 months; sexes combined) in standard deviations below reference (Z scores) (*NCHS/WHO data*)

Age (months)	Weight (kg) Reference	−1 SD	−2 SD	−3 SD	−4 SD	−5 SD
0	3.2	2.8	2.3	1.9	1.4	1.0
1	4.1	3.5	2.9	2.3	1.7	1.1
2	4.9	4.2	3.4	2.7	1.9	1.2
3	5.7	4.9	4.0	3.2	2.3	1.4
4	6.4	5.5	4.6	3.7	2.8	1.9
5	7.0	6.1	5.2	4.3	3.4	2.5
6	7.5	6.6	5.7	4.8	3.9	3.0
7	8.0	7.1	6.2	5.3	4.4	3.5
8	8.5	7.6	6.6	5.7	4.7	3.8
9	8.9	7.9	6.9	5.9	5.0	4.1
10	9.2	8.3	7.3	6.4	5.3	4.3
11	9.6	8.6	7.5	6.5	5.6	4.5
12	9.8	8.8	7.8	6.8	5.8	4.8
13	10.1	9.1	8.0	7.0	5.9	4.9
14	10.3	9.3	8.2	7.2	6.1	5.0
15	10.6	9.5	8.4	7.3	6.2	5.1
16	10.8	9.7	8.5	7.4	6.3	5.2
17	11.0	9.9	8.7	7.6	6.4	5.3
18	11.2	10.0	8.8	7.6	6.5	5.4
19	11.4	10.2	8.9	7.7	6.6	5.5
20	11.5	10.3	9.1	7.9	6.7	5.5
21	11.7	10.5	9.2	8.0	6.8	5.6
22	11.8	10.6	9.4	8.2	7.0	5.8
23	12.0	10.8	9.5	8.4	7.1	5.9
24	12.1	11.0	9.8	8.7	7.2	6.0
25	12.3	11.1	9.9	8.7	7.3	6.1
26	12.5	11.3	10.0	8.8	7.4	6.1
27	12.7	11.5	10.2	9.0	7.5	6.2
28	12.9	11.6	10.3	9.0	7.6	6.2
29	13.1	11.8	10.4	9.1	7.7	6.3
30	13.3	11.9	10.5	9.1	7.8	6.4

Table AP9.2 (Continued)

Age (months)	Weight (kg)					
	Reference	−1 SD	−2 SD	−3 SD	−4 SD	−5 SD
31	13.5	12.1	10.7	9.3	7.9	6.5
32	13.6	12.2	10.8	9.4	8.0	6.6
33	13.8	12.4	10.9	9.5	8.1	6.6
34	14.0	12.5	11.0	9.5	8.1	6.6
35	14.2	12.7	11.2	9.7	8.2	6.7
36	14.4	12.9	11.3	9.8	8.2	6.7
37	14.5	13.0	11.4	9.9	8.3	6.8
38	14.7	13.1	11.5	9.9	8.4	6.8
39	14.9	13.3	11.7	10.1	8.4	6.9
40	15.0	13.4	11.8	10.2	8.5	6.9
41	15.2	13.6	11.9	10.3	8.6	7.0
42	15.4	13.7	12.0	10.3	8.6	7.0
43	15.5	13.8	12.1	10.4	8.7	7.1
44	15.7	14.0	12.3	10.6	8.8	7.1
45	15.9	14.2	12.4	10.7	8.8	7.2
46	16.0	14.3	12.5	10.8	8.9	7.2
47	16.2	14.4	12.6	10.8	9.0	7.3
48	16.3	14.5	12.7	10.9	9.0	7.3
49	16.5	14.7	12.8	11.0	9.1	7.4
50	16.6	14.8	13.0	11.2	9.2	7.4
51	16.8	15.0	13.1	11.3	9.3	7.5
52	16.9	15.1	13.2	11.4	9.4	7.5
53	17.1	15.2	13.3	11.4	9.5	7.6
54	17.2	15.3	13.4	11.5	9.6	7.7
55	17.4	15.5	13.5	11.6	9.7	7.7
56	17.6	15.7	13.7	11.8	9.8	7.8
57	17.7	15.8	13.8	11.9	9.9	7.9
58	17.8	15.9	13.9	12.0	10.0	8.0
59	18.0	16.0	14.0	12.0	10.0	8.0
60	18.2	16.2	14.1	12.1	10.1	8.1

Table AP9.3 Length (height)-for-age for young children (0–60 months; sexes combined) in cm as percentages of reference (*NCHS/WHO data*); figures are for length up to 24 months (100 cm), and height above this age. If the length is measured in children of over 24 months, 2 cm must be subtracted.

Age (months)	Length (cm)				
	Reference	95%	90%	85%	80%
0	50.2	47.7	45.2	42.7	40.2
1	54.1	51.4	48.7	46.0	43.3
2	57.4	54.5	51.7	48.8	45.9
3	60.3	57.3	54.3	51.3	48.2
4	62.8	59.7	56.5	53.4	50.2
5	65.0	61.8	58.5	55.3	52.0
6	66.9	63.6	60.2	56.9	53.5
7	68.5	65.1	61.7	58.2	54.8
8	70.0	66.5	63.0	59.5	56.0
9	71.4	67.8	64.3	60.7	57.1
10	72.7	69.1	65.4	61.8	58.2
11	74.0	70.3	66.6	62.9	59.2
12	75.2	71.4	67.7	63.9	60.2
13	76.4	72.6	68.8	64.9	61.1
14	77.5	73.6	69.8	65.9	62.0
15	78.6	74.7	70.7	66.8	62.9
16	79.7	75.7	71.7	67.7	63.8
17	80.7	76.7	72.6	68.6	64.6
18	81.7	77.6	73.5	69.4	65.4
19	82.6	78.5	74.3	70.2	66.1
20	83.6	79.4	75.2	71.1	66.9
21	84.5	80.3	76.1	71.8	67.6
22	85.4	81.1	76.9	72.6	68.3
23	86.2	81.9	77.6	73.3	69.0
24	85.0	80.8	76.5	72.3	68.0
25	85.9	81.6	77.3	73.0	68.7
26	86.7	82.4	78.0	73.7	69.4
27	87.6	83.2	78.8	74.5	70.1

Table AP9.3 (Continued)

Age (months)	Length (cm) Reference	95%	90%	85%	80%
28	88.4	84.0	79.6	75.1	70.7
29	89.2	84.7	80.3	75.8	71.4
30	89.8	85.3	80.8	76.3	71.8
31	90.7	86.2	81.6	77.1	72.6
32	91.5	86.9	82.4	77.8	73.2
33	92.2	87.6	83.0	78.4	73.8
34	93.0	88.4	83.7	79.1	74.4
35	93.7	89.0	84.3	79.6	75.0
36	94.4	89.7	85.0	80.2	75.5
37	95.1	90.3	85.6	80.8	76.1
38	95.8	91.0	86.2	81.4	76.6
39	96.5	91.7	86.9	82.0	77.2
40	97.2	92.3	87.5	82.6	77.8
41	97.8	92.9	88.0	83.1	78.2
42	98.5	93.6	88.7	83.7	78.8
43	99.2	94.2	89.3	84.3	79.4
44	99.8	94.8	89.8	84.8	79.8
45	100.4	95.4	90.4	85.3	80.3
46	101.1	96.0	91.0	85.9	80.9
47	101.7	96.6	91.5	86.4	81.4
48	102.3	97.2	92.1	87.0	81.8
49	102.9	97.8	92.6	87.5	82.3
50	103.5	98.3	93.2	88.0	82.8
51	104.1	98.9	93.7	88.5	83.3
52	104.7	99.5	94.2	89.0	83.8
53	105.2	99.9	94.7	89.4	84.2
54	105.8	100.5	95.2	89.9	84.6
55	106.4	101.1	95.8	90.4	85.1
56	106.9	101.6	96.2	90.9	85.5
57	107.5	102.1	96.8	91.4	86.0
58	108.1	102.7	97.3	91.9	86.5
59	108.6	103.2	97.7	92.3	86.9
60	109.2	103.7	98.3	92.8	87.4

Table AP9.4 Length (height)-for-age for young people 0–60 months; sexes combined) in cm as standard deviations below reference (Z scores) (*NCHS/WHO data*)

Age (months)	Length (cm) Reference	−1 SD	−2 SD	−3 SD	−4 SD
0	50.2	48.0	45.7	43.5	41.2
1	54.1	51.7	49.3	46.9	44.5
2	57.4	54.9	52.4	49.9	47.4
3	60.3	57.8	55.2	52.7	50.1
4	62.8	60.2	57.6	55.0	52.4
5	65.0	62.4	59.7	57.1	54.4
6	66.9	64.2	61.5	58.8	56.1
7	68.5	65.9	63.2	60.6	57.9
8	70.0	67.4	64.7	62.1	59.4
9	71.4	68.7	66.0	63.3	60.6
10	72.7	70.0	67.3	64.6	61.9
11	74.0	71.3	68.5	65.8	63.0
12	75.2	72.5	69.7	67.0	64.2
13	76.4	73.6	70.8	68.0	65.2
14	77.5	74.7	71.8	69.0	66.1
15	78.6	75.7	72.8	69.9	67.0
16	79.7	76.8	73.8	70.9	67.9
17	80.7	77.7	74.7	71.7	68.7
18	81.7	78.7	75.6	72.6	69.5
19	82.6	79.5	76.4	73.3	70.2
20	83.6	80.4	77.2	74.0	70.8
21	84.5	81.3	78.1	74.9	71.7
22	85.4	82.2	78.9	75.7	72.4
23	86.2	82.9	79.6	76.3	73.0
24	85.0	81.8	78.6	75.4	72.2
25	85.9	82.7	79.4	76.2	72.9
26	86.7	83.4	80.1	76.8	73.5
27	87.6	84.2	80.8	77.4	74.0
28	88.4	85.0	81.5	78.1	74.6
29	89.2	85.7	82.2	78.7	75.2
30	89.8	86.4	82.9	79.5	76.0

Table AP9.4 (Continued)

Age (months)	Length (cm) Reference	−1 SD	−2 SD	−3 SD	−4 SD
31	90.7	87.2	83.6	80.1	76.5
32	91.5	87.9	84.3	80.7	77.1
33	92.2	88.6	84.9	81.3	77.6
34	93.0	89.3	85.6	81.9	78.2
35	93.7	90.0	86.3	82.6	78.9
36	94.4	90.7	86.9	83.2	79.4
37	95.1	91.3	87.5	83.7	79.9
38	95.8	92.0	88.2	84.4	80.6
39	96.5	92.7	88.8	85.0	81.1
40	97.2	93.3	89.4	85.5	81.6
41	97.8	93.9	90.0	86.1	82.2
42	98.5	94.6	90.6	86.7	82.7
43	99.2	95.2	91.2	87.2	83.2
44	99.8	95.8	91.7	87.7	83.6
45	100.4	96.4	92.3	88.3	84.2
46	101.1	97.0	92.9	88.8	84.7
47	101.7	97.6	93.4	89.3	85.1
48	102.3	98.2	94.0	89.9	85.7
49	102.9	98.7	94.5	90.3	86.1
50	103.5	99.3	95.1	90.9	86.7
51	104.1	99.9	95.6	91.4	87.1
52	104.7	100.4	96.1	91.8	87.5
53	105.2	101.0	96.7	92.5	88.2
54	105.8	101.5	97.2	92.9	88.6
55	106.4	102.1	97.7	93.4	89.0
56	106.9	102.6	98.2	93.9	89.5
57	107.5	103.1	98.7	94.3	89.9
58	108.1	103.7	99.2	94.8	90.3
59	108.6	104.2	99.7	95.3	90.8
60	109.2	104.7	100.1	95.6	91.0

Table AP9.5 Weight-for-age (kg) for children aged 5–9.5 years (sexes combined) as percentages of reference (NCHS/WHO data) and as standard deviations

Age (years)	Weight (kg)					
	120%	Reference	80%	+2 SD	Reference	−2 SD
5.0	21.8	18.2	14.6	23.4	18.2	14.1
5.5	22.9	19.1	15.3	24.8	19.1	14.8
6.0	24.1	20.1	16.1	26.4	20.1	15.5
6.5	25.4	21.2	17.0	28.2	21.2	16.2
7.0	26.8	22.3	17.8	30.2	22.3	17.0
7.5	28.3	23.6	18.9	32.5	23.6	17.7
8.0	30.1	25.1	20.1	35.1	25.1	18.5
8.5	31.9	26.6	21.3	37.9	26.6	19.3
9.0	34.0	28.3	22.6	41.0	28.3	20.1
9.5	36.1	30.1	24.1	44.2	30.1	21.0

Table AP9.6 Height-for-age (cm) for children aged 5–9.5 years (sexes combined) as percentages of reference (NCHS/WHO data) and as standard deviations

Age (years)	Height (cm)					
	110%	Reference	90%	+2 SD	Reference	−2 SD
5.0	120.1	109.2	98.3	118.2	109.2	100.1
5.5	123.5	112.3	101.1	121.7	112.3	102.9
6.0	126.9	115.4	103.9	125.1	115.4	105.6
6.5	130.1	118.3	106.5	128.5	118.3	108.1
7.0	133.2	121.1	109.0	131.7	121.1	110.6
7.5	136.3	123.9	111.5	134.9	123.9	112.9
8.0	139.4	126.7	114.0	138.1	126.7	115.3
8.5	142.3	129.4	116.5	141.2	129.4	117.6
9.0	145.4	132.2	119.0	144.4	132.2	120.0
9.5	148.5	135.0	121.5	147.6	135.0	122.5

Table AP9.7 Weight-for-age (kg) of children aged 10–18 years (sexes separate) as percentages of reference (*NCHS/WHO data*)

Age (years)	Weight (kg)					
	Boys			Girls		
	120%	Reference	80%	120%	Reference	80%
10.0	37.7	31.4	25.1	39.0	32.5	26.0
10.5	40.0	33.3	26.6	41.6	34.7	27.8
11.0	42.4	35.3	28.2	44.4	37.0	29.6
11.5	45.0	37.5	30.0	47.0	39.2	31.4
12.0	47.8	39.8	31.8	49.8	41.5	33.2
12.5	50.8	42.3	33.8	52.6	43.8	35.0
13.0	54.0	45.0	36.0	55.3	46.1	36.9
13.5	57.4	47.8	38.2	58.0	48.3	38.6
14.0	61.0	50.8	40.6	60.4	50.3	40.2
14.5	64.6	53.8	43.0	62.5	52.1	41.7
15.0	68.0	56.7	45.4	64.4	53.7	43.0
15.5	71.4	59.5	47.6	66.0	55.0	44.0
16.0	74.5	62.1	49.7	67.1	55.9	44.7
16.5	77.3	64.4	51.5	67.7	56.4	45.1
17.0	79.6	66.3	53.0	68.0	56.7	45.4
17.5	81.4	67.8	54.2	68.0	56.7	45.4
18.0	82.7	68.9	55.1	67.9	56.6	45.3

Table AP9.8 Weight-for-age (kg) of children aged 10–18 years (sexes separate) as standard deviations from reference (*NCHS/WHO data*)

Age (years)	Weight (kg)					
	Boys			Girls		
	+2 SD	Mean	−2 SD	+2 SD	Mean	−2 SD
10.0	46.0	31.4	22.1	49.2	32.5	21.9
10.5	49.3	33.3	23.1	52.8	34.7	23.1
11.0	52.7	35.3	24.1	56.4	37.0	24.5
11.5	56.3	37.5	25.4	60.0	39.2	25.9
12.0	59.9	39.8	26.8	63.3	41.5	27.4
12.5	63.5	42.3	28.4	66.5	43.8	29.1
13.0	67.2	45.0	30.4	69.4	46.1	30.8
13.5	70.9	47.8	32.5	72.1	48.3	32.5
14.0	74.6	50.8	34.9	74.5	50.3	34.2
14.5	78.2	53.8	37.4	76.5	52.1	35.9
15.0	81.6	56.7	39.9	78.3	53.7	37.4
15.5	84.9	59.5	42.4	79.6	55.0	38.7
16.0	87.9	62.1	44.7	80.6	55.9	39.8
16.5	90.7	64.4	46.8	81.2	56.4	40.7
17.0	93.2	66.3	48.6	81.5	56.7	41.3
17.5	95.3	67.8	49.9	81.5	56.7	41.8
18.0	97.0	68.9	50.9	81.3	56.6	42.1

Table AP9.9 Height-for-age (cm) of children aged 10–18 years (sexes separate) as percentages of reference (*NCHS/WHO data*)

Age (years)	Height (cm)					
	Boys			Girls		
	110%	Reference	90%	110%	Reference	90%
10.0	151.3	137.5	123.8	152.1	138.3	124.5
10.5	154.3	140.3	126.3	155.7	141.5	127.4
11.0	157.6	143.3	129.0	159.3	144.8	130.3
11.5	161.0	146.4	131.8	163.0	148.2	133.4
12.0	164.7	149.7	134.7	166.7	151.5	136.4
12.5	168.3	153.0	137.7	170.1	154.6	139.1
13.0	172.2	156.5	140.9	172.8	157.1	141.4
13.5	175.9	159.9	143.9	174.9	159.0	143.1
14.0	179.4	163.1	146.8	176.4	160.4	144.4
14.5	182.8	166.2	149.6	177.3	161.2	145.1
15.0	185.9	169.0	152.1	178.0	161.8	145.6
15.5	188.7	171.5	154.4	178.3	162.1	145.9
16.0	190.9	173.5	156.2	178.6	162.4	146.2
16.5	192.7	175.2	157.7	179.0	162.7	146.4
17.0	193.8	176.2	158.6	179.4	163.1	146.8
17.5	194.4	176.7	159.0	179.7	163.4	147.1
18.0	194.5	176.8	159.1	180.1	163.7	147.3

Table AP9.10 Height-for-age (cm) of children aged 10–18 years (sexes separate) as standard deviations from reference (*NCHS/WHO data*)

Age (years)	Height (cm)					
	Boys			Girls		
	+2 SD	Reference	−2 SD	+2 SD	Reference	−2 SD
10.0	149.7	137.5	125.3	152.0	138.3	124.6
10.5	153.1	140.3	127.6	155.3	141.5	127.6
11.0	156.7	143.3	129.9	158.7	144.8	130.9
11.5	160.5	146.4	132.2	162.0	148.2	134.4
12.0	164.7	149.7	134.6	165.2	151.5	137.9
12.5	168.9	153.0	137.2	168.0	154.6	141.1
13.0	173.0	156.5	139.9	170.5	157.1	143.8
13.5	176.9	159.9	142.8	172.4	159.0	145.7
14.0	180.2	163.1	146.0	173.7	160.4	147.0
14.5	183.0	166.2	149.4	174.7	161.2	147.8
15.0	185.1	169.0	152.9	175.3	161.8	148.3
15.5	186.7	171.5	156.2	175.6	162.1	148.7
16.0	187.9	173.5	159.2	175.7	162.4	149.1
16.5	188.8	175.2	161.5	175.8	162.7	149.7
17.0	189.4	176.2	163.1	175.7	163.1	150.4
17.5	189.8	176.7	163.7	175.7	163.4	151.1
18.0	190.0	176.8	163.6	175.6	163.7	151.8

Table AP9.11 Weight-for-height (in kg and cm) for children (49–120 cm; sexes combined) in 10 per cent levels above and below reference (*NCHS/WHO data*)

	Weight (kg)					
Height (cm)	120%	110%	Reference	90%	80%	70%
49	3.8	3.5	3.2	2.9	2.6	2.2
50	4.1	3.7	3.4	3.1	2.7	2.4
51	4.2	3.9	3.5	3.2	2.8	2.5
52	4.4	4.1	3.7	3.3	3.0	2.6
53	4.7	4.3	3.9	3.5	3.1	2.7
54	4.9	4.5	4.1	3.7	3.3	2.9
55	5.2	4.7	4.3	3.9	3.4	3.0
56	5.5	5.1	4.6	4.1	3.7	3.2
57	5.8	5.3	4.8	4.3	3.8	3.4
58	6.1	5.6	5.1	4.6	4.1	3.6
59	6.4	5.8	5.3	4.8	4.2	3.7
60	6.7	6.2	5.6	5.0	4.5	3.9
61	7.1	6.5	5.9	5.3	4.7	4.1
62	7.4	6.8	6.2	5.6	5.0	4.3
63	7.8	7.2	6.5	5.9	5.2	4.6
64	8.0	7.4	6.7	6.0	5.4	4.7
65	8.4	7.7	7.0	6.3	5.6	4.9
66	8.8	8.0	7.3	6.6	5.8	5.1
67	9.1	8.4	7.6	6.8	6.1	5.3
68	9.5	8.7	7.9	7.1	6.3	5.5
69	9.8	9.0	8.2	7.4	6.6	5.7
70	10.2	9.4	8.5	7.7	6.8	6.0
71	10.4	9.6	8.7	7.8	7.0	6.1
72	10.8	9.9	9.0	8.1	7.2	6.3
73	11.0	10.1	9.2	8.3	7.4	6.4
74	11.4	10.5	9.5	8.6	7.6	6.7
75	11.6	10.7	9.7	8.7	7.8	6.8
76	11.9	10.9	9.9	8.9	7.9	6.9
77	12.1	11.1	10.1	9.1	8.1	7.1
78	12.5	11.4	10.4	9.4	8.3	7.3
79	12.7	11.7	10.6	9.5	8.5	7.4
80	13.0	11.9	10.8	9.7	8.6	7.6
81	13.2	12.1	11.0	9.9	8.8	7.7
82	13.4	12.3	11.2	10.1	9.0	7.8
83	13.7	12.5	11.4	10.3	9.1	8.0
84	13.8	12.7	11.5	10.4	9.2	8.1
85	14.0	12.9	11.7	10.5	9.4	8.2
86	14.3	13.1	11.9	10.7	9.5	8.3
87	14.5	13.3	12.1	10.9	9.7	8.5
88	14.9	13.6	12.4	11.2	9.9	8.7

Table AP9.11 (Continued)

Height (cm)	Weight (kg) 120%	110%	Reference	90%	80%	70%
89	15.1	13.9	12.6	11.3	10.1	8.8
90	15.4	14.1	12.8	11.5	10.2	9.0
91	15.6	14.3	13.0	11.7	10.4	9.1
92	15.8	14.5	13.2	11.9	10.6	9.2
93	16.2	14.9	13.5	12.2	10.8	9.5
94	16.4	15.1	13.7	12.3	11.0	9.6
95	16.8	15.4	14.0	12.6	11.2	9.8
96	17.0	15.6	14.2	12.8	11.4	9.9
97	17.4	16.0	14.5	13.1	11.6	10.2
98	17.8	16.3	14.8	13.3	11.8	10.4
99	18.0	16.5	15.0	13.5	12.0	10.5
100	18.4	16.8	15.3	13.8	12.2	10.7
101	19.0	17.4	15.8	14.2	12.6	11.1
102	19.3	17.7	16.1	14.5	12.9	11.3
103	19.7	18.0	16.4	14.8	13.1	11.5
104	20.0	18.4	16.7	15.0	13.4	11.7
105	20.3	18.6	16.9	15.2	13.5	11.8
106	20.6	18.9	17.2	15.5	13.8	12.0
107	21.0	19.3	17.5	15.8	14.0	12.3
108	21.4	19.6	17.8	16.0	14.2	12.5
109	21.7	19.9	18.1	16.3	14.5	12.7
110	22.1	20.2	18.4	16.6	14.7	12.9
111	22.6	20.7	18.8	16.9	15.0	13.2
112	22.9	21.0	19.1	17.2	15.3	13.4
113	23.3	21.3	19.4	17.5	15.5	13.6
114	23.8	21.8	19.8	17.8	15.8	13.9
115	24.1	22.1	20.1	18.1	16.1	14.1
116	24.6	22.6	20.5	18.5	16.4	14.4
117	25.0	22.9	20.8	18.7	16.6	14.6
118	25.4	23.3	21.2	19.1	17.0	14.8
119	25.9	23.8	21.6	19.4	17.3	15.1
120	26.4	24.2	22.0	19.8	17.6	15.4

Table AP9.12 Weight-for-height (in kg and cm) for children (49–120 cm; sexes combined) in as standard deviations above and below reference (*NCHS/WHO data*)

	Weight (kg)					
Height (cm)	+2 SD	+1 SD	Reference	−1 SD	−2 SD	−3 SD
49	4.1	3.7	3.2	2.9	2.5	2.2
50	4.3	3.9	3.4	3.0	2.6	2.2
51	4.5	4.0	3.5	3.1	2.7	2.3
52	4.7	4.2	3.7	3.3	2.8	2.4
53	5.0	4.5	3.9	3.4	2.9	2.4
54	5.2	4.7	4.1	3.6	3.1	2.6
55	5.5	4.9	4.3	3.8	3.3	2.8
56	5.8	5.2	4.6	4.1	3.5	3.0
57	6.1	5.5	4.8	4.3	3.7	3.2
58	6.4	5.8	5.1	4.5	3.9	3.3
59	6.7	6.0	5.3	4.7	4.1	3.5
60	7.0	6.3	5.6	5.0	4.3	3.7
61	7.3	6.6	5.9	5.3	4.6	3.9
62	7.6	6.9	6.2	5.5	4.8	4.1
63	7.9	7.2	6.5	5.8	5.1	4.4
64	8.2	7.5	6.7	6.1	5.4	4.7
65	8.5	7.8	7.0	6.3	5.6	4.9
66	8.9	8.1	7.3	6.6	5.9	5.2
67	9.2	8.4	7.6	6.9	6.1	5.4
68	9.5	8.7	7.9	7.2	6.4	5.7
69	9.8	9.0	8.2	7.5	6.7	6.0
70	10.1	9.3	8.5	7.7	6.9	6.2
71	10.4	9.6	8.7	8.0	7.2	6.4
72	10.6	9.8	9.0	8.2	7.4	6.6
73	10.9	10.1	9.2	8.4	7.6	6.8
74	11.2	10.4	9.5	8.7	7.8	7.0
75	11.4	10.6	9.7	8.9	8.1	7.2
76	11.7	10.8	9.9	9.1	8.3	7.4
77	11.9	11.0	10.1	9.3	8.5	7.6
78	12.1	11.3	10.4	9.5	8.6	7.7
79	12.4	11.5	10.6	9.7	8.8	7.9
80	12.6	11.7	10.8	9.9	9.0	8.1
81	12.8	11.9	11.0	10.1	9.2	8.3
82	13.0	12.1	11.2	10.3	9.4	8.5
83	13.3	12.4	11.4	10.5	9.6	8.7
84	13.5	12.5	11.5	10.6	9.7	8.8
85	13.7	12.7	11.7	10.8	9.9	9.0
86	13.9	12.9	11.9	11.0	10.1	9.2
87	14.1	13.1	12.1	11.2	10.3	9.4
88	14.4	13.4	12.4	11.5	10.5	9.6

Table AP9.12 (Continued)

Height (cm)	Weight (kg) +2 SD	+1 SD	Reference	−1 SD	−2 SD	−3 SD
89	14.6	13.6	12.6	11.7	10.7	9.8
90	14.8	13.8	12.8	11.8	10.8	9.9
91	15.1	14.1	13.0	12.1	11.1	10.2
92	15.3	14.3	13.2	12.3	11.3	10.4
93	15.6	14.6	13.5	12.5	11.5	10.5
94	15.8	14.8	13.7	12.7	11.7	10.7
95	16.1	15.1	14.0	13.0	11.9	10.9
96	16.4	15.3	14.2	13.2	12.2	11.2
97	16.6	15.6	14.5	13.5	12.4	11.4
98	16.9	15.9	14.8	13.7	12.6	11.6
99	17.2	16.1	15.0	14.0	12.9	11.9
100	17.6	16.5	15.3	14.3	13.2	12.2
101	19.0	17.4	15.8	14.4	13.0	11.6
102	19.3	17.7	16.1	14.7	13.3	11.9
103	19.7	18.1	16.4	15.0	13.5	12.1
104	20.0	18.4	16.7	15.2	13.7	12.2
105	20.3	18.6	16.9	15.5	14.0	12.6
106	20.7	19.0	17.2	15.7	14.2	12.7
107	21.1	19.3	17.5	16.0	14.5	13.0
108	21.4	19.6	17.8	16.3	14.7	13.2
109	21.8	20.0	18.1	16.6	15.0	13.5
110	22.2	20.3	18.4	16.8	15.2	13.6
111	22.6	20.7	18.8	17.2	15.5	13.9
112	23.0	21.1	19.1	17.5	15.8	14.2
113	23.4	21.4	19.4	17.8	16.1	14.5
114	23.9	21.9	19.8	18.1	16.4	14.7
115	24.4	22.3	20.1	18.4	16.7	15.0
116	24.8	22.7	20.5	18.8	17.0	15.3
117	25.4	23.1	20.8	19.1	17.3	15.6
118	25.9	23.6	21.2	19.4	17.6	15.8
119	26.4	24.0	21.6	19.8	18.0	16.2
120	27.0	24.5	22.0	20.2	18.3	16.5

Adults

Data for adult males (25–54 years; 55–74 years) is given in Table AP9.13. Data for adult females (25–54 years; 55–74 years) is given in Table AP9.14.

Arm measurements

Arm circumference

Table AP9.15 gives the arm circumference for young children aged 0–59 months (sexes combined). Table AP9.16 gives the arm circumference for children and adults aged 5–74 years (sexes separate).

Triceps fatfolds

Table AP9.17 gives approximate reference levels for triceps fat folds (mm.) in males and females of different age-groups.

Table AP9.13 Weight-for-height (in kg and cm) for adult males.*

	Weight (kg) of male adults						
Reference I: US males (25–74 years) medium frames, from HANES I and II data sets (Frisancho 1984)				Reference II: US adult males of all frames, Society of Actuaries (1959); Bray (1979)			
	Levels (% of reference median)			Levels			
				Acceptable		Excess	
Height (cm)	120%	100%	80%	Average	Range	Obese	Height (cm)
158	83	69	55	58	51–64	77	158
160	84	70	56	59	52–65	78	160
162	85	71	57	60	53–66	79	162
164	86	72	58	61	54–67	80	164
166	88	73	58	62	55–69	83	166
168	89	74	59	64	56–71	85	168

170	90	75	60	66	58–73	88	170
172	91	76	61	67	59–74	89	172
174	92	77	62	68	60–75	90	174
176	94	78	62	70	62–77	92	176
178	95	79	63	72	64–79	95	178
180	96	80	64	73	65–80	96	180
182	98	82	65	74	66–82	98	182
184	101	84	67	76	67–84	101	184
186	103	86	69	78	69–86	103	186
188	105	88	70	80	71–88	106	188
				82	73–90	108	190
				84	75–93	112	192

Acceptable weight range — lower level for small frame
— upper level for large frame
Acceptable average — lower limit of small frame acceptable weight range
Excess (obese) — 120% of the upper limit of large frame acceptable range
* Two sets of reference data are given as there is uncertainty whether more recent figures (Reference I) are from an overweight, obese population. Assessment in adults must take this in to account, as well as genetic variation. Local references are desirable.

Table AP9.14 Weight-for-height (in kg and cm) for adult females.*

	Weight (kg) of female (25–54 years)						
	Reference I: US females (25–54 years) medium frames, from HANES I and II data sets (Frisancho 1984)			Reference II: US adult females of all frames, Society of Actuaries (1959); Bray (1979)			
	Levels (% of reference median)			Levels			
				Acceptable		Excess	
Height (cm)	120%	100%	80%	Average	Range	Obese	Height (cm)
148	77	64	51	46	42–54	65	148
150	79	66	53	47	43–55	66	150
152	74	62	50	48	44–57	68	152
154	72	60	48	49	44–58	70	154
156	73	61	49	50	45–58	70	156
158	74	62	50	51	46–59	71	158
160	74	62	50	52	48–61	73	160
162	76	63	50	54	49–62	74	162
164	77	64	51	55	50–64	77	164
166	77	64	51	57	51–65	78	166
168	78	65	52	58	52–66	79	168
170	79	66	53	60	53–67	80	170
172	80	67	54	61	55–69	83	172
174	82	68	54	63	56–70	84	174
176	83	69	55	64	58–72	86	176
178	84	70	56	65	59–74	89	178

Weight (kg) of female (55–74 years)

Reference I: US females (55–74 years) medium frames, from HANES I and II data sets (Frisancho 1984)				Reference II: US adult females of all frames, Society of Actuaries (1959); Bray (1979)			
	Levels (% of reference median)			Levels			
				Acceptable		Excess	
Height (cm)	120%	100%	80%	Average	Range	Obese	Height (cm)
148	71	59	47	46	42–54	65	148
150	73	61	49	47	43–55	66	150
152	76	63	50	48	44–57	68	152
154	77	64	51	49	44–58	70	154
156	77	64	51	50	45–58	70	156
158	78	65	52	51	46–59	71	158
160	78	65	52	52	48–61	73	160
162	79	66	53	54	49–62	74	162
164	79	66	53	55	50–64	77	164
166	79	66	53	57	51–65	78	166
168	80	67	54	58	52–66	79	168
170	83	69	55	60	53–67	80	170
172	84	70	56	61	55–69	83	172
174	85	71	57	63	56–70	84	174
176	86	72	58	64	58–72	86	176
178	88	73	58	65	59–74	89	178

Acceptable weight range — lower level for small frame
— upper level for large frame

Acceptable average — lower limit of small frame acceptable weight range

Excess (obese) — 120% of the upper limit of large frame acceptable range

* Two sets of reference data are given as there is uncertainty whether more recent figures (Reference I) are from an overweight, obese population. Assessment in adults must take this in to account, as well as genetic variation. Local references are desirable.

Table AP9.15 Midarm circumference measurements (mm) in young children aged 0–11 months (Wolanski 1964, pers. commun.; Burgess and Burgess 1969) and 12–59 months (data from US NHANES I) (Frisancho 1981) with percentages below reference level. For children aged 12–59 months standard deviations below the reference level are also given

	Midarm circumference (mm)								
		Per cent of median							
Age (months)	Median (100%)	90%	85%	80%	70%	60%	−1 SD	−2 SD	−3 SD
0	104	94	88	83	73	62			
1	113	102	96	90	79	68			
2	123	111	105	98	86	74			
3	133	120	113	106	93	80			
4	139	125	118	111	97	83			
5	144	130	122	115	101	86			
6	147	132	125	118	103	88			
7	150	135	128	120	105	90			
8	152	137	129	122	106	91			
9	154	139	131	123	108	92			
10	156	140	133	125	109	93			
11	157	141	134	126	110	94			
12–23	160	144	136	128	112	96	148	136	124
24–35	163	147	139	130	114	98	151	139	127
36–47	166	149	141	133	116	100	154	142	130
48–59	169	152	144	135	118	101	157	145	133

Table AP9.16 Midarm circumference measurements (mm) in people aged 5–75 years (sexes separate) US NHANES I data) (Frisancho 1981)

Age (years)		Midarm circumference (mm)											
		Males						Females					
		100%	90%	85%	80%	70%	60%	100%	90%	85%	80%	70%	60%
5.5	5	175	158	149	140	122	105	175	158	149	140	122	105
6.5	6	179	161	152	143	125	107	176	158	150	141	123	106
7.5	7	187	168	159	150	131	112	181	163	154	145	127	109
8.5	8	190	171	162	152	133	114	195	176	166	156	137	117
9.5	9	200	180	170	160	140	120	211	190	179	169	148	127
10.5	10	210	189	179	168	147	126	210	189	179	168	147	126
11.5	11	223	201	190	178	156	134	224	202	190	179	157	134
12.5	12	232	209	197	186	162	139	237	213	201	190	166	142
13.5	13	247	222	210	198	173	148	243	219	207	194	170	146
14.5	14	253	228	215	202	177	152	252	227	214	202	176	151
15.5	15	264	238	224	211	185	158	254	229	216	203	178	152
16.5	16	278	250	236	222	195	167	258	232	219	206	181	155
17.5	17	285	257	242	228	200	171	264	238	224	211	185	158
18.5	18	297	267	252	238	208	178	258	232	219	206	181	155
19–24.9	22	308	277	262	246	216	185	265	239	225	212	186	159
25–34.9	30	319	287	271	255	223	191	277	249	235	222	194	166
35–44.9	40	326	293	277	261	228	196	290	261	247	232	203	174
45–54.9	50	322	290	274	258	225	193	299	269	254	239	209	179
55–64.9	60	317	285	269	254	222	190	303	273	258	242	212	182
65–74.9	70	307	276	261	246	215	184	299	269	254	239	209	179

Table AP9.17 Approximate reference levels for triceps fatfolds (mm) in males and females in different age-groups (US NHANES I data). (*Adapted from Frisancho 1981)*

	Triceps fatfolds (mm)					
	Males			Females		
Age in (years)	Low 5th*	Medium 50th*	High 90th*	Low 5th*	Medium 50th*	High 90th*
1–5.9	6	9–10	12–14	6–7	10–11	14–15
6–9.9	5–6	8–10	13–17	6–8	10–13	14–20
10–17.9	4–6	8–11	16–22	7–10	12–19	23–30
18+	4–6	9–12	19–20	10–12	18–25	26–36
Simplified approximations						
1–9.9	5	10	15	5	10	15
10–17.9	5	10	20	10	15	25
18+	5	10	20	10	20	30

* Percentiles and standard deviations are not available from this data.

Appendix 10
Nutritional surveillance systems

Useful reports from conferences in three regions are available from the Cornell Nutritional Surveillance Program, Division of Nutritional Sciences, Cornell University, Ithaca, New York, USA. These conferences were held at Cali, Columbia (Report of the International Workshop on Nutritional Surveillance 1982), Nairobi, Kenya (Social and Nutritional Surveillance in Eastern and Southern Africa 1982), and Bangkok, Thailand (Regional Workshop on Nutritional Surveillance of Asian Countries 1983).

Nutritional surveillance primarily for planning purposes

In Kenya, a nutrition module (anthropometry and feeding habits of young children) was added to the Integrated Rural Surveys done by the Central Bureau of Statistics (Cornell Nutritional Surveillance Program 1984). These are being repeated every 2 years, to assist in the design of programmes at the national and provincial levels.

Costa Rica has used several data sources (Valverde *et al.* 1981*a*, *b* co-ordinated by the SIN (National Information System), Division at the Office of Control of Family Welfare. These sources include an annual national total enumeration by Ministry of Health agents; regular employment/income surveys and a 2–yearly census of school-age entry height done by teachers. The school census is being developed throughout Central America and Panama as a convenient and feasible method to provide a core source of district level and national information for nutrition planning and orientation of programmes (Valverde *et al.* 1985).

Colombia has used regular multipurpose surveys, organized centrally, service data from clinics and hospitals, agricultural census on food production, and seasonal information on crop status (Colombia/FES 1980).

A key activity used in the Philippines for nutritional surveillance is the community weighing programme — Operation Timbang. This involves the twice-yearly weighing of all pre-school age children at local stations. At the national level, data is used to determine priority municipalities for interventions (e.g. food aid allocation) and, at the local level, for programme planning and evaluation (Philippines National Nutrition Council 1979).

Early warning systems

Indonesia is developing a national nutrition surveillance system to predict and prevent food crises at an early stage, so that relief action can be quickly begun. Information may include: rainfall, crop production, unemployment, nutritional status of children, food prices, and agricultural wages. Sources are mainly routine data as well as monthly information at the village level (Maribe 1982; Habicht and Dapice 1984).

Botswana has incorporated biannual weight-for-age results at clinics as well as local rainfall and crop information for specific village-level interventions (primarily food distribution) in the drought relief programme (Maribe 1982; Haaga *et al.* 1983).

Ethiopia established a food and nutrition surveillance system with the Relief and Rehabilitation Commission in 1975. This early warning system included regular rainfall, price, and agricultural reporting. Resources permitting information on the effects of drought can also be sought from satellite photographs.

In addition, a 'disaster area assessment system' used *ad hoc* surveys on crop and livestock conditions, household stocks, market prices, unusual migrations, and nutritional status (Gebre-Mehedin 1979). The surveys relied largely on qualitative information derived from the perception and experiences of settled farmers and pastoralists. Questions included whether rainfall was greater, the same, or less than the preceding periods in prior years; and whether the rains arrived earlier or later than usual.

In the Sahel, a regional centre has been developed near Niamey for broad information on rainfall and crop production in several countries (Vellosa 1979). Recently, a famine early warning system (FEWS) has developed more detailed co-ordinated information for Sahelian countries (Department of Biostatistics and Epidemiology, Tulane University, New Orleans, Louisiana, USA).

On a world-wide scale, the Food and Agriculture Organization of the United Nations issues regular reports for restricted use on national food situations (Food Information Group, ESC, FAO, Rome).

Nutritional surveillance in more technically developed countries

In the USA, the results of clinical examinations (including anthropometry) in selected centres, such as the women, infant, and children (WIC) programme, head-start, and school entrance testing have been used for surveillance. Height and weight data are analysed at the Centers for Disease

Control. Both individual and summary results are then sent back to the clinics of origin via the state public health services (Habicht *et al.* 1978).

In the UK, nutritional surveillance has been instituted through the school system (Rona and Chinn 1982). This has documented over time the relationship between growth, unemployment, and levels of poverty.

Bibliography

The authors' apologies to those of the more than 3000 references and authorities consulted but not included in the bibliography or text because of space limitations.

ACC/SCN Consultation Group on Maternal and Young Child Nutrition (1982). *Food Nutr. Bull.* **4**, 45. Maternal malnutrition.

Aarons, A., Hawes, H., and Gayton, J. (1979). *CHILD-to-child*, Macmillan, London.

Abe, T. (1982). National nutrition survey in Japan. In *Methodologies for human population studies in nutrition related to health* (ed. B. Underwood), National Institutes of Health, Bethesda, Md.

Abbatt, F.R. (1980). *Teaching in better learning: a guide for teachers of primary health care staff.* WHO, Geneva.

Abel, R. (1986). *Trop. Doc.* **16**, 45. Traditional beliefs against weighing children.

Abraham, S., Carroll, M.D., Dresser, C.M., and Johnson, C.L. (1977). *Dietary intake findings, United States, 1971–74.* National Center for Health Statistics, US Department of Health, Education and Welfare, Rockville, Maryland.

——, Johnson, C.L., and Najjar, M.F. (1979). *Weight by height and age for adults 18–74 years, United States, 1971–74.* Department of Health, Education and Welfare, Hyattsville, Maryland.

——, Lowenstein, F.W., and Johnson, C.L. (1975*a*). *Dietary intake and biochemical findings: preliminary findings of the first health and nutrition survey, US, 1971–72.* National Center for Health Statistics, Rockville, Maryland.

——, ——, and —— (1978). *Preliminary findings for the first health and nutrition examination survey, United States, 1971–72. Dietary intake and biochemical findings.* National Center for Health Statistics, US Department of Health, Education, and Welfare, Rockville, Maryland.

——, ——, and O'Connell, D.E. (1975*b*). *Anthropometric and clinical findings: preliminary findings of the first health and nutrition survey, US, 1971–72.* National Center for Health Statistics, Rockville, Maryland.

Abramsom, J.H. (1959). *Br. J. Prev. Soc. Med.* **13**, 67. Observations on the growth and maturation of Indian boys in Durban, South Africa.

——, Gampel, B., Slome, C., and Scotch, N. (1961). *Am. J. Clin. Nutr.* **9**, 217. Sex variations in the nutritional state of urban Zulu adults.

Acheson, K.J., Campbell, I.T., Edholm, O.G., Miller, D.S., and Stock, M.J. (1980). *Am. J. Clin. Nutr.* **33**, 1147. The measurement of food and energy intake in man — an evaluation of some techniques.

Accian, G., Eckroad, J.C., Fajardo, L.F., Munoz, R., de Mercado, R., Pradilla, A., Quintero, G., de Ramirez, B., Victoria, F., and Wilson, D.H. (1977). *Arch. Latimaner. Nutr.* **27**, 359. Comparative analysis of some anthropometric measurements.

Adair, L.S. and Pollitt, E. (1983). *Am. J. Phys. Anthrop.* **62**, 325. Seasonal variation in pre- and postpartum maternal body measurements and infants birth weights.

—— and Mueller, W.H. (1983). *Hum. Biol.* 55, 71. Maternal anthropometric changes during pregnancy and lactation in a rural Taiwanese population.

Addy, D.P. (1986). *Br. Med. J.* **292**, 969. Iron is: happiness.

Afonja, A. and Ademiluyi, A. (1983). *J. Trop. Ped.*, **29**, 252. Heat-labile serum alkaline phosphate as an index of growth in healthy Nigerian infants and children.

Agunda, K.O. (1982). *The integrated rural surveys*, 1976–9. Basic report. Central Burea of Statistics, Nairobi, Kenya.

Ahn, C.H. and MacLean, W.C. (1980). *Am. J. Clin. Nutr.* **33**, 183. Growth of the exclusively breast-fed infant.

Akesode, F.A. (1980). *J. Trop. Pediat.* **26**, 150. Registration of births and deaths in Lagos, Nigeria.

Al-Dabbagh, A. and Ebrahim G.J. (1984). *J. Trop. Pediat.* **30**, 50. The preventable antecedents of childhood malnutrition.

Alisjahbana, A., Widjaya, J., and Sukadi, A. (1984). *J. Trop. Pediat.* **30**, 17. A method of reporting and identifying high risk infants for traditional birth attendants.

Alleyne, G.A.O., Hay, R.W., Picou, D.I., Stanfield, J.P., and Whitehead, R.G. (1977). *Protein–energy malnutrition.* Edward Arnold, London.

Amador, M., Canetti, S., and Cordova, L. (1983). *Rev. Cub. Ped.* **55**, 47. Indices antropometricas para la evaluacion nutricional.

——, Gonzalez, M.E., and Hermelo, M. (1981). *Anthrop. Kozl.* **25**, 3. Energy/protein indices: its usefulness in assessing obesity.

American Journal of Clinical Nutrition (1982). **35**, 1091–1325 (Suppl). Assessment of nutritional status.

American Public Health Association (1981). *Growth monitoring. primary health care issues.* APHA, Washington, DC.

Andersen, K.L., Masironi, R., Rutenfranz, J., and Seliger, V. (1978). *Habitual physical activity and health.* WHO Regional publications, European series No. 6. WHO, Copenhagen, Denmark.

Anderson, C.F. and Wochos, D.N. (1982). *Mayo Clin. Proc.* **57**, 181. The utility of serum albumin values in the nutritional assessment of hospitalized patients.

Anderson, J.E., Ali, J.E., Dakroury, A.H., Said, A.K., Hussein, M.A., El-Ghorab, M.I., Miller, D.C., and Brink, E.W. (1987). *J. Trop. Pedict.* **33**, 57. Use of nutrition surveys for family planning programme education.

Anderson, M.A. (1975). *Am. J. Clin. Nutr.* **28**, 775. Use of height-arm circumference measurement for nutritional selectivity in Sri Lanka school feeding.

—— (1979). *Am. J. Clin. Nutr.* **32**, 2339. Comparison of anthropometric measures of nutritional status in preschool children in five developing countries.

Andre, J. and Holemans, K. (1955). *Ann. Soc. Belge Med. Trop.* **35**, 467. Signification des cheveux rouges chez le nourrisson noir du Kwango.

Andrianosolo, R., Simmons, W.K., Latham, M.C., Gurney, J.M., and D'Souza, A. (1979). *Am. J. Clin. Nutr.* 32, 728. An evaluation of a simplified method for screening hemoglobins in the field.

Aranda-Pastor, J., Menchu, M.T., Teller, C., Sibrian, R., and Salcedo, D. (1983). *J. Trop. Ped.* **29**, 23. Food and nutrition surveillance systems: selected methodological advances.

Arnauld, J., Sizaret, F., and Munoz-Porras, J. (1983). *Food and Nutr.* **9**, 1. Selecting beneficiaries for assistance programs.

Arnhold, R. (1969). *J. Trop. Pediat.* **15**, 243. The QUAC stick: a field measure used by the Quaker service team, Nigeria.

Arroyave, G. and Wilson, D. (1961). *Am. J. Clin. Nutr.* **9**, 170. Urinary excretion of creatinine of children under different nutritional conditions.

Ashcroft, M.T. and Lovell, H.G. (1965). *West. Ind. Med. J.* **14**, 48. Changes in mean size of children in some Jamaican schools.

Auckett, M.A., Parks, Y.A., Scott, P.H., and Wharton, B.A. (1986). *Arch. Dis. Chldh.* **61**, 849. Treatment with iron increases weight gain and psychomotor development.

Austin, J. (1978). *Am. J. Clin. Nutr.* **31**, 2324. The perilous journey of nutrition evaluation.

Austin, J. (1979). *Nutrition programs in the third world*, Oelgesthlager, Gunn and Haln, Cambridge, Massachusetts.

——, Anderson, M.A., Goldman, R., Heimendringer, J., Overholt, C., Pyle, D., Rogers, B., Wray, J., and Zeitlin, M. (1978). Nutrition intervention assessment and guidelines. VN ACC Committee on Nutrition, Rome.

Aykroyd W.R. and Krishnan, B.G. (1941). *Ind. J. Med. Res.* **29**, 703. Infantile mortality in the beriberi area of the Madras presidency.

Aynsley-Green, A. and Macfarlane, J.A. (1983). *Arch. Dis. Childh.* **58**, 535. Method for the earlier detection of abnormal stature.

Babbie, E.R. (1979). *Survey research methods.* Wadsworth Publishing, London.

Babu, D.S. and Chittani, C.S. (1979). *J. Epidemiols. Comm. Hlth.* **33**, 177. Anthropometric indices independent of age for nutritional assessment in schoolchildren.

Backett, E.M., Davies, A.M., and Petros-Barvazian, A. (1984). *The risk approach in health care.* Public Health Paper No. 76. WHO, Geneva.

Baer, E. and Winikoff, B. (1981). *Studies in family planning*, No. 12. Breastfeeding: programs, policy and research issues.

Bagepalli, S., Rao, N., and Nagbhushnan, V.S. (1973). *Life Sci.* **12**, 205. Urinary excretion of 3-methyl histidine in children suffering from protein-calorie malnutrition.

Bailey, K.V. (1975). *Manual on public health nutrition*, WHO, Brazzaville (AFR/NUT/79).

—— (1962). *Trop. Geogr. Med.* **14**, 11. Rural nutrition in Indonesia: (VI) Field surveys of lactating women.

—— (1963*a*). *J. Pediat.* **64**, 97. Dental development of New Guinean infants.

—— (1963*b*). *Trop. Geogr. Med.* **15**, 389. Nutritional status in east New Guinean populations.

Bairagi, R., Aziz, K., Chowdhury, M.K., and Edmonstron, B. (1982). *Demography* **19**, 447. Age misstatement for young children in rural Bangladesh.

Bairagi, R., Edmonston, B. and Khan, A.D. (1987). *Am. J. Publ. Hlth*, **77**, 280. Effects of age misstatement on the utility of methoperative indicators of nutritional status in rural Bangladash.

——, Chowdhury, M.K., Kim. Y.J., and Cunlin, G.T. (1985). *Am. J. Clin. Nutr.* **42**, 296. Alternative anthropometric indicators of mortality.

Bakwin, H. and McLaughlin, S.M. (1964). *Lancet* **2**, 1195. Secular increase in height — is the end in sight?

Baldwin, B.T. (1925). *Am. J. Phys. Anthropol.* **8**, 1. Weight-height standards in metric units for American-born children.

Ballard, J.L., Novak, K.K., and Driver, M. (1979). *J. Pediat.* **95**, 769. A simplified score for assessment of fetal maturation of newly-born infants.

Bantje, H. (1982). *J. Trop. Pediat.* **29**, 50. Seasonal variations in birthweight distribution in Ikwiriri Village, Tanzania.

Barclay, A.J.G., Foster, A., and Sommer, A. (1987). *Brit. Med. J.* 294, 294. Vitamin A supplements and mortality related to measles: a randomized clinical trial.

Barnes, N. (1983). *Arch. Dis. Childh.* **58**, 845. Excessive growth.

Barness, L.A. and György, P. (1962). *World Rev. Nutr. Diet.* **3**, 1. Recent advances in infant nutrition.

Barros, F.C., Victoria, C.G., Vanghan, J.P., Texeira, A.M.B., and Ashworth, A. (1987). *Arch. Dis. Childh.* **6**, 487. Infant mortality in southern Brazil: a population based study of cancer of death.

Bastow, M.D. (1982). *Proc. Nutr. Soc.* **41**, 381. Anthropometrics revisited.

Bauerfiend, J. (ed.) (1986). *Vitamin A deficiency and its control.* Academic Press, New York.

Baumgartner, R.N., Roche, A., and Himes, J.H. (1986). *Am. J. Publ. Hlth.* **43**, 17. Incremental growth tables: supplementary to previously published charts.

Beal, V.A. (1967). *J. Am. Diet. Assoc.* **51**, 426. The nutritional history of longitudinal research.

Beaton, G.H. (1982). *Am. J. Clin. Nutr.* **35**, 1280. Evaluation of nutrition interventions: methodologic considerations.

—— (1985). *Am. J. Clin. Nutr.* **41**, 155. Uses and limits of the use of Recommended Dietary Allowances for evaluating dietator intake data.

—— and Bengoa, J.M. (eds.) (1976). *Nutrition in preventive medicine.* WHO, Geneva.

——, Milner, J., McGuire, V., Feattner, T.E., and Little, J.A. (1983). *Am. J. Clin. Nut.* **37**, 986. Source of variance in 24-hour dietary recall data.

Beck, J. (1979). Nutritional assessment of the adult cancer patient. In *Nutritional management of the cancer patient* (ed. J. Wolland), p.21. Raven Press, New York.

Beck, J.R., Meier, F.A., French, E.E., Brinck-Johnsen, T., and Cornwell, G.G., (1979). *Lancet* **i**, 1080. Serum ferritin.

Belcher, J.C. (1972). *Rural Sociol.* **37**, 208. A cross-cultural household level-of-living scale.

Belizan, J.M., Villar, J., Nardin, J.C., Malamud, J., and Sainz de Vicuna, L. (1978). *Am. J. Obstet. Gynaecol*, **131**, 643. Diagnosis of intrauterine growth retardation by a simple clinical method: measurement of uterine height.

Bender, F.E., Douglass L.W., and Kramer, A. (1982). Statistical methods for food and agriculture. Avi Publishing Co., Westport, Connecticut.

Bengoa, J.M. (1970). *Chron. World Hlth.* **24**, 552. Recent trends in public health aspects of protein-calorie malnutrition.

——, Jelliffe, D.B., and Perez, C. (1959). *Am. Clin. Nutr.* 7, 714. Some indicators for the broad assessment of the magnitude of protein-calorie malnutrition in young children in population groups.

Berg, A. (1981). *Malnourished people: A policy review.* The World Bank, Washington, DC.

Berggren, G.G., Herbert, J.R., and Waternaux, C.M. (1985). *Bull. World Hlth. Org.* **63**, 1141. Comparison of Haitian children in a nutrition intervention programme with children in the Haitian national nutrition survey.

Bernard, H.R., Killworth, P., Kronenfeld, D., and Sailer, L. (1984). *Ann. Rev. Anthrop.* **13**, 495. The problem of informant accuracy: the validity of retrospective data.

Bertrand, W.E. (1985). *World Hlth. Stat. Quart.* **38**, 91. Microcomputer application in health population surveys: experience and potential in developing countries.

Bhan, A., Osborn, A.C., Huang, V.H., and Ratman, S.S. (1985). *J. Trop. Pediat.* **31**, 124. Neonatal anthropometry in relation to ethnic distribution of birth weight in Singapore.

——, Viegas, O.A.C., Huang, H.S., and Ratnam, S.S. (1985). *J. Trop. Pediat.* **31**, 124. Neonatal anthropometry in relation to ethnic distribution of birth weight in Singapore.

Bhargava, S.K., Ramji, S., Kumar, A., Mohan, M., Marwah, J., and Schdey, H.P.S. (1985). *Br. Med. J.* **291**, 1617. Mid-arm and chest circumferences at birth as predictors of low birth weight and neonatal mortality in communities.

Bhatia, B.D., Tyagi, N.K., and Handa, P. (1985). *Ind. J. Med. Res.* **82**, 374. Relation of low birth weight with anthropometry and maternal weight-height indices.

Bhuiya, A., Zimmicki, S., and D'Souza, S. (1986). *J. Trop. Pediat.* **32**, 17. Socioeconomic differentials in child nutrition and morbidity in a rural area of Bangladesh.

Bigwood, E.J. (1939). *Guiding principles for studies of nutrition of populations.* Technical Commission on Nutrition. World Health Organization. League of Nations, Geneva.

Billewicz, W.Z., Kensley, W.F., and Thomson, A.M. (1962). *Br. J. Prev. Soc. Med.* **16**, 183. Indices of adiposity.

—— and McGregor, I.A. (1982). *Ann. Human Biol.* **9**, 309. A birth-to-maturity longitudinal study of the heights and weights in two West African Gambian villages, 1951–1971.

Binkin, N.J., Goldman, H.W., Brown, B.H. and Nieburg, P. (1985). *J. Trop. Pediat.* **31**, 152–157. The weight-for-height chart: Is it accurate enough for field surveys?

Blackburn, G.L. and Harvey, K.B. (1982). *Postgrad. Med.* **71**, 46. Nutritional assessment as a routine in clinical medicine.

——, Bistrian, B.R., Maini, B.S., Schlamm, H.T., and Smith, M.F. (1977). *J. Parent. Enter. Nutr.* **1**, 11. Nutritional and metabolic assessment of the hospitalized patient.

Blankhart, D.M. (1965). *J. Trop. Pediat.* **8**, 18. Measured food intakes in young children in Indonesia.

—— (1971). *J. Trop. Pediat.* **17**, 176. Outline of a survey of the feeding and nutritional status of children under three years of age and their mothers.

Bohdal, M. and Simmons, W. (1969). *Bull. World Hlth. Org.* **40**, 166. A comparison of nutritional indices in healthy African, Asian and European children.

Bondestam, L. (1981). *Fd. Nutr. Bull.* **3**, 1. Understanding hunger and practicing starvation.

Bone, R. (1983). *Approp. Technol.* **9**, 27. Simple haemoglobin screening device.

Borjesson, M. and Hofvander, Y. (1970). *Acta Paed. Scand.* **59**, suppl. 206, 68. Nutrition studies in Tunisia.

Bostock, J. (1962). *Lancet* **i**, 1033. Evolutionary approaches to infant care.

Bouchard, C., Tremblay, A., Leblanc, C., Lortie, G., Savard, R., and Theriault, G. (1983). *Am. J. Clin. Nutr.* **37**, 461. A method to assess energy expenditure in children and adults.

Bouillon, R.A., Auverx, J.H., Lissens, W.D., and Pelemans, W.K. (1987). *Am. J. Clin. Nutr.* **45**, 755. Vitamin D status in the elderly.

Bradfield, R.B. (1974). *J. Pediat.* **84**, 294. Hair tissue as a medium for the differential diagnosis of protein-calorie malnutrition. A commentary.

—— and Jelliffe, E.F.P. (1970). *Nature* **225**, 283. Early assessment of malnutrition.

Brandon, R.N. (1979). *Fed. Proc.* **38**, 2564. Science, senators and uncertainty.

Bray, G.A. (1978). *Intl. J. Obes.* **2**, 99. Definition, measurement and classification of the syndromes of obesity.

—— (1979). *J. R. Soc. Coll. Physic. London* **17**, 1. The health consequences of overweight and obesity.

Briend, A. and Zimicki, S. (1985). *Proc. XIII international congress of nutrition.* Validation of arm circumstance as an indicator of risk of death in one- to four-year-old children.

Bridges, N., Parvin, R.M., and Van Assenfelft, O.W.: (1987). *Am. Clin. Products Rev.*, April issue. Evaluation or a new system for hemoglobin measurement.

British Medical Association (1979). *Epidemiology for the uninitiated.* British Medical Association Press, London.

British Medical Journal (1986). Editorial.

Brooke, O.G. (1980). *Proc. Nutr. Soc.* **39**, 17. Foot and the fetus and neonate.

—— and Butters, E. (1979). *Arch. Dis. Childh.* **54**, 161. Which small-for-dates infants are malnourished?

Brink, E.W., Miller, D.G., and Lane, J.M. (1977). *Trop. Doc.* **7**, 96. Improvised measuring board suitable for the field.

Brown, J.E. and Brown, R.C. (1979*a*). *Finding the causes of child malnutrition. A community handbook for developing countries.* Task Force on World Hunger, Atlanta, Georgia.

—— and —— (1979*b*). *Trans. R. Soc. Trop. Med Hyg.* **73**, 70. An evaluation of nutrition centre effectiveness by measurement of younger siblings.

Brown, K.H., Black, R.E., Becker, S., and Hogue, A. (1982). *Am. J. Clin. Nutr.* **36**, 294. Patterns of physical growth in a longitudinal study of young children in Bangladesh.

Brown, R. and Jelliffe, D.B. (1967). *Am. J. Clin. Nutr.* **20**, 1230. Declining elasticity of the auricular cartilage in Ugandian children with kwashiorkor.

Burgert, S.L. and Anderson, C.F. (1979). *Am. J. Clin. Nutr.* **32**, 1531. A comparison of triceps skinfold values measured by the McGraw and Lange calipers.

Burgess, A. and Dean, R.F.A. (eds.) (1962). *Malnutrition and food habits*. Tavistock Publications, London.

Burgess, H.J.L. and Burgess, A.P. (1969). *J. Trop. Pediat.* **15**, 189. A modified standard for mid-upper arm circumference in young children.

—— and —— (1975). *Am. J. Clin. Nutr.* **28**, 1299. A field worker's guide to a nutritional status survey.

——, Maletnlema, N.T., Burgess, A.P. (1969). *Trop. Geogr. Med.* **21**, 39. The health of children in Kisarawe District, Tanzania.

——, Burgess, A.P., and Wheeler, E.F. (1973). *Trop. Geogr. Med.* **25**, 372. Results and appraisal of a nutritional survey in Malawi.

Burns, J.D., Carriere, R.C., and Rohde, J.E. (1984). *Growth charts: A discussion paper*. UNICEF global growth monitoring meeting, New Delhi, India. Doc. res: 6.

Burns, J.O. (1986). *Scale technologies: issues relating to growth monitoring*. UNICEF, New York.

Buss, D.H. (ed.) (1986). *Proc. Nutr. Soc.* **45**, 345. Symposium on interior recommendations for man: theory and practice.

Butman, M. (ed.) (1982) Prenatal nutrition. A clinical manual. Massachusetts Department of Public Health, Boston, Massachusetts.

Butte, N.F., Garza, C., Smith, E.O., and Nichols, B.L. (1983). *Am. J. Clin. Nutr.* 37, 996. Evaluation of the deuterium dilution technique against the test weighing procedure for the determination of breast milk intake.

Buzina, R. and Uemura, K. (1974). Selection of the minimum anthropometric characteristics to assess nutritional status. In *Nutrition and malnutrition: identification and measurement* (eds. F. Falkner and A. Roche) Plenum Press, New York.

Caird, F.I. (1985). Problems of interpretation of laboratory findings in the old. In *Medicine in old age*, p. 116. British Medical Association, London.

Campbell, J.L., Cutting W.A.M., Elton, R.A., Minton, E.J., and Spreng, J. (1985). *Trans. Roy. Soc. Trop. Med. Hyg.* **70**, 409. A portable Nabarro weight-height anthropetric nutrition assessment chart.

Carr-Hill, R. and Pritchard, C. (1985). The development and exploitation of empirical birth weight standards. London, Macmillan Press.

Caribbean Food and Nutrition Institute (1974). *Food composition tables for use in the English-speaking Caribbean*. CFNI, Jamaica.

Caribbean Food and Nutrition Institute (1977). Nutrient-cost reference tables for use in the Caribbean. CFNI, Jamaica.

Carpenter, Y.A., Barthel, J., and Bruyns, J. (1982). *Proc. Nutr. Soc.* **41**, 405. Plasma protein concentration in nutritional assessment.

—— and Ingenbleek, Y. (1983). *Nutr. Res.* **3**, 617. Serum thyroxine-binding Plasma protein concentration in nutritional assessment.

Carter, E. (1986). *Proc. Nutr. Soc.* **45**, 129A. Comparison of weight-for-height and arm circumference in assessment of acute nutrition.

Casley, D.J. and Lury, D.A. (1981). *Data collection in developing countries*. Oxford University Press, Oxford.

Castle, W. (1979). *Statistics in operation*. Churchill Livingstone, Edinburgh.

Chandler, W.V. (1985). Investing in children. Worldwatch paper No. 64. Worldwatch Institute, Washington, DC.

Chandra, R.K. (1982). *Nutr. Res.* **2**, 543. Nutritional assessment of the individual.

—— and Scrimshaw, N.S. (1980). *Am. J. Clin. Nutr.* **33**, 2694. Immunocompetence in nutritional assessment.

Chavalittamrong, B., Bathakanon, R., Walsripong, R., and Rungrith, W. (1980). *J. Trop. Pediat.* **26**, 139. Height, weight, height velocity and weight velocity in school-age Bangkok children.

Chen, L. and Scrimshaw, N. (eds.) (1982). *Diarrhea and malnutrition: interaction, mechanisms and interventions.* Plenum Press, New York.

Chen, L.C., Chowdhury, A.K.A., and Huffman, S. (1980). *Am. J. Clin. Nutr.* **33**, 1836. Anthropometric assessment of energy-protein malnutrition and subsequent risk of mortality among pre-school aged children.

Chinese Academy of Medical Sciences (1977). *China Med. J.* **3**, 364. Studies on physical development of children and adolescents in New China.

Cnattingius, S., Axelsson, D. and Lindmark, G. (1984). *Acta Oboret. Gynecol. Scand.* **63**, 335. Symphysis-fundus measurement and intranterine growth retardation.

Cobey, J.C. and Cunningham, N. (1968). *J. Trop. Pediat.* **14**, 132. An evaluation of a local calendar used in determining ages of children in a Nigerian village.

Christakis, G. (ed.) (1973). *Am. J. Publ. Hlth.* **63**, Suppl. 1. Nutrition assessment in health programs.

Cochrane, W.J., Klish, W.J., Wong, W.W., Fiorotto, M.L., Klein, P.D., and Nichols, B.L. (1985). *Pediat. Res.* **19**, 216 A. No: 631. The use of total body impedance to determine body composition of infants.

Cohen, M. (1986). *Adv. Int. Mat. Chld. Hlth.* **6**, 148. The influence of street food trade on women and children.

Cole, T.J. (1979). *Ann. Hum. Biol.* **6**, 249. A method for assessing age-standardized weight-for height in children seen cross-sectionally.

—— and Pankin, J.M. (1977). *Trans. R. Soc. Trop. Med. Hyg.* **71**, 196. Infection and its effect on growth: a comparison of the Gambia and Uganda.

Collis, W.F.R., Dema, I., and Omolulu, A. (1962*a*). *Trop. Geogr. Med.* **14**, 140. On The ecology of child health and nutrition in Nigerian villages. 1-Environment, population and resources.

——, ——, and —— (1962*b*). *Trop. Geogr. Med.* **14**, 201. On the ecology of child health and nutrition in Nigerian villages. 2:Dietary and medical surveys.

Colombia/FES (1980). *Nutritional surveillance system: second year progress report.* Mimeo. Cali, Colombia: Nutrition Project.

Conlin, S. and Wiggins, S. (1979). *Rapid rural appraisal.* Land Resources Development Centre, Survey, U.K.

Continua Productions (UK) (1975). *Fred learns basic statistics*, pp. 45–70.

Cook, J.D. and Skifne, B.S. (1982). *Am. J. Clin. Nutr.* **35**, 180. Serum ferritin: a possible model for the assessment of nutrient stores.

—— and Lynch, S.R. (1986). *Am. J. Clin. Nutr.* **43**, 709. Population assessment of iron status.

Contuguera, R.R. and Lopez, C. (1977). *Rev. Cub. Pediat.* **449**, 595. Mortalidad prescolar (1–4 años) en Cuba, 1961–75.

Corless, D. (1985). Diet in the elderly. In *Medicine in old age*, p. 136. British Medical Association, London.

Cornell Nutritional Surveillance Program (1984). Recent advances in nutritional surveillance: A review of Kenya's Experience and Policy Implications. Paper presented at National Workshop on Nutrition and Planning in Kenya, Kisumu, Kenya. January 1984.

Corteguera, R.R. and Lopez, C. (1977). *Rev. Cub. Ped.* **449**, 595. Mortalidad prescolar (1–4 anos) en Cuba, 1961–75.

Cote, J.A. (1984). *Am. Behav. Scient.* **28**, 129. Use of household refuse analysis to measure usual and period-specific food consumption.

Coward, D.G., Sawyer, M.B., and Whitehead, R.G. (1971). *Am. J. Clin. Nutr.* **24**, 940. Microtechniques for the automated analysis of total serum protein and albumin.

Coward, W.A., Cole, T.J., Sawyer, M.B., Prentice, A.M. and Evans, J. (1979). *Lancet* **i**, 13. A new method for measuring milk intake in breast-fed babies.

Cox, P. (1985). Epidemiology and research at low cost. In *Appropriate technology*, p. 28. British Medical Association, London.

Crawford, P.B., Keller, C.A., Hampton, M.C., Pacheco, F.P., and Huenemann, R.L. (1974). *Am. J. Clin. Nutr.* **27**, 706. An obesity index for six-month-old children.

Crosby, W.M., Metcoff, J., Costiloe, J.P., Mameesch, M., Sandstead, H.H., Jacob, R.A., McClain, P.E., Jacobson, G., Reid, W., and Burns, G. (1977). *Am. J. Obstet. Gynaecol.* **128**, 22. Fetal malnutrition: an appraisal of correlated factors.

Crounse, R.G., Bollet, A.J., and Owens, S. (1970). *Nature* **228**, 465. Quantitative measure of human malnutrition using scalp hair roots.

Crue, J.R., Carlssen, B.V.M.H. of vander, Y. Holme, D.T., and Hanson, L.A. (1985). *Acta Paediatr. Scand.* **74**, 338. Studies of human milk II. Concentration of antibodies against Salmonella and Shigella in milk of women from different populations and the daily intake of their breast-fed infants.

Cunningham-Rundles, S. (1982). *Am. J. Clin. Nutr.* **35**, 1202. Effects of nutritional status on immunological function.

Cuthbertson, W.F.J. and Morley, D. (1962). *Trans. R. Soc. Med. Hyg.* **11**, 237. A health and weight chart for children from birth to five.

Cutting, W.A.M. (1980). *Br. Med. J.* **1**, 1188. Growth and growth charts.

Cutting, W.A. (1986). *Trans. R. Soc. Trop. Med. Hyg.* **80**, 665–6. Use of the weight-for-height (Nabarro) chart to screen young children for wasting: a reply.

Daga, S.R., Daga, A.S., Patole, S., Kadam, S., and Mukadain, Y. (1987). *J. Trop. Pediat.* **31**, 61. Foot length measurement from footprint for identifying a number of risks.

Daniels, R.J., Katzeff, H.L., Rasmussin, E., Garrow, J.S., and Danforth, E. (1982). *Am. J. Clin. Nutr.* **35**, 835. Obesity in the Pima Indians: is there a thrifty gene?

Davidson, S., Passmore, R., and Brock, J. (1972). *Textbook of nutrition and dietetics*. Churchill Livingstone, Edinburgh.

——, ——, ——, and Truswell, A.S. (1979). *Human nutrition and dietetics*, 7th edn. Churchill-Livingstone, Edinburgh.

Davis, P.J. and Hersch R. (1986). *Descartes' dream — the world according to mathematics*. Harcourt, Brace and Jovanovich, Orlando, Florida.

Davies, D.P. (1980). *Proc. Nutr. Soc.* **39**, 25. Size at birth and growth in the first year of life of babies who are overweight and underweight at birth.

—— and Leung, S.S.F. (1985). *Early Human Dev.* **11**, 247. Growth of Hong Kong infants during the first two years of life.

—— and Williams, A. (1983). *Br. Med. J.* **286**, 860. Is weighing babies in clinics worthwhile?

Daza, C.H. and Lechtig, A. (1980). *Bull. Pan Am. Hlth. Org.* **14**, 22. Programs to improve the nutrition of pregnant and lactating women.

De Goyet, C de V., Seaman, J., and Geijer, V. (1978). *The management of nutritional emergencies in large populations.* World Health Organization, Geneva.

De Gwynn, E.R. and Sanjur, D. (1974). *Ecol Fd. Nutr.* **3**, 273. Nutritional anthropometry, diet and health-related correlates among pre-school children in Bogota, Columbia.

De Vaquera, M.V., Townsend, J.W., Arroyo, J.J., and Lechtig, A. (1983). *J. Trop. Pediat.* **29**, 167. The relationship between arm circumference at birth and early mortality.

De Sweemer, C., Trowbridge, F.L., Parker, R.L., Brown, K.H., Black, R.E., Reinke, W.A., and Taylor, C.E. (1979). Critical factors in obtaining reliable and accurate data on health in epidemiologic studies. Unpublished document. U.S.–Japan Malnutrition Workshop, July, 1979.

De Wijer, J.F. (1977). *Field guide for the assessment of nutritional health.* ICFSN Nutrition paper no. 2. University of Wageningen, Netherlands.

De Winter, E.R. (1977). *J. Trop. Pediat.* **23**, 111. Measuring weight-gains relation to standard weights-for-age.

De Carvalho, M. and Pittard, W. (1982). *Am. J. Clin. Nutr.* **36**, 963. Breast milk intake: 12 hour versus 24 hour assessment.

Debry, G. (1976). *Ann. Nutr. Alim.* **30**, 115. Validité des methodes d'enquêtes alimentaires.

Delange, F., Bastani, S., and Benmiloud, M. (1986). Classification of goiter size. In *Towards the eradication of endemic goiter* (eds. J.T. Dunn *et al.*). PAHO/WHO Scientific Publication No. 502, Washington, DC.

Delgado, H., Habicht, J.P., Yarbrough, C., Lechtig, A., Martorell, R., Malina, R.M., and Klein, R.E. (1975). *Am. J. Clin. Nutr.* **28**, 216. Nutritional status and the timing of decidous teeth eruption.

Den Hartog, A.P. (1977). *Field guide on food habits.* ICFSN Nutrition paper no. 2, University of Wageningen, Netherlands.

Derman, D.P., Lynch, S.R., Bothwell, T.H., Charlton, R.W., Torrance, J.D., Brink, B.A., Margo, G.M., and Metz, J. (1978). *Br. J. Nutr.* **39**, 383. Serum ferritin as an index of iron nutrition in rural and urban South African children.

Dettwyler, K.A. (1986). *Soc. Sci. Med.* **23**, 651. Infant feeding practices in Mali, West Africa: variation in belief and practice.

Dewey, K.G. (1979). *Ecol. Fd. Nutr.* **8**, 265. Agricultural development, diet and nutrition.

—— (1982). *Am. J. Clin. Nutr.* **37**, 1010. Nutrition survey, Tabasco, Mexico.

——, Daniels, J., Teo, K.S., Hassel, E., and Otow, J. (1986). *Am. J. Clin. Nutr.*

76, 806. Height and weight of Southeast Asian preschool children in northern California.

Dibley, M.J., Goldsby, J.B., Stachling, N.W. and Trowbridge, F.L. (1987). *Am. J. Clin. Nutr.* **46**, 736. Development of normalized curves for international growth reference: historical and technical considerations.

Dibble, M.V., Brin, M., Thiele, V.F., Peel, A., Chen, N., and McMullen, E. (1967). *J. Am. Geriatr. Soc.* **15**, 1031. Evaluation of the nutritional status of elderly subjects, with a comparison between fall and spring.

Disselduff, M.M., Try, G.P., and Berry, W.T.C. (1979). *Fd. Cosmt. Toxi.* **17**, 391. Possible use of dietary surveys to assess intake of food additives.

Donaldson, S.S. and Lenon, R.A. (1979). *Cancer* **43**, 2036. Alteration of nutritional status. Impact of chemotherapy and radiation therapy.

Dorea, J.G., Almeida, I.S., Queiroz, E.F., and Horner, M.E. (1982). *Ecol. Food Nutr.* **12**, 1. Nutritional status and zinc nutriture in infants and children in a poor urban community of Brazil.

Doughty, J. (1979). *Ecol. Fd. Nutr.* **8**, 275. Dangers of reducing the range of food choice in developing countries.

Downs, E.F. (1964). *Am. J. Clin. Nutr.* **15**, 275. Nutritional dwarfing: a syndrome of early protein-calorie malnutrition.

Drake, W.D., Miller, R.I., and Schon, D.A. (eds) (1983). *Nutr. Bull.* 5, 2. Nutrition intervention and evaluation: a call for reflection in action.

Driver, A.G., McAlvey (1980). *Am. J. Clin. Nutr.* **33**, 2057. Creatinine-height index as a function of age.

Dugdale, A.E. (1971). *Am. J. Clin. Nutr.* **24**, 174. An age-independent anthropometric index of nutritional status.

Dugdale, A.E. (1984). *Am. J. Clin. Nutr.* **14**, 59. Nomograms for monitoring nutritional status.

—— (1985). *Lancet* **ii**, 672. Family anthropometry: a new strategy for determining community nutrition.

Duggan, M.B. and Milner, R.D.G. (1986). *Arch. Dis. Childh.* **61**, 436. Energy cost of measles infection.

Durnin, J. and Rahaman, M.M. (1967). *Br. J. Nutr.* **21,** 681. The assessment of the amount of fat in the human body from measurements of skinfold thickness.

—— and Ferro-Luzzi, A. (1982). *Am. J. Clin. Nutr.* **35**, 624. Conducting and reporting studies on human energy intake and output: suggested standards.

Ebomoyi, E. (1986). *Ecol. Fd. Nutr.* **19**, 19. A comparative study of the nutritional status of children in urban and rural Kwara State, Nigeria.

Ebrahim, G.J. (1982). *J. Trop. Pediat.* **28**, ii. Delivery of perinatal care in developing countries.

Edelman, B. and Maller, O. (1982). *Int. J. Obesity.* **6**, 69. Facts and fictions about infantile obesity.

Edwards, L.E., Alton, I.R., Berrada, M.I., and Hatcanson, E.Y. (1979). *Am. J. Clin. Nutr.* **135**, 297. Pregnancy in the underweight woman.

Edwards, D.A.W., Hammond, W.H., Healy, M.J.R., Tanner, J.M., and Whitehouse, R. (1955). *Br. J. Nutr.* **9**, 133. Design and accuracy of calipers for measuring subcutaneous tissue thickness.

Eksmyr, R. and Engsner, G. (1971). *J. Trop. Pediat.* **17**, 110. Skinfold thickness in Ethiopian schoolboys.

Eldridge, E., Salter, C., and Rydjeski, D. (1986). *Disasters* **10**, 189. Towards an early warning system in the Sudan.

El-Lozy, M. (1976). *Am. J. Clin. Nutr.* **29**, 585. Computer simulation of the effects of errors of birth registration on age-independent anthropometric methods.

—— (1978). *Am. J. Clin. Nutr.* **31**, 1718. Programmable calculators in the field assessment of nutritional status.

El-Nofely, A.A. (1978). *Hum. Biol.* **50**, 183. Anthropometric study of growth of Egyptian Nubian children.

El-Sawedy, S.M., Abdel-Tawab, G.A., Zaki, A.M., Zeitoun, M.M., Hamam, M.A., Kantoosh, M.M., and Abdel-Monem, M.A. (1978). *Trans R. Soc. Trop. Med. Hyg.* **72**, 529. The activity of serum ribonuc lease in protein-energy malnutrition.

Essex, B. and Gosling, H. (1987). Nutrition and the community health worker. Guidelines for decision-making. Paper presented at WHO/IUNS Workshop, Caribbean Food and Nutrition Institute, Jamaica (10–18 March 1987).

Elwood, P.C. (1969). *Proc. R. Soc. Med.* **62**, 5. Assessing the functional significance of anaemia.

Enderica, R. (1974). *Arch. Latinamer. Nutr.* **24**, 445. Edad mediana de mortalidad indicador de desarrollo economico-social y como tal componente nutricional.

Eveleth, P.B. and Tanner, J.M. (1976). *World-wide variation in human growth.* Cambridge University Press, Cambridge.

Eveleth, P.B. (1979). Population differences in growth: Environmental and genetic factors. In *Human growth. Vol. 3, Neurobiology and nutrition* (eds. F. Falkner and J.M. Tanner).

Everett, J. (1978). *Obstetric emergencies. A manual for rural health workers.* African Medical Research Foundation, Rural Health Series No: 4, Nairobi, Kenya.

Excler, J.L., Sann, L., Lasne, Y., and Picard, J. (1985). *Early Human Dev.* **11**, 169. Anthropometric assessment of nutritional status in the newborn.

FAO Food and Agriculture Committee on Calorie Requirements (1957). *Calorie requirements*, Rome, Food and Agriculture Organization (FAO Nutritional Studies No. 15).

FAO (1982). *Household food intakes.* FAO, Rome.

FAO/WHO Ad Hoc Expert Committee (1973). *Energy and protein requirements.* World Health Organization Technical Report Series No. 522.

Farthing, M. (1983). *Nutr. Res.* **3**, 619. Serum thyroxine-binding prealbumin may reflect energy and nitrogen intake rather than overall nutritional status in chronic intestinal disease.

——, Mata, L., Urrutia, J.J., and Kronmal, R.A. (1986). *Am. J. Clin. Nutr.* **43**, 395. Natural history of *Giardia* infection of infants.

Favaro, R.M.D., deSouza, N.V., Vannuchi, H., Desai, I.D., and Dutra da Oliveira, J. (1986). *Am. J. Clin. Nutr.* **43**, 940. Evaluation of rose bengal staining test and rapid dark adaptation test in the field assessment of vitamin A status of pre-school children in Southern Brazil.

Feraudi M. and Mejia, L.A. (1987). *Am. J. Clin. Nutr.* **45**, 790. Development of a simplified method to collect blood samples to determine haemoglobin and permotocrit using chromatographic paper discs.

Fernandez, M. and Pelto, G.H. (1981). *Prog. Clin. Biol. Res.* 77, 491. Anthropological studies of nutrition in marginal communities (eds. A.E. Harper and G.K. Davis,) Alan R. Liss Inc., New York.

Ferro-Luzzi, G. (1962). *Metabolism* **11**, 1072. Study on skinfold thickness of schoolchildren in some developing countries. 2 Skinfold thickness in Moroccan boys.

Feuerstein, M. (1979). *Rapid rural appraisal.* Proceedings of a conference. University of Sussex, UK.

Fidanza, F. (1975). *Nutr. Diet.* **21**, 110. Trends in the development of body measurement and body composition.

Fillmore, C.M. and Hussain, M.A. (1984). *Fd. Nutr.* **10**, 2. Agriculture and anthropometry: assessing the impact.

Field, E. and Baber, F. (1973). *Growing up in Hong Kong.* University Press, Hong Kong.

Fisher, M.M. (1976). *Trans. R. Soc. Trop. Med. Hyg.* **70**, 426 Growth of Zambian children.

Flores, M. and Sogondares, L. (1976). *J. Trop. Pediat.* **22**, 277. A guide for the dietary evaluation of pre-school children in the health center.

Foege, W.H. (1976). *Ann. Soc. Belge Med. Trop.* **56**, 305. Epidemiologic surveillance of protein-calorie malnutrition.

Fomon, S.J. (1974). *Infant nutrition*, (2nd edn.) Saunders, Philadelphia, Penn.

—— (1985). Protein requirements in term infants. In *Energy and protein needs in infancy*, p. 55. (eds. S. J. Fomon and W.C. Heird) Academic Press, Orlando, Florida.

—— Haschke, F., Ziegler, E.E., and Nelson, S.E. (1982). *Am. J. Clin. Nutr.* **35**, 1169. Body composition of referency children from birth to age 10 years.

Food and Agriculture Organization. (1977). *Food and Nutrition* **3**, 4. FAO's Food Balance Sheets.

—— (1980). Food balance sheets 1975–77 average. FAO, Rome.

—— (1981). *Guidelines for curriculum content for agricultural training in South-east Asia.* FAO, Rome.

—— (1984). Food balance sheets 1971–81 average. FAO, Rome.

Food and Nutrition Research Institute (1980). Food composition tables recommended for use in the Philippines (Fifth Revision). Manila, Philippines.

Forbes, G.B. and Bruining, G.J. (1976). *Am. J. Clin. Nutr.* **29**, 1359. Urinary creatinine excretion and lean body mass.

Forman, M. (ed.) (1986). *Nutritional aspects of project food aid.* United Nations, New York.

Forse, R.A. and Shizgal, H.M. (1980). *J. Parent. Ent. Nutr.* **4**, 450. Serum albumin and nutritional status.

Forsyth, S.J. (1984). *Food and Nutr. Bull.* **6**, 22. Nutrition education: lack of success in teaching Papua New Guinea mothers to distinguish "good" from "not good" weight development charts.

Foster, G.M. (1952). *Human Org.* **11**, 5. Relationships between theoretical and applied anthropology: a public health program analysis.

Foy, H. and Kondi, A. (1977). *Lancet* **ii**, 401. Haemoglobin measurements in developing countries.

Frankle, R.J. and Owen, A.Y. (1978). *Nutrition in the community: the art of delivering the services.* Mosby, St. Louis, Mo.

Franklin, R.R., Mock, N.B., Malonga, M., Dikassa, L., and Weaver, K. (1984). *Nutr. Rep. Internat.* **30**, 1027. Rapid assessment of urban nutritional status using hospital pediatric records: a case study from Zaire.

Frenk, S., Metcoff, J., Gomez, F., Ramos-Galvan, R., Cravioto, J., and Antonowicz, I. (1957). *Pediat* **20**, 105. Intracellular composition and homeostatic mechanisms in chronic infantile malnutrition. (2) Composition of tissues.

Frerichs, R., Harsha, D.W., and Berenson, G.S. (1979). *Pediat. Res.* **13**, 170. Equations for estimating percentage of body fat in children 10–14 years.

—— (1988). *J. Trop. Ped.* (in press). Rapid microcomputer surveys.

Friedman, P.J. and Hodges, R.E. (1977). *Lancet* **ii**, 1159. Tongue colour and vitamin B deficiencies.

Friel, J.K., Gibson, R.S., Kawash, G.F., and Watts, J. (1985). *J. Pediat. Gastro. Nutr.* **4**, 746. Dietary zinc intake and growth during infancy.

Frisancho, A.R. (1981). *Am. J. Clin. Nutr.* **34**, 254. New norms of upper limb fat and muscle areas for assessment of nutritional status.

—— (1984). *Am. J. Clin. Nutr.* **40**, 808. New standards of weight and body composition by frame size and height for assessment of adults and the elderly.

——, and Flagel, P.N. (1982). *Am. J. Clin. Nutr.* **36**, 967. Relative merits of old and new indices of body mass to skinfold thickness.

—— and Flagel, P. (1983). *Am. J. Clin. Nutr.* **37**, 311. Elbow breadth as a measure of frame size for US males and females.

——, Matos, J. and Flegel, P. (1983). *Am. J. Clin. Nutr.* **38**, 739. Maternal nutritional status and adolescent pregnancy outcome.

Fuchs, R.J., Theis, C.F., and Lancaster, M.C. (1978). *Am. J. Clin. Nutr.* **31**, 673. A nomogram to predict lean body mass in man.

Gabbard, C.P. and Patterson, P.E. (1980). *Ann. Human Biol.* **7**. Relationship and comparison of selected anthropometric measures to muscular endurance and strength in children 3–5 years.

—— and —— (1980). *Ann. Hum. Biol.* **7**, 6. Relationship and comparison of selected anthropometric measures to muscular endurance and strength in children 3–5 years.

Ganguly, C. and Mukherjee, K.L. (1986). *J. Trop. Pediatr.* **32**, 287. Relationship between maternal serum vitamin A and vitamin A status of the corresponding fetuses.

Gammon, A. and Baker, S.J. (1977). *Ind. J. Med. Res.* **65**, 150, Studies in methods of haemoglobin estimations suitable for public health programmes.

Garde, P.M. (1986). *Trop. Doc.* 16, 71. Growth rate score to screen for intrauterine growth retardation.

Garn, S.M. (1962). *Am. J. Clin. Nutr.* **11**, 418. Anthropometry in clinical appraisal of nutritional status.

—— (1978). *Ecol. Fd. Nutr.* 7, 64. Improved prospects for weighing accuracy.

—— (1979). Optimal nutrition. In *Growth and nutrition* (eds. D. and E. Jelliffe), p. 273. Plenum Press, New York.

—— (1983). *Ecol. Fd. Nutr.* **13**, 197. How to use calipers.

—— and Hawthorn, V.M. (1984). *Am. J. Clin. Nutr.* **39**, 490. The 'new' metropolitan weight tables.

—— and Keating, M. T. (1981). *Am. J. Clin. Nutr.* **34**, 115. Hematological status and pregnancy outcomes.

—— Ryan, A. S., and Abraham, S. (1980). *Ecol. Fd. Nutr.* **10**, 69–70. The black-white difference in hemoglobin levels after age, sex and income matching.

—— Smith, N.J., and Clarke, D. (1975). *Am. J. Clin. Nutr.* **28**, 563. The magnitude and the implications of apparent race differences in hemoglobin values.

Garrow, J.S. and Webster, J. (1985). *Int. J. Obes.* **9**, 147. Quetelet's index (W/H^2) as a measure of fatness.

Gebre-Medhin, M. (1977). *Maternal malnutrition and its effects on the offspring.* Uplands Grafiska AB, Uppsala, Sweden.

—— (1979). Nutritional surveillance in developing countries: Ethiopia. In *Human nutrition*, Vol 2: *Nutrition and growth* (eds. D.B. and E.F.P. Jelliffe), Plenum Press, New York.

—— (1982). *Adv. Int. Mat. Chld. Hlth.* **2**, 87. Nutritional rickets: a persisting problem.

Gebre-Medhin, G. and Falk, H. (1980). Body weight changes during pregnancy in Ethiopian women. *Proc. Third European Nutrition Conference*, p. 97. (ed. L. Hambraeus).

Geissler, C.A. and Bates, J.F. (1984). *Am. J. Clin. Nutr.* **39**, 478. The nutritional effect of tooth loss.

Ghassemi, H. (1985). *Growth monitoring of young children.* UNICEF, New York.

—— and Teply, L.J. (1983). Nutrition strategies in UNICEF's perspective. In *Nutrition in the community* (ed. D.S. McLaren). John Wiley, Chichester (West Sussex).

Ghesquière, J.L. and Karvonen, M.J. (1981). *Ann. Hum. Biol.* **8**, 119. Some anthropometric and functional dimensions of the pygmy (Kivu Twa).

Ghosh, S. (1980). *J. Trop. Pediat.* **26**, 266. Growth reference standards for developing countries. (Letter to the Editors.)

Ghosh, S. and Bhargaya, S.K. (1985). *Proc. Asian Pediat. Congress*, Malaysia. A longitudinal study of growth from birth to ten years in an urban cohort.

—— and Mohan, M. (1978). *Lancet* i, 823. Screening for anaemia.

——, ——, and Talib, V.H. (1978). *Ind. Pediat.* **15**, 751. Identification of anaemia with the help of an anaemia recognition card.

——, ——, and Yayathi, T. (1976). *Ind. Pediat.* **13**, 915. Quick nutritional screening by mid-arm circumference bangle.

Gilles, H.M. (1964). *Akufo: an environmental study of a Nigerian village community.* Ibadan, University Press.

Glueck, C.J. (1982). *J. Am. Coll. Nutr.* **1**, 41. Cradle-to-grave atherosclerosis: high density lipoprotein cholesterol.

Goel, K.M., Sweet, E.M., Logan, R.W., Warren, J.M., Arniel, G.C., and Shanks, R.A. (1976). *Lancet* i, 1141. Florid and subclinical rickets among immigrant children in Glasgow.

Golden, M.H.N. (1982). *Am. J. Clin. Nutr.* **35**, 1159. Transport proteins as indices of protein status.

Goldstein, H. (1978). Sampling for growth studies. In *Human growth*, Vol. 2, (eds. F. Falkner and J.M. Tanner), p. 273. Ballière Tindall, London.

—— and Tanner, J.M. (1980). *Lancet* i, 583. Ecological considerations in the creation and use of child growth standards.

Gómez, F., Ramos Galvan, R. Frenk, S., Cravioto, J., Chavez, R., and Vazquez, J. (1956). *J. Trop. Pediat.* **2**, 77. Mortality in second and third degree malnutrition.

Goodman, A.H., Allen, L.H., Hermandez, G.P., Amador, A., Arriola, L.V., Chavez, A., and Pelto, G.H. (1987). *Am. J. Phys. Anthrop.* **72**, 7. Prevalence and age of development of enamel hypoplasias in Mexican children.

Gopalan, C. (1961). *Fed. Proc.* **20**, 177. Nutrition and lactation.

—— (1983). *Future* **8**, 33. Small is healthy?

—— (1984). *Bull. Nutr. Found. India* **5**, 1. "Child survival" and child nutrition.

—— (1986). *Bull. Nutr. Found. India* **7**, 1. The nutritional status of India's children. Has it improved in recent years?

Gopalan, C. (1987*a*). *Bull. Nutr. Found. India* **8**, 1. Growth monitoring: some basic issues.

Gopalan, C. (ed.) (1987*b*). Combating undernutrition: basic issues and practical approaches. Nutrition Foundation of India. Special Publication Series: 3. New Delhi, India.

—— and Chatterjee, M. (1985). *Use of growth charts for promoting child nutrition*: a review of global experience. Special Publication Series: 2. Nutrition Foundation of India, New Delhi.

—— and Jaya Rao, K.S. (1984). *J. Trop. Pediat.* **30**, 7. Classification of undernutrition: limitations and fallacies.

—— and Narasinga Rao, B.S. (1977). *Dietary allowances for Indians*, Spec. Rept. Series No. 60: Indian Council for Medical Research, New Delhi, India.

Gordon, J.E. (1963). *Am. J. Med. Sci.* **246**, 132. Field epidemiology.

——, Chitkara, I.D., and Wyon, J.B. (1963). *Am. J. Med. Sci.* **245**, 129. Weanling diarrhoea.

——, Wyon, J.B., and Ascoli, W. (1967). *Am. J. Med. Sci.* **254**, 121. The second year death rate in less developed countries.

Gortmaker, S.L. and Dietz, W.H., Sobol, M.A., and Wehler, M.S. (1987). *Am. J. Dis. Child.* **141**, 535. Increasing pediatric obesity in the United States.

Gokulnathan, K.S. and Verghese, R.K.P. (1969). *J. Trop. Pediat.* **15**, 118. Sociocultural malnutrition.

Gracey, M. (1987). *World Rev. Nutr. Diet.* **49**, 160. Normal growth and nutrition.

——, Owles, E.N., and Hitchcock, N.E. (1982). *Med. J. Austral.* **2**, 315. Growth standards for Australian infants and children.

Graffar, M. (1956). *Courier* **6**, 455. Une methode de classification sociale d'echantillons de population.

Graham, A.M. (1982). *Proc. Nutr. Soc.* **41**, 343. Assessment of nutritional intake.

Graham, G.G. (1966). Programs for combating malnutrition in the pre-school child in Chile. In *Proceedings of international conference on the prevention of malnutrition in the pre-school child*. National Academy of Sciences, Washington, DC.

Graitcer, P.L. (1981). *A manual for the basic assessment of nutritional status in potential crisis situations*. Center for Disease Control, Atlanta, Georgia.

—— and Genery, E.M. (1981). *Lancet*, **ii**, 297. Measuring children: one reference for all.

——, Goldsby, J.B., and Nichaman, M.Z. (1981). *Am. J. Clin. Nutr.* **34**, 61. Hemoglobins and hematocrits: are they equally sensitive in detecting anemias?

——, Amedee, M., Duckett, E.M., and Nichaman, N.Z. (1979). *Clin. Res.* **27**, 551A. The relationship of nutritional status indicators to recent symptoms of illness, fever and diarrhea.

Grant, A. (1977). *Nutritional assessment for dietitians.* Seattle, Washington.

Grant, J. (1978). *Disparity reduction rates in social indicators.* Overseas Development Council Monograph no: 11.

—— (1987*a*). *State of the world's children. Going for the growth*, p. 64. UNICEF, Oxford University Press, New York.

—— (1987*b*). *Adjustment with a human face.* UNICEF/Oxford University Press, New York.

—— (1988). *The state of the world's children.* UNICEF/Oxford University Press, New York.

Grant, K. and Stone, T. (1986). *J. Trop. Pediat.* **32**, 257. Maternal comprehension of a home-based growth chart and its effect on growth.

Greenfield, H. and Clark, J. (1974). *Nutritional problems associated with pregnancy and lactation.* Papua and New Guinea Institute of Medical Research, 5th Annual Rept. 1973–4.

Greentree, T.R. and Phillips, R. (1979). *Communique* **4**, 1. The PQLI and the DRR: new tools for measuring development programs.

Griffiths, M. (1981). Phillipine Growth Table: Source USAID Mission Phillipines.

—— (1985). *Growth monitoring*, 2nd edn. American Public Health Association, Washington, DC.

—— (1985). *Growth monitoring of pre-school children.* Information for action issue paper. American Public Health Association, Washington, DC.

—— (1987). *Mothers and Children.* **6**, 7. The Bubble Chart.

—— (1987*a*). *The weaning project: new strategies to improve infant feeding practices. Manual for the assessment of weaning practices in Indonesia.* Manoff International, New York.

Grindulis, H., Scott, P., Belton, N.R., and Wharton, B.A. (1986). *Arch. Dis. Childh.* **61**, 843. Combined deficiency of iron and vitamin D in Asian toddlers.

Grounds, J.G. (1964). *E. Afr. Med. J.* **41**, 333. Mortality and wastage rates for East African children in Kenya.

Grivetti, L.E. and Pangborn, R.M. (1973). *J. Nutr. Educ.* **5**, 204. Food habits research: review of approaches and methods.

Guba, E.G. and Lincoln, Y.S. (1981). *Effective evaluation.* Jossey Bass, San Francisco.

Gueri, M., Gurney, J.M., and Jutsum, P. (1980). *Bull. Wrld. Hlth. Org.* **58**, 773. The Gómez classification.

——, Jutsum, P., and Sorhaindo, B. (1982). *Am. J. Clin. Nutr.* **35**, 609. Anthropometric assessment of nutritional status in pregnant women: a reference table of weight-for-height by week of pregnancy.

——, ——, Knight, P., and Hinds, V. (1977). *Arch. Latinam. Nutr.* **27**, 403. The arm circumference at birth and its relation to other anthropometric parameters.

Gurney, J.M. (1969). *J. Trop. Ped.* **15**, 9. A simple tool for assessing the growth of school-age children.

—— (1971). *W. Ind. Med. J.* **20**, 227. Weaning practices from Guyana, rural Trinidad, Grenada, Monserrat and Antigua.

—— (1983). *J. Trop. Pediat.* **29**, 76. Anaemia and the Caribbean.

—— and Jelliffe, D.B. (1973). *Am. J. Clin. Nutr.* **26**, 912. Arm anthropometry in nutritional assessment. Momogram for rapid calculation of muscle circumference and cross-sectional muscle and fat areas.

—— and Jutsum, P.J. (1981). *Am. J. Clin. Nutr.* **34**, 2615. Nutrient-cost nomogram: an appropriate technology.

——, Jelliffe, D.B., and Neill, J. (1972). *J. Trop. Pediat.* **18**, 1. Anthropometry in the differential diagnosis of protein-calorie malnutrition.

Guthrie, D., Haines, H., and Morley, D. (1978). *J. Trop. Pediat.* 24, 1. International year of the Child. Child-to-child programme.

Gwatkin, D., Wilcox, J. and Wray, J. (1980). Can health and nutrition interventions make a difference? Monograph res: 13, Overseas Development Council, Washington, DC.

Gwebu, E.T., Mtero, S., Dube, N., Tangwireyi, J.T., and Mugwagwa, N. (1985). *Centr. Afr. Med. J.* **31**, 193. Assessment of nutritional status in pregnancy: use of a reference table of weight-for-height.

Haaga, J.G., Quinn, V., Mason, J.B., and Williams, K. (1983). Recommendations for development of nutritional surveillance in Botswana. Mimeo. Cornell Nutritional Surveillance Program.

Haas, J.D. (1981). *Fed. Proc.* 40, 2577. Human adaptability approach to nutritional assessment: a Bolivian example.

Habicht, J-P. (1979). *Fed. Proc.* **38**, 2551. Translating science and nutrition findings to social policy.

—— (1980). *Am. J. Clin. Nutr.* **33**, 531. Some characteristics of indicators of nutritional status for use in screening and surveillance.

—— and Dapice, D. (1984). An Indonesian national nutrition surveillance system. Mimeo, R14. Cornell Nutritional Surveillance Program.

—— and Mason, J. (1983). Nutritional surveillance: principles and practice. In *Nutrition in the community* (2nd edn) (ed. D.S. McLaren), pp. 217–244, Wiley, Chichester.

——, Lane, M.J., and McDowell, A.J. (1978). *Fed. Proc.* 37, 1181. National Nutrition Surveillance.

——, Meyers, L.D., and Brownie, C. (1982). *Am. J. Clin. Nutr.* **35** (Suppl.), 1089. Overview: Indicators for identifying and counting the improperly nourished.

——, Yarbrough, C., and Martorell, R. (1979). In *Nutrition and growth* (eds. D.B. and E.F.P. Jelliffe) Plenum Press, New York. Anthropometric field methods: Critical selection.

——, Martorell, R., Yarbrough, C., Malina, R.M., and Klein, R.E. (1974). *Lancet*, Volume No. 611. Height and weight standards for pre-school children. How relevant are ethnic differences in growth potential?

Haenel, H. and Mohr, M. (1974). *Bibl. Nutr. Diet.* **20**, 163. Nutritional status assessment and food consumption surveys carried out in the GDR.

Hall, A. (1981). *Trans. R. Soc. Trop. Med. Hyg.* **75**, 682. Quantitative variability of nematode egg counts in faeces: a study among rural Kenyans.

Hall, J.C. (1983). *Am. J. Clin. Nutr.* **37**, 473. A method for the rapid assessment of sample size in dietary studies.

Hambidge, K.M. (1982). *Am. J. Clin. Nutr.* **36**, 943. Hair analysis: worthless for vitamins, limited for minerals.

Hamill, P.V.V., Drizal, T.A., Johnson, C.L., Reed, R.B., Roche, A.F., and Moore, W.M. (1979). *Am. J. Clin. Nutr.* **32**, 607. National Center for Health statistics percentiles.

Hankin, J.H. (1982). Critical factors in obtaining reliable and accurate food intake data. In *Methodologies for human population studies in nutrition related to health* (ed. B. Underwood). National Institutes of Health, Bethesda, Md.

Hansell, D.T. and Smellie, G.X. (1982). *Br. Med. J.* **ii**, 1012. Cheap and effective method of weighing bed-bound patients.

Harfouche, J.K. (1965). *Growth and illness patterns of Lebanese infants.* Khayat Press, Beirut.

Harijono (1976). *Survey in children under five at Gedang Alas village, Gajah District, Demak Rejeng. Indonesia.* Research and Development Center, Diponegoro University, Semarang, Indonesia.

Harries, A.D., Thomas, J., and Chugh, K.S. (1985). *Human Nutr.* **39c**, 315. Anthropometric cut off points for diagnosis of malnutrition: are they applicable in developing countries?

Harris, K.L. and Lindblad, C.J. (1977). *Post-harvest grain assessment methods.* Office of Nutrition, USAID, Washington, DC.

Harrison, G. and Van Itallie, T.B. (1982). *Am. J. Clin. Nutr.* **35**, 1176. Estimation of body composition: a new approach based on electromagnetic principles.

Harrison, G.A., Weiner, J.S, Tanner, J.M., and Barnicott, N.A. (1964). *Human biology.* Oxford University Press.

Harrison, G.G. (1984). *Fd. Nutr. Bull.* **6**, 18. Application of incremental growth standards.

—— (1985). *Fed. Proc.* **6**, 18. Application of incremental growth standards.

Harsha, D.W., Voors, A.W., and Berenson, G.S. (1980). *Am. J. Phys. Anthrop.* **53**, 333. Racial differences in subcutaneous fat patterns in children aged 7–15 years.

Harvey, K.B., Bothe, A., and Blackburn, G.L. (1979). *Cancer* **43**, 2065. Nutritional assessment and patient outcome during oncological therapy.

Hassan, N. and Ahmad, K. (1984). *Ecol. Fd. Nutr.* **15**, 143. Studies on food and nutrient intake by rural populations of Bangladesh.

Hatchell, D.L. and Sommer, A. (1984). *Arch. Ophth.* 102, 1389. Detection of ocular surface abnormalities in experimental vitamin A deficiency.

Hay, R. and Freeman, R.H. (1978). *Food supply monitoring: a manual.* Oxford University, Oxford.

Heald, F.P. (1985). Nutrition in adolescence. In *The health of adolescents and youths in the Americas*, Sci. Publ. No. 489. Pan American Health Organization, Washington DC.

Hegstedt, D.M. (1972). *Ecol. Fd. Nutr.* **1**, 255. Problems in the use and interpretation of the recommended dietary allowances.

Heimendinger, J. (1964). *Helv. Paed. Acta.* **19**, 406. Gemischt longitudinale messungen von Korperlange, Gewicht, oberem segment, thoraxumfang und kopfumfant bei 1–24 monate alten sauglingen.

Hendrata, L. and Johnson, M. (1978). *Manual for community-based under-fives weighing program, Indonesia.* Yayasan Indonesia Sejehtera, Jakarta.

Hendrickse, R.G. (1984*a*). *Bull. Int. Pediat. Assoc.* **6**, 62. Growth and development in developing countries.

—— (1984*b*). *Trans. R. Soc. Trop. Med. Hyg.* **78**, 427. The influence of aflatoxins on child health in the tropics with particular reference to kwashiorkor.

Herbert, V. (1987*a*). *Am. J. Clin. Nutr.* **45**, 661. Recommended dietary intakes (RDI) of bolate in humans.

—— (1987*b*). *Am. J. Clin. Nutr.* **45**, 671. Recommended dietary intakes (RDI) of vitamin B12 in humans.

Herbert, V. (1987*c*). *Am. J. Clin. Nutr.* **45**, 679. Recommended dietary intakes (RDI) of iron in humans.

Hershko, C., Bar-or, D., Gaziel, Y., Naparstek, E., Konijn, A.M., Grossowicz, N., Kaufman, N., and Izak, G. (1981). *Am. J. Clin. Nutr.* **34**, 1600. Diagnosis of iron deficiency anemia in a rural population. Relative usefulness of serum ferritin, red cell protoporphyrin, red cell indices, and transferrin saturation determinations.

Hessov, I. (1978). *Lancet* **ii**, 1667. Detecting deficient energy and protein intake in hospitalized patients: a simple record method.

Hetzel, B. (1986). *Adv. Int. Mat. Chld. Hlth.* **6**, 79. Iodine deficiency disease a maternal and child health issue.

Hetzel, B.S. (1983). *Lancet* **ii**, 1126. Iodine deficiency disorders (IDD) and their eradication.

Hetzel, I. (1987). *Adv. Int. Mat. Chld. Hlth.* **7**, 79. Iodine deficiency disorders (*IDD*): a maternal and child issue.

Hetzel, B.S., Dunn, J.T., and Stanbury, J.B. (eds.) (1986). *The prevention and control of iodine deficiency disorders.* Elsevier, Amsterdam and New York.

Heymsfield, S.B., Arteaga, C., McManus, C., Smith, J., and Moffitt, S. (1983). *Am. J. Clin. Nutr.* **37**, 478. Measurement of muscle mass in humans: validity of the 24-hour urinary creatinine method.

——, McManus, C., Stevens, V., and Smith, J. (1982). *Am. J. Clin. Nutr.* **35**, 1192. Muscle mass: reliable indicator of protein-energy malnutrition severity and outcome.

——, Olafson, R.P., Kutner, M.H., and Nixon, D.W. (1979). *Am. J. Clin. Nutr.* **32**, 693. A radiographic method of quantifying protein-calorie malnutrition.

Hill, A.G. and Macrae, S. (1985). *UNICEF Soc. Stat. Bull.* **8**, 1. Measuring child mortality levels: a new approach.

Hijazi, S.S. (1977). *Jordan Med. J.* **12**, 26. Mortality patterns of infants and young children in rural Amman.

Hitchcock, N.E. and Gracey, M. (1981). *Lancet* **ii**, 64. Growth of healthy breast-fed infants in the first six months.

Hodges, R.E. (1971). *Am. J. Clin. Nutr.* **24**, 383. What's new about scurvy?

Hojer, B, Gebre-Medhin, M., Sterky, G., Zelterstrom, R., and Daniel, K. (1977). *J. Trop. Pediat.* **23**, 73. Combined vitamin D deficiency rickets and protein-energy malnutrition in Ethiopian infants.

Horton, E. (1982). *Am. J. Clin. Nutr.* **35**, 1228. Effects of low energy diets on work performance.

Hruby, J. (1983). *World Rev. Nutr. Diet.* **41**, 1. Problems of nutrition and food policy.

Huffman, S., Wolff, M., and Lowell, S. (1985). *Am. J. Clin. Nutr.* **42**, 725.

Nutrition and fertility in Bangladesh: nutritional status of non-pregnant women.

Hume, R. (1966). *J. Clin. Path.* **19**, 389. Prediction of lean body mass from height and weight.

Hundley, J.M., Mickelsen, O., Mantel, N., Weaver, R.N., and Taber, R.C. (1955). *Am. J. Publ. Hlth.* **45**, 1455. Height and weight of first grade children as a potential index of nutritional status.

Hunt, I., Murphy, N.J., Cleaver, A.E., Laine, N., and Clark, V. (1983). *Ecol. Food Nutr.* **12**, 235. Protective foods recall as a tool for dietary assessment in the evaluation of public health programs for pregnant Hispanics.

Hurley, L.S. (1980). *Developmental nutrition.* Prentice Hall, New Jersey.

Husaini, Y.K., Husaini, M.A., Sulariman, Z., Jahari, A.B., Barizi, Hudono, S.T. and Karyadi, D. (1986). *Fd. Nutr. Bull.* **8**, 71. Maternal malnutrition, outcome of pregnancy and a simple tool to identify women at risk.

Hytten, F. and Chamberlain, G. (1980). *Clinical physiology in obstetrics.* Blackwell, Oxford.

—— and Leitch, I. (1964). *The physiology of human pregnancy.* Oxford University Press, Oxford.

ICNND (1963). *Manual for nutrition surveys*, US Government Printing Office, Washington, DC.

Illingworth, R.S. (1986). *Arch. Dis. Childh.* **61**, 1151. Anaemia and child health surveillance.

Indian Council of Medical Research. (1972). *In: Growth and development of Indian infants and children.* Tech. Rept. Series No.: 18, ICMR, New Delhi.

Ingenbleek, Y., Visscher, M., and De Nayer, P. (1972). *Lancet* **ii**, 106. Measurement of prealbumin as index of protein-calorie malnutrition.

International Food Policy Research Institute. (1983). *Food and Nutr. Bull.* **5**, 1–41. Household food distribution: a symposium.

International Journal of Epidemiology (1976). *Int. J. Epidemiol.* **3**(1), 3. Editorial: Surveillance.

International Statistical Institute (1975). *Manual on sample designing: Basic document.* World Fertility Survey, Washington, D.C.

International Vitamin A Consultative Group (1975). *Guidelines for the eradication of vitamin A deficiency and xerophthalmia.* Nutrition Foundation, New York.

—— (1982). *Reports of selected methods for the analysis of vitamin A and carotenoids in nutrition surveys.* Nutrition Foundation, Washington, DC.

International Union of Nutritional Sciences (1977). *Am. J. Clin. Nutr.* **30**, 242. Guidelines on the at-risk concept and the health and nutrition of young children.

Jackson, C.M. (1925). *The effects of inanition and malnutrition upon growth and structure.* Blakiston, Philadelphia, Penn.

Jackson, R.T. and Latham, M.C. (1982). *Am. J. Clin. Nutr.* **35**, 710. Anemia of pregnancy in Liberia, West Africa: therapeutic trial.

Jacobson, H.N. (1983). *Birth* **10**, 29. Diet therapy and the improvement of pregnancy outcomes.

Jadhav, M., Webb, J.K.G., Vaishnava, S., and Baker, S.J. (1962). *Lancet* **ii**, 903. Vitamin B_{12} deficiency in Indian infants.

Jain, M.G., Harrison, L., Howe, G.R., and Miller, A.B. (1982). *Am. J. Clin. Nutr.* **36**, 931. Evaluation of a self-administered dietary questionnaire for use in a cohort study.

James, D.K., Drybrough, E.H., and Chiswick, M. (1979). *Arch. Dis. Childh.* **54**, 226. Foot length: a potentially useful measurement in the neonate.

Janes, M.D., Macfarlane, S.B.J., and Moody, J.B. (1981). *Ann. Trop. Pediat.* **1**, 27. Height and weight growth standards for Nigerian children.

Jansen, A.A.J. and T'Mannetje, W. (1982). *J. Trop. Pediat.* **28**, 38. Assessment of nutritional status: a comparison of methods.

Jardin, C. (1967). *History of foods used in Africa*. FAO, Rome.

Jelliffe, D.B. (1954). *Doc. Geogr. Trop. Med.* **5**, 314. Ascaris lumbricoides and malnutrition in tropical children.

—— (1955). *J. Trop. Pediat.* **1**, 39. Hypochromotrichia in Jamaican infants.

—— (1956). *J. Pediat.* 49, 661. Cultural variation and the practical pediatrician.

—— (1957). *Pediat.* **20**, 128. Cultural blocks and protein malnutrition in early childhood in rural West Bengal.

—— (1959). *J. Pediat.* **54**, 277. Protein-calorie malnutrition in tropic pre-school children: a review of recent knowledge.

—— (1966). *The assessment of the nutritional status of the community*. WHO monographs No. 53. Geneva.

—— (1968*a*). *Infant nutrition in the subtropics and tropics, Geneva,* World Health Organization: Monograph series, No. 29, 2nd edn, Geneva.

—— (1968*b*). *J. Trop. Pediat.* **14**, 217. The pre-school child as a biocultural transitional.

—— (1971). *Lancet* ii, 549. An epiphysometer and the community diagnosis of nutritional rickets.

—— (1986). *Med. J. Malaysia.* **41**, 77. Adequacy of lactation: Dysreflaxia vs. maternal nutrition.

—— and Bennett, F.J. (1962). *Fed. Proc.* **20**, 185. Cultural and social factors in infant and maternal feeding.

——, Bras, G., and Stuart, K. (1954). *West Ind. Med. J.* **3**, 43. Kwashiorkor and marasmus in Jamaican infants.

—— and Jelliffe, E.F.P. (1960). *Am. J. Publ. Hlth.* **50**, 1355. The prevalence of protein-calorie malnutrition of early childhood in Haiti.

—— and —— (1961). *J. Pediat.* **59**, 271. The children of the San Blas Indians of Panama.

—— and —— (1968). *J. Trop. Pediat.* **14**, 71. Anthropometry in action. (I) Dental second-year malnutrition.

—— and —— (1971*a*). *Am. J. Clin. Nutr.* **24**, 893. Linear enamel hypoplasia of deciduous incisor teeth in malnourished children.

—— and —— (1971*b*). An assessment of weighing devices for the evaluation of nutritional status of young children in less developed areas. In *Use of growth charts for assessing programs of children and teaching parents*, p. 15. Office of Nutrition, Agency for International Development, Washington, DC.

—— and —— (eds.) (1973). *J. Trop. Pediat.* **19**(2A), 193. Deciduous dental eruption, nutrition and age assessment.

—— and —— (1975). *Am. J. Clin. Nutr.* **28**, 203. The *quipu* in measuring malnutrition.

—— and —— (1978*a*). *Am. J. Clin. Nutr.* **31**, 1421. National policy & young child nutrition.

—— and —— (1978*b*). The socio-economic birth weight quotient. In *Birth weight distribution: An indicator of social development*, p. 41. (eds. G. Sterky and L. Mellander) SAREC Report No. 8, Stockholm.

—— and —— (eds.) (1979*a*). *Nutrition and growth*. New York, Plenum Press.

—— and —— (1979*b*). *Am. J. Clin. Nutr.* **32**, 2058. An evaluation of upper arm measurements used in nutritional assessment.

—— and —— (1981). *J. Trop. Pediat.* **27**, 2. Primary health care workers and family nutrition.

—— and —— (1985*b*). Using growth charts to improve nutrition: A guide for the preparation of decision diagrams for training community health workers. WHO Mimeograph Document, Geneva.

—— and —— (1987). *Asia Pacific J. Publ. Hlth.* **1**, 77. Stimulating action to improve nutrition: how to make community nutritional assessment lead to change.

—— and —— (1989*a*). *Human milk in the modern world* (2nd edn). Oxford, Oxford University Press.

—— and —— (eds.) (1989*b*). Growth monitoring in young children. Selection of methods and techniques of training (in press).

—— and Maddocks, I. (1964). *Clin. Pediat.* **3**, 432. Ecologic malnutrition in the New Guinea Highlands.

——, Symonds, B.E.R., and Jelliffe, E.F.P. (1960). *J. Pediat.* **57**, 922. The pattern of malnutrition in early childhood in Southern Trinidad.

——, Woodburn, J., Bennett, F.J., and Jelliffe, E.F.P. (1962). *J. Pediat.* **50**, 907. The children of the Hadza hunters.

Jelliffe, E.F.P. (1968*a*). *Bull. World Hlth. Org.* **38**, 69. Low birth weight and malarial infection of the placenta.

—— (1968*b*). *Cajanus* **1**, 33. Why do we bother to weigh children?

—— and Jelliffe, D.B. (1964). *Clin. Pediat.* **3**, 604. Children in ancient Polynesian Hawaii.

—— and —— (eds.) (1969). *J. Trop. Pediat.* **15**, 179. The arm circumference as a public health index of protein-calorie malnutrition in early childhood.

—— and —— (eds.) (1973). *J. Trop. Pediat.* **19**, 193. Deciduous dental eruption, nutrition and age assessment.

—— and —— (1988*a*). *Algorithms, growth monitoring and nutritional action.* WHO 8841C, Geneva.

——, ——, Feldon, K., and Ngokwey, N. (1987). *World Rev. Nutr. Diet* **53**, 218. Traditional practices concerning feeding during and after diarrhoea.

—— and —— (eds.) (1988*b*). *Programmes to promote breastfeeding*. Oxford University Press, Oxford.

Jenkins, R. and Guthrie, H. (1984). *J. Nutr. Ed.* **16**, 15. Identification of index nutrients for dietary assessment.

Jerome, N., Kandel, R.F., and Pelto, G.F. (1980). *Nutritional anthropology.* Redgrave, New York.

Jerome, N.W. and Pelto, G.F. (1981). *Fed. Proc.* **40**, 2601. Integrating ethnographic research with nutrition studies.

Johnson, A. (1975). *Ethnol.* **14**, 301. Time allocation in a Machigunenga community.

Johnson, A. and Behrens, C.A. (1982). *Human Ecol.* **10**, 167. Nutritional criteria in Machiguenga food production decisions: a linear programming analysis.

Johnson, M.D., Yamanaka, W.K., and Formacion, C.S. (1984). *J. Trop. Pediat.* **30**, 90. A comparison of anthropometric methods for assessing nutritional status of preschool children: the Philippines study.

Johnston, C. (1982). Selection of methodologies for measuring bone mass in studies of osteoporosis. In *Methodologies for human population studies in nutrition related to health.* (ed. B. Underwood) National Institutes of Health: Bethesda, Md.

Johnston, E.E. (1982). *Hum. Biol.* 54, 221. Relationship between body composition and anthropometry.

——, Bogin, B., MacVean, R.B., and Newman, B.C. (1984). *Hum. Biol.* **56**, 157. A comparison of international standards versus local reference data for the triceps and subscapular skinfolds of Guatemala children and youths.

Jolliffe, N., Goodhart, R.S., Archer, M., Lopez, H., and Diaz, F.G. (1958). *J. Nutr.* **64**, 355. Nutrition status survey of the sixth grade school population in Cuba.

—— (ed.) (1962). *Clinical nutrition*, 2nd edn. Harper, New York.

Jones, E.M. and Munger, S.J. (1978). *Application of a field guide for evaluation of nutrition education to programs in the Philippines.* USAID, Washington, DC.

Jones, R.A.K. and Robertson, R.C. (1986). *Arch. Fis. Child.* **61**, 877. Small for dates babies: are they really a problem?

Jordan, J., Ruben, M., Bendasco, A., De la Vega, R., Jimenez, J.M., Mesa, D. and Hernandez, J. (1978). *Rev. Cub. Ped.* **50**, 425. III. Normas nacionales de peso y tallo.

Jordan, J., Ruben, M., Hernandez, J., Bebelagua, A., Tanner, J.M., and Goldstein, H. (1975). *Ann. Human Biol.* **2**, 153. The 1972 Cuba national child growth study as an example of population health monitoring: design and methods.

Journal of Human Nutrition (1978). October issue, p. 321. Editorial: The assessment of nutritional status.

Joy, J.L. (1973). *J. Agric. Econ.* 24, 165. Food and nutritional planning.

Jyothi, K.K., Dhakshayani, R., Swaminathan, M.C., and Venkatachalam, P.S. (1963) *Trop. Geogr. Med.* **15**, 403. A study of the socio-economic diet and nutritional status of a rural community hear Hyderabad.

Kamath, S.K., Lawler, M., Smith, A.E., Kalat, T., and Olson, R. (1986). *Am. Diet. Assoc. J.* **86**, 203. Hospital malnutrition: a 33-hospital screening study.

Kaminski, M.V. and Jeejeebhoy, K.N. (1979). *J. Surg. Prac.* **8**, 45. Nutritional assessment — diagnosis of malnutrition and selection of therapy.

—— and Ruggiero, R.P. (1979). *Intl. Surg.* **64**, 33. Nutritional assessment: a guide to initiation and efficacy of enteral hyperalimentation.

Kanawati, A.A. (1976). Assessment of the nutritional status of the community. In: *Nutrition in the community* (ed. D.S. McLaren), p. 57. John Wiley and Sons, London.

—— and McLaren, D.S. (1970). *Nature* **228**, 573. Assessment of marginal nutrition.

Kark, S.L. and Steuart, G.W. (1962). *A practice of social medicine.* Churchill Livingstone, Edinburgh.

Karlberg, P., Engstrom, I., Lichtenstein, H., Klackenberg, G., Klackengerg-Larson, I., Stenson, J., and Svennberg, I. (1968). *Acta Paed. Scand.* **57**, Suppl. 87. The development of children in a Swedish urban community.

Kasongo Project Team (1983). *J. Trop. Pediat.* **29**, 69. Anthropometric assessment of young children's nutritional status as an indicator of subsequent risk of dying.

Katch, V.L., Freedson P., Katch, F.I., and Smith, L. (1982). *Am. J. Clin. Nutr.* **36**, 676. Body frame size: validity of self-appraisal.

Keller, W., Donoso, G., and De Maeyer, E.M. (1976). *Nutr. Abstr. Revs.* **46**, 591. Anthropometry in nutritional surveillance: a review based on results of the WHO collaborative study on nutritional anthropometry.

—— and Fillmore, C.M. (1983). *World Hlth. Statis. Quart.* **36**, 129. Prevalence of protein-energy malnutrition.

Kelsey, J.L., Thompson, W.D., and Evans, A.S. (1986). *Methods in observational epidemiology.* Oxford University Press, Oxford.

Kennedy, I. (1982). *Salubritas* **6**, 7. Botswana: midwives use antenatal cards to detect at-risk pregnancies.

Keys, A., Brozek, J., Henschel, A., Michelsen, O., and Taylor, H.L. (1950). *The biology of human starvation*, vols. I and II. University of Minnesota Press, Minneapolis.

——, Fidanza, F., Karvonent, J.J., Kimura, N., and Taylor, H.L. (1972). *J. Chron. Dis.* **25**, 329. Indices of relative weight and obesity.

Khosla, T. (1980). *J. Epidem. Commun. Hlth.* **34**, 143. The plight of female infants in India.

Khanjanasthiti, P., Supachaturas, P., Mekanandha, P., Srimusikapodh, V., Choopanya, K., and Leesuwan, V. (1973). *J. Med. Assoc. Thai.* **56**, 88. Growth of infants and preschool children.

Khosla, T. (1983). *Br. Med. J.* **287**, 736. Sport for tall.

Kielmann, A.A. and McCord, C. (1978). *Lancet* **i**, 1247. Weight-for-age as an index of risk of death in children.

—— and —— (1978). *Lancet* **i**, 1247. Weight-for-age as an index of risk of death in children.

Killeen, J., Vanderburgh, D., and Harlan, W.R. (1978). *J. Chron. Dis.* **31**, 529. Application of height-weight ratios and body indices to juvenile populations.

King, M., King, F., Burgess, L., and Burgess, A. (1972). *Nutrition for developing countries.* Oxford University Press, Oxford.

Kiserud, T. (1986). *Acta Obstet. Gynec. Scand.* **65**, 713. Fundal height growth in rural Africa.

Klein, R.E., Read, M.S., Riecken, H.W., Brown, J.A., Pradilla, A., and Daza, C.H. (1979). *Evaluating the impact of nutrition and health programs.* Plenum Press, New York.

Klepinger, L.L. (1984). *Ann. Rev. Anthrop.* **13**, 75. Nutritional assessment from bone.

Klerks, J.V. (1956). *Berita Kementerian Kesehatan Indonesia,* **5**, 11. Quoted by

Luyken, R. and Luyken-Koning, F.W.M. *Trop. Geogr. Med.* Studies in the physiology of nutrition, IX Somatometrical data. (1961). **13**, 123.

Klevay, L.M. (1970). *Am. J. Clin. Nutr.* **23**, 284. Hair as a biopsy material. (I) Assessment of zinc nutriture.

Klish, W.J., Forbes, G.B., Gordon, A., and Cochran, W.J. (1984). *J. Pediat Gastroent. Nutr.* **3**, 199. A new method of estimation of lean body mass in infants (EMME instrument): validation in non-human models.

Kramer, M.S. (1986). Determinants of intrauterine growth and gestational duration. WHO, Geneva.

Krantzler, N.J., Mullen, B.J., Schutz, H.G., Grivetti, L.E., Holden, C.A., and Meiselman, H.L. (1982*a*). *Am. J. Clin. Nutr.* **36**, 1234. Validity of telephoned diet recalls for assessment of individual food intake.

——, Mullen, B.J., Comstock, E.M., Holden, C.A., Schutz, H.G., Grivetti, L.E., and Meiselman, H.L. (1982*b*). *J. Nutr. Educ.* **14**, 108. Methods of food intake assessment: an annotated bibliography.

Krehl, W.A. and Hodges, R.E. (1965). *Am. J. Clin. Nutr.* **17**, 191. The interpretation of nutritional survey data.

Krenning, L.W. (1983). *Comput. Biol. Med.* **13**, 303. Pocket computer for performing nutritional assessment on hospitalized patients.

Krischer, J. (1980). *Operations Res.* **28**, 97. An annotated bibliography of decision analysis applications to health care.

Krishnamarchari, K.A.V.R. and Krishnaswamy, K. (1974). *Lancet* **ii**, 877. Genu valgum and osteoporosis in an area of endemic fluorosis.

Kumar, V. and Walia, I. (1986). *J. Trop. Pediat.* **32**, 66. Recording of birth weight range by traditional birth attendants (dais) in villages in northern India.

Kune, J.B. (1980). *J. Trop. Pediat.* **26**, 114. Some factors influencing the mortality of under-fives in a rural area of Kenya: a multivariate analysis.

Kushner, R.E. and Schoeller, D.A. (1986). *Am. J. Clin. Nutr.* **44**, 419. Estimation of total body water by bioelectrical impedance analysis.

Kusin, J.A. and Jansen, A.A.J. (1986). *Ann. Trop. Paed.* **6**, 3. Maternal nutrition and built weight: selective review and some results in Machakos, Kenga.

——, Van Rens, M.M., Lakhani, S., and Jansen, A.A.J. (1985). *East Afr. Med. J.*, Vitamin A levels of pregnant and lactating women as assessed by serum Machakos levels in Machakos area, Kenya.

Kuezmarski, R.J., Fanelli, M.T., and Koch, G.G. (1987). *Am. J. Clin. Nutr.* **45**, 717. Ultrasomic assessment of body composition in these adults.

Landicho, B., Lechtig, A., and Klein, R.E. (1985). *J. Trop. Pediat.* **31**, 301. Anthropometric indicators of low birth weight.

Landman, J.P. and Hall, J.S.E. (1988). *J. Trop. Pediat.* (in press). Dietary patterns and nutrition in pregnancy in Jamaica.

——, Jackson, A., Wheeler, E., Grant, P., and McLeod, J. (1979). *J. Trop. Pediat.* **22**, 47. A catch-up growth chart.

Lange, K.O. and Brozek, J. (1961). *Am. J. Phys. Anthron.* **19**, 98. A new model of skinfold calipers.

Lasser, N.L. (1982). Critical factors in the design, management, evaluation and interpretation of epidemiologic studies. In *Methodologies for human population studies in nutrition related to health* (ed. B. Underwood). National Institutes of Health, Bethesda, Md.

Last, J. (ed.) (1983). *Dictionary of epidemiology*. Oxford University Press, Oxford.

Latham, M.C., Stephenson, L.S., Hall, A., Wolgemuth, J.C., Elliott, T.C., and Crompton, D.W.T. (1982). *Trans. R. Soc. Trop. Med. Hyg.* **76**, 734. A comparative study of the nutritional status, parasitic infections and health of male roadworkers in four areas of Kenya.

Laugesen, M. (1975). *Ind. J. Pediat.* **12**, 1261. Child's bangle for nutrition screening.

Leavell, R. (1987). *Adv. Int. Mat. Chld. Hlth.* **7**. Perspectives in vitamin A deficiency and xerophthalmia.

Lechtig, A. (1987). *J. Trop. Pediatr.* **33**, (in press). Predicting risk of delivering low birth weight babies: which indicator is better?

——, Martorell, R., Yarbrough, C., Delgado, H., and Klein, R. (1981). *J. Trop. Pediat.* **27**, 144. Influence of food supplementation on the urinary urea/creatinine (U/C) ratio of the child.

——, Townsend, J.W., Pineda, F., Arroyo, J.J., Klein, R.E., and De Leon, R. (1983). *Adv. Int. Mat. Chl. Hlth.* **3**, 175. SINAPS: the Guatemalan programme of primary health care.

——, Yarbrough, C., Delgado, H., Hebricht, J.J., Martorell, R., and Klein, R.E. (1975). *Am. J. Clin. Nutr.* **28**, 1223. Influence of maternal nutrition on birth weight.

Lederman, C. (1986). *Wives and midwives*. University of California Press, Berkeley, California.

Leevy, C.M. (1980). *Am. J. Clin. Nutr.* **33**, 172. Red cell transketolase as an indicator of nutritional deficiency.

Lees, D.E., Schuette, W. Whang-Peng, J., Atkinson, E.R., and Macnamara, T.E. (1978). *Anaesth. Analg.* **57**, 669. An evaluation of liquid-crystal thermometry as a screening device for intraoperative hyperthermia.

Lew, E.A. (1961). *J. Am. Diet Assoc.* **38**, 323. New data on underweight and overweight persons.

Lewis, B. (1983). *Br. Med. J.* **287**, 1161. The lipoproteins: predictors, protectors and pathogens.

Lewis, C.E., Neumann, C.G., and Preslow, L. (1971). *Ann. Int. Med.* **74**, 146. UCLA interdepartmental conference: The health care system — maligned or malignant?

Lewis, S.M. and Carne, S.J. (1965). *Br. Med. J.* **2**, 1167. Clinical haemoglobinometry: an evaluation of a modified grey-wedge photometer.

Leyland, M.J., Baksi, A.K., Brown, P.J., Kenny, T.W., and Strange, C.A. (1979*a*). *Ann. Trop. Med. Parasit.* 73, 63. Assessment of nutritional anaemia in Northern Nigeria.

——, Harris, H., and Brown, P.J. (1979*b*). *Br. J. Nutr.* **41**, 291. Iron status in a general practice and its relationship to morbidity.

Liljestrand, J. (1985). *Maternal mortality in Mozambique*. Uppsala University, Sweden.

Lindenbaum, J. (1983). *Blood* 61, 624. Status of laboratory testing in the diagnosis of megaloblastic anemia.

Lindner, P. and Lindner, D. (1973). *How to assess degrees of fatness*. Cambridge Scientific Industries, Cambridge, Maryland.

—— and —— (1973). *How to assess degrees of fatness*. Cambridge Scientific Industries, Cambridge, Maryland.

Lloyd, J.K. (1979). The young child: obesity. In *Nutrition and growth* (eds. D.B. and E.F.P. Jelliffe). Plenum Press, New York.

Lockerbie, L. and Lutz, W. (1986). *Questionnaire design: a guide for health workers*. IEA/WHO, Geneva.

Lopes, J., Russell, D.M., Whitewell, J., and Jeejeebhoy, K. (1982). *Am. J. Clin. Nutr.* **36**, 727. Skeletal muscle function in malnutrition.

Lorel, H., de Graaf, J., and Gordon, G. (1984). *Assign. Childr.* **65**, 275. How mothers measure growth.

Loewenson, R., Mason, R.P., and Patterson, B.A. (1986). *Ann. Trop. Paediat.* **6**, 73. Giardiasis and the nutritional status of Zimbabwean school children.

Lowenstein, M.S. and Phillips, J.F. (1973). *Am. J. Clin. Nutr.* **26**, 226. Evaluation of arm circumference measurement for determining nutritional status of children and its use in an acute epidemic of malnutrition: Owerri, Nigeria, following the Nigerian Civil War.

Lozoff, B. and Brittenham, G.M. (1977). Field methods for the assessment of health and disease in pre-agricultural societies. In *Health and disease in pre-agricultural societies*. Ciba Foundation Symposium No: 59 Elsevier Press, Amsterdam.

Lubanski, R.E., Kunzer, M., and Meguid, M.M. (1987). *Am. J. Clin. Nutr.* **45**, 830. Measurement of body composition using bioelectrical impedance analysis.

Lubchenco, L.O., Hansman, C., Dressler, M., and Boyd, E. (1963). *Pediat.* **32**, 793. Intrauterine growth in length and head circumference.

Lucas, V.E. (1978). *Malnutrition in pre-school children in Fiji*. Foundation for the Peoples of the South Pacific, Inc., New York.

Lukaski, H.C. (1987). *Am. J. Cl. Nutr.* **46**, 53. Methods for the assessment of human body composition, traditional and now.

Lutz, W. (1981). *Planning and organizing a health survey: a guide for health workers*. IEA/WHO, Geneva.

—— (1982). *Sampling: how to select people, household and places to study community health*. IEA/WHO, Geneva.

—— (1983). *Finding and using information: a guide for health workers*. IEA/WHO, Geneva.

Lwanga, S. (1983). *Statistical principles of monitoring and surveillance in public health*. Bull. WHO No. 61, p. 713.

—— and Cho-Yook Tye (1986). *Teaching health statistics. Twenty lesson and seminar outlines*. WHO, Geneva.

Magnusson, B. and Proos, L. (1980). *Lakartidningen* **76**, 3192. Vikt-och langdutveckling hos adoptivbarn fran u-lander.

Mahler, H. (1986). *World. Hlth. Chrom.* **40**, No. 3. Appropriate technology — appropriate if used.

Malcolm, L.A. (1970). *Growth and development in New Guinea. A study of the Bundi people of the Madang District*. Madang, Papua-New Guinea Institute of Human Biology, Monograph Res: 1.

——, Balasubramanian, E., and Edwards, G. (1973). *Am. J. Clin. Nutr.* **26**, 479. Effect of protein supplementation on the hair of chronically malnourished New Guinean school children.

Malhotra, R. (1986). *Anthrop. Anz.* **44**, 355. Thoracic adaptation at high altitude.

Malina, R.M., Hamill, P.V.V., and Lemeshow, S. (1973). *Selected body measurements of children 6–11 years.* DHEW publication No. 73–1601. US Government Printing Office, Washington, DC.

Malina, R.M. (1987). *Human Biol.* **59**, 329. Bioelectric methods for estimating body composition: an overview and discussion.

Maloff, C. and Zears, R.W. (1979). *Computers in nutrition.* Artech, Dedham, Massachusetts.

Manetsch, T.J. (1979). *Ecol. Fd. Nutr.* **8**, 209. On strategies and programs for coping with large scale food shortages.

Mankodi, N.A., Maniker, A., Shiddhye, S., and Shah, P.M. (1974). *Trop. Geogr. Med.* **26**, 375. Rickets in pre-school age children in and around Bombay.

Mann, G.V., Roels, O.A., Price, D.L., and Merrill, J.M. (1962). *J. Chron. Dis.* **15**, 341. Cardiovascular disease in African pygmies.

Manoff, R. (1985). *Social marketing.* Praeger Press, New York.

Manshande, U.P. (1980). *Lancet* **i**, 1195. Child growth standards.

——, Vuylsteke, J., Vlientink, R., and Eeckels, R. (1985). *Eur. J. Pediat.* **144**, 32. Arm muscle and fat in the evaluation of nutritional status.

Manson, P. and Zlotkin, S. (1985). *Canad. Med. Assoc. J.* **133**, 186. Hair analysis: a critical review.

Margen, S. (1979). *Med. Clin. N. Amer.* **63**, 1095. Evaluation of nutritional status in the outpatient setting.

Maribe, T.O. (1982). Update of nutrition surveillance in Botswana. In *Report of workshop social and nutritional surveillance in eastern and southern Africa, Nairobi, Kenya, 17–19 May 1982.* UNICEF and Cornell Nutritional Surveillance Program, Ithaca, N.Y.

Marks, R.G. (1987). *Designing a research project.* Van Nostrand Reinhold, New York.

Marr, J.W. and Berry, W.T.C. (1975). *Secular change and food consumption levels.* United Kingdom 9th National Food Survey, 1955–1971.

Marshall, W.A. (1981). *Br. Med. Bull.* **37**, 273. Geographical and ethnic variations in human growth.

—— and Swan, A.V. (1971). *Human Biol.* **43**, 502. Seasonal variation in growth rates of normal and blind children.

Martell, M., Gaviria, J., and Belitzky, R. (1979). *Bull. Pan. Am. Hlth. Org.* **13**, 370. A new method of evaluating postnatal growth in the first two years of life.

Martorell, R. (1982). *Nutrition and health status indicators: suggestions for surveys of the standard of living in developing countries.* LSMS Working Paper No. 13. World Bank, Washington, DC.

——, Habicht, J.P., and Klein, R.E. (1982). Anthropometric indicators of changes in nutritional status in malnourished populations. In *Methodologies for human population studies in nutrition related to health.* (ed.) B. Underwood. National Institutes of Health, Bethesda, Md.

——, Lechtig, A., Yarbrough, C., Delgado, H., and Klein, R.E. (1978). Small stature in developing nations: its causes and implications. In *Progress in human nutrition* (eds. S. Margen and R.A. Ogar), Vol. 2, p. 142. Avi Publ. Co., Westport, Connecticut.

——, Yarbrough, C., Malina, R.M., Habicht, J. P., Lechtig, A., and Klein, R.E. (1975). *J. Trop. Pediat.* **21**, 203. The head circumference/chest circumference ratio in mild-moderate protein-calorie malnutrition.

Mason, J.B. (1978). *Food Nutr.* **4**, 21. Agricultural and economic components of nutritional surveillance.

—— and Mitchell, J.T. (1983). *Bull. World Hlth. Org.* **61**, 1. Nutritional surveillance.

——, Habicht, J.P., Tabatabai, H., and Valverde, V. (1984). *Nutritional surveillance.* WHO, Geneva.

Mason, J. and Stephens, B. (1981). *Housing and health.* Cooperative Housing Foundation, Washington, DC.

Mata, L.J. (1978*a*). *Rev. Biol. Trop.* **26**, 1. Revision de los criterios para evaluar el estado nutricional.

—— (1978*b*). *The children of Santa Maria Cauque. A prospective field study of health and growth.* MIT Press, Cambridge, Massachusetts.

Mathur, A., Tak, S.K., and Kothari, P. (1984). *J. Trop. Pediat.* **30**, 333. Foot length — a newer approach in neonatal anthropometry.

Matthews, D.R. and McPherson, K. (1987). *Br. Med. J.* **294**, 896. Doctors ignorance of statistics.

McArthur, J. (1958). *J. Trop. Med.* **7**, 382. A new concept in microscope design for tropical medicine.

McDowell, I. and King, F.S. (1982). *Arch. Dis. Chldh.* **57**, 292. Interpretation of arm circumference as an indicator of nutritional status.

McFie, J. and Welbourn, H.F. (1962). *J. Nutr.* **76**, 97. Effect of malnutrition in infancy on the development of bone, muscle and fat.

McGregor, I.A., Billewicz, W.A., and Thompson, A.M. (1961). *Br. Med. J.* **2**, 1661. Growth and mortality in children in an African village.

McJunkin, F.E. (1982). *Water and human health.* USAID, Washington, DC.

McKigney, J. (1968). *J. Trop. Pediat.* **14**, 55. The cost-nutrient value of foods.

McIntosh, E.N. and Laurent, L.L. (1983). *Am. Fam. Phys.* **27**, 169. Nutritional assessment of the hospitalized patient.

McLaren, D.S. (1963). *Malnutrition and the eye.* Academic Press, New York.

—— (1981). *Nutrition and its disorders.* Churchill Livingstone, Edinburgh.

—— (1987). *World Rev. Neutr. Diet.* **49**, 87. A fresh look at some perinatal growth and nutritional standards.

—— and Burman, D. (1976). *Textbook of paediatric nutrition.* Churchill Livingstone, Edinburgh.

—— and Kanawati, A.A. (1972). *Am. J. Clin. Nutr.* **25**, 363. A somatic quotient.

—— and Read, W.W.C. (1975). *Lancet* **i**, 533. A simple scoring system for classifying the severe forms of protein calorie malnutrition in early childhood.

McMahon, R., Barton, E., and Piot, M. (1980). *On being in charge: A guide for middle-level management in primary health care.* WHO, Geneva.

McNaughton, J.W. and Sabry, Z.I. (1983). the role of the food policy division of FAO. In: *Nutrition in the community* (ed. D.S. Mclaren), John Wiley and Sons, Chichester.

Meadows, N.J., Till, J., Leaf, A., Hughes, E., Jani, B., and Larcher, V. (1986). *Br. Med. J.* **292**, 1039. Screening for intra-uterine growth retardation using ratio of mid-arm circumference to occipitofrontal circumference.

Mellander, O. and Svanberg, U. (1984). *Adv. Int. Mat. Chld. Hlth.* **4**, 84. Compact calories, malting, and young child feeding.

Mellor, J.W. (1986). *Fed. Proc.* **45**, 2427. Prediction and prevention of famine.

Merritt, R.J., Kalsch, M., Davis, L., Ashley-Mills, J., and Siegel, S. (1983). *J. Am. Coll. Nurs.* **2**, 291. Role of serum albumin in the assessment of pediatric oncology patients.

Messer, E. (1983). *Fd. Nutr. Bull.* **5**, 2. The household focus in international anthropology: an overview.

Metcoff, J. (1980). *Early Human Develop.* **4**, 99. Maternal nutrition and fetal development.

Metress, S.P. and Kart, C.S. (1979). *Nutrition and aging: a bibliographic survey.* Public Administration Series Bibliography p. 309. Vance Bibliographies, Monticello, Illinois.

Micozzi, M. (1978). *Am. J. Publ. Hlth.* **68**, 907. One definition of anemia in pregnancy.

Miles, M.B. and Huberman, A.M. (1984). *Qualitative data analysis: a source book of new methods.* Sage Publications, Beverly Hills, California.

Miller, D.C. (1979). *Proc. Nutr. Soc.* **38**, 197. Prevalence of nutritional problems in the world.

Miller, F.J.W., Court, S.D.M., Walton, W.S., and Knox, F.G. (1960). *Growing up in Newcastle upon Tyne.* Oxford University Press.

Miller, H.C. and Merritt, T.A. (1979). *Fetal growth in humans.* Yearbook Medical Publishers, Chicago.

Miller, R. and Sahn, D. (1984). Built in evaluating systems for supplementary feeding programmes — why and how. In *Methods for the evaluation of the impact of food and nutrition programs* (eds. D. Sahn, R. Lockwood, and N.S Scrimshaw). United Nations University.

Miller, S.A. and Stephenson, M.G. (1985). *Am. J. Clin. Nutr.* **42**, 739. Scientific and public health rationale for the dietary guidelines for Americans.

Milton, R.C. (1982). *Am. J. Clin. Nutr.* **35**, 140. Evaluation of the efficacy of programs to control severe xerophthalmia.

Mitchell, C.O. and Lipschitz, D.A. (1981). *Clin. Res.* **29**, 267A. Nutritional assessment of healthy and malnourished subjects at different ages.

—— and —— (1982). *J. Parent. Ent. Nutr.* **6**, 226. Arm length measurement as an alternative to height in nutritional assessment of the elderly.

Mitchell, F.L., Martinez-Silva, R., Vardhan, H., and Olazabel, D.A.R.R. (1983). *Supply maintenance and repair of health care laboratory equipment in developing countries.* Document LAB/83.8 WHO, Geneva.

Mitzner, K., Scrimshaw, N., and Morgan, R. (1984). *Improving the nutritional status of children during the weaning periods.* M.I.T. Press, Cambridge, Massachusetts.

Mohrs, E. (1978). Evaluation of nutrition in a transitional society. In *Proc. Western Hemisphere Nutr. Congress V*, p. 34. American Medical Association, Chicago.

Montgomerey, E. (1978). *Fed. Proc.* **21**, 61. Towards representative energy data: the Machiguenga study.

Mora, J.A. (1982). Nutritional assessment by anthropometry. In *Malnutrition and behaviour* (eds. J. Brozek and B. Schevech). Nestlé Foundation Publication, Vevey.

Morgan, B.L.G. and Winick, M. (1978). *Br. J. Nutr.* **40**, 529. The effects of supplementation of folic acid during pregnancy in the rats.

Morgan, J. and Mumford, P. (1976). *Proc. Nutr. Soc.* **36**, 47a. Feeding practices and food intake of children under 2 years of age.

Morley, D. (1962). *Am. J. Dis. Childh.* **103**, 230. Factors influencing the growth status of infants and young children in a Nigerian village.

—— (1963). *Trans. R. Soc. Trop. Med. Hyg.* **57**, 79. A health service for under fives in Nigeria.

—— (1968*a*). *Paediatric priorities in the developing world.* Butterworth, London.

—— (1968*b*). *Trop. Geogr. Med.* **20**, 101. Health and weight chart for use in developing countries.

—— (1976). *Int. J. Epidem.* **5**, 51. Nutritional surveillance of young children in developing countries.

—— (1977). *Arch. Dis. Childh.* **52**, 395. Growth charts, 'curative' or 'preventive'?

—— (1978). *Trans. R. Soc. Trop. Med.* **72**, 433. An accurate weighing machine for all ages.

—— (1979). *Am. J. Clin. Nutr.* **32**, 2165. Limitation of film strip and bangle test for identification of malnourished children.

—— (1986). *Bull. Internat. Ped. Assoc.* **38**, 3 Optimal growth and monitoring.

—— and Cutting, W.A. (1983). *Br. Med. J.* **286**, 1823. Weighing babies in clinics.

—— and Woodland, M. (1979). *See how they grow.* Macmillan, London.

Morris, M.D. (1979). *Measuring the condition of the world's poor: the physical quality of life index.* Pergamon Press, New York.

Morrow, H. (1985). *Report on Post-Workshop Projects: mobilizing leadership for primary health care.* International Council of Nurses, Geneva.

Moskowitz, S.R., Georgieff, M.K., Pereira, G.R., and Watkins, J.B. (1983). *J. Am. Coll. Nurs.* 2, 284. Mid-arm circumference ratio (MAC-HC) has an anthropometric measure of protein-calorie deprivation in pre-term infants.

Mueller, W.H. and Malina, R.M. (1987). *Am. J. Physic. Anthrop.* **72**, 437. Relative reliability of circumferences and skinfolds as measures of body fat distribution.

Murphy, E.A. (1976). *Defining the normal.* Johns Hopkins University Press, Baltimore. Md.

Musoke, L.K. (1961). *Arch. Dis. Childh.* **36**, 305. Analysis of admissions to the pediatric division, Mulago Hospital, 1959.

Nabarro, D. and McNab, S. (1980). *J. Trop. Med. Hyg.* 83, 21. A simple new technique for the identification of thin children.

Nadiger, H.A. (1980). *Br. J. Nutr.* 44, 211. Role of vitamin E in the aetiology of phrynoderma (follicular hyperkeratosis) and its relationship with B-complex vitamins.

Naeye, R.L. and Tafari, N. (1985). *Acta Paediat. Scand.* **319**, 164. Biologic bases for international fetal growth curves.

Nammacher, M.A., Bradfield, R.B., and Arroyave, G. (1972). *Am. J. Clin. Nutr.* **25**, 871. Comparing nutritional status methods in a Guatemalan survey.

Natadisastra, G., Wittpenn, J., West, K.P., Muhilal, and Sommer, A. (1987). *Arch. Ophthalm.* **105**, 1224. Impression cytology for detection of Vitamin A deficiency.

National Academy of Sciences (1978*a*). Weight gain in pregnancy 7, 19.

—— (1978*b*). *Laboratory indices of nutritional status in pregnancy*. National Research Council, Washington, DC.

—— (1978*c*). *Postharvest food losses in developing countries*. National Research Council, Washington, DC.

—— (1980). *Recommended dietary allowances*, (9th edn.) Washington DC.

National Dairy Council (1982). Dairy Council Digest **53**. Nutritional epidemiology.

Nelson, G.K. and Dean, R.F.A. (1959). *Bull. World Hlth. Org.* **21**, 779. The electroencephalogram in African children.

Nelson, M. (1986). *Br. J. Nutr.* **55**, 267. The distribution of nutrient intake within families.

Nesheim, R.O. (1982). *Am. J. Clin. Nutr.* **35**, 1292. Overview: Measurement of food consumption — past, present and future.

Nestel, P. and Geissler, C. (1986). *Ecol. F d. Nutr.* **19**, 1. Potential deficiencies of a pastoral diet: A case study of the Masai.

Neumann, A.K., Neumann, C.G., and Ifekwunigwe, A.E. (1973). *Am. J. Clin. Nutr.* **26**, 446. Evaluation of small-scale nutrition programs.

Neumann, C.G. (1982). *Adv. Int. Mat. Chld. Hlth.* **2**, 16. Maternal nutrition and immunocompetence.

—— (1979). Reference data. In *Nutrition and growth* (eds. D.B. and E.F.P. Jelliffe) Plenum Press, New York.

——, Jelliffe, D.B., Zerfas, A.J., and Jelliffe, E.F.P. (1982). *Cancer Res.* suppl. 42, 699. Nutritional assessment of the child with cancer.

——, Lawlor, G.J., Stiehm, E.R., Swenseid, M., Newton, C., Amman, A., and Jacob, M. (1975). *Am. J. Clin. Nutr.* **28**, 89. Immunologic responses in malnourished children.

Nichaman, M.Z. (1979). Nutritional surveillance in an industrialized country. In *Nutrition and growth* (eds. D.B. and E.F.P. Jelliffe) Plenum Press, New York.

—— Lane, J.M., Miller, D.C., Brink, E.W., and Staehling, N.W. (1978). *Am. J. Clin. Nutr.* **31**, 715. Comparison of weight for height and arm circumference variables as anthropometric indicators.

Nicholson, K.G., Metcalf, C.A., Renshaw, A., and Rideout, J.M. (1977). *Lancet* i, 836. A simple technique for measuring haemoglobin.

Nishida, H., Sakamoto, S., and Sakanone, M. (1985). *Acta Paediat Scand.* **319**, 89. New fetal growth curves for Japanese.

Nutrition Center of the Phillipines (1977). *Barangay Nutrition Manual*. Manila, Philippines. Barangay.

Nutrition Reviews (1981). **39**, 394. Interaction of infection and nutrition in children: two studies from Bangladesh.

Nutrition Week (1983). *Nutr. Week* **13** (38). Editional: Nutrition monitoring: has its time come?

O'Brien, R. and Shelton, W.C. (1941). *Women's measurements for garment and pattern construction*. Washington, United States Department of Agriculture (Miscellaneous Publication No. 454).

Oberleas, Caldwell, D.F., and Prasad, A.S. (1972). *Neurobiology of the trace metals zinc and copper*. Academic Press, New York.

Ofosuh-Amaah, S. and Neumann, A.K. (1979). *Danfa Project: Final Report.* University of California, Los Angeles.

Ohlson, M.A., Biester, A., Brewer, W.D., Hawthorne, B.E., and Hutchinson, M.B. (1956). *Hum. Biol.* **28**, 189. Anthropometry and the nutritional status of adult women.

Olson, J.A. (1987*a*). *Am. J. Clin. Nutr.* **45**, 687. Recommended dietary intakes (RDI) of vitamin K in humans.

—— (1987*b*). *Am. J. Clin. Nutr.* **45**, 704. Recommended dietary intakes (RDI) of vitamin A in humans.

—— and Hodges, R.E. (1987). *Am. J. Clin. Nutr.* **45**, 693. Recommended dietary intakes (RDI) of vitamin C in humans.

Olusi, S.O., McFarlane, H., Osunkoya, B.O., and Adeshina, H. (1975). *Clin. Chem. Acta* **62**, 107. Specific protein assays in protein calorie malnutrition.

Oo, T.T. and Naing, K.M. (1982). *Food Nutr. Bull.* **4**, 66. A comparison of milk output of Burmese mothers by three different methods.

Orfanos, C.E., Montagnua, and Stüttgen, G. (1981). *Hair research: status and future aspects.* Springer-Verlag, Berlin.

Ortega, R.G. (1981). Financing food and nutrition plans in Latin America. In *The process of food and nutrition planning* (eds. J. Aranda Pastore and L. Saenz). INCAP, Guatemala.

Ounsted, M.K., Moar, V.A., and Scott, W.A. (1986). *Early Human Dev.* **14**, 49. Growth and proportionality in early childhood.

Owen, G.M. (1982). *Am. J. Clin. Nutr.* **35**, 629. Measurement, recording, and assessment of skinfold thickness in childhood and adolescence: report of a small meeting.

Oyemade, G.A.A. (1977). *J. Trop. Med. Hyg.* **80**, 213. Non-rachitic deformities of the knees in Nigerian children.

Pakrasi, K.I., Desgupta, P., and Desqupta, I. (1986). *Heights and weights of healthy Bengali boys in Calcutta, India.* Indian Statistical Institute, Calcutta.

Pan American Health Organization (1972). *National food and nutrition survey of Barbados.* Sci. Publ. No.: 237. Washington, DC.

—— (1979). *Journal Bull. Pan Am. Hlth. Org.* **13**, 201. Nutritional management of obese pregnant women.

Parillon, C., Valverde, V., Delgado, H.L. and Newman, B. (1987). *Ecol. Fd. Nutr.* **19**, 333. Political and administrative distribution of nutritional status in Panama.

Parent, M.A., Khadraoui, S. and de Shampheleire, I. (1987). *J. Trop Pediat.* **33**, 13. Early clinical rickets and its association with malnutrition.

Pariszkova, J. and Goldstein, H. (1970). *Human Biol.* **42**, 436. A comparison of skinfold measurements using the Best and Harpenden calipers.

—— (ed.) (1978). *Nutrition, physical fitness and health*, University Park Press, Baltimore, Md.

Pearson, C.A. (1978). *Tubercle* **59**, 111. Hypochromia as a clinical sign of tuberculosis in the topics.

Pearson, P.B. and Greenwell, R. (eds.) (1980). *Food, nutrition and man.* University of Arizona Press, Tucson, Arizona.

Pellett, P.L. (1983). *Ecol. Fd. Nutr.* **13**, 115. Changing concepts of world nutrition.

Pelto, G. (1981). *Food Nutr. Bull.* **4**, 21. Methodological issues in nutritional anthropology.

Pelto, G.H. (1984). Intrahousehold food distribution patterns. In *Malnutrition: determinants and consequences* p. 285. Alan Liss, New York.

—— and Pelto, G.H. (1978). *Anthropological research: the structure of inquiry*, 2nd edn. Cambridge University Press, Cambridge.

Perisse, J. (1983). *Fd. and Nutr.* **9**, 14. Heterogeneity in food composition table data.

Peryam, D.R. and Pilgrim, F.J. (1975). *Food Technol.* **11**, suppl. 9–14. Hedonic scale method of measuring food preferences.

Petros-Barvazian, A. and Behar, M. (1978). Low birth weight — a major global problem. In *Birth weight distribution: an indicator of social development.* p. 9. (eds. G. Sterkey and L. Mellander) SAREC Report No. 8, Stockholm.

—— and —— (1978). *Pregnancy and anaemia.* WHO, Geneva.

Pettifor, J.M., Isdale, J.M., Sahakian, J., and Hansen, J.D.L. (1980). *Arch. Dis. Chldh.* **55**, 155. Diagnosis of subclinical rickets.

Pharaon, H.M., Darby, W.J., Shammout, H.A., Bridgforth, E.B., and Wilson, C.S. (1965). *J. Trop. Pediat.* 11, 1 (suppl.). A longitudinal nutrition survey of infants and pre-school children in Jordan.

Philippines National Nutrition Council (1979). *Provincial/city/municipal nutrition planners' manual.* National Nutrition Council, Manila, Philippines.

Phillips, J.L. (1971). Interpreting individual measures. In *Statistical thinking.* W.H. Freeman, San Francisco, Calif.

Pielemeier, N.R. (1985). *J. Trop. Pediat.* **31**, 131. Mothers' knowledge related to child health and nutrition in Ghana and Lesotho.

Pirie, A., Cobby, M., and Yenkatswamy, G. (1976). *Proc. Nutr. Soc.* **36**, 23A. Retinol-binding protein and prealbumin in serum of children with xerophthalmia before and after treatment.

Pitkin, R.M., Kaminetzky, H.A., Neuton, M., and Pritchard, J.A. (1972). *Obstet. Gyn.* **40**, 773. Maternal nutrition. A selective review of clinical topics.

Pizzarello, L.D. (1986). *Arch. Dis. Childh.* **61**, 1100. Age specific xerophthalmia rates among displaced Ethiopians.

Platt, B.S. (1958). *Trans. R. Soc. Trop. Med. Hyg.* **52**, 189. Malnutrition and the pathogenesis of diseases.

——, Eddy, T.P., and Pellett, P.L. (1963). *Food in hospitals.* Oxford University Press, Oxford.

Polacchi, W. (1985). *J. Am. Diet. Assoc.* **85**, 1134. Food composition tables: recommended method for deriving nutritional values in their preparation.

Polacchi, W. (1986) *VNU Fd. Nutr. Bull.* 8, 66. Standardized food terminology.

Pollitt, E., Soemantri, S.G., Yumis, F., and Scrimshaw, N.S. (1985). *Lancet* **i**, 58. Cognitive effects of iron-deficiency anaemia.

Poskitt, E. (1986). *Acta Paed. Scand.* **323**, 24. Obesity in the young child: Whither and whence?

Posner, B.M. (1979). *Nutrition and the elderly: policy development, program planning, and evaluation.* Lexington Books, Lexington, Kentucky.

Powers, P.S. (1980). *Obesity: the regulation of weight.* Williams and Wilkins, Baltimore, Md.

Posner, B.M., Berman, I.C., McCool, A.G., Morgan, J., and Barman, C. (1983). *J. Am. Diet. Assoc.* **82**, 521. Food service and management strategics in nutrition program for older Americans.

Pralhad Rao, N., Mathur, U.C., and Chandra, H. (1973). *J. Trop. Pediat.* **19**, 398. Age assessment of preschool children by 'local event' calendar specifically designed for communities in and around Hyderabad City.

Prasad, A. (1985). *Ann. Rev. Nutr.* 5, 41. Clinical manifestations of zinc deficiency.

Prasad, R., Mathru, P.P., Prasad, J., Sharma, M., and Dayal, R.S. (1982). *J. Trop. Pediat.* **28**, 199. "QUAC-stick" in assessment of nutritional status of preschool children.

Prema, K. (1978). *Ind. J. Med. Res.* **68**, 70. Pregnancy and lactation: some nutritional aspects.

Prentice, A.M., Lamb, W.H., and Bates, C.J. (1983). *Trans. R. Soc. Trop. Med.* 77, 792. A trial of ascorbic acid and multivitamin supplementation on the oral health of West African children.

Presta, E., Casullo, A.M., Costa, R., Slonin, A., and Van Itallie, T.B. (1987). *J. Am. Physiol. Soc.* Body in composition in adolescents: estimation of total body electrical conductivity.

Proc. Nutr. Soc. (1982). **41**, 343. Symposium: the assessment of nutritional status in man.

Program for Appropriate Technology in Health (PATH) (1983). **3**, 1. Assessing nutritional status: practical measures for primary health care.

Prokopec, M. (1977). *J. Human Evol.* **6**, 371. An anthropometric study of the Rembarranga: a comparison with other populations.

Puffer, R.R. and Serrano, C.V. (1970). *Patterns of mortality in childhood.* Sci. Publ. No: 262. Pan American Health Organization, Washington, DC.

Quandt, S.A. (1987). *Am. J. Phys. Anthrop.* **73**, 515. Variation in nutrient intake of infants and implications for collecting reliable data.

Quételet, A. (1836). *Sur l'homme et le dévelopment de ses facultés.* Muquart, Brussels.

Rajalakshmi, R., Subbalakshmi, G., Parekh, B., Dave, I., Bhatt, R.V., and Joshi, S.K. (1978). *Baroda J. Nutr.* **5**, 47. Distribution of birth weight in low and high income groups in India.

Ramachandran, C.R. (1985). *WHO appropriate tech. for hlth.* **17**, 27. Balance for use by traditional birth attendants.

—— (1986*a*). *J. Trop. Pediat.* **32**, 30. Vernier tape for circumferential measurements.

—— (1986*b*). *J. Trop. Pediat.* **32**, 270. A simple device for measurement of foot length in neonates.

——, Kavmar, B.S., Jain, J.K., Tandon, B.M., and Chandi, P.C. (1978). *Am. J. Clin. Nutr.* **31**, 1469. Limitations of film strip and bangle test for identification of malnourished children.

Ramji, S., Marwah, J., Satyanaranya, L., Kapami, V., Mohan, M., and Bhargava, S.K. (1986). *Ind. J. Med. Res.* **83**, 653. Neonatal thigh circumference as an alternative indicator of birth weight.

Ramos-Galvan, R. (1966). Malnutrition in the pre-school child in Mexico — prevalence and programs. In *Proceedings of international conference on the prevention of malnutrition in the pre-school child*, National Academy of Sciences Mexico City.

Rand, W.M. (1985). *J. Am. Diet. Assoc.* **85**, 1081. Food composition data: problem and plans.

Ransome-Kuti, O. (1985). *Acta Paediat. Scand.* **319**, 95. Intra-uterine growth and maturity of the African newborn.

Rask, L., Arundi, H., Bohme, J., Eriksson, U., Fredriksson, A., Nillson, S.F., Ronne, H., Vahlquist, A., and Peterson, P.A. (1980). *J. Clin. Lab. Invest.* **40**, 154. The retinol-binding protein.

Rathje, W.L. and Harrison, G.G. (1978). *Fed. Proc.* **37**, 49. Monitoring trends in food utilization: application of an archaeological method.

Reddy, V., Jagandeesan, V., Ragharamulu, N., Bhaskaran, C., and Srikantia, S.G. (1976). *Am. J. Clin. Nutr.* **29**, 3. Functional significance of growth retardation in malnutrition.

——, Mohanram, M., and Ragharamulu, N. (1979). *Acta Paediat. Scand.* **68**, 65. Serum retinol-binding protein and vitamin A levels in malnourished children.

Reeds, P.J., Jackson, A.A., Picou, D., and Poulter, N. (1978). *Pediat. Res.* **12**, 613. Muscle mass and composition in malnourished infants and children and changes seen after recovery.

Rees, D.G., Henry, C.J., Diskett, P., and Shears, P. (1987). *Lancet* **i**, 87. Measures of nutritional status. Survey of young children in north-east Brazil.

Reh, E. (1962). *Manual on household food consumption surveys.* Food and Agriculture Organization Rome, (FAO Nutritional Studies No. 18).

Reutlinger, S. and Selowsky, M. (1976). *Malnutrition and poverty: Magnitude and policy options.* World Bank Staff Occasional Paper No. 23, Johns Hopkins University Press, Baltimore, Md. and London.

Rideout, J.M., Renshaw, A., and Snook, M. (1978). *Anal. Biochem.* **90**, 744. Swizzle Stick: a novel positive displacement microliter diluting device.

Rivers, J.P.W. (1979). *Proc. Nutr. Soc.* **38**, 225. The profession of nutrition: an historical perspective.

Rizvi, N., Khan, A.D., and Zeitlin, M.F. (1984). *Ecol. Food Nutr.* **15**, 315–321. An interactive dietary assessment method for use in rural Bangladesh, part II: Evaluation.

Roberts, A.B., Roberts, P., Tira, T., and Tulinanu, K. (1981). *J. Trop. Pediat.* **27**, 78. Nutrition and anaemia in Gilbertese pre-school children.

Robinett-Weiss, N.G. (1984). *J. Am. Diet. Assoc.* **84**, 1502. Fogarty tables corrected.

Robson, J.R.K. (1964*a*). *J. Trop. Med. Hyg.* **67**, 46. Seasonal influence on height and weight increments of boys and girls in Tanganyika.

—— (1964*b*). *J. Trop. Med. Hyg.* **67**, 209. Skinfold thickness in apparently normal African adolescents.

—— and El-Tahawi, H.D. (1971). *Brit. J. Nutr.* Hardness of human nail as an index of nutritional status: a preliminary communication.

—— and Wadsworth, G.R. (1977). *Ecol. Fd. Nutr.* **6**, 187. The health and nutritional status of primitive populations.

——, Bazin, M., and Soderstrom, B.S. (1971). *Am. J. Clin. Nutr.* **24**, 864. Ethnic differences in skinfold thickness.

Roche, A.F. and Himes, J.H. (1980). *Am. J. Clin. Nutr.* **33**, 2041. Incremental growth charts.

Roche, A.F. (1984). *Internat. J. Obesity* **8**, 509. Anthropometric methods: new and old, what they tell us.

Roe, D. (1983). *Geriatric nutrition.* Prentice Hall, Englewood Cliffs, New Jersey.

Rohde, J., Ismail, D., and Sustrisno, R. (1975). *J. Trop. Ped.* **21**, 295. Mothers as weight watchers: the road to child health in the village.

——, ——, Sadjimin, T., Suyadi, A., and Tugerin (1979). *J. Trop. Pediat.* **25**, 83. Training course for village nutrition programs.

Rohrer, F. (1921). *Munch. Med. Wchschr.* **68**, 580. Der Index der Korperfulle als Mass des Ernahrungszustandes.

Rona, R.J. and Chinn, S. (1982). *Nutritional and social circumstances of primary school children. In Nutrition and health: a perspective* (ed. M.R. Turner). MTP Press, Lancaster.

Rookus, M.A., Burema, J., Duerenberg, P., and Van der Weil-Wetzels, W.A.M. (1985). *Br. J. Nutr.* **54**, 335. The impact of adjustment of a weight-height index (W/H^2) for frame size on the prediction of body fatness.

Rose, G. and Barker, D.J.P. (1978). *Epidemiology for the uninitiated.* British Medical Association, London.

—— and —— (1979). *Epidemiology for the uninitiated* (see British Medical Association 1979) British Medical Association, London.

Rose, G.A., Blackburn, H., Gillum, R.F., and Prineas, R.J. (1982). *Cardiovascular survey methods* (2nd edition). WHO, Geneva.

Rosenberg, I.H. (ed.) (1985). *Am. J. Clin. Nutr.* **41**, 139. Minisymposium: behind and beyond the "recommended dietary allowances."

Ross, D.A. and Vaughan, J.P. (1986). *Stud. Fam. Pl.* **17**, 78. Health interviews surveys in developing countries: a methodological review.

Rosso, P. (1980). *Fed. Proc.* **39**, 250. Placental growth, development and function in relation to maternal nutrition.

—— (1985). *Am. J. Clin. Nutr.* **42**, 644. A new chart to monitor weight gain during pregnancy.

Royal College of Physicians (1983). *J. R. Coll. Physic. London* **17**, 6. Obesity: a report.

Royston, E. (1982). *Wrld. Hlth. Statist. Quart.* **32**, 52. The prevalence of nutritional anaemia in women in developing countries.

Russell, D.M., Leiter, L.A., Whitwell, J., Marliss, E.B., and Jeejeeboy, K.N. (1983). *Am. J. Clin. Nutr.* **37**, 133. Skeletal muscle function during hypocaloric diets and fasting: a comparison with standard nutritional assessment parameters.

Sackett, D.L. and Holland, W.W. (1975). *Lancet* **ii**, 357. Controversy in the detection of disease.

Sardharwalla, I.B., Lingam, S., and Harvey, D.R. (1986). *Arch. Dis. Childh.* **61**, 411. Prevention of mental handicap in developing countries.

SAREC (1986). *Annual report 1985–6.* Stockholm, Sweden.

Sasanow, S.R., Georgieff, M.K., and Pereira, G.R. (1986). *J. Pediat.* **109**, 311.

Midarm circumference and mid-arm/head circumference ratio.
Satyanarayana, M.B., Naidu, A. Nadamuni, and Rao, N. (1981). *Am. J. Clin. Nutr.* **34**, 161. Studies on the effect of nutritional deprivation during childhood on body composition of adolescent boys: creatinine excretion.
Sauberlich, H.E. (1983). *Surv. Synth. Path. Res.* **2**, 120. Current laboratory tests for assessing nutritional status.
Sauberlich, H.E., Skala, J.H., and Dowdy, R.P. (1974). *Laboratory tests for the assessment of nutritional status.* CRC Press, Cleveland, Ohio, USA.
Sauerborn, R. and Bouyain, G. (1987). *J. Trop. Pediat* **33**, 215. Neonatal mid-upper arm circumference as a valid proxy measure for birth weight.
Scanland, P. (1976). *Publ. Hlth. Rep.* **91**, 360. The age computer. A simple device for improving age determination in censuses and surveys.
Schaffer, B. (1984). Towards responsibility: public policy in concept and practice, p. 142. In: *Room for manoeuvre: an exploration of public policy in agriculture and rural development* (eds. E.J. Clay, and B. Schaffer). Heineman Educational Books, London.
Schofield, S. (1979). *Development and the problems in village nutrition.* Allanheld, Osmund and Co., Montclair, New Jersey.
Scholl, T.O., Johnston, F.E., Cravioto, J., Delicardie, E.R., and Lurie, D.S. (1979). *Am. J. Clin. Nutr.* **32**, 872. The relationship of growth failure.
Schorah, C.J., Zemroch, P.J., Sheppard, S., and Smithalls, R.W. (1978). *Br. J. Nutr.* **39**, 139. Leucocyte ascorbic acid and pregnancy.
Schuftan, C. (1979). *Ecol. Fd. Nutr.* **8**, 29. Household purchasing power deficit: a more operational indicator to express malnutrition.
—— (1981). *J. Trop. Pediat.* **27**, 177. Nutrition Intervention programmes for rural areas, African experiences.
Schwicker, R.E. (1982). *Am. J. Clin. Nutr.* **35**, 1306. Alternative approaches to classic food consumption measurement methods: telephone interviewing and market data bases.
Scott, C., de Andre, P.T.A., and Chander, R. (1980). *Conducting surveys in developing countries.* World Bank, Washington, DC.
Scrimshaw, N.S., Taylor, C.E., and Gordon, J.E. (1959). *Am. J. Med. Sci.* **237**, 367. Interactions of nutrition and infection.
—— (1964). *Am. J. Clin. Nutr.* **14**, 112. Ecological factors in nutritional disease.
—— and Wallenstein, M.B. (1982). *Nutrition policy implementation*, Plenum Press, New York.
——, Taylor, C.E., and Gordon, J.E. (1968). *Interactions of nutrition and infection.* World Health Organization: Monograph Series No. 57, Geneva.
Scrimshaw, S.C.M. and Hurtado, E. (1984). *UNU Food and Nutr. Bull.* **6**, 27. Fieldguide for the study of health-seeking behavior at the household level.
—— and —— (1987). *Rapid assessment procedures for nutrition and primary health: anthropological approaches to program improvement.* UNV, Tokyo; UNICEF, New York; Latin American Studies Center, UCLA, Los Angeles.
eaman, J. (1978). *J. Trop. Pediat.* **24**, 123. Field methods for calculating anthropometric results.
—— and Holt, J.F.W. (1975). *Proc. Nutr. Soc.* **34**, 114A. The Ethiopian famine of 1973–4 (1) Wollo Province.

Segall, M. (1979). *Lancet* **i**, 1352. Growth charts for developing countries.

Sen, A. (1982). *Future*. Fourth quarter, p. 11. Unequal access to food: causes, conflicts, option.

Seltzer, M.H., Bastidas, J.A., Cooper, D.M., Englen, P., Slocum, B., and Fletcher, H.S. (1979). *J. Parent Ent. Nutr.* **3**, 157. Instant nutritional assessment.

Seoane, N. and Latham, M.C. (1971). *J. Trop. Pediat. Env. Chld. Hlth.* **17**, 98. Nutritional anthropometry in the identification of malnutrition in childhood.

Serenius, F., Elidrissy, A., and Dandona, P. (1984). *J. Clin. Path.* **37**, 444. Vitamin D nutrition in pregnancy women at term and in newly born babies in Saudi Arabia.

Shah, K.P. (1978). *J. Ob. Gyn. India* **28**, 1015. Surveillance card for married women for better obstetric performance.

—— (1980) *J. Ob. Gyn. Ind.* **30**, 103. Appropriate technology in primary health care for better midwifery services.

Shah, P.M. (1984). *Physical growth and psychosocial development: an overview*. WHO, unpublished document.

——, Khare, R.D., Rane, A.V., and Bhalerao, V.Y. (1976). *Ind. J. Nutr. Diet.* **13**, 148. The bangle as a tool for assessing malnutrition of under sixes.

Shakir, A. (1979). Anthropometric field methods: simplified methods. In *Nutrition and growth* (eds. D.B. and E.F.P. Jelliffe), p. 389. Plenum Press, New York.

—— and Morley, D. (1974). *Lancet* **i**, 758. Measuring malnutrition.

Sharif, J. and Abitbol, C. (1982). *J. Am. Coll. Nutr.* **1**, 410. Neonatal footprint measurements as an anthropometric index.

Sharman, A. (1970). *J. Dev. Std.* **6**, 77. Nutrition and Social Planning.

Shenkin, A. and Steele, L. (1978). *Proc. Nutr. Soc.* **37**, 95. Clinical and laboratory assessment of nutritional status.

Shiff, C.J. and Day, W.J. (1985). *Adv. Int. Mat. Chld. Hlth.* **5**, 141. Water and child health.

Shumaker, J.D. (1978). Anemia screening at the village level. Unpublished data.

Shorr, I. (1986). How to weigh and measure children. National Household Survey Capability Programme. UN Department of Technical Co-operation for Development and Statistical Office. New York.

Sibert, J.R., Jadhay, M., and Inbaraj, S.G. (1978). *Br. Med. J.* **2**, 1517. Maternal and fetal nutrition in south India.

Sigulem, R.M., Brasel, J.A., Velasco, E.G., Rosso, P., and Winick, M. (1973). *Am. J. Clin. Nutr.* **26**, 793. Plasma and urine ribonuclease as a measure of nutritional status in children.

Siimes, J.M. and Smith, J. (1982). *Proc. Nutr. Soc.* **41**, 115A. Prediction of surgical complications.

Simmonds, S., Vaughan, P., and Bunn, W. (1983). *Refugee community health care*. Oxford University Press, Oxford.

Simmons, W.K., Jutsum, P.J., Fox, K., Spence, M., Gueri, M., Paradis, R., and Burney, J.M. (1982). *Am. J. Clin. Nutr.* **35**, 319. A survey of the anemia status of preschool age children and pregnant and lactating women in Jamaica.

Simner, K., Iles, C.A., Slavin, B., Keeling, P.W.N. and Thompson, R.P.H. (1987). *Hum. Nutr.* 41C, 193. Maternal nutrition and intrauterine growth.

Simopoulos, A. (ed.) (1987). *Am. J. Clin. Nutr.* 45, 1015. Diet and health: scientific concepts and principles. Proceedings of a symposium.

Singh, R.D. (1974). *Am. J. Phys. Anthrol.* **40**, 221. Problems of techniques in anthropometric studies in India.

Sinha, D. (1986). *A system for monitoring nutritional status and actions to improve children's health. A field guide for health workers in the Caribbean.* CFNI/PHO, Kingston, Jamaica.

—— (1987). Personal communication. CFNI, Jamaica.

—— and Bang, F.B. (1973). *Lancet* **ii**, 228. Seasonal variation in signs of vitamin A deficiency in rural West Bengal children.

Smail, P. (1984). *Br. Med. J.* **289**, 1371. Short stature.

Smelser, D.N., Smelser, N.B., Krumdieck, Schreeder, M.T., and Laven, G.T. (1982). *Am. J. Clin. Nutr.* **35**, 342. Field use of hair epilation forceps in nutrition status assessment.

Smith, W.C.S., Tavendale, R. and Tunstall-Pedoe, H. (1986). *Hum. Nutr.* 40, 323. Simplified subcutaneous fat biopsy for nutritional surveys.

Snyder, G., Schneider, L.W., Owings, C.L., Reynolds, H.M., Schork, A.M., and Golomb, D.H. (1977). *Hwy. Res. Inst. Rev.* 7, 1. Physical measurements of US infants, children and teenagers.

Sobolewski, S., Lawrence, A.C.K., and Bagshaw, P. (1978). *J. Clin. Path.* **31**, 1068. Human nails and body iron.

Society of Actuaries (1959). *Build and blood pressure study.* Chicago, vols. I and II.

—— (1980). *Build study, 1979.* New York, NY.

Soeters, R. (1986). *Trop. Doc.* **16**, 173. Pitfalls with weight for height measurements.

Solat, S. (1987). *Xerophthalmia Club Bulletin* **36**, 2. Risk factors of xerophthalmia in young children in Delhua, Uttar Pradesh, India.

Sommer, A. and Lowenstein M.S. (1975). *Am. J. Clin. Nutr.* **28**, 287. Nutritional status and mortality.

—— (1982*a*). *Nutritional blindness: xerophthalmia and keratomalacia.* Oxford University Press, Oxford.

—— (1982*b*). *Field guide to the detection and control of xerophthalmia,* 2nd edn. World Health Organization, Geneva.

—— (1984). *Lancet* i, 347. Vitamin A deficiency and mortality risk.

—— Hussaini, G., Muhilal, Tarwotjo, I., Susanto, D., and Saroso, J.S. (1980). *Am. J. Clin. Nutr.* **33**, 887. History of night blindness: a simple tool for xerophthalmia screening.

—— Tarwotjo, I., Hussaini, G., and Susanto, D. (1983). *Lancet* **ii**, 585. Increased mortality in children with mild vitamin A deficiency.

Spurr, G.B., Barac-Nieto, M., Reina, J.C., and Ramirez, R. (1984). *Am. J. Clin. Nutr.* **39**, 452. Marginal malnutrition in school-aged Colombian boys: efficiency of treadmill walking in submaximal exercise.

Squires, B.T. (1965). *J. Pediat.* **66**, 891. Differential staining of buccal epithelium smears as an indicator of poor nutritional status due to protein-calorie deficiency.

Srikantia, S.G. (1984). *Bull. Nutr. Found. India* 5, 4. Endemic fluorosis in Andra Pradesh.

Srilatha, V.L. (1986). *Bull. Nutr. Found. India* 7, 6. Use of growth charts for promoting child nutrition.

Stallones, R.A. (1982). *Am. J. Clin. Nutr.* **35**, 1290. Comments on the assessment of nutritional status in epidemiological studies and surveys of populations.

Standard, K.L. and Miall, W.E. (1965). *W. Indian Med. J.* **14**, 131. Studies on weight gain in the first year of life.

——, Lovell, H.G., and Garrow, J.S. (1966). *J. Trop. Pediat.* **11**, 100. The validity of certain signs as indices of generalized malnutrition in young children.

Stanfield, J.P. and Donnet, M.L. (1978). Low birthweight in an urban environment in Britain. In: *Birth-weight distribution: an indicator of social development* (eds. G. Sterky and L. Mellander), p. 60. SAREC Report No. 8, Stockholm.

Stein, H. (1975). *Arch. Dis. Childh.* **50**, 146. Maternal protein depletion and small-for-gestational age babies.

Stephenson, G.R., Smith, D.P.B., and Roberts, T.W. (1975). *Beh. Res. Mthds. Inst.* 7, 497. The SSR system: an open format recording system with computerized transcription.

Stephenson, L.S., Latham, M.C., and Oduori, M.L. (1980). *J. Trop. Pediat.* **26**, 245. Costs, prevalence and approaches for control of *Ascaris* infection in Kenya.

——, Crompson, D., Lettam, M.C., Schulpen, T., Neisheim, M.C., and Jansen, A. (1986). *Am. J. Clin. Nutr.* 33, 1165. Relationship between ascaris infection and growth of malnourished pre-school children in Kenya.

Sterky, G. and Mellander, L. (eds.) (1978). *Birth weight distribution*. SAREC Report No. 8, Stockholm.

Steveny, J. (1982). *Trop. Doctor* **12**, 133. Standardized interpretation of under-5 weight curves.

Stini, W.A. (1980). Human adaptability to nutritional stress. In *Food, nutrition and man* (eds. P.B. Pearson and R. Greenwell). University of Arizona Press, Tucson, Arizona.

Stinson, W. (1983). *Information systems, primary health care issues*. Series No. 6, American Public Health Association.

Stoner, H.B. (1982). *Proc. Nutr. Soc.* **41**, 349. Assessment of energy expenditure.

Stuart, H.C. and Stevenson, S.S. (1975). Physical growth and development. In *Textbook of pediatrics* (10th edn) (eds. W.E. Nelson, V.C. Vaughan and R.J. McKay). W.B. Saunders, Philadelphia, Penn.

Sturt, R.J., Muller, H.K.S., and Francis, G.D. (1971). *Med. J. Austral.* **2**, 751. Molluscum contagiosum in villages in the West Sepik District of New Guinea.

Stuff, J.E., Garza, C., Smith, E.O., Nichols, B.L., and Montadon, C.M. (1982). *Am. J. Clin. Nutr.* **37**, 300. A comparison of dietary methods and nutritional studies.

Stuff, J.E., Garza, C. and Nichols, B.L. (1987). *Am. J. Clin. Nutr.* **45**, 838. Growth patterns of breast-fed infants (0–32 weeks).

Sturt, R.J., Muller, H.K.S., and Francis, G.D. (1971). *Med. J. Aust.* **2**, 751. Molluscum contagiosum in villages in the West Sepik District of New Guinea.

Sukmanah, T. (1987). *Growth monitoring as individual and community nutrition education: the Indonesian experience.* WHO/IUNS Workshop, CFNI, Jamaica.

Sundharagiati, B. and Harinasuta, C. (1964). *Trans. Roy. Soc. Trop. Med. Hyg.* **58**, 579. Determination of haemoglobin in dry blood on filter paper.

Suzuki, T. (1981). *J. Human Ergol.* **10**, 13. How great will the stature of Japanese eventually become?

Svensson, W.E., McDermott, E., and O'Gorman, M. (1980). *Br. Med. J.* **1**, 1188. Growth and growth charts.

Swaminathan, M.C., Jyothi, K.K., Singh, R., Madhavan, S., and Gopalan, C. (1964). *Ind. J. Ped.* **1**, 255. A semi-longitudinal study of growth of Indian children and related factors.

Sweeney, E.A., Saffir, A.J., and DeLeon, R. (1971). *Am. J. Clin. Nutr.* **24**, 29. Linear hypoplasia of deciduous teeth in malnourished children.

Tafari, N. (1981). *Adv. Int. Mat. Chld. Hlth.* **1**, 105. Low birth weight: an overview.

Taffal, S.M. and Keppel, K.G. (1986). *Am. J. Publ. Hlth.* **76**, 1396. Advice about weight gain in pregnancy and actual weight gain.

Tai, M. (1982). *Chin. Med. J.* **95**, 962. High-iodine endemic goiter.

Takaishi, M. (1986). *Proc. XVIII Congress of Pediatrics* Abstr. 549. Secular trend of physical growth in Japan: a consideration for growth standards.

Tanner, J.M. (1962). *Growth at adolescence*, 2nd edn. Blackwell Scientific Publications, Oxford.

—— (1976). *Arch. Dis. Childh.* **51**, 1. Population differences in body size, shape and growth rate: a 1976 view.

——, Whitehouse, R.H., and Takaishi, M. (1966). *Arch. Dis. Childh.* **41**, 454. Standards from birth to maturity for heights, weights, height velocity and weight velocity: British children, 1965.

——, Hayashi, T., Preece, M.A. and Cameron, N. (1982). *Ann. Human Biol.* **9**, 411. Increase in length of leg relative to trunk in Japanese children and adults from 1957 to 1977: comparison with British and Japanese Americans.

Telwar, P.P. (1975). *Am. J. Publ. Hlth.* **65**, 1170. Developing indices of nutritional level from anthropometric measurements in women and young children.

Thompson, A.M. (1965). *Practition* **194**, 743. Diet in pregnancy.

—— and Billewicz, W.Z. (1957). *Brit. Med. J.* **i**, 243. Clinical significance of weight trends in pregnancy.

Thornton, S.P. (1977). *Ann. Ophth.* **9**, 731. A rapid test for dark adaption.

Tibrewalla, S.N. and Shah, K.P. (1978). *Baroda Med. J.* **5**, 43. The use of the arm circumference as an indicator of body weight in adult women.

Timmreck, T.C. (1977). *Geriatrics*, October, 137. Nutrition problems: a survey of the rural elderly.

Tjon, A., Ten, W.E., Kusin, J.A., and de With, C. (1985). *J. Trop. Pediat.* **31**, 249. Fundal height as an antenatal screening method.

Tomkins, M., Drasar, B.S., Bradley, A.K., and Williamson, A. (1977). *Proc. Nutr. Soc.* **36**, 141A. Water supplies and nutritional status in rural northern Nigeria.

Torun, B., Young, V.R., and Rand, W.M. (eds.) (1981). Protein-energy requirements of developing countries: evaluation of new data.

Tremlett, G., Lovel, H., and Morley, D. (1983). *Assign. Chldr.* **61**, 143. Guidelines for the design of national weight-for-age growth charts.

Trotter, M. and Glaser, G. (1951). *Am. J. Phys. Anthrop.* **9**, 311. The effect of ageing on stature.

Trowbridge, F.L. and Newton, L.H. (1979). *Am. J. Trop. Med. Hyg.* **28**, 135. Some seasonal changes in malnutrition and diarrheal disease among preschool children in El Salvador.

—— and Staehling, N. (1980). *Am. J. Clin. Nutr.* **33**, 687. Sensitivity and specificity of arm circumference indicators in identifying malnourished children.

—— and Stetler, H.C. (1980). *Bull. World Health. Org.* **58**, 327. Nutritional surveillance in El Salvador.

——, Hand, K.A., and Nichaman, M.Z. (1975). *Am. J. Clin. Nutr.* **28**, 712. Findings related to goiter and iodine in the ten state nutrition survey.

——, Hiner, C.D., and Robertson, A.D. (1982). *Am. J. Cl. Nutr.* **36**, 691. Arm muscle indicators and creatinine excretion in children.

Trowell, H.C., Davis, J.N.P., and Dean, R.F.A. (1954). *Kwashiorkor*. Edward Arnold, London.

Truswell, A.S. (1983*a*). *J. Am. Diet. Assoc.* **35**, 498. The development of dietary guidelines.

—— (1983*b*). *Nutr. Abstr.* **53**, 939. Recommended dietary intakes around the world.

Tuchman, B. (1982). *Practicing history: collected essays*. Ballantine Books, New York.

Tukei, P.M. (1963). *J. Trop. Med. Hyg.* **65**, 42. A calendar for the assessment of the ages of young Baganda children.

US Agency for International Development (1972). *Evaluation handbook* (2nd edn.). AID Office and Program Evaluation, Washington, DC.

US Agency for Nutritional Development (1971). *Office of Nutrition: Use of growth charts for assessing progress of children and teaching of parents.* Washington, DC.

US Food and Nutrition Board (1981). *Food consumption practices*. National Academy of Sciences, Washington, DC.

Ugalde, A. (1970). *Rural Soc.* **35**, 512. Measuring wealth in a semi-cash economy.

Underwood, B.A. and Hofvander, Y. (1982). *Acta. Paediat. Scand.* suppl. 294. Appropriate timing for complementary feeding of the breast-fed infant.

—— and —— (1984). *Acta Paed. Scand.*, Suppl. No. 294. Appropriate timing for complementary feeding of the breast fed infant. A review.

UNICEF (1984). *Salter weighing balance: Instruction book*. UNICEF/ROSCA, New Delhi.

UNICEF (1986). *Monitoring and promotion of child growth*. New Delhi, May 7–9.

United Nations High Commissioner for Refugees (1982). *Handbook for emergencies*. UNHCR, Geneva.

UN High Commissioner for Refugees (1987). Operational guidelines for health and nutrition programmes in refugee settings. UNHCR, Geneva.

US Department of Agriculture (1975*a*). *Composition of foods: raw, processed, prepared.* Agricultural Handbook No: 8. Washington, DC.

—— (1975*b*). *Nutritive value of American foods in common units.* Agriculture Handbook No: 456. Washington, DC.

US Department of Health and Human Services (1985). Cholesterol counts. NIH Publication No 85–2699 Washington, DC.

—— (1986). *Maternal weight gain and outcome of pregnancy, U.S., 1980.* National Center for Health Statistics Series 21, No. 44, Hyattsville, Md.

US National Academy of Sciences (1970).

—— (1986). *Nutrient adequacy: assessment using food consumption surveys.* National Academy Press, Washington, DC.

US National Research Council (1980). Recommended dietary allowances. Washington, DC.

Valcovic, V. (1977). *Trace elements in human hair.* Garland STPM Press, New York and London.

Valverde, V., Vargas, W., Payne, P., and Thomson, A. (1981). *Food policy.* February, pp. 19–26. Data requirements and use in nutrition planning in Costa Rica.

——, Delgado, H., Flores, R., Sibrian, R., and Palmieri, M. (1985). *Fd. Nutr. Bull.* 7, 32. The school as a data source for food and nutrition surveillance in Central America and Panama.

——, ——, Flores, R., Sibrian, R., and Palmieri, M. (1985). *Fd Nutr. Bull.* 7, 32–37. Food and nutrition surveillance in Central American Schools.

——, Rojas, Z., Vinocur, P., Payne, P., and Thomson, A. (1981). *Fd. Nutr.* 7, 32. Organization of an information system for food and nutrition programmes in Costa Rica.

——, Delgado, H., Martorell, R., Belizan, J.M., Mejia-Pivaral, V., and Klein, R.E. (1982). *Arch Latinoam. Nutr.* **3**, 521. Seasonality and nutritional status.

Van Esterik, P. (1984). Intrafamilial food distribution: its relevance for maternal and child nutrition. *Cornell Nutritional Surveillance Program* Working Paper No. 31. Cornell University, Ithaca, New York.

Van Loan, M. and Mayclin, P. (1987). *Am. J. Clin. Nutr.* **45**, 181. A new TOBEC instrument and the procedure for assessment of body composition.

Van Loon, Saverys, U., Vuylstecke, J.P., Vlietinck, R.F., and Eeckels, R. (1986). *Annal. Hum. Biol.* **13**, 347. Local vs. universal growth standards: the effect of using NCHS as universal reference.

Van Slyke, D.S., Phillips, R.P., Dole, V.P., Hamilton, P.B., Archibald, R.M., and Plazin, J. (1950). *J. Biol. Chem.* **183**, 349. Calculation of haemoglobin from blood specific gravities.

Vandiviere, T., Dale, A., Driess, R.D., and Watson, K.A. (1971). *Arch. Env. Hlth.* **23**, 61. Hair shaft diameter as an index of protein-calorie malnutrition.

Velloso, J. (1979). *Ceres* May/June, pp. 25–27. Under surveillance.

Velbezoear, M.I., Selwyn, B.J., Sargent, F., Pollitt, E., and Delgardo, H. (1983*a*). *J. Trop. Pediat.* **29**, 135. Evaluation of arm circumference as a public health index of protein energy malnutrition in early childhood.

——, ——, ——, ——, and —— (1983*b*). *J. Trop. Pediat.* **29**, 159. The use of the arm circumference in simplified screening for acute malnutrition by minimally trained health workers.

Venkatachalam, P.S. (1962). *Bull World Hlth. Org.* **26**, 193. Maternal nutritional status and its effect on the newborn.

—— (1975). *PAG Bulletin* **5**, 27. Nutritional nuances of the term 'preschool child' and the need for precise terminology.

—— Shankar, K., and Gopalan, C. (1960). *Ind. J. Med. Res.* **48**, 511. Changes in body composition during pregnancy.

Victoria, C.G. and Coelho, V.H. (1983). *J. Trop. Pediat.* **29**, 133. Volume of household measures.

Villar, J. and Belizan, J.M. (1981). *Lancet* **ii**, p. 621. Breast-feeding in developing countries.

——, ——, and Klein, R.E. (1982). *Am. J. Clin. Nutr.* **35**, 271. Heterogeneous postnatal growth patterns of intrauterine growth retarded infants (IUGR).

Vir, S.C. and Love, A.H.G. (1980). *Gerontol.* **26**, 1. Anthropometric measurements in the elderly.

Visweswara Rao, K. and Singh, D. (1970). *Am. J. Clin. Nutr.* **23**, 83. An evaluation between nutritional status and anthropometric status.

——, Reddy, P.J., and Narayanan, T.P. (1978). 17, 25. *Ind. J. Nutr. Diet.* A comparison of arm and calf circumferences as indicators of protein-calorie malnutrition in early childhood.

——, Susheela, T.P., and Swaminathan, M.C. (1973). *J. Trop. Pediat.*, **19**, 193. Association of growth status and dental eruption among rural Indian children.

Viteri, F.E. and Alvarado, J. (1970). *Pedialics* **46**, 696. The creatinine height index: its use in the estimation of the degree of protein depletion and repletion in protein calorie malnourished children.

—— and Torun, B. (1974). *Clin. Haemat.* **3**, 609. Anaemia and physical work capacity.

Voorhoeve, H.W.A. (1983). *Courier* **35**, 451. The mid-arm circumference in child health: to measure under- and overnutrition.

Vorster, B.J. and Milner, L.V. (1979). *Lancet* **i**, 1295. Colour-blind laboratory technicians.

Waldmann, E. (1976). *Ecol. Fd. Nutr.* **5**, 133. Early Bapedi growth in Sekhukuniland, Transvaal, South Africa.

Walravens, P.A., Krebs, N.F., and Hambridge, K.M. (1983). *Am. J. Clin. Nutr.* **39**, 195. Linear growth of low income preschool children receiving a zinc supplement.

Warner, W.L., Meeker, M., and Eels, K. (1960). *Social class in America.* Social Torchbooks, New York.

Waterlow, J.C. (1948). Fatty liver disease in infants in the British West Indies. *Spec. Rep. Med. Res. Coun.* No. 263, London.

—— (1972). *Br. Med. J.* **3**, 566. Classification and definition of protein-calorie malnutrition.

—— (1973) *Lancet* **ii**, 87. Note on the assessment and classification of protein-energy malnutrition in children.

Waterlow, J.C. (1978) Anthropometric and biochemical findings in marginal malnutrition. In: *Proc. W. Hemisph. Nut. Congress* V. p. 273. American Medical Association.

—— (1979). *Lancet* **ii**, 250. Anthropometric assessment of malnutrition in children.

——, Ashworth, A., and Griffiths, M. (1980). *Lancet* **ii**, 1176. Faltering in growth in less developed countries.

——, Buzina, R., Keller, W., Lane, J.M., Nichaman, M.Z., and Tanner, J.M. (1977). *Bull. Wrld Hlth. Org.* **55**, 489. The presentation and use of height and weight data for comparing the nutritional status of groups of children under the age of 10 years.

Waterston, A. and Nhambe, M. (1984). *Central Afr. Med. J.* **30**, 97. Causes of malnutrition in Harare — a hospital case-control study.

Watson, R. (ed.) (1985). *Handbook for nutrition in the aged.* CRC Press, Cleveland, Ohio.

Webb, E.J., Campbell, D.T., Schwartz, R.D., and Sechrest, L. (1972). *Unobstrusive measures: non-reactive research in the social sciences.* Rand McNally, Chicago.

Weiner, J.S. and Lourie, J.A. (eds.) (1981). *Practical human biology.* Academic Press, New York.

Weisell, R.C. and Francois, P.J. (1982). *Food Nutr.* **8**, 12. Reference weight-for-heights: an easier approach to computerization.

Welbourn, H.F. (1954). *E. Afr. Med. J.* **31**, 332. Signs of malnutrition among Baganda children attending child welfare clinics.

Welham, W.C. and Behnke, A.K. (1942). *J. Am. Med. Assoc.* **118**, 498. The specific gravity of healthy man.

Wenlock, R.W. (1977). *Br. J. Nutr.* **38**, 239. Hydroxyproline indices as a tool for nutrition status surveys in malarial regions.

Werner, D. and Bower, B. (1982). *Helping health workers to learn.* Hesperian Foundation, Palo Alto, California.

Wharton, B.A. (1985). *Acta Paed. Scand.* Suppl. 319, 120. Sorrento studies of birthweight. Case for international references data.

Whitehead, R.G. (1965). *Lancet* **2**, 567. Hydroxyproline creatinine ratio as an index of nutritional status and rate of growth.

—— and Dunn, P.D. (eds.) (1985). *Acta Paed. Scand.*, Suppl. 319. The question for an international standard of reference.

—— (1986). *Proc. Nutr. Soc.* **45**, 361. Principles involved in assessing energy, protein and micronutrieur needs in infancy.

—— and Dean, R.F.A. (1964). *Am. J. Clin. Nutr.* **14**, 320. Serum amino-acids in kwashiorkor. 2-An abbreviated method of estimation and its application.

——, Frood, J.D.L., and Poskitt, E.M.E. (1971). *Lancet* **ii**, 287. Value of serum albumin measurements in nutritional surveys: a reappraisal.

——, Paul, A.A., and Ahmed, E.A. (1986). *Acta Paediat. Scand.* **323**, 14. Weaning practices in the United Kingdom and variations in anthropometric variation.

WHO (World Health Organization) (1970). The prevention of perinatal mortality and morbidity. *Tech. Rep. Ser. No. 457.* WHO, Geneva.

—— (1972*a*). *Tech. Rep. Ser. No. 405*, WHO, Geneva.

—— (1972*b*). Nutritional anaemias. *Tech. Rep. Ser. No. 503.* WHO, Geneva.

—— (1976). Methodology of nutritional surveillance. *Tech Rep. Ser. No. 593.* WHO, Geneva.

—— (1977*a*). *International classification of diseases. Manual of the international* *statistical classification of diseases, injuries, and causes of death*. WHO, Geneva.

—— (1977*b*). *Oral health surveys. Basic methods*. (Second Edition). WHO, Geneva.

—— (1978*a*). *A growth chart for international use in maternal and child care: guidelines for primary health care personnel*. WHO, Geneva.

—— (1978*b*). *Lay reporting of health information*. WHO, Geneva.

—— (1979). *Principles of design, supply, and usage of clinical laboratory equipment for primary health care in developing countries. July, 1978*. WHO, Geneva.

—— (1981). *Development of indicators for monitoring progress toward health for all by the year 2000*. WHO, Geneva.

—— (1983*a*). *Measuring change in nutritional status. Guidelines for assessing the nutritional impact of supplementary feeding programmes for vulnerable groups*. WHO, Geneva.

—— (1983*b*). Training in recording the child's growth. Document EPI/PHW/83/TM.1/Rev. 2. WHO, Geneva.

—— (1985*a*). *A guide to curriculum review for basic nursing education: orientation of primary health care and community health*. WHO, Geneva.

—— (1985*b*). Energy and protein requirements. *Tech. Rep. Ser. No. 724*. WHO, Geneva.

—— (1985*c*). *Iodine deficiency disorders in South-east Asia*. WHO SEARO, New Delhi.

—— (1986*a*). *Growth performance. Decision-making skills for selecting appropriate actions*. WHO, Genera.

—— (1986*b*). *Intersectoral action for health*. WHO, Geneva.

—— (1986*c*). *Methods recommended for essential clinical chemical and haematological tests for intermediate hospital laboratores*. Doc. LAB/86.3 WHO, Geneva.

—— (1986*d*). *Report of Working Group on Scales and Related Technologies for Weighing Pregnant Women, Newborns, Infants and Children*. WHO/MCH/86.5.

—— (1986*e*). *The growth chart. A tool for use in infant and children care*. WHO, Geneva.

—— (1986*g*). *Bull. Wrld. Hlth. Org.* **64**, 929. Use and interpretation of anthropometric indicators of nutritional status.

Wiersinga, A. and Korte, (1970). *East Afr. Med. J.* **47**, 14. A cytological study of buccal smears as an indicator of nutritional status.

—— and Van Rens, M.M. (1973). *J. Trop. Pediat.* **19**, 141. The simultaneous effect of protein-calorie malnutrition on weight and height velocity.

Willcocks, J. (1977). *Proc. Nutr. Soc.* **36**, 1. The assessment of fetal growth.

Wilcox, A.J. (1983). *Early Human Dev.* **8**, 189. Intrauterine growth resondetion: beyond birth weight criteria.

Wilkinson, K.N. (1982). *Trans. R. Soc. Trop. Med. Hyg.* **76**, 77. A damping system for under-fives weighing scales.

Williams, C.D. (1933). *Arch. Dis. Childh.* **8**, 434. A nutritional disease of children associated with a maize diet.

——, Baumslag, N., and Jelliffe, D.B. (1985). *Mother and child health: delivering the services* (2nd edition). Oxford University Press, Oxford.

Wills, V.G. and Waterlow, J.C. (1958). *J. Trop. Pediat.* **3**, 167. The death rate in the age group 1–4 years as an index of malnutrition.

Wilson, C.S. (1964). *J. Trop. Pediat* **20**, 9. Child following: a technique for learning food and nutrition intakes.

—— (1979). *J. Nutr. Ed.* **11**, 4, Suppl. 1. Food, custom and nurture.

——, Schaefer, A.E., Darby, W.J., Bridgforth, E.B., Pearson, W.N., Combs, G.F., Leatherwood, E.C., Greene, J.C., Teply, L.J., Plough, I.C., McGanity, W.J., Hand, D.B., Kertesz, Z.I., and Woodruff, C.W. (1964). *Am. J. Clin. Nutr.* **15**, 29. A review of methods used in nutrition surveys conducted by the interdepartmental committee on nutrition for national development (ICNND).

Winick, M. (ed.) (1979). *Hunger disease.* Wiley, New York.

Winikoff, B. (1978). *Nutrition and national policy*, MIT Press. Cambridge, Mass.

Wishik, S.M. and Van der Vynckt, S. (1976). *PAG Bulletin* **5**, 11 Nutrition, mother's health and fertility: the effects of child-bearing on health and nutrition.

Wit, J.M., Davies, C., and Molthof, J. (1984*a*). *Trop. Doctor* **14**, 36. Introduction of home- and clinic based growth chart in Dominica.

——, Van t'Hof, A., and Rouede, M.J. (1984*b*). *Growth* **48**, 370. Reference curves for biceps, triceps and supra-iliac skinfold in Dutch children from 7–14 years.

Woelk, G.B., Moyo, I.M., and Mehlomakhuhr, M.N. (1986). *Cent. Afr. Med. J.* **32**, 71. Knowledge of weight-for-height growth curves and maternal childhood immunisations of mothers attending children's clinics in Harare.

Woodland, M. and Kelly, M. (1979). *J. Trop. Pediat.* **25**, 139. Nurses study growth charts.

Wood, C.S. and Gans. L.P. (1984). *J. Trop. Pediat.* **30**, 104. Some hematological findings in children of Western Samoa.

Woods, H.F. (1982). *Proc. Nutr. Soc.* **41**, 419. Biochemical methods in nutritional assessment.

World Federation of Public Health Associations (1983*a*). *Training community health workers.* UNICEF, New York.

—— (1983*b*). *Synopses of CHW trained in selected projects.* UNICEF, New York.

World Health Organization Expert Committee on Dental Health (1962). Standardization of reporting of dental disease and condition. *Tech. Rep. Ser. No. 242.* WHO, Geneva.

Wrigley, E.S. (1984). *J. Am. Diet. Assoc.* **84**, 417. Average? ideal? desirable? A brief overview of height-weight tables in the United States.

WuLeung, W.T., Butrum, R.R., and Chang, F. (1972). *A selected bibliography on East Asian foods.* U.S. Department of Health, Education and Welfare, Washington, DC, and FAO, Rome.

Yang, Y.P. (1971). *Fact-finding with rural people: Sampling and other statistical methods.* FAO, Rome.

Yearick, E.S. (1978). *J. Geront.* **33**, 657. Nutritional status of the elderly: anthropometric and clinical findings.

——, Wang, M.L., and Pisias, S.J. (1980). *J. Geront.* **35**, 663. Nutritional status of the elderly: dietary and biochemical findings.

Yee, V.S. (1985). *Guidelines for the design and organization of health sector nutritional status surveillance.* International nutrition unit technical report series. Office of International Health. Rockville, Md.

Yi-Ling, Y. and Bei-Jun, W. (1982). *Am. J. Publ. Hlth.* **72**, 41. An anthropometric study of school children in Shanghai.

Yip, R., Bridges, N., Van Assenfeldft, O., Gove, S.S., and Hassan, B.F. (1987). *Proc. Am. Publ. Hlth. Assoc. Conference* (rear or leans). Rapid field survey with a portable haemoglobinometer. APHA, Washington, DC.

Yost, D.A. and Pust, R.E. (1987). *J. Trop. Pediat.* **34**, 275. Arm circumferences an index of protein energy malnutrition in 6–11 months.

Young, G.A. and Hill, G. (1978). *Am. J. Clin. Nutr.* **31**, 429. Assessment of protein-calorie malnutrition in surgical patients from plasma proteins and anthropometric measurements.

Zeitlin, M.F. (1979). *Hum. Biol.* **51**, 11. The derivation of a reference standard for maximum thigh circumference of preschool children, aged 0–5 years.

Zeitlin, M.F., Briser A. and Weld, L. (1987*b*). *Policy implications of a project to investigate misclassification errors in growth monitoring, in press.*

——, Inciong, M.B., Lacuna, R., and Opena, M. (1981). *J. Trop. Pediat* **27**, 267. The advantages of using a thigh circumference tape analogous to the Shakir strip for detection of malnutrition in pre-school children.

——, Mansour, M., and Bajrai, J.D. (1987*a*). *Adv. Int. Mat. Chld. Hlth.* **7**, 94. Positive deviance in nutrition: an approach to child health whose time has come.

——, Pyle, D.F., Austin, J.E., Sempore, G., and Gouba, E. (1982). *J. Trop. Pediat.* **28**, 62. Circumference growth charts for community level workers with little or no formal schooling.

——, Rizvi, N., and Khan, A.D. (1984). *Ecology of Food and Nutrition* **15**, 299–313. An interactive dietary assessment method for use in rural Bangladesh part I: Methodology for instrument development.

Zerfas, A. (1979). Anthropometric field methods: general. In *Nutrition and growth* (eds. D.B. and E.F.P. Jelliffe), p. 339. Plenum Press, New York.

—— (1975). *Am. J. Clin. Nutr.* **28**, 782. The insertion tape: a new circumference tape for nutritional assessment.

—— (1985). *Checking decisions for action based on growth charts.* School of Public Health, UCLA, Los Angeles, Calif.

—— (1986). *Decisions for health interventions. A manual for trainers and supervisors.* LTS/International Nutrition Unit, Rockville, Md.

——, Browdy, B., Clay, W.D., Shorr, I.J., Jelliffe, D.B., and Jelliffe, E.F.P. (1982). *Adv. Int. Mat. Chld. Hlth* 2. Focused national nutrition surveys in developed countries (with special references to young children.

——, ——, and —— (1985). *Adv. Int. Mat. Child. Hlth. 5*, 155. Assessing child nutrition: epidemiological insights.

——, Shorr, I., and Neumann, C.G. (1977). *Pediat. Clin. N. Amer.* **24**, 253. Office assessment of nutritional status.

Addendum 1988

Scope (p. 1)

The following is very recent information and follows the same sequence as the main chapters. Recent publications continue to emphasize the significance of *vitamin A deficiency* (Eastman 1987; Mason 1989) and the use of ocular impression cytology as an early pre-clinical test (Eastman 1987; Tarwotjo *et al.* 1987). The geometric speed of population growth including migration to urban slums, continues to increase in most parts of the world. The quest for '*food security*' remains precarious in many less technically developed countries because of post-harvest losses (Bourne 1987), and man-made and 'natural' famines. *General reviews* of the world situation have been made recently by Scrimshaw (1985), Gopalan (1988), and Bender (1988).

The two 'extremes' of methods of nutritional assessment — from simplified and approximate to detailed epidemiological — are indicated by varying methods of predicting low birth weight (Kestler *et al.* 1987; Mardones-Restat and Jones 1987), and short- and long-term functional effects of nutrient deficiency and excess. Pressure to use uniform *SI (Système Internationale) units* for clinical laboratory data (Young 1987) has increased. This will help ultimately, although certainly with some confusion initially. The role of *simplified methods* of nutritional assessment, as approximate but practical approaches, has been given attention, as with 'rapid rural appraisal' (Longhurst 1987*a*). A 1989 issue of the *International Journal of Epidemiology* is currently in preparation on 'rapid epidemiological assessment', and a new booklet has been published by WHO (Beghin *et al.* 1988.)

Direct assessment (p. 13)

Little additional information has been obtained concerning *clinical signs*, except for revival of interest in blue sclerae as suggesting iron deficiency (Kalra *et al.* 1986). McLaren's *Atlas* (1981) needs belated mention as a useful teaching tool. Increased concern with *trace elements* is evidenced by the appearance of a new journal — the *Journal of Trace Elements in Experimental Medicine* (1988) (published by Alan Liss). The biophysical test of the moment remains *ocular impression cytology* for pre-clinical avitaminosis A (Amedee-Manesme *et al.* 1988), which is under trial in several countries.

Major attention continues to be focused on *anthropometry*,* including a re-

*Catalogues and list of equipment, with up-to-date prices, are given by Geissler *et al.* (1988), CMS Equipment Ltd. (18 Camden High St, London NW1 OJH, UK) and the Illinois Dept. of Health, Springfield, Illinois, USA.

look at the value of simple weight-for-age measurements (Popkin and Yamamoto 1985; Jansen *et al.* 1985). Considerable emphasis has been given to body size and composition, and to the usefulness and limitations of arm circumference measurements. With regard to *body size and physique*, McLaren (1988) notes that obvious normal variation in body build ('somatotypes') are not given much consideration nowadays. The question of *frame size* has been touched on occasionally, as with the development of a 'frameter' (measuring elbow breadth) by Frisancho (1988). *Body composition* studies have focused on fat, including the different *patterning in pregnancy* (Johnson *et al.* 1988). A relatively new book has been written on the subject, edited by Norgan (1985). Most attention seems to be given to the estimation of body fat by *electrical impedance* (Abu Khaled *et al.* 1988: Brown *et al.* 1988; Cordain *et al.* 1988). However, it has been pointed out that the body is made up of numerous 'compartments' (Steen 1988), which make interpretation more difficult than is often recognized. Controversies concerning *growth monitoring* have come to the forefront in children (Yee and Zerfas 1987; Rohde 1988; Jelliffe and Jelliffe 1989) and, increasingly, in pregnancy. Greater appreciation of difficulties and significance have emerged, especially training (CRS/CARITAS 1988).

The need for low-cost light-weight *height-measuring equipment* continues, and a new *relatively* economical plastic apparatus has been developed, the 'Accustat' (Roche *et al.* 1988). *Secular trends* in height have been reported recently from various parts of the world. These have been upwards in Korea (Ko 1987) and in Japan (Zachmann 1987) (where it may be continuing); but have shown no change in forty years in poor urban Indian women (National Institute of Nutrition of India 1986). Differences in genetic *patterning and tempo of growth* have again been noted, whether through dramatic examples such as the absence of the pubertal growth spurt among Pygmies (Mann 1987), or through less striking differences in the growth pattern of well-fed young Chinese children in Hong Kong (Davies and Leung 1985).

Considerable attention has been paid to the significance of diminished linear growth (stunting) (Waterlow 1986) and the usefulness and limitations of the *arm circumference (AC)*. It has been found to be sensitive, specific, and with positive and negative predictive value in young children (Briend *et al.* 1987). Yost and Pust (1988) noted that in fact the AC does not vary much between 6 and 11 months, so that a mid-point reference level can be used for screening. They suggest 12.5 cm as a lower level rather than 13.5 cm for children aged 12–59 months. Detailed longitudinal studies have been reported by Sann *et al.* (1988) of changes in arm muscle and fat area in the first year of life. Much discussion has arisen as a result of modern technological analysis, using computerized tomography and cross-sectional electric impedance of the components making up the arm circumference. It has been emphasized (as was already known) that the mid-arm is not circular, but elliptical, that the underlying muscle is 'clover-leaf' in shape, that the humerus can vary slightly in size, that the subcutaneous fat varies from the triceps to the biceps areas, and that the 'pinch' of the calipers used can give measurements 20–40 per cent below the true fatfold (Forbes *et al.* 1988). For these reasons, Heymsfield *et al.* (1982) suggested an addition to mid-arm area calculations of 10 cm for adult males and 6.5 cm for adult females. It needs emphasizing that all body measurements are exposed to similar criticisms.

Despite such scientifically meticulous investigations, the mid-arm circumference measurement remains a simple, approximate, economical method of categorizing malnutrition in the newborn, in young children, and in pregnant women. It is feasible and affordable for community health workers in less technically developed countries, as a 'muscle-fat' proxy. However, as re-emphasized by Gayle *et al.* (1988), use of this measurement does not give exactly the same rates of 'thinness' as does the weight-for-height; nor would this be expected.

The need for exchange of information between those working in less technically developed countries and those largely in hospital nutritional assessment remains very great, as indicated by the completely different pictures of kwashiorkor and marasmus given in various text-books (Weinser and Butterworth 1981).

Health statistics (p. 128)

A more cautious attitude has rightly developed in correlating such statistics too exclusively with protein-energy malnutrition, as so many variables are also involved. Probably the most significant new emphasis has been on the fact that other nutrient deficiencies than protein and energy (calories) can influence mortality in children, including iron, probably zinc, and certainly vitamin A. For example, in India mild clinical avitaminosis A is associated with a two-fold increase in severe respiratory tract infections in young children (Milton *et al.* 1987). Also, recent community data from Indonesia indicate that the pre-school age mortality is three times as high in those with pre-clinical vitamin A deficiency (Tarwotjo *et al.* 1988).

Partly as a result of problems with obtaining and interpreting infant growth charts, increased attention is moving to practical indicators of *materno-fetal malnutrition*, especially anaemia (and minor haemorrhage) in pregnancy (WHO 1987*a*), and the incidence of low birth weight babies, preferably differentiated into pre-term and 'light-for-dates' (acute and chronic).

Lastly, there seems an increased use of selected components of the health services as 'sentinel' units, exemplified by recent accounts of 'clinic-based' nutritional surveillance.

Ecological variables (p. 142)

Probably the two most emphasized variables are the unresolved issues of dramatic increases in overall population in many Third World countries and of the 'urban avalanche' in particular (Food and Nutrition Bulletin 1987). The impact of infections has also received much deserved attention, especially diarrhoea (Bairagi *et al.* 1987) and its dietary management. Ever-increasing recognition of the importance of cultural influences is indicated by the publication of a new journal *Nutritional Anthropology* (John Wiley).

The complexity of different causes (Pellet 1987) (including, for example, mycotoxins and a wide range of infections, often seasonal) has led a considerable output of factually correct, but complex, diagrams, which can tend to bemuse rather than to offer practical assistance. The need for a system for sorting out priorities — which problems are the most serious and realistically preventable —

has evolved into the concept of *risk-factor assessment* (Backett *et al.* 1984). This needs to be an exercise blending science with common sense.

Recent research and publications on various aspects of the food chain re-emphasize the difficulties in assessment: uncertainties, inevitable approximations, difficulties of assessment at every link in the chain. These include *very considerable variation in RDA (RDI)* in different countries (Truswell 1982), *data on food composition* (Stewart 1983), and *considerations or nutritional adequacy* (WHO 1985) in relation to individual and community variation, to body proportions, to levels of activity, and to the influence of chronic or intermittent infections.

The '*food frequency approach*' can be of assistance as a practical, focused method, especially when limited to local items that are rich in nutrients known to be deficient in the diet of the particular community. The start of INFOODS (International Network of Food Data Systems) (Food and Nutrition Bulletin 1983) will be most helpful in different parts of the world in stimulating action into food consumption analysis and in exchanging information between research centres.

Estimating food availability in different circumstances needs to take into account special considerations. In *extreme food shortages or famines*, the cost of basic foods increases greatly, the selling price of animal stock falls (to buy essential foods), and the use of edible, usually culturally despised, often semi-wild 'non-foods' increases (Longhurst 1987*b*).

With dietary recall studies, a '*nutrient data base*' — that is information on the nutrient content — is needed for locally used cooked items. In many populations, this will be a small list, as the diet does not vary much.

Conversely, in more technically developed countries, a very large number of processed items are available, and in order to identify those produced by manufacturers in different countries a '*factored food vocabulary*' (FFV) has been introduced which enables foods to be compared. This lists twelve factors: (A) product types, (B1) food source, (B2) part of plant on animal, (C) physical state, shape, or form, (D1) degree of preparation, (D2) cooking method, (D3) treatment applied, (D4) preservation method, (E1) packing medium, (E2) container or wrapping, (E3) food contact surface, (F) user group. The real value of this system remains to be seen.

At another level, the influence of the *street food trade* on women and children has become recognized increasingly as a previously underemphasized part of the food chain in many countries (Cohen 1986).

Interpretation in different age-groups (p. 226)

There has been a much increased and overdue emphasis on *materno-fetal malnutrition*, recently reviewed by Soysa (1987). From very many parts of the world, the variability and adaptation of nutrient needs in pregnancy and lactation have been important findings, including conservation of energy (Forsum *et al.* 1988). However, low birth weight can result from maternal malnutrition, often from a pre-gravid inadequacy *plus* a deficient intake during pregnancy. This has been described, for example, as occurring during the 'hungry' or 'lean' pre-harvest season in West Africa (Prentice *et al.* 1987). In Latin America, maternal malnutrition, infections, continued lactation during pregnancy, and possibly even frequent prolonged exposure to smoke in kitchens, have been considered responsible alone or in various combinations (Martorell and Gonzalez-Cossio 1987).

Monitoring maternal nutrition during pregnancy is being investigated all over the world — for both mother and newborn. In addition to different weight charts and measuring the uterine height (Munjanjo *et al.* 1987), various means have been used as potential risk indicators for subsequent low birth weight, ranging from complex statistically based scores (Kestler *et al.* 1987) to simple 'suggesters' such as the mother's arm circumference ($\geq$ 28.5 cm in Central America) (Lechtig 1988), or using fundal height in parts of Africa (Munjanjo *et al.* 1987). As yet little considered is the need to differentiate the *various types of low birth weight babies* (pre-term *and* acute and chronic small- or light-for-dates). This can be done by knowledge of the length of gestation (from the last menstrual period, if known), and of the reflex development achieved by the neonate, and by anthropometry at birth (usually weight and length). This is important, as it can usually give insight into causation, and, in addition, various types of low-weight neonates have different immediate and long-term problems and risks (Haas *et al.* 1987; International Pediatric Association 1988), including ability for catch-up growth if well-fed in infancy.

In over-fed countries, the opposite issue of maternal obesity is occurring, with increased numbers of large newborns (macrosomia) and obstetrical risks (Lucas *et al.* 1988).

In *young children* (p. 259) the question of transplacental HIV virus infection needs to be included in the differential diagnosis of marasmus and accompanying opportunistic infections, as this is how AIDS can present in this age-group. Also, in breastfed babies, the deuterium oxide research method, when the D_2O is given to the mother, has been shown to give similar results as regards volume of milk produced as carefully supervised 24-hour test-weighing (Butte *et al.* 1988).

With regard to kwashiorkor, the old Latin American title '*sindrome pluricarencial*, may be more apt than previously recognized, as deficiency of one or more nutrients, such as iron, riboflavin, vitamin A, etc., is almost always present at the same time as lack of calories and protein. Also, Golden (1988) considers that kwashiorkor (as opposed to marasmus) may be partly due to 'superimposition of various noxae'. This presumably includes aflatoxin, in areas of the worlds in which this fungal infection of grain and cereals occurs (Hendrickse 1986), but also the newly recognized production of 'free radicals' in the body (Golden 1988).

In *school age children and adolescents* (p. 329) the problem of obesity is increasing in relatively affluent families around the world, as is *adolescent pregnancy*. The later presents special problems with regard to nutritional assessment, because of the young mother's own incomplete growth, reproductive immaturity (size of the uterus and pelvis), possible nutrient deficiencies as a result of 'fad diets', and sometimes the effects of behavioural considerations, such as cigarette-smoking, alcohol consumption, and the use of drugs (Stevens-Simon and McAnarney 1988). In the general *adult population* (p. 339), obesity (with its associated later mortality from diabetes, hypertension, etc.) predominates in regions where food is easily accessible, especially in the form of compact calories. This has been categorized as follows: Grade III $W/H^2 > 40$; Grade II 30–40;

Grade I 25–29.9 (Garrow 1981). In middle-aged, post-menopausal women, osteoporosis is often common. It is partly dietary in origin (calcium, vitamin D) and partly hormonal, related to decreased secretion of oestrogens.

In *sick adults* (p. 348) a major issue can be estimating body-weight in those who are non-ambulatory, especially the *elderly* (p. 352). Various anthropometric formulas have been devised to estimate body weight (Chumlea *et al.* 1988). As a simplified approximation, the mid-arm circumference has been used, and reference levels have been developed (Faciglia *et al.* 1988). Such estimations are needed for various purposes, including the difficult problem of effective, but non-toxic, dosage of medical drugs.

Data collection (p. 335)

A limited number of longitudinal studies have been reported, as for example in the PDR of Yemen (Bågenholm 1988). Various types of rapid assessment have been employed experimentally in the last few years. One of these — 'Rapid Rural Appraisal' — is based on using existing information, selecting limited 'key indicators': (species of food plants available, birth weights, type of housing, inventories in shops and markets of selected items) using village-level researches, key informants, and group interviews, with emphasis on direct observation ('taking time to walk and look' and acquiring local, indigenous technical knowledge) (Longhurst 1987*a*). Essentially, this approach is a mixture of limited, focused prevalence studies with anthropological-type observation and discussion. Items included need careful selection for the population concerned. Information obtained will necessarily be approximate and superficial.

Another recent development has been termed 'Rapid Survey Methodology', using battery-operated lap-top computers which can be used for field work in rural areas (Frerichs 1988). This has enabled a limited range of information gathered by questionnaire during home-visiting to be entered into the computer at the end of each day, so that final results can be made available immediately at the end of the survey. The speed of this process and its technological appeal are positive factors. So far, limitations are cost (initial and for repairs), and the questions included have been important, but mostly limited to basic factual information. The method's actual role needs further trial as one component of community assessment, and will vary with circumstances, as with every other method. It will always need complementary in-depth information obtainable, focus group interviews, key informants, and other anthropological techniques (p. 165).

Data entry and analysis have been facilitated by publicly available software for microcomputers, including a module for anthropometric conversions.*

Implementation (p. 384)

This aspect of the subject is sometimes obscured by the specialized languages of the epidemiologist, the statistician, and computer experts. A glossary has been included to help readers through the verbal maze (Appendix 4) (p. 508).

*Available from S. Lee, Tulane School of Public Health, New Orleans, Louisiana, USA.

With regard to *sampling*, there is 'no single design that is ideal for all surveys' (Rothenburg *et al.* 1985). As noted earlier (p. 405), the limiting factors are 'statistical confidence', time, funds, and the purpose of the investigation. Often '*simplified cluster sampling*' is employed, as particularly emphasized in WHO assessment of immunization programmes (Henderson and Sundarasan, 1982). However, it may be noted that these are intended for relatively simple questions of the 'yes/no' variety.

Nutritional surveillance remains to the forefront of assessment both in mainly well-nourished communities, such as the USA (Forbes 1987), in the continuing activities of the National Nutritional Monitoring Board in India (Srikantia 1988, 1987*b*) and in famine-warning systems in areas at risk (Longhurst 1987*b*). In Central Africa, Brown (1987) has found the QAC stick a useful appropriate technology in young children, as one component of surveillance. Overall methods have been reviewed by the UNAC/SNN in a manual entitled 'Nutrition in Times of Disaster' (1989).

Nutritional indicators for example, anthropometry — are being increasingly used in large-scale surveys — for instance, Demographic Health Surveys (Westinghouse, IRD, Columbia, Maryland) have replaced earlier World Fertility Surveys.

Essentially, the overall need is for caution in interpretation and in the nutrition assessment studies, including *national cross-sectional surveys* (as in Pakistan 1985–7) (Nutrition Division 1988) or '*impact evaluation of programmes*'. 'Triangulation' of information from several quite different methods is increasingly appreciated.

Bibliography 1988

Abu Khaled, A., McCutcheon, M.J., Reddy, S., Pearman, P.L., Hunter, G.R., and Weinser, R.L. (1988). Electrical impedance in assessing human body composition: the BIA method. *Am. J. Clin. Nutr.*, **47**, 789.

Amedee-Manesme, O., Luzeau, R., Wittepen, J.R., Hanck, A., and Sommer, A. (1988). Impression cytology detects subclinical vitamin A deficiency. *Am. J. Clin. Nutr.* **47**, 875.

Andersen, A.F. (1985). *Practical comprehensive treatment of anorexia nervosa and bulimia.* Johns Hopkins University Press, Baltimore, Md.

Austin, J.E. and Zeitlin, M.F., (ed.) (1981). Nutrition intervention in developing countries. Oelgeschlager, Gunn, and Hain, Cambridge, Mass.

Backett, E.M., Davies, A.M., and Petros-Barvazian, A. (1984). *The risk approach in health care.* Publ. Hlth Paper No. 76. WHO, Geneva.

Bågenholm, G. (1988). Feeding patterns, growth and morbidity among pre-school children in PDR Yemen. Dept. of Pediatrics, Gothenburg University, Sweden.

Bairagi, R., Chowdhury, M.K., Kim, Y.J., Curlin, G.T., and Grary, R.H. (1987). The association between malnutrition and diarrhoea in rural Bangladesh. *Int. J. Epidem.* **16**, 477.

Beghin, I., Cape, M., and Dujardin, B. (1988). A guide to nutritional assessment. WHO, Geneva.

Bender, A.E. (1988). Some recent advances in nutrition. *J. R. Soc. Health* **108**, 191.

Bender, F.E., Douglas, L.W., and Kramer, A. (1982). *Statistical methods for food and agriculture.* Avi Publishing Co., Westport, Connecticut.

Bourne, M.C. (1987). Postharvest food losses in developing countries. *L.I.F.E.* 20, 1.

Bridges, N., Parvin, R.M., and Van Assendelft, O.W. (1987). Evolution of a new system for hemoglobin measurement. *Am. Clin. Product Rev.* April issue.

Briend, A., Wojtyniak, B., and Rowland, M.G. (1987). Arm circumference and other factors in children at high risk of death in rural Bangladesh. *Lancet* **ii**, 725.

Brown B.H., Karatzas, T., Nakielny, R., and Clarke, R.G. (1988). Determination of upper arm muscle and fat areas using electrical impedance measurements. *Clin. Phys. Physical Meas.* **9**, 47.

Brown, R.C. (1987). Nutrition surveillance by QUAC stick. *Trans. R. Soc. Trop. Med. Hyg.* **81**, 1038.

Butte, N.F., Wong, W.W., Patterson, B.W., Garza, C., and Klein, P.D. (1988). Human milk intake measured by deuterium oxide to the mother: a comparison with the test-weighing technique. *Am. J. Clin. Nutr.* **47**, 815.

Callaway, D. (ed.) (1982). *Assessing the nutritional status of the elderly state of the art.* Reprt of Third Ross Round Table on Medical Issues. Columbus, Ohio.

Chadwick, S.J.D., Sim, A.J.W., and Dudley, D.A.T. (1986). Changes in fibronetin during acute deprivation in healthy human subjects. *Br. J. Nutr.* 55, 7.

Chandra, R.K. (1980). *Immunology of nutritional disorders.* Edward Arnold, London.

—— (1988). Nutrition and community. *Papua New Guinea Med. J.*, **30**, 97.

Chumlea, W.C., Roche, A.F., and Steinbaugh, A. (1988). *J. Am. Diet. Assoc.* **85**, 564. Prediction of body weight in the non-ambulatory elderly from anthropometry.

Chwang, L., Soemantri, A.G., and Pollitt, E. (1988). Iron supplementation and physical growth of rural Indonesian children. *Am. J. Clin. Nutr.* **47**, 496.

Cohen, M. (1986). *Adv. Intl. Mac. Chld. Hlth.* **6**, 148. The influence of street food trade on women and children.

Cordain, L., Whicken, R.E., and Johnson, J.E. (1988). Body composition determination in children using bioelectrical impedance. *Growth Dev. Aging,* **52**, 37.

CRS/CARITAS (1988). *Growth monitoring and nutrition education.* Office of Nutrition USAID, Washington, DC 20523.

Daga, S.R., Daga, A.S., Patole, S., Kadam, S., and Mukadam, Y. (1988). Foot length measurement from footprint for identifying a newborn at risk. *J. Trop. Pediatr.*, **34**, 16.

Davies, D.P. and Leung, S.S.F. (1985). *Early Human Dev.* **11**, 247. Growth of Hong Kong infants.

Eastman, S.J. (1987). Vitamin A deficiency and xerophthalmia. Recent findings and some programme implications. *Assignment children*, No. 3.

Faciglia, G., O'Connor, J. and Gedling, E. (1988). *J. Am. Diet Assoc.* **88**, 569. Circumference norms in elderly white subjects.

Food and Agriculture Organization (1984). *Food harvest losses in quality of food grain.* Paper No. 29. FAO, Rome.

Food and Nutrition Bulletin (1982). Special issues: post harvest food losses. *Food Nutr. Bull.*, **4**, 1.

—— (1983). Special INFOODS issue. *Food Nutr. Bull.,* **5**, 15.

Food and Nutrition Bulletin (1987). Special issue: nutrition and urbanization. *Food Nutr. Bull.*, **9**, 1.

—— (1988). Women and nutrition. *Food Nutr. Bull.*, **10**, 3–54.

Forbes, A.L. (ed). (1987). ASCN public policy forum — Federal monitoring of the nation's nutritional status. *Am. J. Clin. Nutr.,* **47**, 318.

Forbes, G.B., Brown, M.R., and Griffiths, H.J.L. (1988). Arm muscle plus bone area: anthropometric and CAT scan compared. *Am. J. Clin. Nutr.,* **47**, 729.

Forsum, E., Sadurskis, A., and Wagen, J. (1988). Resting metabolic rate and body composition of healthy Swedish women during pregnancy. *Am. J. Clin. Nutr.* **47**, 942.

Foundation for the Advancement of Knowledge of Mother and Child in Developing Countries (1987). Infant nutrition and growth, Proceedings of a workshop. Arnhem, Netherlands.

Frisancho, A.R. (1988). *J. Am. Diet Assoc.* **47**, 929 Arm muscle plus bone area.

Frerichs, R.R. (1988). Rapid microcomputer surveys. *J. Trop. Pediatr.*, **34**, 147.

Ganguly, C. and Mukherjee, K.L. (1986). Relationship between maternal serum vitamin A and vitamin A status of the corresponding fetuses. *J. Trop. Pediatr.*, **32**, 287.

Garrow, J.S. (1981). *Treat obesity seriously*. Churchill Livingstone, Edinburgh.

Gayle, H.D., Binkin, N.J., Staehling, N.W., and Trowbridge, F.L. (1988). Arm circumference vs weight-for-height in nutritional assessment: are the findings comparable? *J. Trop. Pediatr.*, **34**, 207.

Geissler, C., Saravanabevandan, P., and Crook, S. (1988). *Field equipment for nutrition and health studies*. Dept. of Food and Nutrition, Kings College, University of London, Campden Hill Road, London W8 7AH.

Golden, M. (1988). The effects of malnutrition in the metabolism of children. *Trans. R. Soc. Trop. Med. Hyg., 82*, 3.

Gopalan, C. (1988). Nutrition problems and programmes in Southeast Asia. *J. Trop. Pediatr.*, **34**, 139. (WHO Regional office for Southeast Asia, New Delhi, India.)

—— (ed.) (1988). Profiles in undernutrition and underdevelopment. *Nutr. Found. India Sci. Rep.*, No. 8. (New Delhi, India.)

Haas, J.D., Balcazar, H., and Caulfield, L. (1987). Variation in early neonatal mortality for different types of fetal retardation. *Am. J. Phys. Anthropol.*, **73**, 467.

Henderson, R.H. and Sundarasan, T. (1982). Cluster sampling to assess immunization average: a review of experience with a simplified sampling method. *Bull. WHO*, **60**, 253.

Hendrickse, R.G. (1984). *Trans. R. Soc. Trop. Med. Hyg.* **78**, 427. The influence of aflatoxins on child health in the tropics

Heymsfield, S.B. McManus, C., Stevens, V., and Smith, J. (1982). *Am. J. Clin. Nutr.* **35**, 1192. Muscle mass: reliable indicator of protein–energy malnutrition severity and outcome.

Husaini, Y.K., Husaini, M.A., Sulainan, Z., Jahari, A.B., Barizi, S.T., Hudono, and Karyadi, D. (1986). Maternal malnutrition, outcome of pregnancy and a simple tool to identify women at risk. *Food Nutr. Bull.*, **8**, 71.

International Pediatric Association (1988). Report of IPA/UNICEF/WHO Symposium of prevention of pre-term delivery and low birth weight. *Bull. Int. Pediatr. Assoc.*, **9**, 7.

Jansen, A.A.J., Thiuri, B., and t'Mannetje, W. (1985). The predictive and retrospective values of weight and height measurements of below fives. *J. Trop. Pediatr.*, **31**, 320.

Jelliffe, D.B. and Jelliffe, E.F.P. (ed.) (1988). *Programmes to promote breastfeeding*. Oxford University Press.

—— and —— (1989). *Growth monitoring in young children*. Oxford University Press, New York. (In press.)

Jerome, N., Kandel, R.F., and Pelto, G.H. (ed.) (1980). *Nutritional anthropology*. Redgrave Publishing Co., New York.

Johnson, F.E., Wadden, T.A., Stunkard, A.J., Pena, M., Wang, J., Pierson, R.N., and Van Italie, T.E. (1988). Body fat deposition in adult obese women. (I) Patterns of fat distribution. *Am. J. Clin. Nutr.* **47**, 225.

Johnston, F.E., (ed.), (1987). *Nutritional anthropology*. Alan Liss Inc., New York.

Journal of Nutrition Science and Vitaminology (1987). Symposium on assessment of marginal nutritional status. *J. Nutr. Sci. Vitaminol.* **33** (complete volume).

Kalra, L., Harnlyn, A.N., and Jones, B.J.M. (1986). Blue sclera: a common sign of iron deficiency? *Lancet* ii, 1267.

Kestler, E., Dorgan, J., Sibrian, R., Aquino, O., and Villan, J. (1987). Epidemiologic identification of infants with low birth weight in urban areas of Latin America. *PAHO Bull.*, **21**, 369.

Ko, K. (1987). Studies on the secular trends of growth in Korean children in three decades. *Acta Paediatr. Jpn* **29**, 91.

Lechtig, A. (1988). Predicting risk of delivering low birthweight babies: which indicator is best? *J. Trop. Pediatr.*, **34**, 34.

Lohman, T.G., Roche, A.F., and Martorell, R. (ed.) (1988). *Anthropometric standardization reference manual.* Human Kinetics Books, Champaign, Illinois.

Longhurst, R. (1987*a*). Rapid rural appraisal: an improved means of information gathering for rural development and nutrition projects. *Food Nutr.* **13**, 44.

—— (1987*b*). Famines, food, and nutrition: issues and opportunities for policy and research. *Food Nutr. Bull.*, **9**, 30.

Lucas, A., Morley, R., Cole, T.J., Baumford, M.F., and Pearse, R. (1988). Maternal fatness and viability of preterm infants. *Br. Med. J.*, **296**, 1495.

Mann, G.V. (1987). The riddle of pygmies. *New Engl. J. Med.*, **317**, 709.

Mardones-Restat, F. and Jones, G. (1987). Prediction of poor infant growth. *PAHO Bull.*, **21**, 341.

Martorell, R. and Gonzalez-Cossio, T. (1987). Maternal nutrition and birthweight. *Yearb. Phys. Anthropol.*, **30**, 195.

McBean, L. (ed.) (1988). Nutrition and the school-age child. *Dairy Council Digest (USA)*, **59**, 7.

McLaren, D.S. (1981). *A colour atlas of nutritional disorders.* Wolfe Medical Publications, London.

—— (1988). Body composition methods. *Am. J. Clin. Nutr.*, **47**, 1087.

Milton, R.C., Reddy, V., and Naido, A.W. (1987). Mild vitamin A deficiency and childhood morbidity — an Indian experience. *Am. J. Clin. Nutr.* **46**, 827.

Munjanjo, S.P., Masona, D., Maxwell, M., and Mahomed, M.M. (1987). A symphysial – fundal height nomogram for Central Africa. *Cent. Afr. Med. J.*, **33**, 29.

Natadisastra, G., Wittpenn, J., West, K., Muhilal, and Sommer, A. (1987). Impression cytology for detection of vitamin A deficiency. *Arch. Opthalmol.*, **105**, 1224.

National Academy of Sciences (1978). *Post-harvest food losses in developing countries.* The Academy, Washington, DC.

National Institute of Nutrition of India (1986). *Annual Report 1985–6*, p. 134. Indian Council of Medical Research, Hyderabad, India.

Neumann, C.G., and Bwibo, N. (1987). *Report of Collaboratives Research Program on Food Intake and Human Function*: Kenya Project. USAID, Washington, DC.

Norgan, N.G. (ed.) (1985). *Human body composition and fat distribution.* (Euro-Nut. Rep. 8.) Koninklyijke Biblioteek, Den Haag, Netherlands.

Nutrition Division (1988). *National Nutrition Survey 1985–7.* National Institute of Health, Islamabad, Pakistan.

Pellett, P.L. (1987). The determinants of nutritional status. *Food Nutr.*, **13**, 2.

Pennington, J.A.T., Smith Holden, J.M., Soergel, D., and Wiley, R.C. (1988). FDA's factored food vocabulary for food product consumption. *Am. J. Diet. Assoc.*, **88**, 336.

Popkin, B.M. and Yamamoto, M.E. (1985). A comparison of anthropometric classifications for nutritional status determination: a case study in the Philippines. *J. Trop. Pediatr.*, **31**, 311.

Prentice, A.W., Cole, T.J., Foord, F.A., Lamb, W.H., and Whitehead, R. (1987). Increased birth weight after prenatal dietary supplementation in rural African women. *Am. J. Clin. Nutr.*, **46**, 912.

Roche, A.F., Guo, S., Baumgartner, R.N., and Falls, R.A. (1988). The measurement of stature. *Am. J. Clin. Nutr.*, **47**, 922.

Roe, D.A. (1987). *Geriatric nutrition.* Prentice-Hall, Englewood Cliffs, NJ.

Rohde, J. (ed.) (1988). Growth monitoring and promotion: symposium. *Ind. J. Pediatr.*, **Suppl. 1**.

Rothenberg, R.B., Lobanov, A., Singh, K.B., and Stroh, G. (1985). Validity of clinic based nutritional surveillance for prevalence estimation of undernutrition. *Bull. WHO.*, **65**, 529.

Rowland, M.G.M., Rowland, S.G.J., and Cole, T.J. (1988). Impact of infection in the growth of children from 0–2 years in an urban West African community. *Am. J. Clin. Nutr.*, **47**, 134.

Sann, L., Durand, M., Picard, J., Lasne, Y., and Bethenad, M. (1988). Arm fat and muscle areas in infancy. *Arch. Dis. Child.*, **63**, 256.

Scrimshaw, N.S. (1985). Realistic approaches to world hunger: policy considerations. *Food Nutr. Bull.*, 7, 1.

Soysa, P. (1987). Women and nutrition. *World Rev. Nutr. Diet.*, **52**, 1.

Spyckerelle, Y., Guegnen, R., Guellernot, M., Tosi, E., and Deschamps, J.P. (1988). Adiposity indices and clinical opinion. *Ann. Hum. Biol.*, **15**, 45.

Srikantia, S.G. (1988). The National Nutrition Monitoring Bureau. *Nutr. Found. India Bull.*, **9**, (2), 1.

Steen, B. (1988). Body composition and ageing *Nutr. Rev.*, **46**, 45.

Stevens-Simon, C. and McAnarney, E.R. (1988). Adolescent maternal weight gain and low birth weight: a multifactorial model. *Am. J. Clin. Nutr.*, **47**, 948.

Stewart, K.K. (1983). The state of food composition data: an overview with some suggestions. *Food Nutr. Bull.*, **5**, 54.

Tanner, J.M. (1987). Growth as a mirror of the condition of society: secular trends and class distinctions. *Acta Paediatr. Jpn*, **29**, 96.

Tarwotjo, I., Sommer, A., West, K.P., Djunaedi, E., Mele, L., Hawkins, B., and the ACEH Study Group (1987). Influences of participation on mortality in a randomized trial of vitamin A prophylaxis. *Am. J. Clin. Nutr.* **45**, 1466.

Truswell, A.S. (ed.) (1982). RDI and allowances around the world: an introduction. *Food Nutr. Bull.*, **34**, 34.

Tulchinsky, T.H., Acker, C., El Malki, K., Socolar, R.S., and Reshef, A. (1985). Use of growth charts as a simple epidemiological monitoring system of nutritional status of children. *Bull. WHO.* **63**, 1137.

UN Administrative Committee for Co-ordination, Subcommittee on Nutrition (ACC/SCN) (1989). *Nutrition in times of disaster.* WHO/UNHCR, Geneva.

Valverde, V., Delgado, H., Flores, R., Sibrian, R., and Palmieri, M. (1986). Uses and constraints of school children's height/data for planning purposes: national experiences in Central America. *Food Nutr. Bull.*, **8**, 42.

Waterlow, J.C. (ed.) (1986). *Linear growth retardation in less developed countries.* Raven Press, New York.

Weinser, R.L. and Butterworth, C.E. (1981). *Handbook of clinical nutrition.* Mosby, St. Louis, Mo.

Whitehead, R.G. and Paul, A.A. (1984). Growth charts and the assessment of infant feeding practices in the Western world and developing countries. *Early Hum. Dev.*, **9**, 187.

Winick, M. (ed.) (1987). *Nutritional disorders of American women.* John Wiley, New York.

World Health Organization (1985). *Energy and protein requirements.* Tech. Rep. Ser. 724. WHO, Geneva.

—— (1987*a*). *Studying maternal mortality in developing countries. Rates and causes. A guidebook.* Dec. WHO/FHE/87, 7.

—— (1987b). *Oral health surveys*, (3rd edn). WHO, Geneva.

Yee, V. and Zerfas, A.J. (1987). Issues in growth monitoring. Unpublished mimeo: LTS, 47th St., Chevy Chase, MD 20815, USA.

Yost, D.A. and Pust, R.E. (1988). Arm circumference as an index of protein – energy malnutrition in six-to-eleven-month-old rural Tanzanian children. *J. Trop. Pediatr.*, **34**, 15.

Young, D.S. (1987). Implementation of SI units for clinical laboratory data: style specifications and emversion tables. *Ann. Intern. Med.*, **106**, 114.

Zachmann, M. (1987). Japanese growth standards in a Swiss journal. *Helv. Paediatr. Acta.*, **42**, 109.

Index

Page references suffixed 'n' refer to footnotes on those pages.